Surgical Techniques in Veterinary Medicine

Surgical Techniques in Veterinary Medicine

Editor: Maria Muray

MURPHY & MOORE
www.murphy-moorepublishing.com

Murphy & Moore Publishing,
1 Rockefeller Plaza,
New York City, NY 10020, USA

Visit us on the World Wide Web at:
www.murphy-moorepublishing.com

ISBN: 978-1-63987-509-2 (Hardback)

Cataloging-in-Publication Data

Surgical techniques in veterinary medicine / edited by Maria Muray.
p. cm.
Includes bibliographical references and index.
ISBN 978-1-63987-509-2
1. Veterinary surgery--Technique. 2. Veterinary medicine. I. Muray, Maria.
SF911 .S87 2022
636.089 7--dc23

Table of Contents

Preface

This book has been an outcome of determined endeavour from a group of educationists in the field. The primary objective was to involve a broad spectrum of professionals from diverse cultural background involved in the field for developing new researches. The book not only targets students but also scholars pursuing higher research for further enhancement of the theoretical and practical applications of the subject.

Veterinary medicine is a branch of medicine which deals with the diagnosis and prevention of diseases, disorders and injuries related to animal species. It is widely practiced using either veterinary drugs or surgical procedures, or both. The discipline helps in controlling and preventing the transmission of causative agents or zoonotic diseases to humans. Surgical procedures performed by veterinarians fall under three broad categories, orthopaedics, soft tissue surgery and neurosurgery. Common veterinary surgery includes non-emergency elective procedures such as castration, a sterilization procedure. Other surgical procedures involve cardiology surgery, caesarean surgery, dental surgery, cystotomy, wound repair, surgery for gastric dilatation volvulus, ophthalmic surgery and cancer surgery. This book elucidates new techniques and their applications in a multidisciplinary manner. It provides significant information of surgical techniques in veterinary medicine to help develop a good understanding. For all those who are interested in veterinary medicine, this book can prove to be an essential guide.

It was an honour to edit such a profound book and also a challenging task to compile and examine all the relevant data for accuracy and originality. I wish to acknowledge the efforts of the contributors for submitting such brilliant and diverse chapters in the field and for endlessly working for the completion of the book. Last, but not the least; I thank my family for being a constant source of support in all my research endeavours.

Editor

A surgical approach in the treatment of preputial gland abscesses in mice

Henri G. M. J. Bertrand[1*], Aurelie A. Thomas[1], Yvette C. Ellen[1,2], Robert S. Dorward[2] and Paul A. Flecknell[1,3]

Abstract

Background: Preputial gland infection is a common occurrence in non-breeder male mice and can lead to abscesses. This report describes a surgical approach to treating and preventing this condition.

Results: Surgical removal of the glands was undertaken in 258 male C3H/HeNHsd mice. The glands were successfully removed in all of the animals with a low rate of post-surgery complications. Abscess recurrence due to incomplete gland resection occurred in 2.3 % of animals. Surgical wound opening (3.1 %) and infection of the surgical site (2.3 %) also occurred but were treated successfully.

Conclusion: In the study described here, early intervention was successful in preventing intercurrent infection compromising both animal welfare and the outcome of the study.

Keywords: Refinement, Preputial, Gland, Surgery, Abscess

Background

Preputial glands are accessory glands of the reproductive system of the male mouse and play a role in reproduction and dominance behavior [1, 2]. Inflammation and infection of these glands can lead to abscess formation. This health issue occurs more frequently in some mouse strains such as B6C3F1 [3, 4] however the incidence is usually quite low in C3H mice [5, 6]. The usual presentation of preputial gland inflammation is a uni- or bilateral subcutaneous swelling on either side of the prepuce. This develops to form a palpably hard mass and the overlying skin can be inflamed. In the worst case the abscesses can ulcerate and purulent exudate can be visible on the coat (Fig. 1). During a long-term (12 month) study in our facility, a high incidence of abscesses were noted, and the principal investigator was concerned at the impact of chronic infection and antibiotic treatment on both mouse welfare and the scientific goals of the study. To try to resolve the problem, a procedure to remove the glands surgically was developed, and this was used both to treat established abscesses, and as a preventive measure.

* Correspondence: henri.bertrand@ncl.ac.uk
[1]Comparative Biology Centre, Newcastle University, Framlington Place, Newcastle Upon Tyne NE2 4HH, UK
Full list of author information is available at the end of the article

Results

No complications related to the anaesthesia protocol occurred. In a small number of animals minor bleeding from the fatty tissue around the gland occurred but this was easily managed by applying pressure on the tissue with a dry swab. Given the location, perforation of the abdominal muscle layer or trauma to the penis could occur, but in our cases none of these complications occurred. The most common complication was re-opening of the surgical wound. Eight mice (3.1 %) removed skin sutures within 24 h post surgery, and the wound was closed again under general anaesthesia. Infection of the surgical wound, with obvious exudate occurred in six mice (2.3 %) within 24–48 h post surgery. Antibiotics were administered until infection resolved (typically 72 h). Recurrence of an abscess at the surgical site was noted in six mice (2.3 %).

Discussion

The incidence of preputial gland inflammation or abscess are influenced by several factors. Mouse strain, age and microbiological flora are considered to be of importance [3–10] but also environmental condition such as group housing have been considered to increase the incidence of the condition [2]. In this case report, the high prevalence of this condition in C3H/HeNHsd mice was considered to be due to the high fat diet and the sugar water regimen

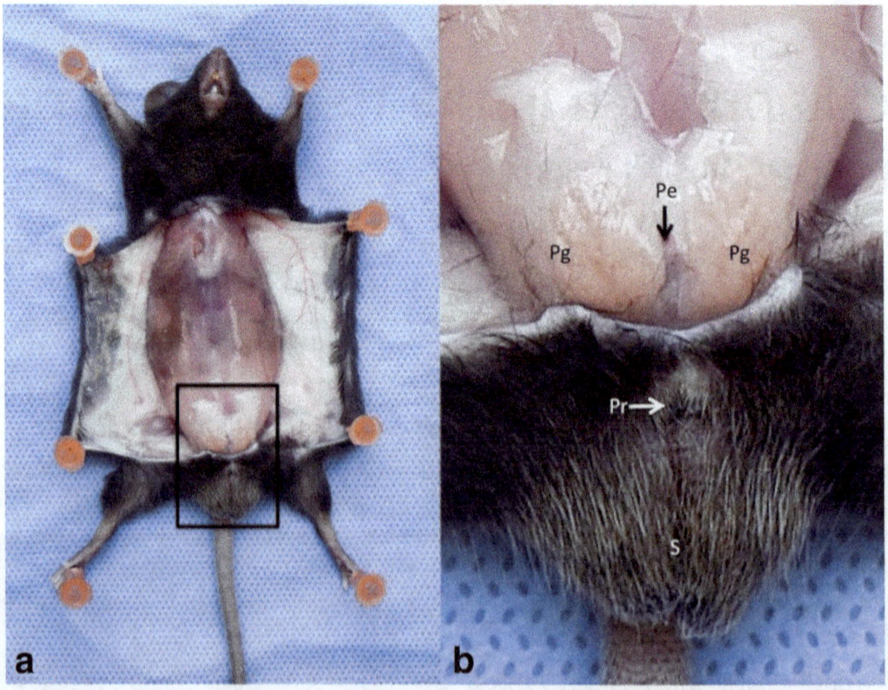

Fig. 1 Anatomic Region of the preputial glands. **a** General view. The abdominal skin layer has been reclined to expose the muscle layer and the preputial glands region. The black frame represents the area enlarged in the next picture. **b** Enlarged view of the preputial glands region. (S = Scrotum; Pr = Prepuce; Pg = Preputial gland; Pe = Penis)

used for the main study but no bacterial culture was performed to identify an infectious agent, as this would not have impacted our treatment approach. No histopathology exam was performed to confirm the diagnosis of abscess. This diagnosis was only based on the clinical signs observed and the similar progression of clinical signs in all animals. The treatment suggested in the literature is to lance the abscess and administer antibiotics to the animals [1, 7, 11]. However, in our experience the recurrence rate was high (95 %) when using this treatment regimen. This might be due to the multilobular structure of the gland preventing complete drainage of the abscess. The recurrence of these abscesses therefore represents a welfare cost for mice, as it may be associated with pain, fever and can lead to systemic amyloidosis [10]. Both a surgical procedure and repeated antibiotic therapy can impact on the welfare of the mice [12, 13]. The surgical procedure described has the advantages of preventing infection, and resolving established abscesses. It was associated with a low level of complication (in total 20 mice, 7.7 %). However this procedure is more technically demanding and time consuming than the previously documented treatment regimen. Like other surgical procedures, principles of good aseptic technique should be followed and a non-sterile assistant should be available to prepare the animal for surgery, monitor the anaesthesia and assist the surgeon. The time taken to perform each individual surgery was not recorded but in our experience each surgery required just under 10 min. Isoflurane was considered to be the anaesthetic of choice for this procedure as it provides a fast and smooth induction and recovery and also reliably produces a surgical plane of anaesthesia [14]. The other issue with this procedure, which was not investigated, is the potential impact on reproductive function since these glands play a role during the mating [1]. As a consequence, we only advise surgical removal of the preputial glands if a high incidence of the condition appears associated with a specific study, and when other means of reducing the incidence of the condition have been considered.

Conclusion

In the study described here, early intervention was successful in preventing intercurrent infection compromising both animal welfare and the outcome of the study.

Methods

Ethical statement

Animals were housed in a Home Office (UK authority) accredited facility and in compliance with the Animal Scientific Procedure Act 1986 and the European Directive 2010/63/EU. Newcastle University Animal Welfare and Ethic Review Body and the Home Office approved research protocols. The procedure was performed under the United Kingdom Veterinary Surgeon's Act 1969 with

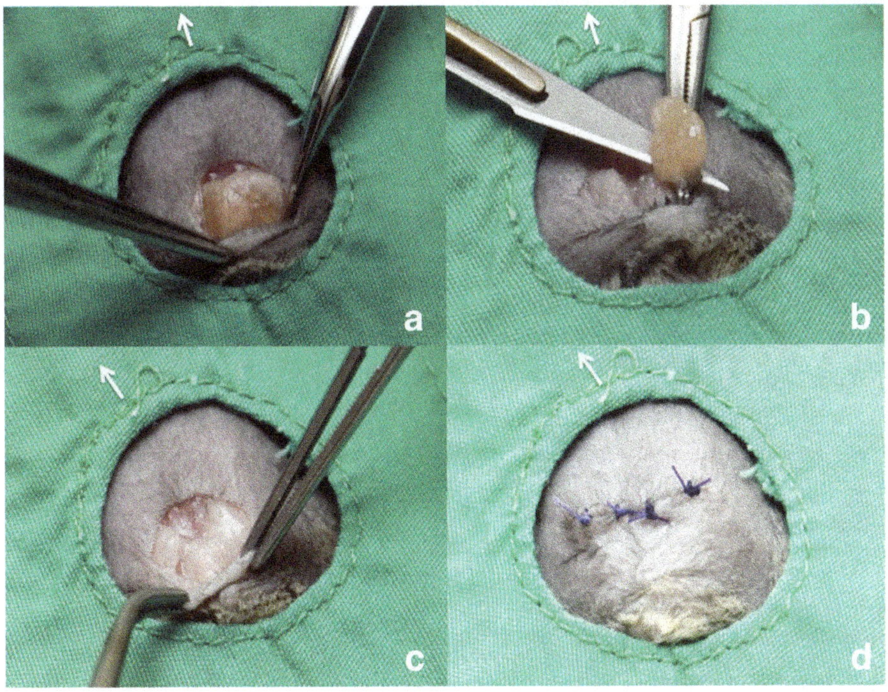

Fig. 2 Ablation surgery of preputial glands. **a** Preputial glands exposed (**b**) Gland ablation after haemostat was placed on the duct (**c**) Surgical site after glands are removed (**d**) Interrupted pattern suture to close surgical site. The withe arrow indicates the direction of the head

the agreement of the principal investigator and the Home Office.

Animals and husbandry

This report is based on treatment of 258 male mice C3H/HeNHsd (from Harlan Laboratories, UK) involved in a study of the effect of several diets on the formation of liver fibrosis. Animals were aged from 6 to 10 weeks at the start of the study and the first signs of gland inflammation were noted between 18 and 20 weeks of age. In total, 56 mice (21.7 %) developed at least one gland abscess. The mice were housed in Individually Ventilated Cages (580 cm^2, 226 mm × 419 mm × 147 mm, Arrowmight, UK), with 20 air cycles per hour. The day-night cycle was 12–12 h and the temperature was maintained at 22+/− 2 °C. During the study, an increasing number of mice presented with inflammation of their preputial glands. Because of the large number of affected animals, and because medical management of similar cases had proved unsuccessful, surgical removal of the gland was proposed.

Surgical procedure and perioperative cares

Anaesthesia was induced with 5 % and maintained with 2.5 % of isoflurane (IsoFlo 100 % w/w Inhalation Vapour, Abbott Laboratories, Maidenhead, UK), in 100 % oxygen. Anaesthesia was maintained for no more than 10 min. Body temperature was maintained with a heat pad set at 38 °C (Homeothermic Blanket system, Harvard Apparatus, Cambridge, UK). Meloxicam (5 mg/g s/c) (Metacam, Boehringer Ingelheim Limited, Bracknell, UK) was administered 10 min prior to surgery for pain relief and enrofloxacin (10 mg/kg s/c)(Baytril 2.5 % solution for injection, Bayer plc, Newbury, UK) as prophylactic antibiotic therapy. The preputial region was prepared for aseptic surgery (http://www.procedureswithcare.org.uk/aseptic-technique-in-rodent-surgery/). A 15 mm transverse skin incision was made cranial to the prepuce using a number 11 scalpel blade. The subcutaneous tissues were gently dissected forward to the prepuce with Metzenbaum scissors and Debakey forceps, without touching the penis. The healthy gland appeared as a flattened circular structure with a cream to light brown colouration (Fig. 1). In contrast the infected gland appeared larger and thin walled with a yellow-red colouration [15]. When a gland was infected, pus was often visible in one lobe of the gland or disseminated throughout. Some glands were embedded in fatty tissue, necessitating its isolation by gentle manipulation with a sterile cotton bud or a swap. Each gland was removed using a hemostat is placed on the ventral side of its duct, followed by cutting proximally with a scalpel blade 11. In animals with abscessation of the gland, adhesions with the skin necessitated very careful dissection before removal. If the gland ruptured during this dissection the surgical wound was thoroughly flushed with sterile saline and an additional dose of enrofloxacin administered at 24 h post-surgery. The skin was closed with polyglactin 910, 4/0 suture (Coated VicrylEthicon, Johnson&Johnson international, Diegrem, Belgium) with an interrupted pattern and skin glue (Indermil xfine, Henkel, Dublin, Ireland) to reinforce the closure (Fig. 2).

Competing interests

None of the authors of this paper has a financial or personal relationship with other people or organizations that could inappropriately influence or bias the content of the paper. The authors declare that they have no competing interests.

Authors' contributions

HB, AT and PF developed the surgical procedure and collected the data. HB and AT performed the surgery and YE and RD provided anaesthesia and perioperative cares support. The final version of the manuscript was read and approved by all authors of this study.

Author details

[1]Comparative Biology Centre, Newcastle University, Framlington Place, Newcastle Upon Tyne NE2 4HH, UK. [2]School of Veterinary Medicine and Science, Nottingham University, Nottingham, UK. [3]Institute of Neurosciences, Newcastle University, Newcastle Upon Tyne, UK.

References

1. Laber-Laird K, Swindle M, Flecknell PA. Handbook of Rodent and Rabbit Medicine. Oxford: Elsevier Science; 1996.
2. Tanabe M, Kimura T. Aggression and preputial gland of male mice affected by the presence of other males. J Ethol. 1995;13:63–8.
3. Ward JM, Goodman DG, Squire RA, Chu KC, Linhart MS. Neoplastic and nonneoplastic lesions in aging (C57BL/6N x C3H/HeN)F1 (B6C3F1) mice. J Natl Cancer Inst. 1979;63:849–54.
4. Holtfreter S, Radcliff FJ, Grumann D, Read H, Johnson S, Monecke S, et al. Characterization of a mouse-adapted staphylococcus aureus strain. PLoS One. 2013;8:e71142.
5. Rowlatt C, Chesterman FC, Sheriff MU. Lifespan, age changes and tumour incidence in an ageing C57BL mouse colony. Lab Anim. 1976;10:419–42.
6. Hong CC, Ediger RD. Perputial gland abscess in mice. Lab Anim Sci. 1978;28:153–6.
7. Fox JG, Anderson LC, Loew FM, Quimby FW. Laboratory Animal Medicine. 2nd edition. San Diego: Elsevier Science; 2002.
8. Marchlewska-Koj A, Ponchron E, Sliwowska A. Salivary glands and preputial glands of males as source of estrus-stimulating pheromone in female mice. J Chem Ecol. 1990;16:2817–22.
9. Needham JR, Cooper JE. Bulbourethral gland infections in mice associated with Staphylococcus aureus. Lab Anim. 1976;10:311–5.
10. Radaelli E, Manarolla G, Pisoni G, Balloi A, Aresu L, Sparaciari P, et al. Suppurative adenitis of preputial glands associated with corynebacterium mastitidis infection in mice. J Am Assoc Lab Anim Sci. 2010;49:69–74.
11. Harkness JE, Turner PV, VandeWoude S, Wheler CL. Harkness and Wagner's Biology and Medicine of Rabbits and Rodents. 5th edition. Ames, IA: Wiley-Blackwell; 2013.
12. Miller AL, Wright-Williams SL, Flecknell PA, Roughan JV. A comparison of abdominal and scrotal approach methods of vasectomy and the influence of analgesic treatment in laboratory mice. Lab Anim. 2012;46:304–10.
13. Davis JN, Courtney CL, Superak H, Taylor DK. Behavioral, clinical and pathological effects of multiple daily intraperitoneal injections on female mice. Lab Anim (NY). 2014;43:131–9.
14. Flecknell P. Laboratory Animal Anaesthesia. 4th edition. Oxford: Elsevier Science; 2015.
15. Donnelly TM, Walberg J. Enlarged mouse preputial glands. Lab Anim (NY). 2011;40:69–71.

2

Total intravenous anaesthesia in a goat undergoing craniectomy

Verónica Vieitez[1*], Ignacio Álvarez Gómez de Segura[2], Víctor López Rámis[1], Massimo Santella[1] and Luis Javier Ezquerra[1]

Abstract

Background: Cerebral coenurosis is a disease of the central nervous system in sheep and goats, and is usually fatal unless surgical relief is provided. Information regarding neuroanaesthesia in veterinary medicine in goats is scant.

Case presentation: We describe anaesthetic management of an intact female goat (2 years; 16 kg) presented for craniectomy. The goat was sedated with xylazine (0.05 mg kg^{-1}, i.m.) and morphine (0.05 mg kg^{-1}, i.m.). General anaesthesia was induced 20 min later with propofol and maintained with a constant rate infusion of propofol (0.2 mg kg^{-1} min^{-1}). A cuffed endotracheal tube was placed and connected to a rebreathing (circle) system and mechanical ventilation with 100% oxygen was initiated. A bolus of lidocaine (1 mg kg^{-1}), midazolam (0.25 mg kg^{-1}) and fentanyl 2.5 μg kg^{-1} was delivered via the intravenous route followed immediately by a constant rate infusion of lidocaine (50 μg kg^{-1} min^{-1}), midazolam (0.15 mg kg^{-1} h^{-1}) and fentanyl (6 μg kg^{-1} h^{-1}) administered via the intravenous route throughout surgery. Craniectomy was undertaken and the goat recovered uneventfully.

Conclusion: Total intravenous anaesthesia with propofol, lidocaine, fentanyl and midazolam could be an acceptable option for anaesthesia during intracranial surgery in goats.

Keywords: Goat, Propofol, Fentanyl, Lidocaine, Midazolam, Craniectomy, Total intravenous anaesthesia

Background

Cerebral coenurosis is a disease of the central nervous system (CNS) in sheep and goats. Due to development of the cyst in brain, the animal starts showing nervous signs that include circling, visual defects, gait abnormalities, hyperesthesia, and paraplegia [1]. Surgical removal is the only available treatment. However, there are few reports of surgical treatment [1–4] and only brief descriptions of anaesthetic management. In those studies, goats were sedated [3] or controlled manually by an assistant [2] while surgery was undertaken under local anaesthesia. Only Merbl et al. [1] described two cases of constant rate infusion (CRI) of propofol and fentanyl.

Anaesthesia for intracranial neurosurgical procedures must provide haemodynamic stability, maintain cerebral perfusion pressure (CPP), reduce the cerebral metabolic rate (CMR), preserve cerebral autoregulation and avoid an increase in intracranial pressure (ICP) [5]. Anaesthesiologists must plan for smooth emergence, rapid awakening, and early neurological assessment of the patient in the postoperative period [6].

Volatile and intravenous anaesthetic agents are used for the maintenance of anaesthesia during neurosurgical procedures. Which type of anaesthetic (inhalational or intravenous) is preferable for a craniectomy is controversial. Volatile anaesthetics are dose-dependent cerebral vasodilators that affect cerebral autoregulation and ICP [7]. However, most intravenous anaesthetic, analgesic and sedative agents maintain a linear relationship between a reduction in cerebral blood flow (CBF) and CMR, autoregulation of cerebral perfusion and CO_2 responsiveness, and have minimal effects on ICP [7].

In human medicine propofol does not interfere with CBF regulation [8] and decreases CMR, which stimulates vasoconstriction and results in decreased ICP in rats [9]. Clinical studies have suggested that propofol alone or in combination with alfentanil can aid the maintenance of anaesthesia during craniotomy in human beings [10].

Pure mu-agonist opioids (e.g. fentanyl) are commonly used for analgesia in balanced total intravenous anaesthesia

* Correspondence: vvieitez@gmail.com
[1]Veterinary Teaching Hospital, University of Extremadura, Avda, Universidad s/n, 10003 Cáceres, Spain
Full list of author information is available at the end of the article

(TIVA) and can attenuate nociceptive signals from noxious stimuli at subcortical levels of the CNS [11]. In goats, fentanyl has been shown to be effective against thermal and mechanical stimuli using a model of nociception [12].

Benzodiazepines such as midazolam contribute to TIVA through sedation and muscle relaxation [13]. Midazolam has been reported to be a potent sedative drug [14] that can be administered during the pre-anaesthetic period to reduce the dose of propofol required for induction of general anaesthesia in goats [15].

Intravenous lidocaine has been used as a supplement to general anaesthesia, and its perioperative administration reduces postoperative pain. Intravenous lidocaine has been shown to reduce the minimum alveolar concentration of isoflurane in dogs [16], cats [17], horses [18] and goats [19].

There is limited information regarding neuroanaesthesia in veterinary medicine. Moreover, goats are anaesthetised rarely, so information on the efficacy of anaesthetic drugs in this species is scant [13]. Maintenance of anaesthesia using propofol administered by CRI in combination with other injectable drugs or inhalation agents has been reported in goats [19–21]. Fentanyl, midazolam [21] and ketamine [20] have been shown to be anaesthetic-sparing agents that lower the propofol dose required for the maintenance of anaesthesia.

Here, we describe anaesthetic management in a goat undergoing resection of an intracranial coenurosis. Concurrent use of propofol, fentanyl, lidocaine and midazolam in goats has not been reported.

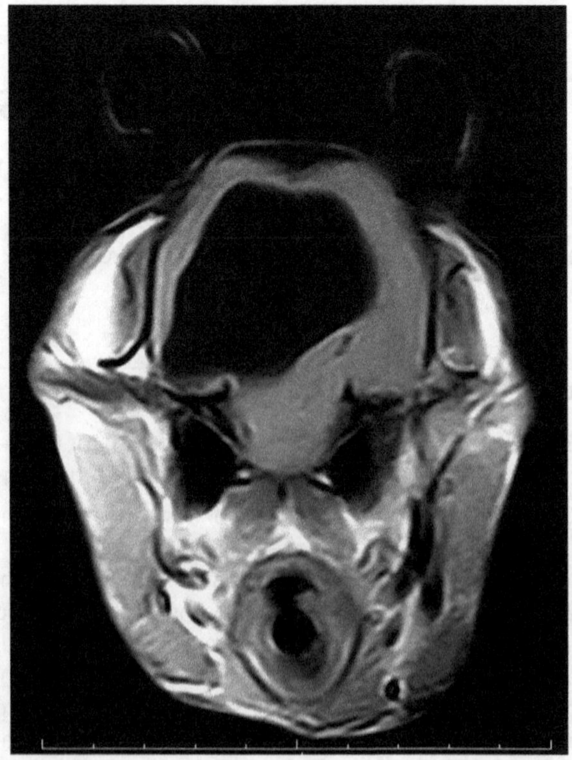

Fig. 1 Axial T1 magnetic resonance image showing a hypointense lesion occupying most of the right hemisphere suspected to be a cerebral cyst

Case description

An intact female goat (2 years old; 16 kg) was admitted to hospital for investigation of neurological signs. Behavioural disturbances, standing apart from other goats, and disorientation were observed. Furthermore, it seemed to be very easy to chase and catch the goat.

General physical examination was unremarkable. However, upon neurological examination, an absent left-sided menace response, alert mentation and head tilt were noted. No other abnormalities were noted and the results of haematology and blood biochemistry were unremarkable. Magnetic resonance imaging (MRI; Vet-MR Grande; Esaote S.A., Barcelona, Spain) of the brain revealed a cystic lesion at the level of the right cerebral hemisphere (Fig. 1). The goat was scheduled for resection of this lesion.

The goat was anaesthetised for surgery. Food (but not water) was withheld 12 h before anaesthesia. The goat was pre-medicated with xylazine (0.05 mg kg^{-1}, i.m.; Rompun 2% soluble injection; Bayer, Barcelona, Spain) and morphine (0.05 mg kg^{-1}, i.m.; Morfina 1%; Fresenius Kabi España S.A., Barcelona, Spain) 20 min before the induction of anaesthesia. A 20-G catheter (BD Insyte; Becton Dickinson Medicals Pte. Ltd., Singapore) was inserted into the cephalic vein for the administration of drugs and intravenous fluids. An antibiotic (ampicillin, 20 mg kg^{-1}, i.v.; Britapen, 500-mg soluble injection; Reig Jofre S.A., Madrid, Spain) was given and administration repeated every 90 min throughout the surgical procedure. The auricular artery in the left ear was catheterised using a 24-G catheter. Five minutes before the induction of anaesthesia, the goat underwent pre-oxygenation via a facemask with 100% oxygen. Before the induction of anaesthesia, the degree of sedation was moderate. Propofol (Vetofol, 10 mg mL^{-1}; Esteve, Barcelona, Spain) was administered initially as a bolus at 2 mg kg^{-1} over 30 s, followed by incremental doses at 0.5 mg kg^{-1} every 15 s, until the goat was anaesthetised sufficiently to allow endotracheal intubation (total dose, 50 mg). A cuffed, 6.5-mm ID endotracheal tube was placed and connected to a rebreathing (circle) system. Intermittent positive pressure ventilation (IPPV) with 100% oxygen was initiated using a pressure-cycled mechanical ventilator (ABC; Stephan GmbH, Gackenbach, Germany). Peak inspiratory pressure (PIP) was set at 8–10 cmH_2O, and the respiratory rate (f_R) adjusted to maintain a partial pressure of expired carbon dioxide ($PE'CO_2$) at 33–35 mmHg.

The goat was placed in sternal recumbency for preparation of the surgical site with the head elevated at 30°.

Occlusion of the jugular vein was avoided throughout the procedure. The goat was connected to a multi-parameter anaesthesia monitor (S/5; Datex-Ohmeda, Inc., Madison, WI, USA), which displayed continuously a lead-II electrocardiogram, heart rate (HR), f_R, $PE'CO_2$, inspired fraction of oxygen, tidal volume, invasive blood pressure (IBP), PIP, dynamic respiratory system compliance and plethysmographic oxygen saturation (SpO_2). The catheter in the auricular artery was connected to an electronic pressure transducer (Deltran DPT-200; Utah Medical Products, Inc., Midvale, UT, USA) zeroed at the level of shoulder joint to measure IBP. Body temperature was measured using an intra-oesophageal temperature probe and displayed continuously on the multi-parameter monitor.

A CRI of propofol (6 mg kg^{-1} h^{-1}) was started immediately after the induction of anaesthesia. Additionally, a bolus of lidocaine (1 mg kg^{-1}; Lidocaína 2% soluble injection; B. Braun Medical S.A., Barcelona, Spain), midazolam (0.25 mg kg^{-1}; Dormicum 5 mg mL^{-1} soluble injection; Roche Farma S.A., Madrid, Spain) and fentanyl (2.5 μg kg^{-1}, Fentanest 0.05 mg mL^{-1} soluble injection; Kern Pharma, Barcelona, Spain) were delivered (i.v.) by hand over 60 s, followed immediately by a CRI of lidocaine (50 μg kg^{-1} min^{-1}), midazolam (0.15 mg kg^{-1} h^{-1}) and fentanyl (6 μg kg^{-1} h^{-1}) administered via the intravenous route throughout the surgical procedure. Propofol and fentanyl for CRI were drawn up to fill a 20-mL syringe (Perfusor Compact; B. Braun Medical S.A.), whereas 600 mg of lidocaine and 30 mg of midazolam were mixed in 1 L of lactated Ringer's solution (Ringer Lactato; B. Braun Medical S.A.) and infused together with a volumetric pump (Niki: C.M.E. Ltd., Lichtenstein, Germany) at 5 mL kg^{-1} h^{-1}.

The criteria used to assess the depth of anaesthesia were HR, IBP, attempts to breathe against the ventilator and spontaneous movement. According to clinical signs, CRI of propofol was increased to 12 mg kg^{-1} h^{-1} 10 min after the induction of anaesthesia. Lactated Ringer's solution was infused via the intravenous route during surgery at 5 mL kg^{-1} h^{-1}. A bolus of propofol (0.5 mg kg^{-1}, i.v.) was administered if voluntary movement occurred. The infusion rate of propofol was recorded every 5 min, along with all physiological parameters displayed on the multi-parametric monitor.

Samples of arterial blood were collected anaerobically from the arterial catheter. They were analysed immediately and 45 min after the induction of anaesthesia to ensure blood gases remained within established reference ranges ($PaCO_2$, 39.5 mmHg; PaO_2, 475 mmHg; HCO_3, 29.5 mmol L^{-1}; base excess, 5 mmol L^{-1}; SaO_2, 100%; pH 7.481; lactate, 0.88 mmol L^{-1}).

TIVA provided adequate cardiovascular stability (HR, 76–96 bpm) and adequate arterial blood pressure (Fig. 2) throughout anaesthesia (mean arterial blood pressure (MAP), 75–90 mmHg). Regurgitation, hyper-salivation and tympany were not observed. Oesophageal temperature decreased gradually over the period of anaesthesia but hypothermia (36.1 °C) was not corrected until the end of the procedure.

Craniectomy was undertaken to remove the cyst. Five minutes before completion of surgery, a bolus of dexamethasone (0.3 mg kg^{-1}, i.v.; Cortesona 2 mg mL^{-1} soluble injection; Laboratorios Syva, León, Spain) and acepromazine (0.02 mg, i.v.; Equipromacina 5 mg mL^{-1} soluble injection; Labiana Life Sciences, S.A., Barcelona, Spain) were administered to ensure a smooth recovery. After skin closure, all CRI was stopped (total dose of propofol, 310 mg). IPPV was continued until attempts were made to breathe spontaneously. Then, the goat was moved in sternal recumbency to the recovery room. To avoid complications associated with the digestive tract and respiratory system, the goat was supported in sternal recumbency and the endotracheal tube removed only after return of the swallowing reflex (20 min after the end of the surgery). Total anaesthesia time (from the induction of anaesthesia to TIVA cessation) was 90 min. The goat recovered uneventfully from anaesthesia and could stand and eat <24 h after surgery.

Assessment of pain and physiological variables was conducted every hour until hospital discharge: no abnormalities were detected. Immediate postoperative care comprised administration of dexamethasone (0.1 mg kg $^{-1}$, i.v.) every 24 h, buprenorphine (0.005 mg kg^{-1}, i.v.; Buprecare 0. 3 mg mL^{-1} soluble injection; Group Divasa-Farmavic, Barcelona, Spain) every 8 h, head elevation, intravenous fluid therapy (Sterovet; B. Braun Vetcare S.A., Barcelona, Spain) to maintain normotension and regular evaluation of neurological status. Neurological examination was done 24 h after surgery and revealed no worsening of neurological deficits. Neurological signs improved within 5 days and resolved upon hospital discharge (14 days after surgery).

Discussion

Wider availability of imaging methods (e.g. MRI) to veterinary surgeons and the growing popularity of having goats as domestic pets have resulted in more goats requiring surgery that involves general anaesthesia. Recommendations for patients with intracranial neoplasms have not been determined and management has been extrapolated from studies in head-trauma patients [22]. Many methods for anaesthesia in animals with CNS disease have been reported, but their cerebrovascular effects are unknown.

The main aim of any anaesthetic method used for intracranial surgery is preservation of neuronal function [22]. The latter is dependent upon adequate CBF, which

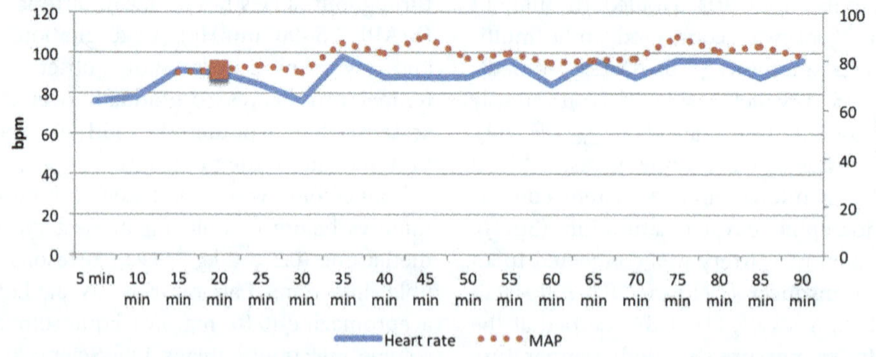

Fig. 2 Heart rate (bpm) and mean arterial blood pressure (mmHg) in a goat undergoing craniectomy anaesthetized with TIVA of propofol, lidocaine, fentanyl and midazolam. Square marks the beginning of surgery

in turn is dependent on the CPP and cerebral vascular resistance (CVR). CPP is defined as the difference between MAP at the level of the base of the brain and ICP. In patients with increased intracranial pressure, it is vital to consider the changes that a decrease in blood pressure may have in CPP [23], so maintaining adequate and stable cardiovascular function is essential.

Tracheal intubation can stimulate coughing and gagging, as well as a reflex sympathetic pressor response, which results in an elevated HR and blood pressure in humans [24], dogs [25] and cats [26]. This reflex may have adverse effects in patients with increased ICP.

Intravenous lidocaine has been used in humans at 1.5–2.5 mg kg^{-1} at least 3 min before the induction of anaesthesia to blunt the haemodynamic and coughing responses to tracheal intubation [27]. In this case, lidocaine administration before intubation to minimise the pressor response to intubation (as has been described in humans) was not done, but non-significant changes were observed in the HR or MAP after intubation. In this case, propofol provided a smooth induction of anaesthesia with no apnoea or myoclonus, as have been reported elsewhere [15, 28].

The position of the head can aid or worsen the control of ICP. Head elevation by 15–30° can improve cerebral venous drainage and limit cerebral venous congestion, thereby reducing ICP without reducing CPP or CBF [29]. Therefore, maintenance of this position is recommended if an increase in ICP is suspected. Occlusion of the jugular vein can impair venous drainage to cause increased ICP. Jugular catheterisation of patients at risk of raised ICP is controversial [29], so we avoided measuring CVP in this case.

In this case, we preferred lactated Ringer's solution to ensure electrolyte balance despite being a slightly hypotonic fluid and could therefore cause oedema. The MRI did not show evidence of oedema in the surrounding tissue, for this reason we avoided using mannitol preoperatively (as has been recommended). However we used corticosteroids perioperatively to maintain adequate CPP by reducing peri-cyst oedema after surgery, as has been described in the treatment of brain tumours [30].

In the absence of direct monitoring of ICP, it is recommended that a MAP of 80–100 mmHg be maintained to ensure adequate CPP [31]. Maintenance of an adequate depth of anaesthesia to avoid hypotension is very important. In this case, MAP was >80 mmHg most of the time (Fig. 2). Elevated ICP could be a problem until reduction in ICP occurs after durotomy, but no treatment was initiated to increase MAP. Because of the positioning of the animal for surgery, the eye position, jaw tone and palpebral reflexes could not be used to assess the depth of anaesthesia. Furthermore, the usefulness of MAP and HR in the assessment of the depth of anaesthesia is confounded by the effects of anaesthetic agents on cardiovascular function [22]. Despite such difficulties in the assessment of the depth of anaesthesia, the goat started to breathe against the ventilator and received a bolus of propofol only once. In human medicine, electroencephalography is useful for monitoring the adequacy of sedation and anaesthesia during neurosurgery, but an electroencephalograph was not available in our hospital.

The $PaCO_2$ is an important factor for the control of CVR and CBF. An acute rise in $PaCO_2$ can cause a decrease in arteriolar pH, which results in decreased CVR and which increases CBF. In contrast, hypocapnia results in intracranial vasoconstriction and decreased cerebral perfusion [29]. IPPV is mandatory in neurosurgical patients to prevent increases in $PaCO_2$ as well as the associated vasodilatation and increased ICP [32]. Improvements in MAP and CPP may also be achieved by limiting the detrimental effects of IPPV upon venous return and cardiac output [22]. IPPV can increase central venous pressure (CVP) and decrease venous drainage from the head, thereby leading to venous congestion, increased ICP and further reductions in CPP [32]. Court et al. [33] proposed that this effect could be minimised by using neuromuscular blocking agents that increase thoracic compliance and thus decrease the intrathoracic pressure required to ventilate the animal adequately. In this case, we avoided neuromuscular blocking agents but muscle relaxation was sufficient to ensure adequate IPPV with no apparent cardiovascular effects.

Interest in TIVA for neuroanaesthesia has been well documented in the literature on human medicine [10]. Research on TIVA in goats has become increasingly popular over the past few years [13, 21, 34]. However, information on TIVA protocols applicable to goats is very scarce [34].

Pharmacokinetic studies in various species have revealed that propofol has a large volume of distribution, rapid metabolism and rapid clearance if given by repeated doses or continuous intravenous infusion [28, 35, 36]. The rapid onset, short duration of action and rapid recoveries make this drug potentially useful in ruminants, in which these features are particularly desirable [37]. Plasma clearance of propofol in goats is rapid and exceeds the rate clearance in dogs, horses and humans [36]. Propofol has been used as a continuous intravenous infusion to achieve and maintain general anaesthesia in goats [1, 19–21].

The minimum infusion rate of propofol to prevent purposeful movement of the extremities in response to a standardised noxious stimulus in non-premedicated goats is 0.45 mg kg^{-1} min^{-1} [38]. In studies undertaken by Dzikiti et al. [39] and Larenza et al. [20], infusion rates of propofol of 0.2 and 0.3 mg kg^{-1} min^{-1}, respectively, were reported. Both studies co-administrated anaesthetic-sparing agents (fentanyl, midazolam [39]; ketamine [20]), to lower the infusion rates of propofol required to maintain anaesthesia. Nevertheless, Carroll et al. [40] reported a higher dose rate (0.52 mg kg^{-1} min $^{-1}$) in pre-medicated (detomidine and butorphanol) goats undergoing orchiectomy and ovariectomy, perhaps because surgical stimulation may exceed the standardised supramaximal stimulus applied in research studies. In our case, the CRI of propofol was 0.2 mg kg^{-1} min^{-1}, this can be explain for co-administration of lidocaine, midazolam and fentanyl CRI.

Midazolam produces a rapid onset of short-duration, dose-dependent sedation in goats [14, 15] and decreases the induction doses of propofol required [15]. It is associated with minimal adverse cardiovascular effects if administered as pre-anaesthetic medication [15] and at 0.1–0.9 mg kg^{-1} h^{-1} for an adjunctive role to general anaesthetic drugs in goats [21, 39]. Midazolam produces marked reductions in drug requirements for general anaesthesia in inhalation and intravenous anaesthesia in goats [21, 39, 41]. Sedative effects of midazolam in goats are dose dependent, therefore, in this case, a higher dose of midazolam might have been used to further decrease the dose of propofol required for maintenance.

Lidocaine was infused immediately after intubation throughout surgery to elicit neuroprotective and analgesic effects. Lidocaine may reduce secondary brain injury by preventing sodium influx into ischemic neurons [42]. Evidence suggests that infusion of an antiarrhythmic dose (1.5–2 mg kg^{-1}) after the onset of brain ischemia reduces the risk of death of neuronal cells and improves neurologic outcome [43].

The synthetic μ-opioid agonist fentanyl is used for the treatment of moderate-to-severe pain. Fentanyl administered via the intravenous route as CRI after a bolus dose could be a useful analgesic adjunct to general anaesthesia in goats [39]. Fentanyl causes minimal adverse effects on cardiopulmonary function in goats, but has been associated with restlessness, increased vocalisation and exaggerated tail wagging during recovery from anaesthesia [39]. Although we used a low dose of fentanyl, to avoid these possible adverse effects and to ensure a smooth recovery and more compliant animal in the postoperative period, a small dose of acepromazine was administered at the end of the surgery. Despite that acepromazine should cause hypotension and vasodilatation and presumably decrease of CPP, we believe that the effects of an excited recovery would be even more damaging in this goat.

In our case, the recovery time was short and adverse effects such as myoclonus (which has been reported in goats recovering from a single dose of propofol [15]) was not observed, unlike in studies were CRI of propofol was used to maintain anaesthesia [21]. One important feature of a neuroanaesthetic protocol is rapid recovery from anaesthesia to allow prompt neurological assessment [10]. Rapid predictable recovery with minimal excitement regardless of the duration of anaesthesia is required to identify postoperative complications (e.g. haemorrhage, increased ICP) and prevent severe neurological impairment and death [23]. Moreover, rapid recovery from anaesthesia is important in ruminants because they are prone to tympany and regurgitation of ruminal contents, which increases the risk of hypoxemia and aspiration of regurgitated ruminal contents [37].

Conclusion

We reported on anaesthetic management in a goat undergoing surgical treatment for cerebral coenurosis. This is the first report of CRI of propofol, lidocaine midazolam and fentanyl in goats. TIVA (achieved by co-administration of propofol, lidocaine, midazolam and fentanyl) for the maintenance of anaesthesia in a ventilated oxygen-supplemented goat undergoing craniectomy resulted in satisfactory anaesthesia with minimal negative impact on cardiopulmonary function as well as good recovery. This method could be an acceptable option for anaesthesia during intracranial surgery in goats.

Abbreviations

CBF: Cerebral blood flow; CMR: Cerebral metabolic rate; CNS: Central nervous system; CPP: Cerebral perfusion pressure; CRI: Continuous rate infusion;

CVP: Central venous pressure; CVR: Cerebral vascular resistance; f_R: Respiratory rate; HR: Heart rate; IBP: Invasive blood pressure; ICP: Intracranial pressure; IPPV: Intermittent positive pressure ventilation; MAP: Mean arterial blood pressure; PIP: Peak inspiratory pressure; SpO_2: Plethysmographic oxygen saturation; TIVA: Total intravenous anaesthesia; $PE'CO_2$: Partial pressure of expired carbon dioxide

Author details

[1]Veterinary Teaching Hospital, University of Extremadura, Avda, Universidad s/n, 10003 Cáceres, Spain. [2]Department of Animal Medicine and Surgery, Veterinary Faculty, University Complutense of Madrid, Avda. Puerta de Hierro, 28040 Madrid, Spain.

Authors' contributions

All authors were implicated in the clinical management of the case. VV drafted the manuscript and provided the figures. All authors revised it critically, provided helpful discussions and final corrections on the manuscript. They read and approved the final version of this manuscript.

Competing interests

The authors declare that they have no competing interests.

Author details

[1]Veterinary Teaching Hospital, University of Extremadura, Avda, Universidad s/n, 10003 Cáceres, Spain. [2]Department of Animal Medicine and Surgery, Veterinary Faculty, University Complutense of Madrid, Avda. Puerta de Hierro, 28040 Madrid, Spain.

References

1. Merbl Y, Shilo-Benjamini Y, Chai O, Chamisha Y, Anglister N, King R, Horowitz I, Aizenberg Z, Shamir MH. Taenia multiceps brain cyst removal in two wild Nubian ibex (Capra nubianas). J Zoo Wildl Med. 2014;45(1):193–6.
2. Amin MN, Hashim MA, Hossain MA, Al-Sultan II. Coenurus cerebralis infection (Gid disease) in Black Bengal goats; Effects on certain blood values after surgical treatment. JABPA. 2013;3(1):1–7.
3. Biswas D. Ultrasound diagnosis and surgical treatment of coenurosis (GID) in bengal goat (Capra hircus) at chittagong metropolitan area, Chittagong, Bangladesh. Sci J Vet Adv. 2013;2:68–75.
4. Komnenou A, Argyroudis S, Giadinis N, Dessiris A. Surgical treatment of coenurosis (gid) in sheep. Vet Rec. 2000;147(9):242–4.
5. Weglinski MR, Perkins WJ. Inhalational versus total intravenous anes- thesia for neurosurgery: Theory guides, outcome decides. J Neurosurg Anesthesiol. 1994;6:290–3.
6. Banevičius G, Rugytė D, Macas A, Tamašauskas A, Stankevičius E. The effects of sevoflurane and propofol on cerebral hemodynamics during intracranial tumors surgery under monitoring the depth of anesthesia. Medicina (Kaunas). 2010;46(11):743–52.
7. Matta BF, Heath KJ, Tipping K, Summors AC. Direct cerebral vaso- dilatory effects of sevoflurane and isoflurane. Anesthesiology. 1999;91:677–80.
8. Matta BF, Lam AM, Strebel S, Mayberg TS. Cerebral pres- sure autoregulation and carbon dioxide reactivity dur- ing propofol-induced EEG suppression. Br J Anaesth. 1995;74(2):159–63.
9. Souter MJ, Andrews PJD, Piper IR, Miller JD. Effects of alfentanil on cerebral haemodynamics in an experimental model of traumatic brain injury. Br J Anaesth. 1997;79:97–102.
10. Coles JP, Leary TS, Monteiro JN, Brazier P, Summors A, Doyle P, Matta BF, Gupta AK. Propofol anesthesia for cra- niotomy: A double-blind comparison of remifentanil, alfentanil, and fentanyl. J Neurosurg Anesthesiol. 2000;12:15–20.
11. Bouillon TW, Bruhn J, Radulescu L, Andresen C, Shafer TJ. Pharmacodynamic interaction between propofol and remifentanil regarding hypnosis, tolerance of laryngoscopy, bispectral index, and electroence- phalographic approximate entropy. Anesthesiology. 2004;100:1353–72.
12. Valverde A, Gunkel CI. Clinical practice review: pain management in horses and farm animals. J Emerg Crit Care. 2005;15:295–307.
13. Dzikiti TB, Ndawana PS, Zeiler G, Bester L, Dzikiti LN. Determination of the minimum infusion rate of alfaxalone during its co-administration with midazolam in goats. Vet Rec Open. 2015 Feb 25;2(1):e000065. https://doi.org/10.1136/vetreco-2014-000065.
14. Stegmann GF, Bester L. Sedative-hypnotic effects of midazolam in goats after intravenous and intramuscular administration. Vet Anaesth Analg. 2001;28:49–55.
15. Dzikiti TB, Stegmann GF, Hellebrekers LJ, Auer RE, Dzikiti LN. Sedative and cardiopulmonary effects of acepromazine, midazolam, acepromazine-butorphanol and midazolam- butorphanol on propofol anaesthesia in goats. J S Afr Vet Assoc. 2009;80(1):10–6.
16. Valverde A, Doherty TJ, Hernandez WD. Effect of intravenous lidocaine on isoflurane MAC in dogs. Vet Anaesth Analg. 2004;31:264–71.
17. Pypendop BH, Ilkiw JE. The effects of intravenous lidocaine administration on the minimum alveolar concentration of isoflurane in cats. Anesth Analg. 2005;100:97–101.
18. Dzikiti TB, Hellebrekers LJ, van Dijk P. Effects of intravenous lidocaine on isoflurane concentration, physiological parameters, metabolic parameters and stress-related hormones in horses undergoing surgery. J Am Vet Med Assoc. 2003;50:190–5.
19. Doherty T, Redua MA, Queiroz-Castro P, Egger C, Cox SK, Rohrbach BW. Effect of intravenous lidocaine and ketamine on the minimum alveolar concentration of isoflurane in goats. Vet Anaesth Analg. 2007;34:125–31.
20. Larenza MP, Bergadano A, Iff I, Doherr MG, Schatzman U. Comparison of the cardiopulmonary effects of anaesthesia maintained by continuous infusion of ketamine and propofol with anaesthesia maintained by inhalation of sevoflurane in goats undergoing magnetic resonance imaging. Am J Vet Res. 2005;66:2135–41.
21. Dzikiti TB, Stegmann FG, Dzikiti LN, Hellebrekers LJ. Total intravenous anaesthesia (TIVA) with propofol–fentanyl and propofol–midazolam combinations in spontaneously breathing goats. Vet Anaesth Analg. 2010; 37:519–25.
22. Raisis AL, Leece EA, Platt SR, Adams VJ, Corletto F, Brearley J. Evaluation of an anaesthetic technique used in dogs undergoing craniectomy for tumour resection. Vet Anaesth Analg. 2007;34:171–80.
23. Bruder NJ. Awakening management after neuro- surgery for intracranial tumours. Curr Opin Anaes- thesiol. 2002;15:477–82.
24. Gurulingappa AMA, Awati MN, Adarsh S. Attenuation of cardiovascular responses to direct laryngoscopy and intubation — A comparative study between IV bolus fentanyl, lignocaine and placebo (NS). J Clin Diagn Res. 2012;6:1749–52.
25. Jolliffe CT, Leece EA, Adams V, Marlin DJ. Effect of intravenous lidocaine on heart rate, systolic arterial blood pressure and cough responses to endotracheal intubation in propofol-anaesthetized dogs. Vet Anaesth Analg. 2007;34:322–30.
26. Tomori Z, Widdicombe JG. Muscular, bronchomotor and cardiovascular reflexes elicited by mechanical stimulation of the respiratory tract. J Physiol. 1969;200:25.
27. Sun L, Guo R, Sun L. The impact of prophylactic intravenous lidocaine on opioid-induced cough: A meta-analysis of randomized controlled trials. J Anesth. 2014;28:325–33.
28. Bettschart-Wolfensberger R, Semder A, Alibhai H, Demuth D, Aliabadi FS, Clarke KW. Cardiopulmonary side-effects and pharmacokinetics of an emulsion of propofol (Disoprivan) in comparison to propofol solved in polysorbate 80 in goats. J Vet Med A Physiol Pathol Clin Med. 2000;47:341–50.
29. Armitage-Chan EA, Wetmore LA, Chan DL. Anesthetic management of the head trauma patient. J Vet Emerg Crit Care. 2007;17:5–14.
30. Jellinek DA, Freeman R. Perioperative care. In: Kaye AH, McL BP, editors. Operative Neurosurgery. Edinburgh: Churchill Livingstone; 2000. p. 15–32.
31. Cornick JL. Anesthetic management of patients with neurological abnormalities. Compend Cont Ed Pract Vet. 1992;14:163–73.
32. Walters FJM. Neuro anaesthesia – a review of the basic principles and current practices. Cent Afr J Med. 1990;36:44–51.
33. Court MH, Dodman NH, Norman WM, Seeler DC. Anaesthesia and central nervous system disease in small animals part I: general considerations. Br Vet J. 1990;146:285–95.
34. Dzikiti TB. Intravenous anaesthesia in goats: a review. J S Afr Vet Assoc. 2013;84:1–8.
35. Langley MS, Heel RC. Propofol. A review of its pharmacodynamic and pharmacokinetic properties and use as an intravenous anaesthetic. Drugs. 1988;35:334–72.

36. Reid J, Nolan AM, Welsh E. Propofol as an induc- tion agent in the goat: a pharmacokinetic study. J Vet Pharmacol Therap. 1993;16:488–93.
37. Prassinos NN, Galatos AD, Raptopoulos D. A comparison of propofol, thiopental or ketamine as induction agents in goats. Vet Anaesth Analg. 2005;32:289–96.
38. Ferreira JP, Ndawana PS, Dzikiti LN, Dzikiti BT. Determination of the minimum infusion rate of propofol required to prevent purposeful movement of the extremities in response to a standardized noxious stimulus in goats. Vet Anaesth Analg. 2015; https://doi.org/10.1111/vaa.12327.
39. Dzikiti TB, Stegmann GF, Dzikiti LN, Hellebrekers LJ. Effects of midazolam on isoflurane minimum alveolar concentration in goats. Small Rumin Res. 2011; 97:104–9.
40. Carroll GL, Hooper RN, Slater MR, Hartsfield SM, Matthews NS. Detomidine-butorphanol-propofol for carotid artery transloca- tion and castration or ovariectomy in goats. Vet Surg. 1998;27:75–82.
41. Ndawana PS, Dzikiti TB, Zeiler GE, Dzikiti NL. Determination of minimum infusion rate (MIR) of alfaxalone required to prevent purposeful movement of the extremities in response to a standardised noxious stimulus in goats. Vet Anaesth Analg. 2015;42:65–71.
42. Hemmings HC Jr. Neuroprotection by Na channel blockade. J Neurosurg Anesthesiol. 2004;16:100–1.
43. Lei B, Popp S, Capuano-Waters C, Cottrell JE, Kass IS. Effects of delayed administration of low-dose lidocaine on transient focal cerebral ischemia in rats. Anesthesiology. 2002;97:1534–40.

3

Serum concentration of ketamine and antinociceptive effects of ketamine and ketamine-lidocaine infusions in conscious dogs

Ubedullah Kaka[1,2], Bullo Saifullah[3], Adamu Abdul Abubakar[1], Yong Meng Goh[4,5], Sharida Fakurazi[6,7], Asmatullah Kaka[1,9], Atique Ahmed Behan[8,9], Mahdi Ebrahimi[4] and Hui Cheng Chen[1*]

Abstract

Background: Central sensitization is a potential severe consequence of invasive surgical procedures. It results in postoperative and potentially chronic pain enhancement. It results in postoperative pain enhancement; clinically manifested as hyperalgesia and allodynia. N-methyl-D-aspartate (NMDA) receptor plays a crucial role in the mechanism of central sensitisation. Ketamine is most commonly used NMDA-antagonist in human and veterinary practice. However, the antinociceptive serum concentration of ketamine is not yet properly established in dogs. Six dogs were used in a crossover design, with one week washout period. Treatments consisted of: 1) 0.5 mg/kg ketamine followed by continuous rate infusion (CRI) of 30 μg/kg/min; 2) 0.5 mg/kg ketamine followed by CRI of 30 μg/kg/min and lidocaine (2 mg/kg followed by CRI of 100 μg/kg/min); and 3) 0.5 mg/kg ketamine followed by CRI of 50 μg/kg/min. The infusion was administered up to 120 min. Nociceptive thresholds and ketamine serum concentrations were measured before drug administration, and at 5, 10, 20, 40, 60, 90, 120, 140 and 160 min after the start of infusion.

Results: Maximum concentration recorded was 435.34 ± 26.18 ng/mL, 582.34 ± 227.46 ng/mL and 733.77 ± 133.6 ng/mL for K30, KL30 and K50, respectively. The concentration at 120 min was 250.87 ± 39.87, 221.73 ± 91.03 and 343.67 ± 63.21 ng/mL at 120 min in K30, KL30 and K50, respectively. All the three infusion regimes maintained serum concentrations above 200 ng/mL. The thresholds returned towards baseline values within 20 min, after cessation of infusion.

Conclusion: Serum concentration to produce mechanical antinociceptive effects in dogs is between 100 and 200 ng/mL. All the three infusion regimes in this study provided antinociceptive effects throughout the infusions. In this study, we found that the serum concentration of ketamine to produce mechanical antinociceptive effects in dogs is above 200 ng/mL. All three infusion regimes provided antinociceptive effects throughout the infusions without causing harmful effects. Further studies are recommended in a clinical setting.

Keywords: Ketamine, NMDA receptor, Nociceptive mechanical thresholds, Dog, Lidocaine

* Correspondence: chen@upm.edu.my
[1]Department of Veterinary Clinical Studies, Faculty of Veterinary Medicine, Universiti Putra Malaysia, 43400 Serdang, Selangor, Malaysia
Full list of author information is available at the end of the article

Background

The glutamate-activated *N-methyl-D-aspartate* (NMDA) receptor plays a crucial role in the development of central sensitization. Some of the characteristics associated with central sensitization are manifested clinically by a painful sensation from a non-painful stimulus (allodynia) and augmented pain sensation from previously painful stimuli (hyperalgesia) [1–5].

Association of the NMDA receptor with postoperative pain ushered a new chapter in the exploration of NMDA-antagonists for postoperative analgesia protocol. Ketamine is well established NMDA- antagonist. It is commonly used as an anaesthetic agent in children and animals. It is useful for its anti-nociceptive properties in acute pain, and can be used for chronic and neuropathic pain as well [4]. Ketamine has prevented hyperalgesia, improved analgesia [6–8] and decreased postoperative opioid consumption [8–10] in surgical patients.

The analgesic dose range of ketamine for use in dogs has not been properly established. As a consequence, analgesic benefits of ketamine are not yet fully recognized in dogs. The effective dose range of ketamine in human surgical patients has been established at a loading dose of 0.5 mg/kg, followed by continuous rate infusion (CRI) of 2 to10 μg/kg/min [7, 10–12]. In the absence of appropriate analgesic dose range, the doses used in studies of dogs [13–15] have been taken from human studies [16, 17]. This has resulted in reporting inconclusive results. Moreover, most of the studies were clinical. Consequently, the use of opioids pre and postoperatively in these studies might have masked the analgesic effects of ketamine. Apart from this, various scoring scales used in these studies have not been validated for reliability, specificity or linearity. Most importantly these scales were based on subjective assessment of behaviour [18, 19], which can be biased by inter-observer variability. Furthermore, none of these studies correlated effects with serum concentrations of ketamine.

So far, only one study reported plasma concentration versus antinociceptive actions in dogs [20]. In this study, ketamine was administered at 0.5 mg/kg, followed by 10 μg/kg/min for 59 min in dogs, antinociceptive effect was demonstrated only for the first four minutes, at which time the plasma concentration was >100 ng/mL. Plasma concentration of ketamine declined to <100 ng/mL after 5 min [20]. Further analysis revealed that the plasma concentrations of ketamine at pseudo-steady state were five times lower than the expected concentrations to that in humans receiving the same CRI. They concluded that this dose was insufficient to maintain the analgesic concentration of the ketamine. This also suggests that ketamine pharmacokinetics in dogs may differ from that in humans, and that may warrant the use of higher infusion rates in dogs.

Lidocaine is commonly used as a local anaesthetic and anti-arrhythmic agent in veterinary and human medicine. With the mechanism based approach combination of lidocaine acting on sodium channels, which play a part in generation and transmission of nociceptive impulses [1] and ketamine acting on NMDA receptors would be better strategy to manage postoperative pain, compared to conventional method of administering single drug for post operative pain management. The major benefit of combining lidocaine and ketamine is to prevent the development of central sensitization during surgical intervention [21], which may reduce pain and discomfort in the postoperative period. The combination of ketamine and lidocaine has been reported to decrease the minimum alveolar concentration (MAC) of inhalant anaesthetics in dogs [22–25]. It has been suggested that the MAC reducing effect may be due to analgesic or sedative effect or both [22, 24, 25]. The analgesic effects of the combination of lidocaine and ketamine in conscious dogs have not been reported.

This study therefore, aimed to correlate the serum concentrations of ketamine to the antinociceptive effects using two infusion rates of ketamine. Furthermore, this study also evaluated the clinical and antinociceptive effects of incorporation of lidocaine infusion to ketamine in a controlled, repeatable situation.

Methods

Animals and treatments

Six adult healthy mix-breed female dogs weighing 17.2 ± 2.2 kg (Mean ± SD) with the age of 2 to 10 years old were used in this study. Animals were obtained from a local stray animal holding facility following informed consent. These animals were acclimatized for one month, during this period they were kept under observation for any disease or abnormality. Dogs were judged healthy based on physical examination, hematology, and blood biochemistry, and have not been showing any sign of illness during one month of previous observation. Animals were brought daily to the experimental room, which was adjacent to the kennels, in order to familiarise them with the experimental station. Experiments were conducted in animal experimental station in a quiet environment with minimum number of observers. Experiments were conducted in day time, starting at 8:00 am. The study was approved by the Universiti Putra Malaysia Animal Care and Utility Committee (Reference Number UPM/IACUC/AUP-R023/2013).

All six dogs were subjected to three treatment protocols in a randomized crossover design with one-week washout period between the treatments. Treatment protocols were: 1) 0.5 mg/kg ketamine (NARKETAN®-10, 100 mg/mL, Vetoquinol UK Limited, Buckingham, UK) followed by continuous rate infusion (CRI) of 30 μg/kg/

min (K30); 2) Combination of ketamine (0.5 mg/kg followed by CRI of 30 µg/kg/min) and lidocaine hydrochloride (Xylocaine® 2 % AstraZeneca, France) 2 mg/kg followed by CRI of 100 µg/kg/min (KL30); and 3) 0.5 mg/kg ketamine followed by CRI of 50 µg/kg/min (K50).

The loading doses of K30, KL30 and K50 were mixed in normal saline to a final volume of 3 mL and injected over one minute. Ketamine was diluted with normal saline to 5 mg/mL and lidocaine 16.66 mg/mL for infusion. Infusions were delivered for 120 min through a precision syringe pump (Omnifuse, Graseby medical limited, United Kingdom). Right and left cephalic veins were catheterized with 20 G indwelling catheters (Vasofix® Braunule®, B. Braune Melsungen AG 34209 Melsungen, Germany) for blood sampling and infusion of drugs, respectively. Prior to the actual study, the infusion regimens were tested in two of the six dogs.

Algometer device

Wagner algometer (FPX 25, Wagner Instruments, Greenwich CT, USA) with a modified tip was used in this study.

Nociceptive mechanical thresholds

The nociceptive mechanical thresholds were recorded in duplicates from the carpal pad, metacarpal footpad, tibia and femur of right limbs, and the abdomen. Thresholds were determined before treatment as baseline and then after start of treatment at 10, 20, 40, 60, 90, 120, 140 and 160 min. These body points were selected based on models used in the previous studies [26–28] conducted in dogs. The carpal pad and metacarpal pad were tested by applying the tip of the algometer at midpoint of these pads. The tibia was tested on the distal latero-dorsal surface where bone could be palpated through the skin. The femur was tested on the distal latero-dorsal surface, where the bone could be palpated through the skin by displacing the muscle with little pressure applied with fingers. The abdomen was tested on the midline at the midpoint between umbilicus and pubis. The order of testing was firstly the metacarpal pad, followed by carpal pad, femur, tibia, and finally, the abdomen. At each testing point, the tip was placed perpendicular to the surface area. The pressure was increased gradually until the dog responded. The entire threshold recording was performed by the same researcher. During thresholds determination, the operator did not look at the reading of the algometer as he applied consistent force. Instead, he concentrated on the dogs' response and immediately stopped at response. The end-points were cross-checked by another observer who took note of both the algometer readings and dogs' response. The most common response identified during the preliminary trial was clear withdrawal reflex of the limb, vocalization, withdrawal of the limb accompanied with vocalization and guarding of the abdomen. According to Le Bars et al. (2001), in order to avoid tissue damage, cut-off pressure should be set at three times the thresholds of control [29]. Preliminary trials and the baseline thresholds on body points tested in this study were 5 to 6 Newtons (N). Thus, the cut-off pressure was set at 18 N for this study. If no reaction was perceived before the cut-off limit, this value (18 N) was recorded as the mechanical nociceptive threshold. One of the dogs did not respond to application of the algometer up to the cut-off point of 18 N at its abdomen, thus, was not tested at abdomen for all treatment groups.

Sedation score and side effects

A composite sedation score and a behavioural chart adopted from Bergadano et al. (2009) were used to evaluate the psychomimetic side effects of ketamine at the measurement time points [20]. The sedation score on a 0 (no sedation) to 12 (deep sedation) scale, was assigned by adding the ranking of different descriptors (Table 1). The incidence of psychomimetic signs (disorientation, lateral head movements, fixed eyes, apneustic respiration, salivation, tremors and hyperactivity) was noted for each treatment group. The person involved in scoring sedation and side effects was blinded to the treatments.

Blood sampling

Blood samples were taken before administration of treatment as baseline, and then at 1, 5, 10, 20, 40, 60, 90, 120 and 140 min after the start of infusion. At each time points, 2 mL of blood was sampled and kept in plain sampling tubes (BD Vacutainer®, BD Franklin Lakes NJ USA), and immediately placed on ice. Samples were centrifuged and serum was harvested, and then frozen at - 80 °C until analysis.

Table 1 Sedation score scale used in this system (Adopted from Bergadano et al. 2009)

Score	Consciousness	Eye	Responsiveness	Relaxation
0	Awake	Not rotated	Respond to voice	Moves spontaneously
1	Aware	Moderate rotation	Respond to gentle touch	Relaxed, no shivering
2	Not aware but arousable	Rotated	Does not respond to touch	Very Relaxed
3	Not aware and not arousable	Nystagmus	Hyperexcitable	Hypertonous

High performance liquid chromatography analysis

Ketamine concentration in serum was determined using high performance liquid chromatography (HPLC). In brief, the system consisted of Waters HPLC 2695 separation module, an Agilent C18 column (5 µm particle size; 4.6 × 150 mm), photodiode array (PDA) detector and a computer equipped with Empower software (Waters, Milford, MA, USA).

Extraction of drug from serum

The ketamine was extracted from serum by the method reported earlier (Doherty et al. 2007). Briefly, the frozen serum samples were thawed followed by vortex mixing and transferred to 1 mL of glass test tube containing 25 µL of (internal standard, 50 µg/mL) trimethoprim. Further, 200 µL of 1 molar solution (1 M) of sodium hydroxide (NaOH) and 5 mL methylene chloride (CH_2Cl_2) were added to above samples. Tubes were vortex mixed again and then centrifuged for 20 min at 1500 g. The organic layer was separated and placed in clean tube evaporated with gentle stream of nitrogen till dryness. Finally, samples were reconstituted with 1 mL of mobile phase and 100 µL was injected for HPLC analysis.

Sample analysis

In brief, freshly prepared isocratic mixture of 0.02 M potassium dihydrogen phosphate (KH_2PO_4) pH 4.5, adjusted with phosphoric acid and acetonitrile (ACN) (ACN:KH_2PO_4 (40:60) was used as mobile phase with flow rate of 1.0 mL/min. Calibration curves for serum analysis were prepared by spiking the dog serum with ketamine. A linear concentration range of 25–1500 ng/mL was established with r^2 value of 0.99.

Statistical analysis

Data are presented as mean ± standard deviation. Statistical analysis was performed using the SAS software package, version 9.3 (SAS Institute Inc., Cary, NC, USA). Prior to the analysis, data were checked for their conformance to the normal distribution using Kolmogrov-Simirnov test. Changes in mechanical thresholds and serum concentrations over time and across treatment groups were compared using the repeated-measures ANOVA model. Bonferroni adjusted P values were used when indicated by a significant F test ($P < 0.05$). Correlation between the mechanical thresholds and serum concentrations of ketamine was calculated with Pearson test. Effects of treatment over time on sedation score were analyzed using Friedman's test. Overall significance was set at a value of $P < 0.05$. The observed power for the current study was determined to be 80.53 % for 1-Way ANOVA, and 90.75 % for Repeated Measure ANOVA. This was based on an effect size value of 0.8165, obtained by calculating the serum ketamine concentrations 1 min after administration (peak value), and at 120 min after administration. Power calculations were performed using G*Power Software, version 3.1.9.2 [30].

Results

The experiments were well tolerated by all the dogs. Changes in behavior due to recognized psychomimetic effects of ketamine were mild and harmless. The behavioral changes disappeared within 20 min after the end of infusion, and the dogs resumed their activity immediately after the end of experiment. The algometer device was well tolerated by all the animals. Transient dimples were observed at the carpal pad, metacarpal footpad, and abdomen, which disappeared within 1 min, before the replicate measurement. There was no sign of redness, swelling, bleeding, exudates, and lameness during, immediately after, and 24 h after the experiment.

Serum concentrations of ketamine

The serum concentrations (Mean ± SD) of K30, KL30 and K50 across time points are illustrated in Fig. 1. Maximum concentration was observed at 1 min for K30 (435.34 ± 26.18 ng/mL), KL30 (582.34 ± 227.46 ng/mL), and K50 (733.77 ± 133.6 ng/mL), which remained stable for 20 min, and declined gradually reaching around 250.87 ± 39.87, 221.73 ± 91.03 and 343.67 ± 63.21 ng/mL at 120th min in K30, KL30 and K50, respectively. The serum concentration decreased rapidly to less than 100 ng/mL within 20 min following the end of infusions in all three treatments. Between 1 and 40 min, serum concentration of K50 was higher than K30, while concentration of KL30 lied in between K50 and K30. By 60th min, the three groups were not statistically different.

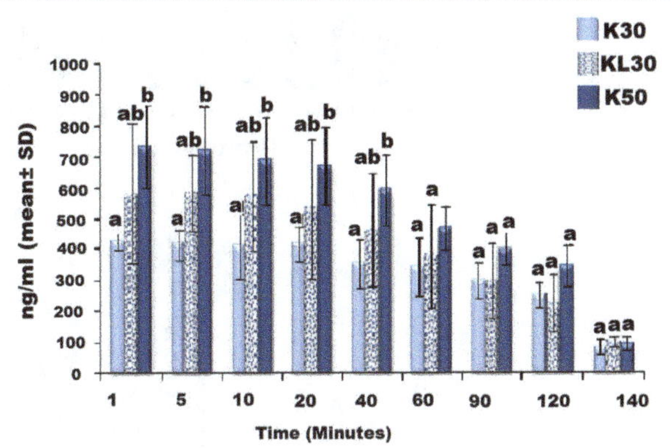

Fig. 1 Comparison (Mean ± SD) between serum concentration of K30, KL30 and K50 in 6 dogs during and after CRI. K30 = Ketamine 0.5 mg/kg loading dose followed by 30 µg/kg/min, KL30 = Ketamine 0.5 mg/kg loading dose followed by 30 µg/kg/min and lidocaine 2 mg/kg loading dose followed by 100 µg/kg/min, K50 = Ketamine 0.5 mg/kg loading dose followed by 50 µg/kg/min CRI. At each time point, groups with similar alphabet are not different ($P < 0.05$)

Nociceptive mechanical thresholds

There was no significant difference among the baseline mechanical thresholds at carpal pad, metacarpal foot pad, tibia, femur and abdomen in all treatment groups (Fig. 2a-e). All the three treatments increased thresholds significantly ($P < 0.05$) throughout the infusion up to 120 min. Mechanical thresholds returned to baseline within 20 min of the end of CRI at 140th min. Overall, nociceptive mechanical thresholds were higher in KL30 than in K30 and also higher in K50 than in KL30, and some significant differences between groups were recorded. There was weak positive correlation between serum concentration of K30 with mechanical thresholds at carpal pad (r-0.24 $P = 0.141$), metacarpal footpad (r-0.32, $P = 0.053$), tibia (r-0.33, $P = 0.047$), femur (r-0.30, $P = 0.075$) and abdomen (r-0.35, $P = 0.053$). Likewise, weak positive correlation of K50 with mechanical thresholds at carpal pad (r-0.29 $P = 0.080$), metacarpal footpad (r-0.38, $P = 0.020$), tibia (r-0.18, $P = 0.330$), femur (r-0.22, $P = 0.185$) and abdomen (r-0.12, $P = 0.527$) were observed.

Heart rate, body temperature and respiration

Baseline heart rates were not different amongst all treatments. Heart rates increased significantly from baselines in all treatments during the 120 min of treatment infusions. Following cessation of infusions, heart rates decreased, but remained higher than baselines in KL30 and K50. Heart rates between K30 and KL30 were not different, while K50 resulted in higher heart rates compared to K30 at 40 to 60 min and KL30 at 40 to 120 min (Table 2). Body temperatures increased significantly from baselines throughout the 160-minute study period in K30 and KL30 groups, and up to 120 min in K50 (Table 3). This increase in body temperature was within the normal range. The change in respiration was insignificant in K30, while KL30 and K50 resulted in increased respiratory rates at 120 to 160, and 20 to 160 min, respectively.

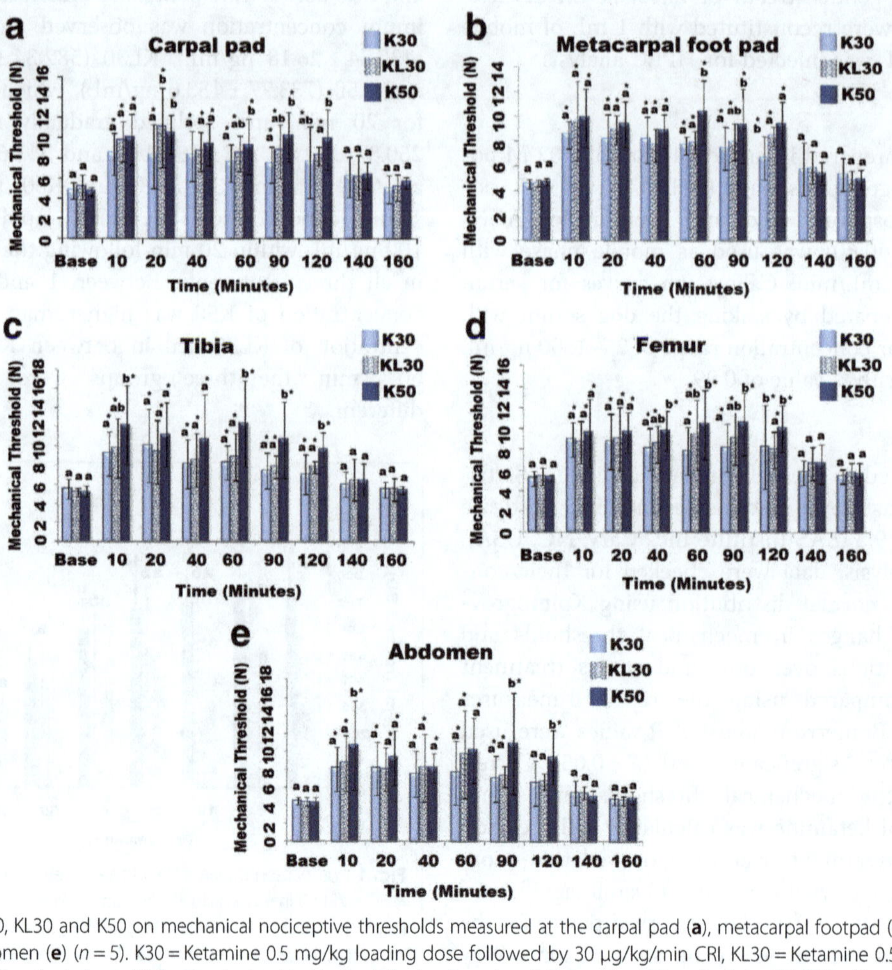

Fig. 2 Effects of K30, KL30 and K50 on mechanical nociceptive thresholds measured at the carpal pad (**a**), metacarpal footpad (**b**), tibia (**c**), femur (**d**) ($n = 6$) and abdomen (**e**) ($n = 5$). K30 = Ketamine 0.5 mg/kg loading dose followed by 30 μg/kg/min CRI, KL30 = Ketamine 0.5 mg/kg loading dose followed by 30 μg/kg/min and lidocaine hydrochloride 2 mg/kg loading dose followed by 100 μg/kg/min CRI, K50 = Ketamine 0.5 mg/kg loading dose followed by 50 μg/kg/min CRI,. Data are expressed as mean ± SD. * denotes significant difference from baseline within treatment, at each time point, groups with similar alphabet are not different ($P < 0.05$)

Table 2 Effects of K30, KL30 and K50 on heart rates (Mean ± SD) measured in 6 dogs using crossover design

	K30	KL30	K50
Baseline	79 ± 6	77 ± 7	81 ± 6
20 min	113 ± 24[a]	101 ± 19[a]	113 ± 22[a]
40 min	104 ± 16[a]	99 ± 18[a]	123 ± 19[abc]
60 min	105 ± 15[a]	104 ± 260[a]	124 ± 23[abc]
90 min	113 ± 15[a]	107 ± 21[a]	127 ± 25[ac]
120 min	106 ± 19[a]	98 ± 20[a]	114 ± 14[ac]
140 min	93 ± 20	93 ± 12[a]	99 ± 15[a]
160 min	86 ± 14	94 ± 11[a]	102 ± 25[ab]

K30 Ketamine 0.5 mg/kg loading dose followed by 30 μg/kg/min CRI, *KL30* Ketamine 0.5 mg/kg loading dose followed by 30 μg/kg/min and lidocaine hydrochloride 2 mg/kg loading dose followed by 100 μg/kg/min CRI, *K50* 0.5 mg/kg loading dose followed by 50 μg/kg/min CRI. [a]denotes significant difference from baseline within same treatment, [b]denotes significant difference from K30 at corresponding values, [c]denotes significantly different from KL30 at corresponding time points. Overall significance was set at a value of $P < 0.05$

Respiratory rate increased from 33 ± 7 at baseline, to as much as 93 ± 5 breaths per minute in KL30, and from 29 ± 7 at baseline, to as much as 93 ± 5 breaths per minute in K50 during infusion of treatment.

Sedation and side effects

Sedation score and side effects are presented in Tables 4 and 5. There was significant difference in the sedation score between K30, KL30 and K50 groups. The median sedation scores were 0 throughout the 160-minute study period in K30 and KL30. In contrast, median score in K50 were 3 between 1 and 20 min, and reduced to 1 between 40 and 90 min. Most of the dogs exhibited one or more side effects such as disorientation, swaying of the head, salivation and hyperactivity. These effects were observed throughout the duration of 120 min infusion and disappeared at 140th min, which is within 20 min after the end of infusions. The side effects were less severe in K30 and KL30 compared to K50.

Table 3 Effects of K30, KL30 and K50 on body temperatures (Mean ± SD) measured in 6 dogs using crossover design

	K30	KL30	K50
Baseline	38.6 ± 0.4	38.7 ± 0.3	38.8 ± 0.2
20 min	39.0 ± 0.5[a]	39.1 ± 0.6[a]	39.2 ± 0.6[a]
40 min	39.1 ± 0.6[a]	39.0 ± 0.5[a]	39.3 ± 0.5[a]
60 min	39.2 ± 0.4[a]	39.1 ± 0.4[a]	39.3 ± 0.5[a]
90 min	39.2 ± 0.4[a]	39.1 ± 0.4[a]	39.0 ± 0.4[a]
120 min	39.1 ± 0.5[a]	39.1 ± 0.5[a]	39.0 ± 0.3[a]
140 min	39.3 ± 0.5[a]	39.2 ± 0.4[a]	39.0 ± 0.3
160 min	39.0 ± 0.4[a]	39.1 ± 0.5[a]	39.0 ± 0.3

K30 Ketamine 0.5 mg/kg loading dose followed by 30 μg/kg/min CRI, *KL30* Ketamine 0.5 mg/kg loading dose followed by 30 μg/kg/min and lidocaine hydrochloride 2 mg/kg loading dose followed by 100 μg/kg/min CRI, *K50* 0.5 mg/kg loading dose followed by 50 μg/kg/min CRI [a]denotes significant difference from baseline within same treatment. Overall significance was set at a value of $P < 0.05$

Table 4 Sedation score in median (IQR) values across each time points of the each group after administration of K30, K50, and KL30 in 6 dogs

Time (minutes)	K30	KL30	K50[a]
0	0 (0–0)	0 (0–0)	0 (0–0)
01	0 (0–0)	0 (0–0)	3 (0–3)
05	0 (0–0)	0 (0–0)	3 (0–3)
20	0 (0–0)	0 (0–0)	3 (0–3)
40	0 (0–0)	0 (0–0)	1 (0–3)
60	0 (0–0)	0 (0–0)	1 (0–3)
90	0 (0–0)	0 (0–0)	1 (0–3)
120	0 (0–0)	0 (0–0)	0 (0–0)
140	0 (0–0)	0 (0–0)	0 (0–0)
160	0 (0–0)	0 (0–0)	0 (0–0)

K30 ketamine 0.5 mg/kg loading dose followed by 30 μg/kg/min, *K50* 0.5 mg/kg loading dose followed by 50 μg/kg/min, *KL* = ketamine 0.5 loading dose followed by 30 μg/kg/min + lidocaine 2 mg/kg loading dose followed by 100 μg/kg/min. Overall significance was set at a value of $P < 0.05$. [a]K50 is significantly different from K30 and KL at $P < 0.003$ (Friedman test)

Discussion

The concentrations of ketamine in the present study were 435.34 ± 26.18 ng/mL for K30, 582.34 ± 227.46 ng/mL for KL30 and 733.77 ± 133.6 ng/mL for K50 at 1 min and 250.87 ± 39.87, 221.73 ± 91.03 and 343.67 ± 63.21 ng/mL at 120 min for K30, KL30 and K50, respectively. The serum concentrations of ketamine produced by all the 3 CRI regimens in this study could be maintained above 100 ng/mL during the 120- min infusions. Furthermore, nociceptive thresholds at most body points were raised above baseline values during the 120 min of infusions. The nociceptive thresholds returned towards baseline values within 20 min after cessation of infusions, at which point, serum levels were found to be lower than 100 ng/mL. Results from this study suggested that the minimum concentration of ketamine to produce analgesia in dogs is between 100 as observed at 140 min and 200 ng/mL during infusion. This concurred with findings in humans, where serum concentration of 100–200 ng/mL of ketamine was reported to be analgesic with minimal side effects [11, 31].

Effective analgesic concentration of ketamine has not been reported in dogs. The only study reporting the analgesic concentration of ketamine versus its antinociceptive action in dogs has been conducted by Bergadano et al. [20]. They found that the analgesic effect only lasted for the first four minutes at plasma concentration of 220–370 ng/ mL. No further analgesic effect was observed thereafter for up to 59 min, when plasma concentration was found to be below 100 ng/mL. They selected

Table 5 Frequency of side effects (number of dogs out of six showing a specific psychomimetic sign)

		0 min	1 min	5 min	20 min	40 min	60 min	90 min	120 min	140 min	160 min
Disorientation/confused	K30	0	5	5	4	3	3	3	3	0	0
	K50	0	5	5	6	6	6	5	6	0	0
	KL30	0	4	5	5	5	5	5	5	0	0
Lateral head movements	K30	0	3	3	2	2	2	2	2	0	0
	K50	0	5	5	6	6	6	5	5	0	0
	KL30	0	3	4	4	4	4	4	4	0	0
Glazy Eyes	K30	0	0	0	0	0	0	0	0	0	0
	K50	0	0	0	0	0	0	0	0	0	0
	KL30	0	0	0	0	0	0	0	0	0	0
Apneustic respiration	K30	0	0	0	0	0	0	0	0	0	0
	K50	0	0	0	0	0	0	0	0	0	0
	KL30	0	0	0	0	0	0	0	0	0	0
Salivation	K30	0	4	4	4	4	4	4	4	0	0
	K50	0	4	4	4	4	4	4	4	0	0
	KL30	0	4	4	4	4	4	4	4	4	0
Tremors	K30	0	0	0	0	0	0	0	0	0	0
	K50	0	0	0	0	0	0	0	0	0	0
	KL30	0	0	0	0	0	0	0	0	0	0
Hyperactivity	K30	0	1	1	1	1	1	1	1	0	0
	K50	0	3	3	3	3	3	3	3	0	0
	KL30	0	2	2	2	1	1	0	0	0	0

K30 ketamine 0.5 mg/kg loading dose followed by 30 μg/kg/min, K50 0.5 mg/kg loading dose followed by 50 μg/kg/min, KL30 ketamine 0.5 loading dose followed by 30 μg/kg/min + lidocaine 2 mg/kg loading dose followed by 100 μg/kg/min

a ketamine dose of 0.5 mg/kg and 10 μg/kg/min from the human studies [16, 17, 31, 32]. However, these dosages had difficulties to sustain a desired plasma ketamine concentration (i.e. above 100–200 ng/mL) to produce antinociceptive effect conscious dogs. The authors suggested that this variation was due the difference in pharmacokinetics of ketamine between human and dogs, in addition to inter-species an intra species difference has also been reported in dogs [33]. Various factors could contribute to the individual variations within the species; these include age, body weight, lean-to-fat body ratio and genetics [34–36]. Although there is no data reporting the influence of genetic factors on the disposition of ketamine in dogs, its potential role cannot be excluded. In this study, we selected the ketamine dose based on the prior results reported by Bergadano et al. [20] . We used similar loading dose of 0.5 mg/kg, but increased the CRI to 30 and 50 μg/kg/min, doses 3 and 5 times higher than that used by Bergadano. Both the doses maintained serum concentration above the level required to raise the mechanical nociceptive thresholds up to 120 min. Our study showed that the mechanical nociceptive threshold in dogs can be raised through ketamine infusion. In order to maintain this plasma concentration and have an antinociceptive effect over 120 min, higher infusions rates than previously employed by Bergadano et al. in dogs (20) are deemed necessary. A time of 120 min was selected in our study to simulate a multimodal analgesic approach that could provide pre-intra and post-operative antinociception for a potential surgery of 45 min. This period covers the time before, during and after surgery up to recovery. Thus, results of this study confirmed the need for higher infusion rates of ketamine in dogs than that previously employed by Bergadano in dogs [20].

In the present study, the concentration of ketamine was higher during first 10–20 min of adminsitration, and declined gradually thereafter. The initial hike and maintenance of the higher serum concentrations were likely contributed by the loading dose. Since ketamine is a high clearance drug, it requires continuous infusion for at least five half lives, which is approximately 10 h to maintain steady state [37]. Ketamine also increases sympathetic nervous system activity, resulting in increased cardiovascular functions and hepatic blood flow [38, 39]. Thus, the elevated heart rates in the present study are likely a reflection of sympathetic stimulation by ketamine.

Nociceptive mechanical thresholds increased significantly compared to baseline after administration of the K30, KL30 and K50 groups and remained elevated throughout the 120-minutes of infusion. The thresholds returned to baseline at 140 min, that is, within 20 min after the end of infusion. Mechanical thresholds have been used in previous studies in animals [14, 26–28, 40–45] for the objective quantification of pain and to evaluate the analgesic efficacy of drugs. The analgesic effect of the test drug reported by these studies was either increase in the mechanical thresholds at the site of test compared to baseline [26, 28] or concurrent rise in the mechanical thresholds equal to that produced by positive control analgesic or dose used to compare with [40, 45] or equal rise in mechanical thresholds at the site of surgery by the same drug compared for two routes of administration [40, 44]. Kukanich et al. (2005) and Kaka et al. (2015) reported increase in mechanical thresholds after administration of intravenous morphine at 1 mg/kg [26, 28]. The increase in mechanical thresholds compared to baseline in these studies was suggestive of analgesic action of morphine. In the present study mechanical thresholds increased significantly compared to baseline in K30, KL30 and K50 treatments throughout the infusion period of 120 min and returned to baseline within 20 min after the end of infusion. The rise in mechanical thresholds suggests the antinociceptive actions of K30, KL30 and K50 throughout the duration of infusion. The modified algometer and technique used in this study have been validated previously in our lab [28]. In this study, conscious vocalization may not be a good indicator of nociceptive threshold as it occurred only in 2 of subjects, and therefore we depended on algometer readings, even though vocalization has been accepted as part of the pain study protocol in human beings.

Mechanical pressure for quantification of surgical pain or hyperalgesia is termed as "algometry". Algometry has been used to identify abnormal pain thresholds and to monitor response to analgesic treatment in animals and humans [46–49]. Algometry has also been used to evaluate the analgesic effects of drugs in dogs [26, 27, 40]. Rate of force of application plays a crucial part on the reliability of this method. Application of force at a faster rate may provoke a low false threshold reading [50]. In a study of reliability and validity of algometer Kinser et al. (2009) concluded that this is highly reliable and valid method [51]. The authors suggested that with some practice, an individual becomes reliable in applying force with an algometer. In this study researcher who operated the algometer has sufficient practice in applying the rate of force of application during preliminary experiments, which have been demonstrated as consistent results in saline treatment during validation of the method [28]. Similarly, in this study no significant difference in mechanical thresholds between control and 140 min indicates the reliability of results. Thus, the results of the above studies suggest that algometry is reliable and valid technique for the quantification of mechanical nociceptive thresholds. It should be noted that despite an open label approach of the current study, potential operator bias was minimized by blinding the operator of the algometer to the threshold values. Only another nearby observer who was not operating the algometer was entrusted to record the readings displayed on the LCD screen. It should be noted that the operator of the algometer, cannot see the values projected on the LCD screen. We are aware that open label studies have the limitation that results could be refined and biased [51], however, we tried to minimise the bias by blinding to the treatment the investigator who evaluated sedation and side effects of the infusions, and the investigator operating the algometer to the values recorded.

Ketamine has been reported to increase body temperature in dogs [23]. Effects of body temperature on mechanical thresholds in dogs have not been reported. In this study body temperatures increased significantly from baseline throughout study, however, this increase was within the normal range. The increase in mechanical thresholds throughout infusion and decrease in the mechanical thresholds after the end of infusion, at which time the temperature was still higher than baseline suggests that increase in temperatures did not affect the mechanical thresholds.

Ketamine is well known for its psychomimetic effects in dogs; these effects range from hypersalivation to excitability and delirium. The dose regimens used in this study did produce such side effects; however they were harmless and ceased within 20 min of ending the infusions. Furthermore, side effects were less intense and occurred less frequently in K30 and KL30 compared to K50. The sedation score recorded in this study was as low as 0 in K30 and KL30, and as high as 3 in K50, which is mild and comparable to the scores reported by Bergadano et al. [20].

Commonly used potent analgesics reduce the minimum alveolar concentration (MAC) of inhalant anaesthetics in dogs and humans [52, 53] ; the reduction in MAC of inhalant anaesthetic has been suggested either due to analgesic or sedative effects of the drug. Hence, if a drug decreases the MAC, it should be tested for its analgesic effects in awake patients [54]. The dosage of lidocaine selected in this study was based on MAC studies in dogs under anaesthesia [25] and studies in conscious dogs [55]. In the study on conscious dogs, lidocaine CRI of 100 µg/kg/min up to four hours did not produce any side effect [55]. Therefore, lidocaine at 2 mg/kg loading dose and CRI 100 µg/kg/min was combined to ketamine in this study. This combination of lidocaine and ketamine in present study was tested in preliminary study on two dogs before actual experiments. The major benefit of combining lidocaine and ketamine is to decrease the drug related side effects [56], decrease opioid requirement [57] intensity of pain in postoperative period due to central sensitization during surgical intervention [21]. The addition of lidocaine at 2 mg/kg loading dose and CRI of 100 μg/kg/min to ketamine infusion in this study resulted in higher mean nociceptive threshold values only at carpal pad and metacarpal footpad. Whereas, no difference in the serum concentration between K30 and KL 30 as well as KL 30 and K50 was observed due to addition of lidocaine to ketamine. The inherent high individual variability in these parameters would require large sample size to demonstrate statistical difference, which was not feasible in this study.

In this study, overall nociceptive thresholds were relatively higher in K50 than K30. Suggesting that K50 provided slightly more analgesia than K30. On the other hand, there was no such difference between KL30 and K50. Thus, K 50 and KL30 demonstrated more or less similar effect on nociceptive thresholds than K30. Nevertheless, all the three regimens significantly raised nociceptive thresholds from baseline thresholds, suggesting significant analgesic effects demonstrated by the three regimens used. Further studies are required to investigate the analgesic effects of these three doses in dogs undergoing surgical procedures.

Conclusions

All the three treatment regimes in this study maintained serum concentrations of ketamine above 200 ng/mL and raised mechanical nociceptive thresholds at most body points during the 120 min of infusions. A linear correlation between the mechanical thresholds and serum concentrations of ketamine was found. Results from this study suggested that the minimum concentration of ketamine to produce analgesia in dogs is between 100 and 200 ng/mL. All the three treatments provided antinociceptive effects throughout the infusions. In this setting the addition of lidocaine to ketamine increased mechanical thresholds without any further side effect. Clinical studies are encouraged to evaluate the analgesic effects of ketamine CRI and combination of lidocaine and ketamine at these dose regimens.

Acknowledgments
The authors are very grateful to the Faculty of Veterinary Medicine, Universiti Putra, Malaysia and Sindh Agriculture University Tandojam, Pakistan.

Funding
No funding resources for this study.

Authors' contributions
UK and CHC contributed to original idea and design of the study. AAA, AK, UK and AAB conducted the experiments and collected the data. UK, BS and SF performed HPLC analysis. UK, ME and YMG performed statistical analysis. All authors were involved in the manuscript preparation and approved the final manuscript.

Competing interests
The authors declare that they have no competing interests.

Consent for publication
Not applicable.

Author details
[1]Department of Veterinary Clinical Studies, Faculty of Veterinary Medicine, Universiti Putra Malaysia, 43400 Serdang, Selangor, Malaysia. [2]Department of Surgery and Obstetrics, Faculty of Animal Husbandry & Veterinary Sciences, Sindh Agriculture University Tandojam, Sindh 70060, Pakistan. [3]Material Synthesis and characterization laboratory, Institute of Advanced technology, Universiti Putra Malaysia, 43400 Serdang, Selangor, Malaysia. [4]Department of Veterinary Preclinical Sciences, Faculty of Veterinary Medicine, Universiti Putra Malaysia, 43400 Serdang, Selangor, Malaysia. [5]Institutes of Tropical Agriculture, Universiti Putra Malaysia, 43400 Serdang, Selangor, Malaysia. [6]Laboratory of Vaccines and Immunotherapeutics, Institute of Bioscience, Universiti Putra Malaysia, 43400 Serdang, Selangor, Malaysia. [7]Department of Human Anatomy, Faculty of Medicine and Health Science, Universiti Putra Malaysia, 43400 Serdang, Selangor, Malaysia. [8]Department of Animal Sciences, Faculty of Agriculture, Universiti Putra Malaysia, 43400 Serdang, Selangor, Malaysia. [9]Faculty of Animal Husbandry & Veterinary Sciences, Sindh Agriculture University Tandojam, Sindh 70060, Pakistan.

References

1. Babos MB, Grady B, Wisnoff W, McGhee C. Pathophysiology of pain. Dis Mon. 2013;59(10):330–58.
2. Schaible HG, Ebersberger A, Natura G. Update on peripheral mechanisms of pain: beyond prostaglandins and cytokines. Arthritis Res Ther. 2011;13(2): 210.
3. Tao YX. Dorsal horn alpha-amino-3-hydroxy-5-methyl-4-isoxazolepropionic acid receptor trafficking in inflammatory pain. Anesthesiology. 2010;112(5): 1259–65.
4. Zhuo M. Plasticity of NMDA receptor NR2B subunit in memory and chronic pain. Mol Brain. 2009;2(4):1756–6606.
5. Wilder-Smith OH, Arendt-Nielsen L. Postoperative hyperalgesia: its clinical importance and relevance. Anesthesiology. 2006;104(3):601–7.
6. De Kock MF, Lavand'homme PM. The clinical role of NMDA receptor antagonists for the treatment of postoperative pain. Best Pract Res Clin Anaesthesiol. 2007;21(1):85–98.
7. Stubhaug A, Breivik H, Eide P, Kreunen M, Foss A. Mapping of punctuate hyperalgesia around a surgical incision demonstrates that ketamine is a powerful suppressor of central sensitization to pain following surgery. Acta Anaesthesiol Scand. 1997;41(9):1124–32.
8. Zakine J, Samarcq D, Lorne E, Moubarak M, Montravers P, Beloucif S, et al. Postoperative ketamine administration decreases morphine consumption in major abdominal surgery: a prospective, randomized, double-blind, controlled study. Anesth Analg. 2008;106(6):1856–61.
9. Aida S, Yamakura T, Baba H, Taga K, Fukuda S, Shimoji K. Preemptive analgesia by intravenous low-dose ketamine and epidural morphine in gastrectomy: a randomized double-blind study. Anesthesiology. 2000;92(6):1624–30.
10. Fu ES, Miguel R, Scharf JE. Preemptive ketamine decreases postoperative narcotic requirements in patients undergoing abdominal surgery. Anesth Analg. 1997;84(5):1086–90.
11. Domino EF, Zsigmond EK, Domino LE, Domino KE, Kothary SP, Dominof SE. Plasma levels of ketamine and two of its metabolites in surgical patients using a gas chromatographic mass fragmentographic assay. Anesth Analg. 1982;61(2):87–92.
12. Javery KB, Ussery TW, Steger HG, Colclough GW. Comparison of morphine and morphine with ketamine for postoperative analgesia. Can J Anaesth. 1996;43(3):212–5.

13. Sarrau S, Jourdan J, Dupuis-Soyris F, Verwaerde P. Effects of postoperative ketamine infusion on pain control and feeding behaviour in bitches undergoing mastectomy. J Small Anim Pract. 2007;48(12):670–6.
14. Slingsby LS, Waterman-Pearson AE. The post-operative analgesic effects of ketamine after canine ovariohysterectomy—a comparison between pre-or post-operative administration. Res Vet Sci. 2000;69(2):147–52.
15. Wagner AE, Walton JA, Hellyer PW, Gaynor JS, Mama KR. Use of low doses of ketamine administered by constant rate infusion as an adjunct for postoperative analgesia in dogs. J Am Vet Med Assoc. 2002;221(1):72–5.
16. Richebe P, Rivat C, Rivalan B, Maurette P, Simonnet G. Low doses ketamine: antihyperalgesic drug, non-analgesic. Ann Fr Anesth Reanim. 2005;24(11-12): 1349–59.
17. Schmid RL, Sandler AN, Katz J. Use and efficacy of low-dose ketamine in the management of acute postoperative pain: a review of current techniques and outcomes. Pain. 1999;82(2):111–25.
18. Hansen BD. Assessment of pain in dogs: veterinary clinical studies. Ilar Journal. 2003;44(3):197–205.
19. Holton LL, Scott EM, Nolan AM, Reid J, Welsh E, Flaherty D. Comparison of three methods used for assessment of pain in dogs. J Am Vet Med Assoc. 1998;212(1):61–6.
20. Bergadano A, Andersen OK, Arendt-Nielsen L, Theurillat R, Thormann W, Spadavecchia C. Plasma levels of a low-dose constant-rate-infusion of ketamine and its effect on single and repeated nociceptive stimuli in conscious dogs. Vet J. 2009;182(2):252–60.
21. Muir WW, Woolf CJ. Mechanisms of pain and their therapeutic implications. J Am Vet Med Assoc. 2001;219(10):1346–56.
22. Matsubara LM, Oliva VN, Gabas DT, Oliveira GC, Cassetari ML. Effect of lidocaine on the minimum alveolar concentration of sevoflurane in dogs. Vet Anaesth Analg. 2009;36(5):407–13.
23. Solano AM, Pypendop BH, Boscan PL, Ilkiw JE. Effect of intravenous administration of ketamine on the minimum alveolar concentration of isoflurane in anesthetized dogs. Am J Vet Res. 2006;67(1):21–5.
24. Valverde A, Doherty TJ, Hernández J, Davies W. Effect of lidocaine on the minimum alveolar concentration of isoflurane in dogs. Vet Anaesth Analg. 2004;31(4):264–71.
25. Wilson J, Doherty TJ, Egger CM, Fidler A, Cox S, Rohrbach B. Effects of intravenous lidocaine, ketamine, and the combination on the minimum alveolar concentration of sevoflurane in dogs. Vet Anaesth Analg. 2008; 35(4):289–96.
26. KuKanich B, Lascelles BDX, Papich MG. Assessment of a von Frey device for evaluation of the antinociceptive effects of morphine and its application in pharmacodynamic modeling of morphine in dogs. Am J Vet Res. 2005;66(9): 1616–22.
27. Lascelles BD, Cripps PJ, Jones A, Waterman AE. Post-operative central hypersensitivity and pain: the pre-emptive value of pethidine for ovariohysterectomy. Pain. 1997;73(3):461–71.
28. Kaka U, Chen HC, Goh YM, Abubakar AA, Fakurazi S, Ebrahimi M. Validation of a modified algometer to measure mechanical nociceptive thresholds in awake dogs. Biomed Res Int. 2015;2015:7. doi:10.1155/2015/375421.
29. Le Bars D, Gozariu M, Cadden SW. Animal models of nociception. Pharmacol Rev. 2001;53(4):597–652.
30. Faul F, Erdfelder E, Lang A-G, Buchner A. G* Power 3: A flexible statistical power analysis program for the social, behavioral, and biomedical sciences. Behav Res Methods. 2007;39(2):175–91.
31. Clements JA, Nimmo WS, Grant IS. Bioavailability, pharmacokinetics, and analgesic activity of ketamine in humans. J Pharm Sci. 1982;71(5):539–42.
32. Arendt-Nielsen L, Petersen-Felix S, Fischer M, Bak P, Bjerring P, Zbinden A. The effect of N-methyl-D-aspartate antagonist (ketamine) on single and repeated nociceptive stimuli: a placebo-controlled experimental human study. Anesth Analg. 1995;81(1):63–8.
33. Pypendop BH, Ilkiw JE. Pharmacokinetics of ketamine and its metabolite, norketamine, after intravenous administration of a bolus of ketamine to isoflurane-anesthetized dogs. Am J Vet Res. 2005;66(12):2034–8.
34. Evans WE, Johnson JA. Pharmacogenomics: the inherited basis for interindividual differences in drug response. Annu Rev Genomics Hum Genet. 2001;2(1):9–39.
35. Palmer SN, Giesecke NM, Body SC, Shernan SK, Fox AA, Collard CD. Pharmacogenetics of anesthetic and analgesic agents. Anesthesiology. 2005; 102(3):663–71.
36. Spielberg SP. N-acetyltransferases: pharmacogenetics and clinical consequences of polymorphic drug metabolism. J Pharmacokinet Biopharm. 1996;24(5):509–19.
37. Wagner JG. A safe method for rapidly achieving plasma concentration plateaus. Clin Pharmacol Ther. 1974;16(4):691.
38. Adams HR, Parker JL, Mathew BP. The influence of ketamine on inotropic and chronotropic responsiveness of heart muscle. J Pharmacol Exp Ther. 1977;201(1):171–83.
39. Virtue R, Alanis J, Mori M, Lafargue R, Vogel J, Metcalf D. An anesthetic agent: 2-orthochlorophenyl, 2-methylamino cyclohexanone HCl (CI-581). Anesthesiology. 1967;28(5):823.
40. Buhari S, Hashim K, Yong Meng G, Mustapha NM, Gan SH. Subcutaneous Administration of Tramadol after Elective Surgery Is as Effective as Intravenous Administration in Relieving Acute Pain and Inflammation in Dogs. Sci World J. 2012;2012:564939.
41. Hardie EM, Lascelles BDX, Meuten T, Davidson GS, Papich MG, Hansen BD. Evaluation of intermittent infusion of bupivacaine into surgical wounds of dogs postoperatively. Vet J. 2011;190(2):287–9.
42. Haussler KK, Erb HN. Mechanical nociceptive thresholds in the axial skeleton of horses. Equine Vet J. 2006;38(1):70–5.
43. Lascelles BDX, Cripps PJ, Jones A, Waterman-Pearson AE. Efficacy and kinetics of carprofen, administered preoperatively or postoperatively, for the prevention of pain in dogs undergoing ovariohysterectomy. Vet Surg. 1998;27(6):568–82.
44. Moak P, Hosgood G, Rowe E, Lemke K. Evaluation of intra-articular and subcutaneous administration of meloxicam for postoperative analgesia following stifle surgery in dogs. Vet Comp Orthop Traumatol. 2011;24(1):32.
45. Slingsby LS, Taylor PM, Murrell JC. A study to evaluate buprenorphine at 40 μg kg – 1 compared to 20 μg kg – 1 as a post-operative analgesic in the dog. Vet Anaesth Analg. 2011;38(6):584–93.
46. Chambers J, Waterman A, Livingston A. Further development of equipment to measure nociceptive thresholds in large animals. Vet Anaesth Analg. 1994;21(2):66–72.
47. Haussler K, Erb H. Pressure algometry for the detection of induced back pain in horses: a preliminary study. Equine Vet J. 2006;38(1):76–81.
48. Nussbaum EL, Downes L. Reliability of clinical pressure-pain algometric measurements obtained on consecutive days. Phys Ther. 1998;78(2):160–9.
49. Wylde V, Palmer S, Learmonth ID, Dieppe P. Somatosensory abnormalities in knee OA. Rheumatology. 2012;51(3):535–43.
50. Jensen K, Andersen HØ, Olesen J, Lindblom U. Pressure-pain threshold in human temporal region. Evaluation of a new pressure algometer. Pain. 1986;25(3):313–23.
51. Kinser AM, Sands WA, Stone MH. Reliability and validity of a pressure algometer. J Strength Cond Res. 2009;23(1):312–4.
52. Ko JC, Weil AB, Inoue T. Effects of carprofen and morphine on the minimum alveolar concentration of isoflurane in dogs. J Am Anim Hosp Assoc. 2009;45(1):19–23.
53. Machado CE, Dyson DH, Grant MM. Effects of oxymorphone and hydromorphone on the minimum alveolar concentration of isoflurane in dogs. Vet Anaesth Analg. 2006;33(1):70–7.
54. Boscan P, Monnet E, Mama K, Twedt DC, Congdon J, Eickhoff JC, et al. A dog model to study ovary, ovarian ligament and visceral pain. Vet Anaesth Analg. 2011;38(3):260–6.
55. MacDougall LM, Hethey JA, Livingston A, Clark C, Shmon CL, Duke-Novakovski T. Antinociceptive, cardiopulmonary, and sedative effects of five intravenous infusion rates of lidocaine in conscious dogs. Vet Anaesth Analg. 2009;36(5):512–22.
56. Woolf CJ, Salter MW. Neuronal plasticity: increasing the gain in pain. Science. 2000;288(5472):1765–8.
57. Kehlet H, Dahl JB. The value of "multimodal" or "balanced analgesia" in postoperative pain treatment. Anesth Analg. 1993;77(5):1048–56.

4

Intraperitoneal implantation of life-long telemetry transmitters in three rehabilitated harbor seal pups

Markus Horning[1,2*], Martin Haulena[3], Justin F. Rosenberg[3] and Chad Nordstrom[3]

Abstract

Background: Pinnipeds, including many phocid species of concern, are inaccessible and difficult to monitor for extended periods using conventional, externally attached telemetry devices that are shed during the annual molt. Archival satellite transmitters were implanted intraperitoneally into three stranded Pacific harbor seal pups (*Phoca vitulina richardii*) that completed rehabilitation, to evaluate the viability of this surgical technique for the deployment of life long telemetry devices in phocids. The life history transmitters record information throughout the life of the host and transmit data to orbiting satellites after extrusion following death.

Results: Surgeries were performed under general anesthesia and a single transmitter was inserted into the ventrocaudal abdominal cavity via a 7–8 cm incision along the ventral midline between the umbilicus and pubic symphysis or preputial opening in each animal. Surgeries lasted from 45 to 51 min, and anesthesic times ranged from 55 to 79 min. All animals recovered well, were released into dry holding pens overnight, and were given access to water the following day. All three animals exhibited an expected inflammatory response, with acute phase responses lasting approximately three to four weeks. All three animals were tracked via externally attached satellite transmitters after release at 58 to 78 days following surgery, and minimum post-release survival was confirmed through continued movement data received over 278 to 289 days.

Conclusion: The initial findings of low morbidity and zero mortality encountered during captive observation and post-release tracking periods support the viability of this surgical technique for the implantation of long-term telemetry devices in phocids.

Keywords: Life history transmitter, LHX tag, Telemetry, Vital rate, Implant surgery, Pinniped

Background

The determination of vital rate data essential to the effective management and conservation of many pinniped species is empirically challenging, especially for those phocid species that do not congregate and breed on specific haulouts or rookeries [1–6]. Essential data include seasonal and age-specific survival, causes and locations of mortality, and age at primiparity and pupping rates in females. Survival and reproductive data are also crucial for the assessment of success and impact of stranded animal rehabilitation programs [7].

* Correspondence: markush@alaskasealife.org
[1]Alaska SeaLife Center, 301 Railway Avenue, Seward, AK 99664, USA
[2]Oregon State University, 2030 SE Marine Science Drive, Newport, OR 97365, USA
Full list of author information is available at the end of the article

Every year, thousands of rehabilitated pinnipeds are released back into the wild in North America [8]. However, no published studies have been able to accurately determine post-release survival beyond four months, nor the social and reproductive behavior, reproductive success, or potential effects on wild populations. The few extant studies have relied on external and internal VHF radio-transmitters, external Argos satellite transmitters, flipper tags, hot-iron branding, color markings and photo-identification. Gaydos and collaborators [9] compared the movement behavior of ten rehabilitated harbor seal pups to ten wild pups. Rehabilitated pups were tracked for a mean of 76.5 days and wild pups for a mean of 132.7 days. No survival rate analysis was conducted. Lander and Gulland [10] tracked three rehabilitated Steller sea lions for 1–4 months, and no other analyses were reported. Lander and collaborators [11] compared the post-release movement and dive behavior between 29 rehabilitated harbor seal pups to and 24 wild pups using VHF transmitters. Animals were tracked for varying periods in different years, up to 179 days. Survival rates were compared up to 14 weeks after release, and were found lower in rehabilitated than wild animals. Morrison and collaborators [12] tracked six rehabilitated harbor seal pups after release using Argos satellite transmitters, and five wild pups for an average of 122 days (rehabilitated) and 150 days (wild). Norris and collaborators [13] used satellite-relayed GPS trackers on six rehabilitated and three wild Hawaiian monk seals for average durations of 91 days (rehabilitated) and 230 days (controls). Vincent and collaborators [14] marked 92 rehabilitated juvenile grey seals via flipper tags, color markings, photo identification satellite tags, or head tags. The photo identification approach allowed the longest periods of resight observation up to five years. Satellite tracking of four of these seals covered periods up to 80 days. 52% of the seals released were never resighted. None of these studies were able to accurately estimate age-specific survival beyond four months after release. The short tracking durations, wide pup dispersal and low visual observation rates also did not allow the determination of social or reproductive behavior.

In marine vertebrates, recent advances in telemetry technology have revolutionized our ability to monitor behavior and movement of individual animals [15]. However, direct telemetric measures of survival and reproduction have been labeled as 'empirically intractable' and remain largely elusive [16]. In wild pinnipeds, social behavior, reproductive rates and survival have been accurately documented primarily via mark re-sight approaches using hot-iron branding or natural markings, and often in conjunction with remote video observation systems [17]. These efforts require a large investment in marking and consistent, multi-year re-sight efforts, or the installation, maintenance and operation of remote imaging systems [17, 18]. Such systems have only been used in comparably accessible locations, and on otariid species with a high degree of site fidelity. Such systems are not practicable for phocid species such as harbor seals [19–22]. Reproductive rates for otariids have also been estimated from aerial survey photographic counts of pups in relation to non-pups. Such age ratios can be used to predict population trajectories, or to estimate vital rates such as natality or juvenile survival to inform management decisions for exploited or threatened terrestrial or marine mammals. However, the reliability of such indicators to accurately reflect the underlying dynamics of a population has been criticized [23] and has not been evaluated for marine mammals, and these approaches cannot provide reproductive data on phocids.

Telemetry technology has been tested in a few cases to study survival rates in wild pinnipeds. Externally attached transmitters are not an option due to limited transmitter retention resulting from the annual molt [1, 6, 24]. Subcutaneously implanted transmitters have been used in two studies of harbor seals. Blundell and collaborators [24] used subcutaneous VHF transmitter implants with a battery life of at least three years in 277 harbor seals in Alaska. Transmitters were locally tracked primarily via shore-based VHF receiving data loggers and satellite-linked relay transmitters. These efforts were supplemented via small aircraft VHF scanning flights in the region. As a result of a number of trans-cutaneous tag extrusions observed, combined with tag failures and technical difficulties experienced in tracking the implanted transmitters, the authors concluded that this type of telemetry study using sub-cutaneous VHF transmitters was not suited for the determination of survival rates via electronic mark-recapture studies in harbor seals. Manugian and collaborators [25, 26] used the same type of subcutaneous VHF transmitters implanted into 32 wild harbor seals in California to estimate survival rates. Re-sight effort was conducted via spatially constrained small aircraft VHF scanning survey. However, emigration and possible effects of implants on survival were not evaluated, and tag failure as well as tag loss by extrusion – while observed – were not accounted for. Thus, the reported local apparent survival rates are likely underestimating actual survival by an unknown amount. Prevailing electronic telemetry approaches also do not provide data on birth events in females.

To overcome these constraints and provide vital rate data from pinnipeds in remote, difficult to observe regions, we specifically developed the Life History Transmitter (LHX tag, [27]) in collaboration with Wildlife Computers Inc. (Redmond, WA, USA). LHX tags are intraperitoneally implanted under general gas anesthesia using aseptic surgical procedures [28]. LHX tags record sensor data throughout the life of their host, and have a projected life span of at least 10 years. Summary data are transmitted post-mortem via the Argos satellite data system that provides global coverage with multiple daily uplink opportunities (CLS America, Ltd) only after the tags are liberated from the decomposing, dismembered, or digested carcass [29]. Thus, LHX tags provide the equivalent of end-of-life, known-fate data with spatially and temporally unrestricted data recovery, for at least 10 years. The recommended experimental design using two implants per animal allows the estimation of tag failure rates and data return probabilities. LHX tags store and process data from multiple sensors, including temperature and light. First generation LHX1 tags also incorporated a proprietary sensor to categorize surrounding medium into tissue, water or air [27]. Second generation LHX2 tags (see below) no longer include this sensor and instead incorporate a tri-axial accelerometer sensors used to detect motion and activity. Mortality is determined when temperature falls below a preset threshold. Sensor data is evaluated via a heuristic algorithm to determine state of the host animal, and transmissions are only initiated when tag extrusion has been determined as likely [27]. Two types of data are then transmitted: 48 h of original temperature, light and activity data spanning the detected mortality event, and the parameters of a logistic fit to temperature curves used to detect parturition events, as well as time stamps of detected events. Parturition events are inferred from body core temperature patterns via a modified method first proposed by T. Tinker, as described in [30]. From these transmitted data, exact dates and times of mortality can be obtained, as well as locations of tag emergence via the positioning information provided by the Argos system. From a detailed analysis of transmitted data, inferences may be made on the causa mortis [29, 31]. In some instances of predation resulting in immediate liberation of tags from dismembered hosts, inferences on the nature of predators involved in specific mortality events could be made [31]. If however emergence of tags is delayed and tags cool within an intact carcass, body mass of the deceased animal can be estimated from algor mortis models we previously parameterized for pinnipeds [29]. LHX tags have been used successfully to determine survival and predation rates in juvenile Steller sea lions in the Gulf of Alaska [29, 31, 32].

First generation LHX1 tags were comparably large with a diameter of 42 mm, length of 127 mm, and a mass of 117 g. This limited applications to large animals such as California sea lions (*Zalophus californianus*) and Steller sea lions (*Eumetopias jubatus*). From 2004 through 2014 single or dual LHX tags were implanted into four California sea lions (single tags: 66 and 118 kg, dual tags: 140 and 195 kg) and 45 Steller sea lions (single tags: 109 and 119 kg, dual tags: range 89 to 190 kg, mean 123.6 kg +/− 26 kg S.D.).

In 2014 we completed the development of 2nd generation LHX2 tags that are smaller to allow for applications in smaller species (Fig. 1). Here we report on the surgery, post-operative monitoring, and post-release tracking of single LHX2 tags implanted into three harbor seal pups that completed rehabilitation, at the Vancouver Aquarium's Marine Mammal Rescue Centre in 2014. These are the first intraperitoneal telemetry implants in a phocid seal.

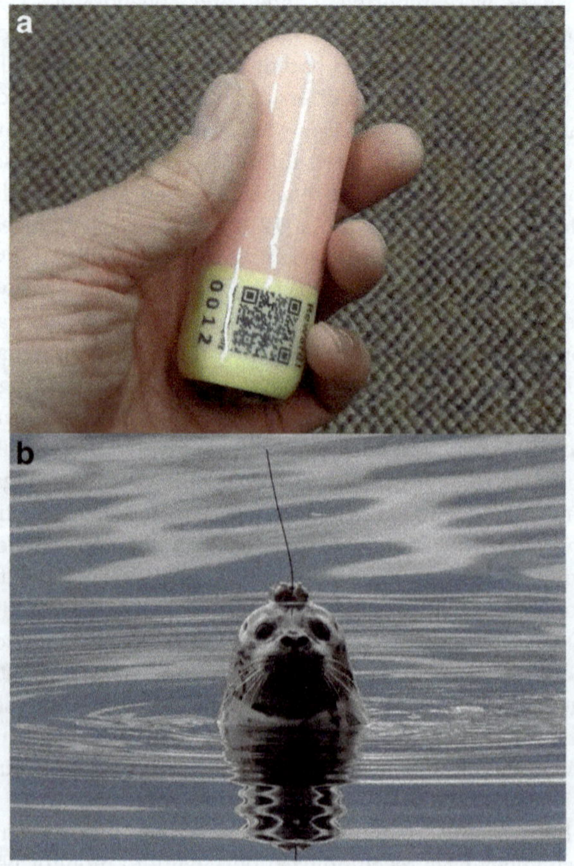

Fig. 1 **a** A 2nd generation implantable Argos-compatible satellite-linked life history transmitter (LHX2 tag, Wildlife Computers Inc., Redmond, WA). Exterior dimensions are 97 mm length by 33 mm diameter. The tag mass is 54 g, buoyancy is 0.26 N. The device is coated in Epo-Tek 302-3 M resin, a material certified under the USP Class 6 standard for biological reactivity. The QR code links to information on the tag, project and rewards for return (Photo © Markus Horning). **b** A location-only satellite linked transmitter (SPOT5 tag, Wildlife Computers Inc.) glued onto the head fur via 5-min epoxy, on the just released animal Pv14–123. Exterior dimensions: 70 mm length, 41 mm width, 23 mm height. Tag mass: 72 g (Photo © Sheanna Steingass)

Methods

Study area

This study was conducted in British Columbia, Canada, between September 2014 and September 2015. Young of the year Pacific harbor seals (*Phoca vitulina richardii*) were implanted at the Vancouver Aquarium Marine Mammal Rescue Centre and were released at Porteau Cove north of Vancouver on November 22, 2014. Seals were subsequently tracked using conventional satellite telemetry for 10 months as they made use of the waters in Howe Sound and the northern portion of the Salish Sea.

Telemetry transmitters

The 2nd generation Life History Transmitters used in this study have a cylindrical shape with hemispherical ends, with a length of 97 mm, a diameter of 33 mm and a mass of 54 g. Tags are positively buoyant in saltwater (buoyancy 0.26 N). The tags have a pressure rating of >2000 m, and are individually tested to 1000 m. The tags are completely coated in Epo-Tek® 302-3 M medical grade epoxy (Epoxy Technology, Billerica, MA, USA) certified to USP Class VI standards for biological reactivity with implantation in non-cured and polymerized states. Epo-Tek 302-3 M has the lowest moisture absorption amongst Class 6 certified resins, and has exceptionally high resistance to solvents, acids and bases, as well as long-term stability. This material prevents adhesion to connective tissue or omentum. Tags were sterilized in ethylene oxide gas (Anprolene®, Andersen Products Inc., Haw River, NC, USA). The LHX2 transmitters were programmed to transmit abdominal temperatures for postoperative monitoring, every other hour for periods of 12 days following implantation, to a nearby handheld UHF receiver.

For post-release tracking, location only SPOT5 type satellite transmitters (model 287c, Wildlife Computers, WA, USA) were employed using the Argos satellite system for remote data relay. SPOT5 tags measured 70 mm long, 41 mm wide, and 23 mm high and weighed 72 g in air. SPOT5 transmitters were not duty cycled (e.g., they were programmed to transmit whenever possible) but outgoing transmissions were delayed until receiving satellites were predicted to be overhead and transmissions were slowed when seals were hauled-out on land. Animal positions were estimated by Argos CLS America (Maryland, USA) by computing the Doppler shift obtained when satellites passed over transmitting SPOT5 tags and employed a Kalman filter algorithm. Latitudes, longitudes, and quality scores for each derived location were downloaded from the Argos web portal at regular intervals during the tracking period and continued until all tags ceased transmitting. Quality scores reflected the number of satellites in range and the number of successive connections between the transmitting tags and satellites during a given pass with stated accuracies ranging from 250 m to several km (Argos User Manual v. 1.6.6, 2016). Given that the devices were not expected to be recovered and the goal was to maximize deployment longevity, no other parameters were logged or transmitted in order to extend battery capacity for as long as possible.

Tracks for each seal were reconstructed using the trip package [33] and R statistical software [34]. The straight-line distance between successive positions was calculated after outliers were removed from each seal track using a course speed filter set at 5 m per sec (twice the maximum expected speed of 2.5 m per sec for harbor seals) and using locations scored as class 'B' or higher. Given the error associated with Argos locations and the inherent gaps in the data record from tags transmitting from diving animals, the distance values reported here should be considered minimum estimates and are solely intended to describe the general movements of the seals in the year following surgery.

Subjects, anesthesia, and radiographs

Three female harbor seal pups were selected in 2014 that had completed rehabilitation and were deemed releasable based on standard rehabilitation program criteria [35, 36]. Data from a fourth animal (Pv14–099) that did not receive an implant, but was released and tracked at the same time as the three subjects are included here. All four animals were originally admitted as neonates in poor body condition. One animal (Pv14–073) additionally had multiple purulent wounds on both hind flippers, and one (Pv14–062) exhibited monocytosis likely due to chronic inflammation.

Surgeries were performed in a clean, heated shed adjacent to animal holding areas. Starting on the day before surgery and for the following 5 days, subjects were administered a single daily oral dose of the non-steroidal anti-inflammatory drug carprofen (25 mg). Starting on the day after surgery and for the next three days, subjects were orally administered the opioid tramadol (25 mg) twice daily. Subjects were fasted on surgery days, were fed 50% of their normal diet on the day following surgery, and their normal diet was resumed thereafter. Animals were restricted from water access immediately after surgery until the next afternoon, for approximately 18 to 24 h.

Animals were mildly sedated with 0.1 mg/kg midazolam and 0.1 mg/kg butorphanol via intravenous injection into the intervertebral extradural vein. Subjects were then masked with 5% isoflurane (AErrane®, Fort Dodge Animal Health, Fort Dodge, CO, USA) in 100% oxygen for induction of anesthesia [37]. Animals were intubated with a 6.0 mm diameter cuffed endotracheal tube and anesthesia maintained with 1% to 3% isoflurane in 100% oxygen delivered via a semi-closed, partially rebreathing circuit. Depth of anesthesia was assessed based on respiratory rate and tidal volume, response to stimuli, palpebral reflex, capillary refill time, and jaw and muscle tone. Respiratory rate, heart rate, oxygen saturation of hemoglobin (SpO_2), end-tidal carbon dioxide ($EtCO_2$), and deep rectal body temperature were monitored during anesthetic procedures. Animals were provided with mechanically assisted ventilation through a volume regulated ventilator (Model 2000, Hallowell EMC, Pittsfield, MA, USA) at a rate of six to ten breaths per minute and a volume of approximately 15–20 ml/kg/breath if prolonged apnea occurred. A local lidocaine block (5 ml of 5 mg/ml) was performed around the surgical site post-induction. After surgery, isoflurane was discontinued and animals were maintained on 100% oxygen via endotracheal tube during initial recovery. Two view abdominal radiographs were taken for two seals (Pv14–062 and Pv14–073) during recovery. Animals were extubated once jaw tone and the swallowing reflex had returned and they were able to hold their heads up. Recovery occurred within 1 h for all animals, and they were then allowed to recover overnight in dry pens.

Surgeries

Subjects were positioned in dorsal recumbency and the area from umbilicus to pubis was shaved and prepared with povidone iodine scrub / 70% isopropyl alcohol / povidone iodine solution. A sterile, fenestrated drape was placed over the surgical site and secured with towel clamps. A longitudinal skin incision of approximately 7 cm was made along the ventral midline, caudal to the umbilicus, with a No.10 scalpel. A combination of sharp and blunt dissection through blubber and subcutaneous tissues was utilized to expose the linea alba. The linea alba was then lifted with forceps and incised via stab incision and sharply dissected to expose the peritoneal cavity while avoiding the abdominal contents, to a length sufficient to insert the transmitter (approximately 5 cm). The peritoneum was visualized, incised, and manually expanded. A single, sterilized LHX transmitter was activated, removed from the sterilization peel pouch, rinsed in sterile saline, and inserted into the caudal abdomen through the previously described incision. Bleeding was controlled when necessary with hemostatic forceps and ligatures of 2–0 PDS II absorbable monofilament suture (Ethicon®, Inc., Somerville, NJ, USA). The surgical incision was closed in multiple layers using PDS II sutures. A simple interrupted cruciate pattern with 3–0 PDS II was utilized to close the body wall, ensuring that the external rectus sheath was incorporated into every bite. The thick blubber layer was closed with a simple continuous pattern using 3–0 PDS II. A simple continuous intradermal suture pattern with 3–0 PDS II apposed the skin edges. On two animals only (Pv14–062, Pv14–073), external skin sutures were placed with 3–0 PDS II using interrupted cruciates. The third animal (Pv14–123) did not receive any external skin sutures. Anesthetic times (masking to extubation) and surgical times (incision to completion of sutures) were 66/45, 79/51 and 55/50 min, respectively.

Postoperative monitoring

Following implantation surgeries, all three seals were closely monitored for 59 to 79 days before release (Table 1). Animals received periodic health screenings and two abdominal view radiographs prior to release to confirm implant positioning. Blood samples were analyzed by a commercial laboratory (IDEXX Laboratories, Delta, B.C., Canada) for hematology and differentials, biochemistry, as well as fibrinogen and haptoglobin concentrations. One day prior to release, animals were sedated with butorphanol and midazolam (each 0.15 mg/kg IV), induced and maintained via mask with isoflurane as described above, and the external SPOT5 satellite transmitters were glued to the head fur using 5-min epoxy (Devcon®, MA, USA).

The three implanted seals, and one additional seal (Pv14–099) not carrying an LHX transmitter but carrying a SPOT5 external tag were transported via truck to the release location in Porteau Cove approximately 35 km north of Vancouver in portable kennel cages, and released simultaneously.

Reference hematology data and descriptive statistics

Reference values for all blood analytes were obtained from the pre-release health examination blood screening records of rehabilitated female harbor seal pups that were released from the Vancouver Aquarium Marine Mammal Rescue Centre in 2014 (n = 34) and 2015 (n = 28). However, fibrinogen and haptoglobin are not a standard assay on the pre-release exam, and no reference data for harbor seal pups is available. To test for significant effects of surgeries, peak and minimum values for all three experimental animals (the highest and lowest post-surgical value for each individual animal) were compared to the reference values using Student's two-sample t-test in Systat (Version 10.1). All tests were two-tailed, except leukocytes (1-tailed). Test results are reported as the two-sample t-value$_{(\text{degrees freedom})}$, and p-value for alpha = 0.05. Since harbor seal pups continue physiological maturation through the first three months of life (see [38–40]), peaks and minima from weeks one through four after surgery were compared to reference values from pups released prior to three months of age, and peaks and minima for

Table 1 Identifiers, dates and body mass of three implanted and one non-implanted female harbor seal pups through rehabilitation and release

Identifier	Admit date	Admit mass (kg)	Admit condition	Surgery date	Surgery mass (kg)	Release date	Release mass (kg)	Days tracked post release
Pv14–073	07/25/14	7.45	poor body condition, wounds	09/02/14	13.00	11/20/14	35.60	278
Pv14–062	07/21/14	7.5	poor body condition, monocyt.	09/02/14	12.45	11/20/14	30.70	289
Pv14–123	08/19/14	8.8	poor body condition	09/22/14	14.30	11/20/14	35.75	284
Pv14–099	08/07/14	5.7	poor body condition, wounds	N/A	N/A	11/20/14	33.65	272

weeks five through 11 after surgery were separately compared to reference values from pups released after three months of age.

Results

Body mass, temperatures and general observations

All three neonates gained body mass at an average rate ranging from 0.19 to 0.29 kg/d between intake and release. Mass gain rates from intake to surgery were 0.11, 0.15 and 0.16 kg/d. Surgeries occurred at 164, 173 and 160% of intake mass, and release at 409, 478 and 406% of intake mass, respectively (Table 1, Fig. 2). All three subjects briefly lost mass during the pre-surgery and surgery days as a result of restricted diet, and gained mass during the week following surgery at 0.28, 0.24 and 0.20 kg/d.

As a result of technical complications, no transmitted temperatures were recorded from the first two animals for the first three post-operative days. Recorded post-operative temperatures ranged from 36.8 °C to 39.6 °C, and averaged 37.99, 37.91 and 38.11 °C, respectively (Fig. 3).

Incisions measured 75, 78 and 70 mm in length immediately after surgery, and 65, 65 and 60 mm prior to release. Fig. 4 illustrates the progression of incision healing across the three subjects, from surgery to 78 days after surgery just prior to release. One of the two animals with external skin sutures (Pv14–062) exhibited minor swelling and minor purulent discharge from the incision by the end of the first postoperative week (Fig. 4c). Skin sutures were removed 9 days after surgery. The incision was well apposed with no visible evidence of infection, with some granulation apparent by day 9 and good granulation by the end of the second week, and in most cases no visible dehiscence of the skin layer. The incision appeared healed by the 6th week (Fig. 4e, g). The second animal with skin sutures (Pv14–073) exhibited pressure necrosis from these sutures with some purulent discharge by the end of the first week, when skin sutures were removed, and with more discharge observed by day 9. On day 18, the incision was moderately well apposed with a few areas of dehiscence no more than 3 mm at the widest. By 2 weeks, granulation was apparent with some areas of dehiscence (approx. 10 mm) and some discharge. By 24 days, granulation was progressing, but small amounts of discharge persisted through day 46. The incision was mostly healed by day 48 with only 2 small areas remaining to fully close (1–2 mm diameter), and was fully healed by release (Fig. 4h). The animal without skin sutures (Pv14–123) exhibited minor swelling after 1 week, and some discharge on the 2nd week. By the end of the second week small amounts of discharge continued, and a small amount of dehiscence (2–3 mm) was observed (Fig. 4d). By 4 weeks healing had progressed nicely with good granulation, only very minor discharge and a small amount of dehiscence (1–3 mm) on the caudal aspect of the incision (Fig. 4f). This persisted through the release exam on day 58 after surgery, but did not preclude the animal from release.

In the immediate post-operative abdominal radiographs collected from two animals, the implanted transmitters are positioned just rostral of the pelvis and have a relative length of about 4 vertebrae (Fig. 5a, b). In pre-release radiographs of all three animals the transmitters have moved towards the diaphragm, and have a relative length of about 3 vertebrae (Fig. 5c, d).

Hematology and clinical chemistry

All data from analyses of blood samples are available in Additional file 1. CBC and differentials were unremarkable

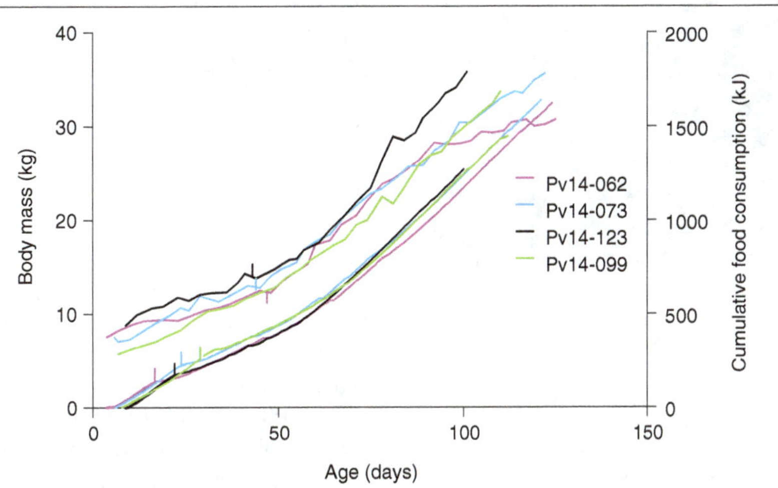

Fig. 2 Body mass and cumulative food consumption of four rehabilitated harbor seal pups from admission to release. The transition from formula to whole fish is marked by vertical bars for all four pups on the lower lines showing food consumption. The implant surgeries for three of four subjects are marked by vertical bars on the upper lines showing body mass

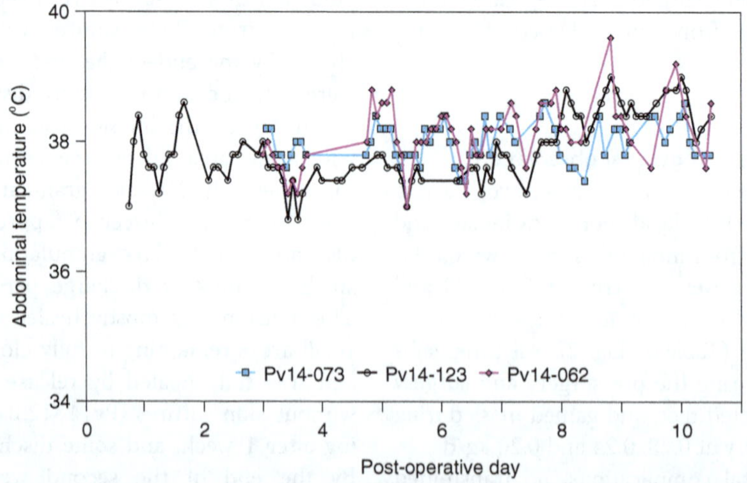

Fig. 3 Abdominal temperatures transmitted from the telemetry transmitters intraperitoneally implanted into three rehabilitated harbor seal pups, and received by a nearby telemetry receiver, for up to 10 days after surgery. Due to technical complications, no data were recorded from two of the three animals for the first two days

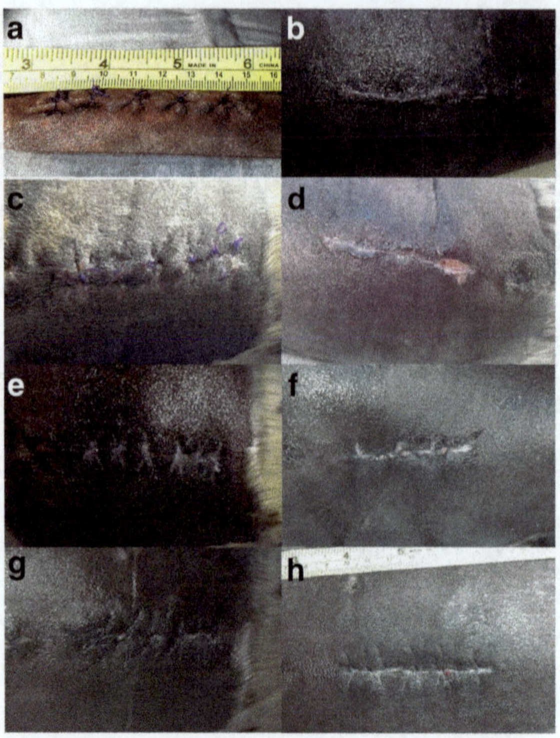

Fig. 4 Photos of surgical incisions in three harbor seal pups at varying intervals from surgery to release. **a** Pv14–062 immediately after surgery. External, interrupted cruciate sutures are visible. **b** Pv14–123 on day 4 after surgery. This animal did not receive external skin sutures. **c** Pv14–062 on day 6 after surgery, and before the external sutures were removed. **d** Pv14–123 on day 14 after surgery. There is about a 10 mm section of the incision where the outermost skin layer is separated and not fully apposed after removal of external sutures. **e** Pv14–062 on day 24 after surgery. **f** Pv14–123 on day 28 after surgery. **g** Pv14–062 on day 48 after surgery. **h** Pv14–073 on day 78, prior to release

on surgery days. Clinical chemistry markers were considered normal for age and diet. Surgeries were completed without complications, and the animals recovered from anesthesia as expected. On the days following surgery, all animals exhibited appetite and consumed all food offered (50% of normal allocation on the day after surgery, 100% thereafter).

During the first four weeks following surgeries, all three animals exhibited inflammatory and acute phase responses (Figs. 6, 7 and 8, data in Additional file 1). Leukocytes ($t_{(2,41)} = -5.745$, $p < 0.0001$), neutrophils ($t_{(2,41)} = -5.9623$, $p < 0.0001$) and monocytes ($t_{(2,41)} = -7.2105$, $p < 0.0001$) exhibited significant peaks compared to reference values (Fig. 5a, b). Eosinophils ($t_{(2,41)} = -1.236$, $p > 0.22$), lymphocytes ($t_{(2,41)} = -1.268$, $p > 0.21$) and platelets ($t_{(2,41)} = -0.413$, $p > 0.68$) tended to increase overall following surgery, but with considerable variance (Fig 6). Fibrinogen and haptoglobin could not be compared to reference values. Fibrinogen exhibited no overall trends when compared to the considerable variance. Haptoglobin levels first increased and then dropped to pre-surgical values by about week three (Fig. 7). Levels of the positive acute phase protein globulin ($t_{(2,41)} = -1.9302$, $p = 0.0602$) increased relative to reference values without exhibiting a significant peak. The negative acute phase protein albumin exhibited significant post-surgical minima ($t_{(2,41)} = -4.24303$, $p = 0.00012$) (Fig. 7). Creatinine concentrations exhibited significant minima following surgery ($t_{(2,41)} = 3.4708$, $p = 0.0012$), and creatinine kinase activity exhibited substantial variation with a single pronounced peak in each animal at distinct times following surgery, resulting in significant peaks compared to the reference pool ($t_{(2,41)} = -4.475$, $p < 0.0001$). Blood urea nitrogen (BUN) overall increased after surgery, and values for the first four

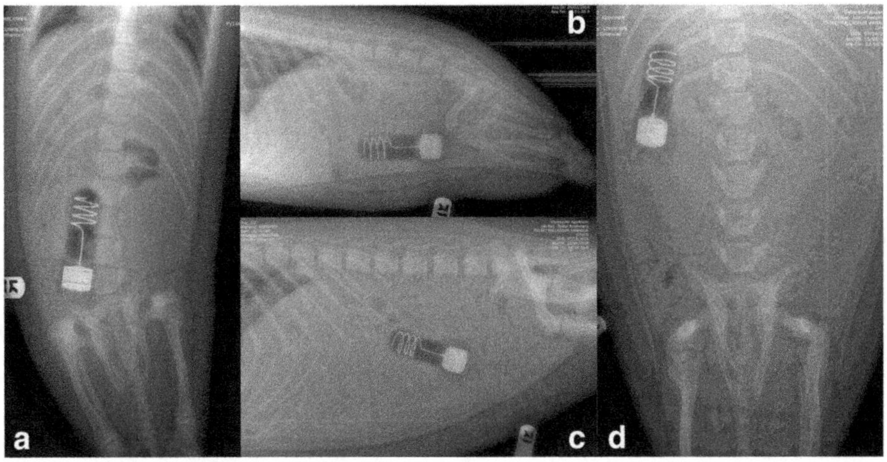

Fig. 5 Abdominal radiographs of female harbor seal pup Pv14–062. Immediately after surgery (**a**: dorsoventral, **b**: lateral view) the LHX tag (98 mm length × 33 mm diameter) has a relative length of about 4 vertebrae. 78 days after surgery (**c**: lateral, **d**: dorsoventral view) the LHX tag has a relative length of about 3 vertebrae

weeks were higher than for weeks five, seven and nine. However, all early post-surgical values were low compared to the reference pool (minima: $t_{(2,41)} = 2.6812$, $p = 0.0104$). The BUN to creatinine ratio increased sharply after surgery, and dropped by the 5th week, but with considerable variance in subjects and reference pool neither peaks nor minima were significant (Fig. 8).

During weeks five to 11 after surgery, only BUN exhibited significant minima (during weeks five and seven: ($t_{(2,20)} = 2.2342$, $p = 0.036$), and a single extreme value in creatine kinase in week five resulted in significant peaks compared to controls ($t_{(2,20)} = -3.161$, $p = 0.0045$). No other analytes exhibited significant peaks or minima compared to the reference values for animals older than three months.

Post-release telemetry

Animals were tracked for an extended period following release (range = 272 to 289 days). Overall, LHX instrumented seals moved at a mean rate of 27.0 km/d (SE = 1.10, 95% CI = 24.85–29.15) over the course of the deployment (November 2014 to August/September 2015) while Pv14–099 (without the internal transmitter) travelled a nearly identical 26.8 km/d on average over the same time period (SE = 2.70, 95% CI = 21.5–32.1).

Monthly movements were tabulated for each LHX seal to look for any patterns that could indicate difficulty adjusting to life in the wild (e.g., extended at-sea travel, repetitive long-distance movements, or alternatively restricted movements near urban areas such as marinas or docks). No such behaviors were observed other than some long distance movements following the initial release period. However, some individual tendencies were apparent. Pv14–123 routinely travelled less per day (22.9 km, SE = 1.49) than either Pv14–062 (27.9 km, SE = 1.55) or Pv14–073 (29.822.9 km, SE = 1.94) when averaged on a monthly scale. As a result, movements above or below the group's 95% confidence interval could not be used to generalize inter-animal differences for the three seals. For example, Pv14–123's movements would be considered less than expected in 8 out of 10 months rather than being within his established range, given this animal's tendency to move less than the other implanted seals. Instead, a focused search for intra-animal variation and months when multiple seals collectively moved more or less than their established norms was conducted. Specifically, a confidence interval for the monthly average distance traveled per day for each seal was calculated, after removing months with less than 20 days of data (typically the first and last months of the deployment; Table 2). When the average movement in any given month was exceptional for that particular animal the average movement of other implanted seals was considered. Movements in 53% of cases exceeded an individual seal's confidence interval but no regular patterns were apparent among seals beyond a tendency to travel more in the first two months after leaving the relatively protected waters of Howe Sound. The exception was the month of July where all 3 seals moved in an atypical manner but while two animals moved slightly more than expected, the third moved notably less than its established average. Similarly, no patterns were observed when movements were examined by season with mean rates changing little over time and ranging from 24.9 km/day (summer) to 26.4 km/day (spring).

All four external satellite tags ceased transmitting within 17 days of each other, indicating that the instruments likely exhausted their batteries or fell off during the annual molt.

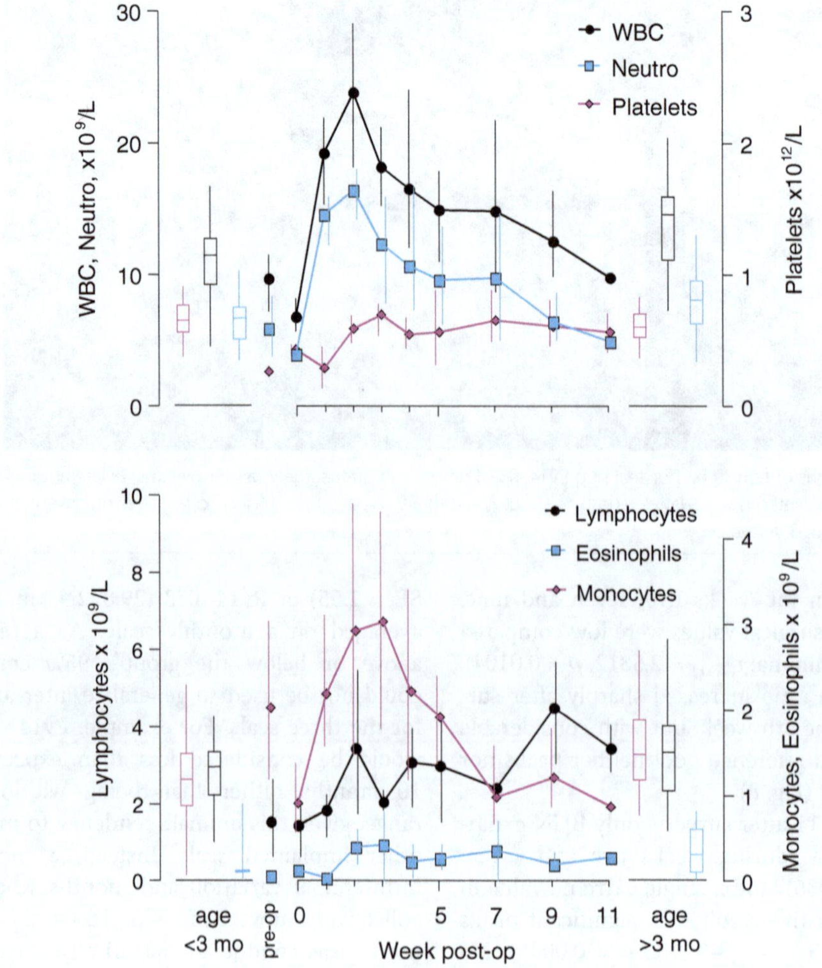

Fig. 6 Inflammatory response to implant surgery in three female harbor seal pups. White cell counts (WBC), neutrophils and platelets (upper panel), as well as lymphocytes, monocytes and eosinophils (lower panel) from surgery at approximately 6 weeks of age through release 11 weeks after surgery. Samples were collected at surgery, and at weeks 1, 2, 3, 4, 5, 7, 9 and 11. Pre-surgery values were averaged from available samples collected approximately 4 weeks before surgery. Data points are averages from available samples, and vertical lines connect highest and lowest sample at each week. Reference values for female harbor seal pups under three months of age (whisker boxes on left side of each panel, from n = 42 animals), and over three months of age (whisker boxes on right side of each panel, from n = 21 animals) were calculated from available data as described under methods

Through February 2017, no data returns from the implanted LHX tags were received.

Discussion

The three subjects were admitted into the Vancouver Aquarium Marine Mammal Rescue Centre as neonates less than one week old. Intake body mass was below the 11.2 kg average reported for wild newborn harbor seal pups in the study region [41]. All three pups completed rehabilitation procedures and were deemed releasable when they were selected for implantation surgery. Growth rates during the rehabilitation period averaged 0.14 kg/d, which is below the rate reported for wild harbor seal pups in the region of 0.39 kg/d [41], but within the range of 0.04 to 0.55 kg/d reported for harbor seal pups in rehabilitation [42]. Surgery occurred at an age of a little over 6 weeks, by which time wild harbor seal pups are typically weaned [41]. At this age harbor seal pups still grow and develop, and continue to undergo physiological maturation and adjustments. Weight gain for the week following surgery averaged 0.24 kg/d, which was also the overall average weight gain from admit to release. This suggests that within the constraints imposed by stranding and rehabilitation, food intake, digestion, assimilation, and the resulting growth rates were not affected by the surgeries or the implanted telemetry devices.

Physiologically, the three pups exhibited the expected immunological and acute phase responses.

White blood cell counts increased one week after surgery, peaked at two weeks and then declined. Levels

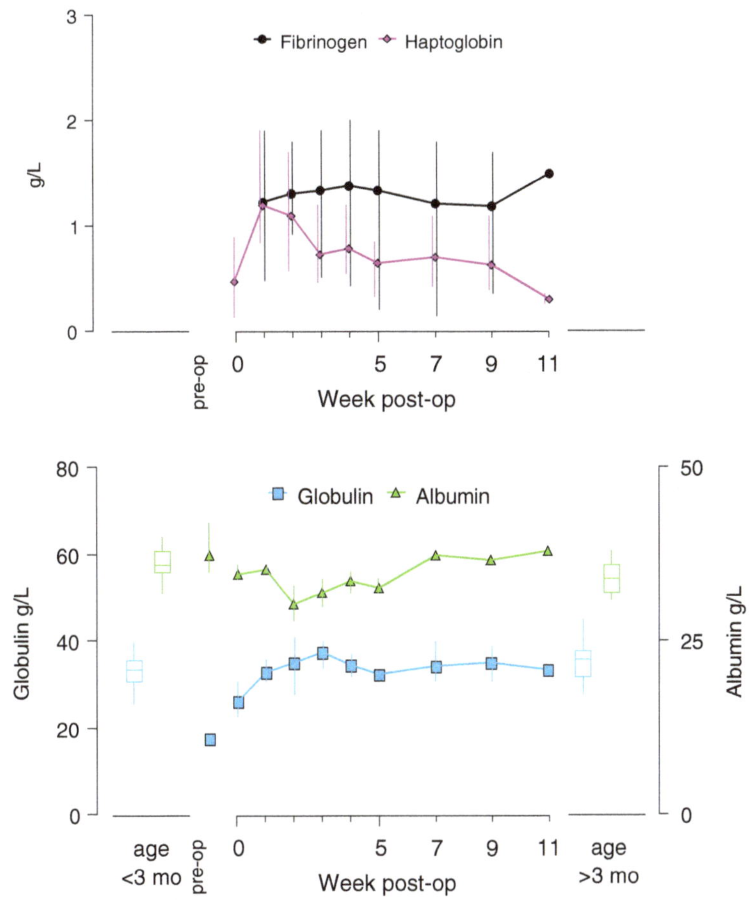

Fig. 7 Acute phase response to implant surgery in three female harbor seal pups. Fibrinogen and haptoglobin concentrations (upper panel), as well as globulin and albumin concentrations (lower panel) from surgery at approximately 6 weeks of age through release 11 weeks after surgery. Samples were collected at surgery, and at weeks 1, 2, 3, 4, 5, 7, 9 and 11. No fibrinogen assays were conducted on surgery days. Pre-surgery values were averaged from available samples collected approximately 4 weeks before surgery (lower panel only). Data points are averages from available samples, and vertical lines connect highest and lowest sample at each week. Reference values for female harbor seal pups under three months of age (whisker boxes on left side of each panel, from n = 42 animals), and over three months of age (whisker boxes on right side of each panel, from n = 21 animals) were calculated from available data as described under methods (lower panel only)

had declined to within the reference range by week five, and had returned to normal at the time of release at week 11. This appeared largely driven by mature neutrophils (absolute values) and monocytes, which showed an identical pattern. Eosinophils also increased after surgery but with considerable variance between samples and individuals. Platelets increased in all three subjects, but with considerable variance, and remained elevated but within reference ranges throughout the observation period. Lymphocytes increased overall and varied considerably, but remained within reference ranges. The two subjects that received skin sutures exhibited two peak lymphocyte values each above normal ranges, whereas the third subject did not.

The acute phase protein response was qualitatively as expected. The positive response protein haptoglobin increased and peaked at one week post-operative, after which values declined. Pre-operative values were only obtained from two animals. Comparable post-operative values were reached in week three. No pre-operative fibrinogen values were obtained, the post-operative values showed no clear trend within large variance. Pre-operative levels of globulin (a positive response protein) were below reference values, increased to within reference range with a peak at three weeks, and then declined slightly but remained within the reference range. The negative response protein albumin declined only during the 2nd week, after which values gradually increased.

Creatinine concentrations dropped following surgery and some values were below reference ranges for pups younger than three months. Values returned to pre-surgery levels by week five, and further increased up until release. By release, values were highest, but still within the reference range for pups older than three months. The decrease in creatinine could be related to temporarily reduced food intake, reduced activity in the

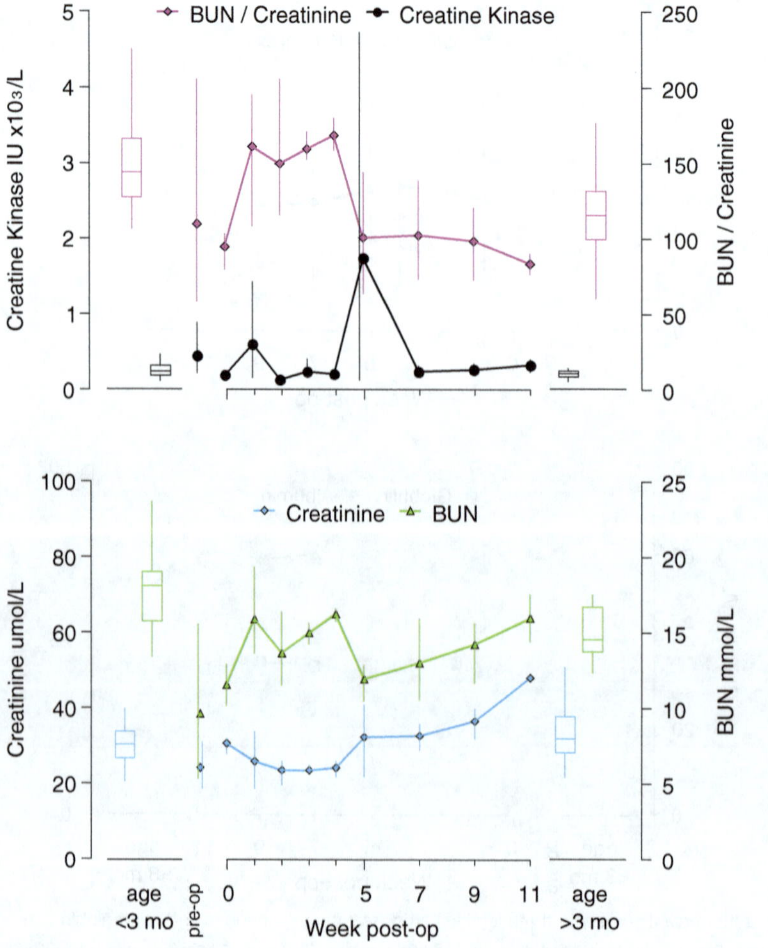

Fig. 8 BUN to creatinine ratios and activity of creatine kinase (upper panel), as well as creatinine and BUN concentrations (lower panel) from surgery at approximately six weeks of age through release 11 weeks after surgery. Samples were collected at surgery, and at weeks 1, 2, 3, 4, 5, 7, 9 and 11. Pre-surgery values were averaged from available samples collected approximately four weeks before surgery. Data points are averages from available samples, and vertical lines connect highest and lowest sample at each week. Reference values for female harbor seal pups under three months of age (whisker boxes on left side of each panel, from n = 42 animals), and over three months of age (whisker boxes on right side of each panel, from n = 21 animals) were calculated from available data as described under methods

small intestine and pancreas, or less likely due to increased kidney function. All three animals exhibited highly varying levels of creatine kinase (CK), with each showing a pronounced peak at one, three, and five weeks after surgery, respectively. In one animal (Pv14–073) the CK peak at one week preceded a drop in creatinine, and in two animals the peaks coincided or preceded increases in creatinine levels. Increased CK levels may be indicative of damage to tissue with already high normal levels of CK (such as muscles) and were likely secondary to surgery, or possibly from hematomas due to multiple weekly venipunctures. No other analytes from the animals exhibiting these single high CK values at those times were concerning, suggesting that these isolated high values were not clinically relevant. Blood urea nitrogen increased, and the BUN to creatinine ratio

Table 2 Identifiers and summary statistics (mean, standard deviation, standard error, and 95% confidence intervals) for the monthly averaged daily movements (km) of three implanted and one non-implanted harbor seal pups post-release

Identifier	Mean daily km per month	SD	SEM	CI	Lower CI	Upper CI
Pv14–073	29.8	5.83	1.94	3.81	25.96	33.57
Pv14–062	27.9	4.66	1.55	3.04	24.93	30.92
Pv14–123	22.9	4.21	1.49	2.92	19.94	25.77
Pv14–099	26.8	8.11	2.70	5.30	21.51	32.11

increased sharply after surgery, and dropped by the 5th week (Fig. 8). However, BUN values were below the reference range just prior to surgery and then increased to within this range. While an increase in BUN/creatinine could be indicative of kidney injury or gastrointestinal bleeding, or due to the processing of large hematomas, this is unlikely given the overall low values. A possible cause of the generally low BUN values prior to surgery and around week five may be in the combination of temporarily reduced food intake prior to surgery, and possibly reduced exercise after surgery. Generally, BUN, creatinine and CK values appeared to vary considerably but remained broadly within the wide reference ranges and were not deemed related to clinically relevant complications.

Overall, the observed biochemical changes appear more reflective of a response to surgery, tag insertion and inflammation, rather than an immune response. Electrolytes were unremarkable and exhibited age and high protein diet-related changes. The initial, acute response lasted through approximately week four, by which time acute response proteins had largely returned to pre-surgery values. Similarly, the initial inflammatory response peaked between the second and third week, after which some levels normalized. Following this acute response phase, all analytes with a few isolated exceptions did not indicate the persistence of a protracted, chronic response to surgery or implants.

The post-release tracking data confirms that all three pups survived at least their first year post surgery. Despite individual differences in the movement rates among LHX seals, the mean daily and seasonal movement rates were nearly identical to the non-surgical seal from the same cohort that was tracked simultaneously, and were generally within the range observed in rehabilitated harbor seal pups released by the Rescue Centre in 2013 (*Haulena unpub data*). In contrast, movement rates were much greater than rehabiliated pups and wild pups instrumented further south in the adjacent waters of Puget Sound in Washington State [9]. However, given that transmission duration was also at least twice as long for our deployments further north in the more open areas of the Salish Sea, it's more likely that differences in movements are more reflective of geography than of a result of the LHX implantation procedure. The extended deployments allowed the opportunity to assess coarse changes in seal movements over nearly a year but few patterns were apparent on a monthly or seasonal basis. Movement rates were highly individualistic which prevented us from describing any trends or potential development in the movements of the rehabilitated pups. Nevertheless, the movements of all seals did slow during the final months of the recorded deployments when compared to their previous months (August or September). Reduced activity is associated with the late summer/early fall molting period but in our case the results were confounded by incomplete monthly records (as the tags were likely shed before recording most of the final month).

The absence of post-mortem transmissions from LHX tags further suggests a high likelihood that all three animals survived through their second year. However, the reliability of these 2nd generation LHX2 tags has not yet been empirically validated in wild animals. Three of nine 2nd generation LHX2 tags deployed in combination with 1st generation tags in 9 weaned female Steller sea lions in 2014 transmitted after their host died, demonstrating their functionality. 1st generation LHX1 tags deployed in 36 weaned, juvenile Steller sea lions in the Gulf of Alaska between 2005 and 2014 had a 87% individual tag probability of uplinking to the Argos satellite system after the host animal had died [31]. If data return probability of 2nd generation tags is comparable, this would indicate a very high probability that all three pups were still alive two years following implantation surgery.

Despite significant recent advances in anesthesia and veterinary surgical techniques, abdominal surgeries in pinnipeds are still considered a rare option for treatment of captive or rehabilitated animals, or for deployment of internal telemetry transmitters [43]. To date, Steller sea lions are the only pinniped species in which intraperitoneal implants have been conducted on a larger scale (45 animals), and where the impact of implants has been studied in detail both before and after release [28, 29, 31, 44–50]. Based on the analysis of blood samples from the initial six sea lions, an acute inflammatory postoperative response was observed, primarily in the form of an increase in haptoglobin concentrations. This response lasted through five weeks, with a return to presurgery levels by the 6th week [45, 47]. From this, the authors derived a six week study inclusion criterion for studies based on LHX implants: survival has to be demonstrated to six weeks for data to be included in vital rate studies. Post-operative body core temperatures transmitted from the implants of all 45 sea lions ranged from 36 to 38.2 °C, though in a few instances a response to localized inflammations at the incision led to temperatures as high as 39.4 °C [28, 31]. By comparison, postoperative temperatures in the three harbor seal pups averaged at the upper end of the normal temperature range observed for Steller sea lions. A similar peak temperature of 39.6 was observed. In Steller sea lions, a comparison between a subset of 35 of the implanted animals, and 27 free-ranging control animals revealed no difference in cumulative survival from ages 14 months to 5 years, though due to the small sample sizes the power of the comparison was very low [50].

In phocids, no intraperitoneal implants have been used prior to this study. Four different types of subcutaneous implants have been tested through extended postoperative monitoring in 10 harbor seals [51]. However, no detailed longitudinal health assessments were reported other than CBC and serum biochemistry values that were within normal ranges 1 week after surgery for 9 of the 10 subjects. From visual observations of tissue reaction and wound healing, the authors concluded that one type of wax coated implant led to fewer tissue reactions and was preferable for long-term studies. Another five wild harbor seals received this type of implant and were released without extended postoperative monitoring. As described in the background section, two studies used subcutaneous implants to determine survival rates in wild harbor seals. One study on 32 seals did report apparent survival rates but without correcting for emigration, tag failures and extrusion, or tag effects on survival [25, 26]. The second study on 277 seals concluded that this technique was not suited to the estimation of survival rates via telemetric mark re-sight experiments. Conversely, a much smaller sample size of 45 Steller sea lions implanted with dual LHX tags delivering known fate data via temporally and spatially unrestricted satellite transmissions with a better than 98% post-mortem data return probability (for dual tag deployments), has already led to findings on survival and causes of mortality that could not otherwise be obtained in pinnipeds [29, 31, 32].

Conclusions

The low post-operative morbidity, expected clinical effects of surgeries and implants, and zero mortality during at least the first year after release illustrate the survivability of implantation surgery and intraperitoneal telemetry transmitters in phocid seals. This in turn suggests LHX tags as a viable technology to study vital rates in phocid seals, and to evaluate the efficacy and impact of rehabilitation programs. Additional studies with a larger sample size, possibly on non-rehabilitated animals, could lead to a greater statistical power on the nature and duration of the acute phase inflammatory response, and may yet reveal other tag effects not apparent here. This may also allow the establishment of a shorter study inclusion criterion than the five to six weeks suggested by these initial results, for vital rate studies in phocids using LHX tag technology. Any additional studies using LHX tags in harbor seals should furthermore continue to monitor for any long-term effects on behavior, reproduction and survival.

Abbreviations

BUN: Blood urea nitrogen; CBC: Complete blood count; CK: Creatine kinase; LHX: Life History Transmitter; UHF: ultra high frequency; VHF: very high frequency

Acknowledgements

We thank the staff and volunteers at the Vancouver Aquarium Marine Mammal Rescue Centre – in particular Shanie Fradette, Emily Johnson and Lindsaye Akhurst for their invaluable support.

Funding

This project received financial support from the National Science Foundation (U.S.) through awards #0964253 and #1556495 to M. Horning, from Oregon State University's Marine Mammal Institute, from the Vancouver Aquarium, from the Alaska SeaLife Center, from the Gordon and Patricia Gray Animal Welfare Foundation, and from Joanne and Stuart Watts. The funders had no role in the design of the study, data collection, analysis and interpretation of data, or writing of the manuscript.

Authors' contributions

MHorning designed and built transmitters in collaboration with Wildlife Computers, designed study, analyzed pre-release telemetry and clinical data, drafted manuscript; MHaulena designed study, developed implant surgery protocol, led implant surgeries, assisted in manuscript preparation; JR participated in implant surgeries, supervised post-operative husbandry and monitoring, assisted in manuscript preparation; CN developed satellite transmitter protocols and conducted attachments, compiled post-release telemetry data, analyzed Argos tracking data, participated in manuscript preparation. All authors read and approved the final manuscript.

Competing interests

The lead author (MH) is the co-developer of LHX tag in collaboration with Wildlife Computers, Inc. (Redmond, WA). Development of LHX tags was funded by the National Science Foundation (US), and a stated goal of the development grant is the future commercial availability of LHX tags to the general user community.

Consent for publication

Not applicable.

Author details

[1]Alaska SeaLife Center, 301 Railway Avenue, Seward, AK 99664, USA. [2]Oregon State University, 2030 SE Marine Science Drive, Newport, OR 97365, USA. [3]Vancouver Aquarium, 845 Avison Way, Vancouver, BC V6G 3E2, Canada.

References

1. Cooke SJ, Hinch SG, Wikelski M, Andrews RD, Kuchel LJ, Wolcott TG, et al. Biotelemetry: a mechanistic approach to ecology. Trends Ecol Evol. 2004;19:334–43.
2. Hooker SK, Biuw M, McConnell BJ, Miller PJO, Sparling CE. Bio-logging science: logging and relaying physical and biological data using animal-attached tags. Deep-Sea Res II. 2007;54:177–82.
3. Cooke SJ. Biotelemetry and biologging in endangered species research and animal conservation: relevance to regional, national, and IUCN red list threat assessments. Endang Species Res. 2008;4:165–85.
4. Small RJ, Boveng PL, Byrd VG, Withrow DE. Harbor seal population decline in the Aleutian archipelago. Mar Mamm Sci. 2008;24:845–63.
5. Womble JN, Pendleton GW, Mathews EA, Blundell GM, Bool NM, Gende SM. Harbor seal (*Phoca vitulina richardii*) decline continues in the rapidly changing landscape of Glacier Bay National Park, Alaska 1992–2008. Mar Mamm Sci. 2010;26:686–97.
6. Hazen EL, Maxwell SM, Bailey H, Bograd SJ, Hamann M, Gaspar P, et al. Ontogeny in marine tagging and tracking science: technologies and data gaps. Mar Ecol Prog Ser. 2012;457:221–40.
7. Moore MG, Early G, Touhey K, Barco S, Gulland F, Wells R. Rehabilitation and release of marine mammals in the United States: risks and benefits. Mar Mamm Sci. 2007;23:731–50.
8. Simeone CA, Gulland FMD, Norris T, Rowles TK. 2015. A systematic review of changes in marine mammal health in North America, 1972-2012: the need for a novel integrated approach. PLoS one;2015:10(11):e0142105.

9. Gaydos JK, Ignacio Vilchis L, Lance MM, Jeffries SJ, Thomas A, Greenwood V, et al. Postrelease movement of rehabilitated harbor seal (*Phoca vitulina richardii*) pups compared with cohort-matched wild seal pups. Mar Mamm Sci. 2013;29:282–94.
10. Lander ME, Gulland FMD. Rehabilitation and post-release monitoring of Steller Sea lion pups raised in captivity. Wildl Soc Bull. 2003;31(4):1047–53.
11. Lander ME, Harvey JT, Hanni KD, Morgan LE. Behavior, movements, and apparent survival of rehabilitated and free-Ranging Harbor seal pups. J Wildl Manag. 2002;66(1):19–28.
12. Morrison C, Sparling C, Sadler L, Charles A, Sharples R, McConnell B. Postrelease dive ability in rehabilitated harbor seals. Mar Mamm Sci. 2012; 28(2):E110–23.
13. Norris TA, Littnan CL, Gulland FMD. Evaluation of the captive Care and post-release behavior and survival of seven juvenile female Hawaiian monk seals (*Monachus schauinslandi*). Aquat Mamm. 2011;37(3):342–53.
14. Vincent C, Ridoux V, Fedak A, Hassan S. Mark-recapture and satellite tracking of rehabilitated juvenile grey seals (*Halichoerus grypus*): dispersal and potential effects on wild populations. Aquat Mamm. 2002;28(2):121–30.
15. Hussey NE, Kessel ST, Aarestrup K, Cooke SJ, Cowley PD, Fisk AT, et al. Aquatic animal telemetry: a panoramic window into the underwater world. Science. 2015;348:1255642.
16. Crossin GT, Cooke SJ, Goldbogen JA, Phillips RA. Tracking fitness in marine vertebrates: current knowledge and opportunities for future research. Mar Ecol Prog Ser. 2014;496:1–17.
17. Maniscalco JM. The effects of birth weight and maternal Care on survival of juvenile Steller Sea lions (*Eumetopias jubatus*). PLoS One. 2014;9(5):e96328.
18. Altukhov AV, Andrews RD, Calkins DG, Gelatt TS, Gurarie ED, Loughlin TR, et al. Age specific survival rates of Steller Sea lions at rookeries with divergent population trends in the Russian far east. PLoS One. 2015;10(5):e0127292.
19. Harwood J, Rohani P. The population biology of marine mammals. In: Floyd RB, Sheppard AW, De Barro PJ, editors. Frontiers of population ecology. Melbourne: CSIRO Publishing; 1996. p. 173–90.
20. Pistorius PA, Bester MN, Lewis MN, Taylor FE, Campagna C, Kirkman SP. Adult female survival, population trend, and the implications of early primiparity in a capital breeder, the southern elephant seal (*Mirounga leonina*). J Zool (Lond). 2004;263:107–19.
21. Bowen WD, McMillan JI, Blanchard W. Reduced population growth of gray seals at Sable Island: evidence from pup production and age of primiparity. Mar Mamm Sci. 2007;23:48–64.
22. Rotella JJ, Link WA, Chambert T, Stauffer GE, Garrott RA. Evaluating the demographic buffering hypothesis with vital rates estimated for Weddell seals from 30 years of mark–recapture data. J Anim Ecol. 2012;81:162–73.
23. Caughley G. Interpretation of age ratios. J Wildl Manag. 1974;38(3):557–62.
24. Blundell GM, Hoover-Miller AA, Schmale CA, Berngartt RK, Karpovich SA. Efficacy of subcutaneous VHF implants and remote telemetry monitoring to assess survival rates in harbor seals. J Mammal. 2014;95:707–21.
25. Manugian S, Van Bonn W, Harvey JT. Modified technique for the subcutaneous implantation of radio transmitters in harbour seals (*Phoca vitulina richardii*) under field conditions. Vet Rec Case Rep. 2015;3:e000154.
26. Manugian S, Greig D, Lee D, Becker BH, Allen S, Lowry MS, et al. Survival probabilities and movements of harbor seals in central California. Mar Mam Sci. 2017;33:154–71.
27. Horning M, Hill R. Designing an archival satellite transmitter for life-long deployments on oceanic vertebrates: the life history transmitter. IEEE J Ocean Eng. 2005;30:807–17.
28. Horning M, Haulena M, Tuomi P, Mellish J. Intraperitoneal implantation of life-long telemetry transmitters in otariids. BMC Vet Res. 2008;4:51.
29. Horning M, Mellish JE. Spatially explicit detection of predation on individual pinnipeds from implanted post-mortem satellite data transmitters. Endang Species Res. 2009;10:135–43.
30. Esslinger GG, Bodkin JL, Breton AR, Burns JM, Monson DH. Temporal patterns in the foraging behavior of sea otters in Alaska. J Wildl Manag. 2014;78(4):689–700.
31. Horning M, Mellish JE. In cold blood: evidence of Pacific sleeper shark (*Somniosus pacificus*) predation on Steller sea lions (*Eumetopias jubatus*) in the eastern Gulf of Alaska. Fish Bull. 2014;112:297–310.
32. Horning M, Mellish JE. Predation on an upper Trophic marine predator, the Steller Sea lion: evaluating high post-weaning mortality in a density dependent conceptual framework. PLoS One 2012;7(1):e30173 .
33. Sumner MD. trip: Tools for the Analysis of Animal Track Data. R package version 1.1-21.2015; https://CRAN.R-project.org/package=trip . Accessed 9 Feb 2017.
34. R Core Team. R: A language and environment for statistical computing. Vienna, Austria: R Foundation for Statistical Computing; 2016. https://www.R-project.org/ . Accessed 9 Feb 2017.
35. Dierauf LA, Gulland FMD. CRC handbook of marine mammal medicine. 2nd ed. Boca Raton, FL: CRC Press; 2001.
36. Geraci JR, Lounsbury VJ. Marine mammals ashore – a field guide for Strandings. 2nd ed. National Aquarium Baltimore: Baltimore, MD; 2005.
37. Haulena M: Otariid seals. In: West G, Heard D, Caulkett N. Ames, editors. Zoo animal and Wildlife immobilization and anesthesia. Iowa: Blackwell Publishing; 2007:469-478.
38. Lander ME, Harvey JT, Gulland FM. Hematology and serum chemistry comparisons between free-ranging and rehabilitated harbor seal (*Phoca vitulina richardsi*) pups. J Wildl Dis. 2003;39:600–9.
39. Greig DJ, Gulland FMD, Rios CA, Hall AJ. Hematology and serum chemistry in stranded and wild-caught harbor seals in central California: reference intervals, predictors of survival, and parameters affecting blood variables. J Wildl Dis. 2010;46:1172–84.
40. Frouin H, Haulena M, Akhurst LMF, Raverty SA, Ross PS. Immune status and function in harbor seal pups during the course of rehabilitation. Vet Immunol Immunopathol. 2013;155:98–109.
41. Cottrell PE, Jeffries S, Beck B, Ross PS. Growth and development in free-ranging harbor seal (*Phoca vitulina*) pups from southern British Columbia. Canada Mar Mamm Sci. 2002;18:721–33.
42. MacRae AM, Haulena M, Fraser D. The effect of diet and feeding level on survival and weight gain of hand-raised harbor seal pups (*Phoca vitulina*). Zoo Bio. 2010;29:1–10.
43. Higgins JL, Henrickson DA. Surgical procedures in Pinniped and cetacean species. J Zoo Wildl Medicine. 2013;44(4):817–36.
44. Mellish JE, Calkins DG, Christen DR, Horning M, Rea LD, Atkinson SK. Temporary captivity as a research tool: comprehensive study of wild Pinnipeds under controlled conditions. Aq Mamm. 2006;32:58–65.
45. Mellish JE, Thomton J, Horning M. Physiological and behavioral response to intra-abdominal transmitter implantation in Steller sea lions. J Exp Mar Biol Ecol. 2007;351:283–93.
46. Petrauskas L, Atkinson S, Gulland F, Mellish J, Horning M. Monitoring glucocorticoid response to rehabilitation and research procedures in California and Steller sea lions. J Exp Zool. 2008;309A:73–82.
47. Thomton JD, Mellish JE. Haptoglobin concentrations in freerange and temporarily captive juvenile steller sea lions. J Wildl Dis. 2007;43:258–61.
48. Thomton J, Mellish J, Hennen D, Horning M. Juvenile Steller sea lion dive behavior following temporary captivity. Endang Species Res. 2008;4:195–203.
49. Walker K, Horning M, Mellish J, Weary D. Behavioral responses of juvenile Steller sea lions to abdominal surgery: an assessment of post-operative pain. Appl Anim Behav Sci. 2009;120:201–7.
50. Shuert C, Horning M, Mellish J. The effect of novel research activities on long-term survival of temporarily captive Steller Sea lions (*Eumetopias jubatus*). PLoS One. 2015;10:e0141948.
51. Lander ME, Haulena M, Gulland FMD. Implantation of subcutaneous radio transmitters in the harbor seal (*Phoca vitulina*). Mar Mamm Sci. 2005;21:154–61.

5

Degenerative changes of the canine cervical spine after discectomy procedures, an in vivo study

Peter Grunert[1,2], Yu Moriguchi[1], Brian P. Grossbard[3], Rodolfo J. Ricart Arbona[4], Lawrence J. Bonassar[5] and Roger Härtl[1*]

Abstract

Background: Discectomies are a common surgical treatment for disc herniations in the canine spine. However, the effect of these procedures on intervertebral disc tissue is not fully understood. The objective of this study was to assess degenerative changes of cervical spinal segments undergoing discectomy procedures, in vivo.

Results: Discectomies led to a 60% drop in disc height and 24% drop in foraminal height. Segments did not fuse but showed osteophyte formation as well as endplate sclerosis. MR imaging revealed terminal degenerative changes with collapse of the disc space and loss of T2 signal intensity. The endplates showed degenerative type II Modic changes. Quantitative MR imaging revealed that over 95% of Nucleus Pulposus tissue was extracted and that the nuclear as well as overall disc hydration significantly decreased. Histology confirmed terminal degenerative changes with loss of NP tissue, loss of Annulus Fibrosus organization and loss of cartilage endplate tissue. The bony endplate displayed sclerotic changes.

Conclusion: Discectomies lead to terminal degenerative changes. Therefore, these procedures should be indicated with caution specifically when performed for prophylactic purposes.

Keywords: Canine spine, Discectomy, Degeneration, Disc herniation, Disc fenestration, Nucleus pulposus, Annulus fibrosus, Quantitative MRI

Background

Discectomies are a commonly performed surgical procedures for the treatment of disc herniations in the canine spine [1, 2] and essentially describe an extraction of intervertebral disc (IVD) tissue out of the disc space. They are either performed independently using a ventral approach to treat simple disc protrusions without significant disc material extruding into the spinal canal [3] or in conjunction with a ventral slot procedure [1, 2]. Discectomies in the form of fenestration procedures are also performed prophylactically to reduce recurrence of disc herniation at the index segment or prevent further herniation at the adjacent levels above and below [4, 5]. The term discectomy and fenestration can

* Correspondence: roger@hartlmd.net
[1]Department of Neurological Surgery, Weill Cornell Medicine, New York-Presbyterian Hospital, Weill Cornell Brain and Spine Institute|, 525 East 68th Street, Box 99, New York, NY 10065, USA
Full list of author information is available at the end of the article

Discectomies comprise removal of the Nucleus Pulposus (NP) through a "window" or defect created in the Annulus Fibrosus (AF) via various approaches [6, 7]. The AF is only partially removed. Despite its crucial physiological function, such as maintaining disc height, and segmental stability [8–10] the extracted disc tissue is usually not replaced with an interbody device (e.g. cage, prosthesis or bone grafts) as done routinely in humans [11]. Removal of the disc and subsequent altered segmental functionality [8, 10, 12] could enhance degenerative changes [9, 13], which is why several authors advocate not to perform discectomies especially for prophylactic purposes [14, 15]. However, the correlation of discectomy procedures and segmental degenerative changes is somewhat hypothetical as it has not been studied in vivo. To fill this knowledge gap we studied radiological and histological changes of beagles undergoing ventral cervical discectomy procedures in vivo. Our goal was to evaluate direct postoperative changes within the first 16 weeks according to established diagnostic parameters. Specifically, we assessed qualitative and quantitative MR imaging to study morphological changes of spinal segments as well as residual Nucleus Pulposus size and hydration. Radiographs were performed ex vivo to assess for disc and foraminal height as well as probable fusion or osteophyte formation. Histological sections of discectomized segments were analyzed to evaluate degenerative changes of the Annulus Fibrosus, the Nucleus Pulposus, endplate cartilage and vertebral endplate bone.

Methods

Study design

All experimental procedures were reviewed and approved by the Institutional Animal Care and Use Committee at Weill Cornell Medicine (ethic's protocol number: 2013–0110). Animals were housed in a facility accredited by the Association for the Assessment and Accreditation of Laboratory Animal Care (AAALAC) in compliance with applicable NY State, and Federal regulations.

This study is a subgroup analysis of an in vivo study evaluating tissue engineered intervertebral discs implanted in the beagle cervical spine [16] after undergoing a discectomy procedure. In this report we only include the control group of the main study which simply underwent a discectomy procedure without disc implantation.

Six skeletally mature male, sexually intact, purpose-bred beagles were included. They were obtained from Covance Research Products. At the time of surgery, the animals were 1 to 1.5 years old weighing between 15 and 25 kg.

All animals were assessed with magnetic resonance imaging (MRI) at 4, 8 and 16 weeks post surgery. After 16 weeks all animals were euthanized and specimens were harvested for ex vivo histology and radiographic analysis.

Discectomy procedure

All animals were sedated with acepromazine hydromorphone cocktail given intramuscularly (IM). Anesthesia was induced with ketamine/midazolam cocktail given intravenously (IV), and maintained with a combination of IV fentanyl/lidocaine/ketamine and inhaled isoflurane. After endotracheal intubation, animals were placed in dorsal recumbency with the neck carefully extended supporting the nasal bridge. The surgical site was prepared by clipping hair and alternating chlorhexidine with alcohol solution three times. Each animal was preoperatively given acefazolin IV and repeated 2 h later during the surgical procedure.

A ventral midline incision was made from the base of the larynx to the sternum. The paired sternocephalicus and sternohyoideus muscles were separated by blunt dissection, exposing the trachea. Retractors were then positioned to retract the carotid sheath laterally and the trachea, and esophagus medially. The surgical level was identified by palpation of the prominent transverse process of C6. Small curved hemostats were used to separate the longus coli muscle overlying the ventral AF at C5-C6. The subsequent steps were carried out with a surgical microscope. After the ventral part of the AF has been incised (about 5 mm length) and resected with a scalpel and a Kerrison rongeur, the NP was completely extracted using a small tartar scraper, a 4–0 bone curette, and a Kerrison rongeur. Lastly, muscle fascia, subcutaneous tissue and skin were sutured.

Qsualitative magnetic resonance imaging

We used a sagittal T2 sequence (TR = 2200 ms, TE = 66 ms, slice thickness = 2 mm) for qualitative MRI assessments (Siemens Tim TRIO 3 Tesla MRI Scanner, Erlangen, Germany). Images were obtained at week 8 and 16. Intervertebral disc (IVD) degenerative changes were evaluated according to the well established Pfirrmann grading scale [17], which outlines five grades of degeneration as defined by NP signal intensity, homogeneity and loss of disc height (Table 1). In addition, the canine specific grading scheme of Seiler et al. was used for evaluation. This classification takes NP signal intensity as well as AF morphology, possible disc herniation and spondylosis formation into account [18]. MRIs were further used to evaluate possible compression of nerve roots and the spinal cord.

T1 flash sequences (TR = 3 ms, TE = 4.9 ms, slice thickness = 0.9 mm) with high bone contrasts were used

Table 1 Pfirrmann MRI grading [17]

Grade	Structure	Distinction of Nucleus Pulposus	Signal intensity	Height of intervertebral disc
I	Homogeneous, bright white	Clear	Hyperintense, isointense to cerebrospinal fluid	Normal
II	Inhomogeneous with or without horizontal bands	Clear	Hyperintense, isointense to cerebrospinal fluid	Normal
III	Inhomogeneous, gray	Unclear	Intermediate	Normal to slightly decreased
IV	Inhomogeneous, gray to black	Lost	Intermediate to hypointense	Normal to moderately decreased
V	Inhomogeneous, black	Lost	Hypointense	Collapsed disc space

to evaluate possible kyphotic or lordodic deformity changes of the operated segments. All discectomized discs were compared to adjacent levels control levels C6/C7.

Quantitative magnetic resonance imaging

NP hydration and size were assessed with quantitative MRI using sagittal multislice multiecho pulse sequence (TR = 2000 ms, TE = 12 ms, NEX = 2, number of echoes = 12, echo spacing = 12 ms, slice thickness = 1 mm, and matrix size = 320 × 320, resolution: 125 μm × 125 μm × 1 mm). Images were obtained at week 4, 8 and 16.

NP hydration was assessed by its average T2 relaxation time, NP size by the amount of MRI NP voxels it is composed of.

The following algorithm previously developed by our group [19] was used for radiological segmentation of the NP:

A standard region of interest (ROI) measuring approximately 4 mm^2 (comprising 300 voxels) was drawn within the center NP of the healthy disc proximal to the experimental segments. The average T2-relaxation time (T2-RT) of that ROI was measured, and this value minus 3 standard deviations was used to set a subtraction threshold for all voxels in that slice. Voxels with T2 values lower than the threshold were subsequently subtracted. As a result, only voxels with T2 values representing NP tissue remained in the disc space [19]. Subsequently, NP size was calculated by the amount of NP voxels it is composed of. The NP hydration was calculated by measuring the average T2 relaxation time of those NP voxels.

Histological assessment

Animals were euthanized 16 weeks post-surgery by pentobarbital overdose IV. Cervical spines were harvested from C4-C7 and fixed using 10% neutralized formalin supplemented with 1% cetylpyridinium chloride (CPC). Spinal segments were decalcified, cut in a mid-sagittal plane and transferred to 75% ethanol. Subsequently segments were embedded in paraffin, cut to 5-μm thickness, and stained with Picrosirius Red, Safranin-O and Alcian Blue.

Degenerative changes were graded using the Bergknut classification which was established specifically for canine spine. The NP and AF are graded according to their staining characteristics, cell composition and endplate morphology [20, 21] (Table 2). Stained slides were observed under polarized light to evaluate the AF structure. Discectomized discs were compared to C6/C7 healthy control discs.

Radiographic measurements

Radiographic images were performed in a digital radiographic cabinet (Faxitron). They were obtained 16 weeks

Table 2 Histological degenerative grading according to Bergknut et al. [20]

Morphology of annulus fibrosus (AF)	Chondrocyte metaplasia of AF	Tears and cleft formation	Chondrocyte proliferation of nucleus pulposus	Presence of notochordal cells in nucleus pulposus
0 Well-organized, half ring-shaped, collagen lamellae 1 Mild disorganized; some loss of half ring-shaped structure, most lamellar layer, still distinguishable (<25%) 2 Moderately disorganized; partly ruptured AF, loss of half ring-shaped structure (25–75%) 3 Completely ruptured AF; no or	0 No chondrocyte morphology, just spindle-shaped fibroblasts 1 Mild chondrocyte proliferation (i.e. limited to inner most AF layers) 2 Moderate chondrocyte proliferation (i.e. chondroid cells in up to half of the AF) 3 Marked chondrocyte proliferation (i.e. chondroid cells up to outer layers of the AF)	0 Absent 1 Rarely present 2 Present in intermediate amounts 3 Abundantly present 4 Scar/tissue defects	0 No proliferation 1 Increased chondrocyte-like cell density 2 Connection of two chondrocytes 3 Small size clones (i.e., several chondrocytes group together, i.e. 2–7 cells) 4 Moderate size clones (i.e. >8 cells) 5 Huge clones (i.e. >15 cells) 6 Scar/tissue defects	0 Abundantly present (>50%) 1 Present (1–50%) 2 Absent

Matrix staining of the nucleus pulposus with Alcian blue/Picrosirius red staining	Endplate morphology	New bone formation	Subchondral bone sclerosis
0 Blue stain dominates 1 Mixture of blue and red staining 2 Red stain dominates	0 Regular thickness; homogeneous structure 1 Slightly irregular thickness 2 Moderately irregular thickness 3 Severely irregular thickness with interruption of the endplate	0 Absent 1 Minor new bone formation 2 Moderate amounts of new bone formation 3 Abundant new bone formation; tendency towards bridging/complete bridging	0 No sclerosis (<2 _ the thickness of the dorsal vertebral cortex) 1 Mild sclerosis (2–4 _ the thickness of the dorsal vertebral cortex) 2 Moderate sclerosis (>4 _ the thickness of the dorsal vertebral cortex) 3 Severe subchondral bone irregularities

post discectomy ex vivo directly after the cervical spine was collected for histological analysis. Images were used for disc height and foraminal height measurements. The IVD height was expressed as a disc height index, calculated by dividing disc height by adjacent vertebral body height on the basis of the modified method of Lu et al. [22]. Foraminal height was measured in pixels using the software pixel stick. Height of the discectomized segments is presented in percentage of the distal healthy adjacent segment (C6/C7). In contrast to quantitative MR imaging, we used the distal adjacent segment as a control for radiographic measurements. This is because two specimens were harvested at the C4/C5 disc space instead of the C4 vertebral body. Thus, this level could not be used for radiographic assessments in all specimens.

Data analysis and statistics

For the analyses for continuous outcomes in disc height index, NP size, and NP hydration, generalized estimating equation (GEE) models were used to assess main effects and interaction factors of disc group and longitudinal assessment of time. Statistical analysis was performed with IBM SPSS Statistics 22 (SPSS, Chicago, IL, USA). P values <0.05 were considered statistically significant.

Results

Radiographic imaging

Healthy control discs showed no signs of degenerative changes on radiographs. Average DHI of healthy discs was 0.15 at week 16. Discectomized segments appeared collapsed at 16 weeks (Fig. 1a, b), showing a significantly lower DHI of 0.06 (<0.05) compared to adjacent control segments. This represents a 60% percent drop in disc height compared to adjacent controls.

Disc height reduction led to a subsequent decrease in neuroforaminal height (Fig. 1a, b).At 16 weeks the average height was 24% less in discectomized segments (C5/C6) compared to adjacent healthy controls at C6/C7.

Morphological changes included endplate sclerosis (Fig. 1c). Discectomized endplates became more radiopaque compared to healthy segments making the trabecular pattern of the endplate cancellous bone significantly less distinct. Discectomized segments also showed signs of spondylosis, ventrally at the the cranial vertebral body of the operated segment (Fig. 1c).

There was no significant angulation or kyphotic deformity present at operated segments. No fusion occurred according to radiographic images.

Qualitative MR imaging

After 16 weeks, healthy adjacent discs (C6/C7) showed no signs of degenerative changes. Five discs displayed a Pfirrmann degeneration grade I, indicating a completely healthy disc with a homogenous bright hyperintense Nucleus Pulposus on T2 weighted images (Fig. 2a). The hypointense AF showed a clear border to the nucleus. No bulging of the AF was present. One specimen showed a Pfirrmann grade of II which represents a healthy disc with a less homogenous bright NP showing a nuclear cleft,

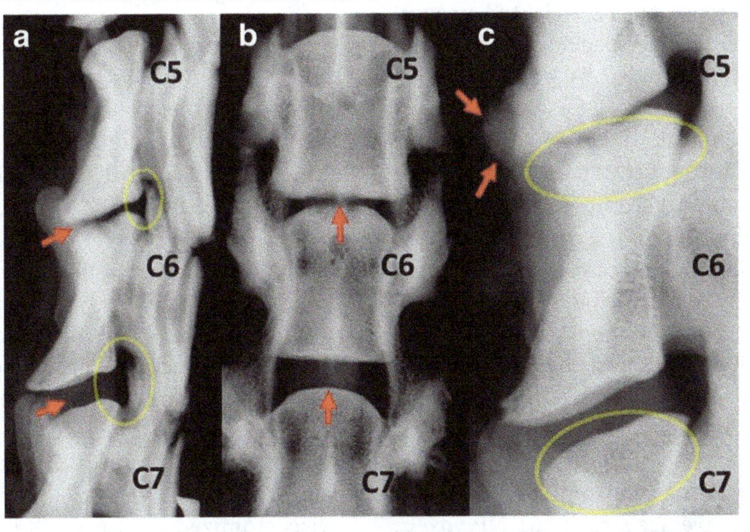

Fig. 1 Radiograph of the lower cervical spine. **a** Lateral view, discectomy segment C5/C6 compared to adjacent healthy control C6/C7. *Red arrow* marks both disc spaces. The discectomy segment is almost completely collapsed. The neuroforamen of both segments are marked with a yellow ellipse. Loss in disc height subsequently lead to a loss of foraminal height. Both segments show no signs of kyphotic or lordotic deformity. **b** Ventro-dorsal view of the same specimen. *Red arrow* points to the disc space which is significantly narrowed at C5/C6. **c** Lateral view of different specimen. Bony endplates are marked with yellow ellipse. The healthy endplate at C6/C7 shows trabecular bone pattern. Sclerotic changes of the degenerated bony endplate at C5/C6. Endplate is more radio dense indicating increased cortical bone and decreased trabecular bone. *Red arrow* marks an osteophyte which formed ventrally at the C5 vertebral body

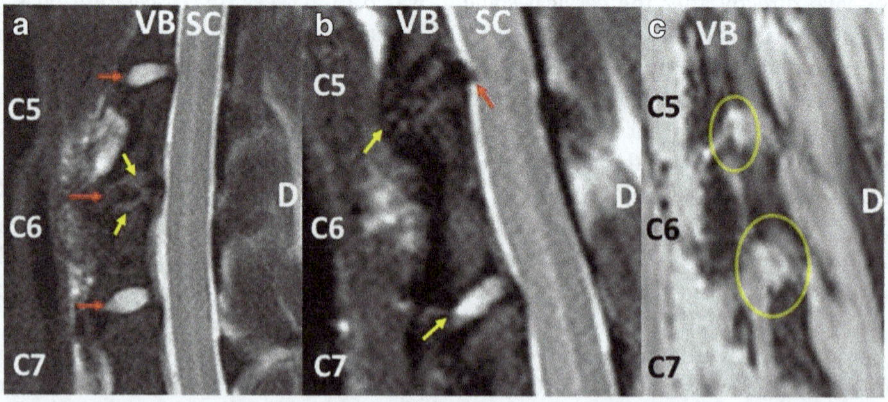

Fig. 2 Sagittal T2 weighted MR images of the lower cervical spine. Right side of each slide is dorsal (D) **a** *Red arrows* point to the intervertebral discs between the vertebral bodies (VB) which are ventral to the spinal canal (SC). Healthy control discs at C6/C7 demonstrate a bright hyperintense, homogenous NP. The hyperintensity indicates normal NP tissue hydration. There is a clear border to the hypointense AF without loss of disc height. The endplates are hypointense. In contrast, the discectomy segment C5/C6 shows a black disc sign. There is complete loss of nuclear hyperintensity. The disc space is collapsed. The endplates (*yellow arrow*) are hyperintense which is indicative of type II Modic degenerative changes. **b** Different specimen. *Yellow arrows* point to disc space. *Red arrow* points to extruded disc at the discectomy segment. There is no significant spinal cord compression present. **c** Lateral view to the neuroforamen (*marked by yellow ellipse*). The C5/C6 discectomy segment shows a narrower foramen compared to the healthy C6/C7 segment. However, the nerve root (hypointense structure within foramen) appears not to be compressed at the discectomy segment

which is a horizontal gray band representing fibrous tissue dissecting the nucleus [18]. According to the canine specific Seiler grading, adjacent discs (C6/C7) of five animals were evenly graded as I indicating completely healthy discs. One specimen was graded as II for displaying a nuclear cleft.

At week 16 all discectomized IVDs (C5/C6) showed a Pfirrmann grade of V, representing terminal degenerative changes with a completely collapsed discs space and "black disc" sign (hypointense on T2 weighted images) (Fig. 2a). According to the canine specific Seiler grading all C5/C6 discs were evenly graded as V indicative of progressed degenerative changes.

In contrast to healthy endplates (C6/C7) which appear hypointense (dark) on T2 weighted images, endplates in discectomized discs became hyper intense which is indicative of type II Modic changes.

Disc protrusions without significant spinal cord or nerve root compression were also visible (Fig. 2b).

The collapsed disc space also led to a decrease in size of the neuroforamen which narrowed the space for the exiting nerve root (Fig. 2c). However, a clear sign of nerve root impingement was not visible.

Quantitative MR imaging

Healthy nuclei showed an average size of 361 NP voxels. Average T2 relaxation time (correlating to NP hydration) was 372 ms. Both did not significantly change over 16 weeks.

Discectomized discs showed a significant decrease in NP size compared to healthy disc with an average NP voxel count of 16 ($p < 0.05$) (4 specimen were 0) by week 4 and 2,25 ($p < 0.05$) (4 specimen were 0) by week 16 (Fig. 3a, b). Compared to healthy discs, hydration of the residual NP decreased by 4 weeks as T2 relaxation time decreased to an average of 113 ms ($p < 0.05$). The average T2 relaxation time on week 16 was further reduced to an average of 42 ms ($p < 0.05$).

High bone contrast MR imaging

No significant kyphotic or lordotic deformity was observed after discectomy procedures at 16 weeks.

Histology

After 16 weeks, healthy C6/C7 discs showed no signs of degenerative changes. The AF was composed of lamellar parallel aligned fibers and spindle shaped fibroblasts and appeared well organized (Fig. 4a). The Nucleus Pulposus was predominantly composed of notochordal cells. The nucleus stained intensively with Safranin O for proteoglycans. The endplates had a regular homogenous thickness and cartilage structure with chondrocytes embedded in a proteoglycan rich matrix (indicated by intense Safranin O staining) (Fig. 4a). The average Bergknut degeneration grading score was 0 out of 24 indicating no degenerative changes.

Discectomized C5/C6 discs in contrast showed progressed signs of degeneration after 16 weeks. The AF was partially ruptured; cleft formation was present (Fig. 4b). The AF appeared less organized, displaying alterations of its lamellar structure under polarized light (Fig. 5). The AF cell composition changed from fibroblasts to chondrocytes, a typical degenerative change

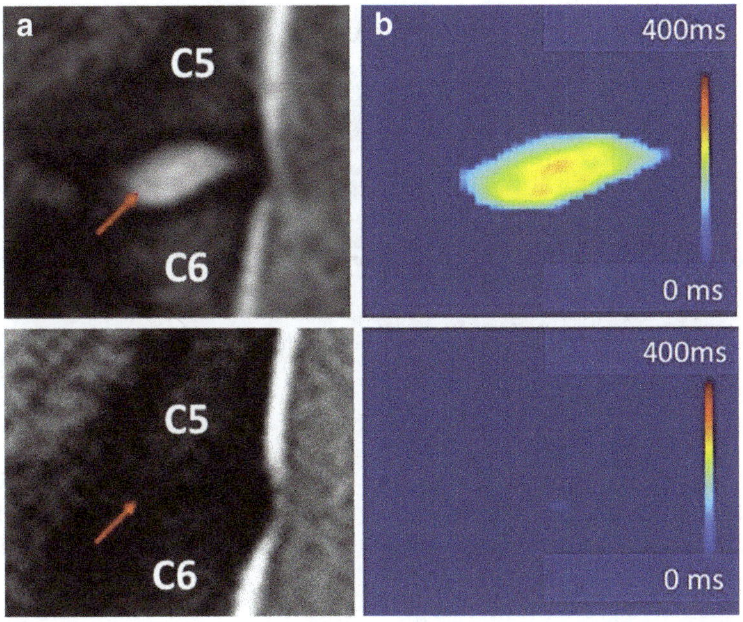

Fig. 3 Display of quantitative MR imaging for nuclear size and hydration measurements. **a** Sagittal T2 weighted MR image of a healthy (top) and degenerated disc (bottom). **b** Corresponding T2 relaxation time of the NP displayed as a heat map. Red colors represent high T2 relaxation time (high tissue hydration), *blue colors* low T2 times (low tissue hydration). All MRI voxels not representing NP tissue according to their T2 relaxation time were subtracted leaving only MR voxels representing nuclear tissue in the slide. The size of the nucleus was measured by the amount of NP voxels it was composed of. The degenerated disc on the bottom shows no residual NP voxels indicating that there is no nuclear tissue present on that slide

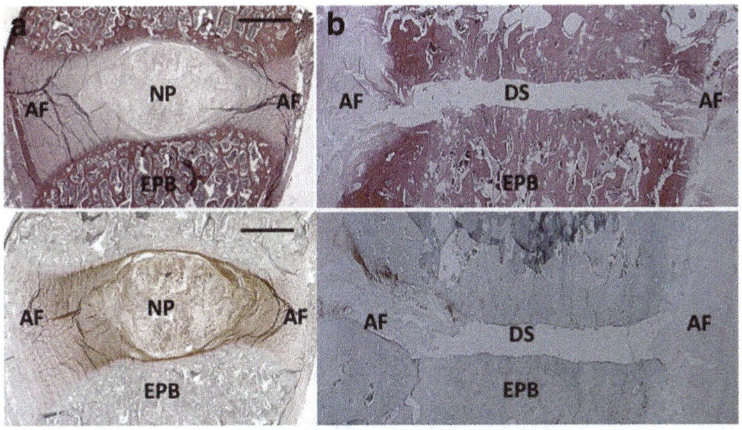

Fig. 4 Histology sections of explanted cervical segments (×2 magnification). **a** Healthy discs. Top Picrosirius red stain (stains for collagen), bottom Safranin-O stain (stains for proteoglycans). Both discs show a well organized AF composed of lamellar aligned collagen fibers which stain intense for Picrosirius *red*. There is a clear border to the NP which appears as a homogenous structure. It stains with Safranin-O indicating proteoglycan rich matrix. The cartilaginous endplate (*black arrow*) forms a border between the NP to the endplate bone (EPB). It stains intensively with Safranin-O indicating high proteoglycan content. **b** Discectomy discs. Top Picrosirius red, bottom Safranin-O stain. The annulus is disrupted and disorganized on both sides. Annular Picrosirius red staining is less intense. There is no NP tissue left in the disc space (DS). The cartilaginous endplate completely disappeared. The Endplate bone is sclerotic indicated by dense cortical bone structure and decreased trabecular bone. The collapse of the disc space is visible on histological sections

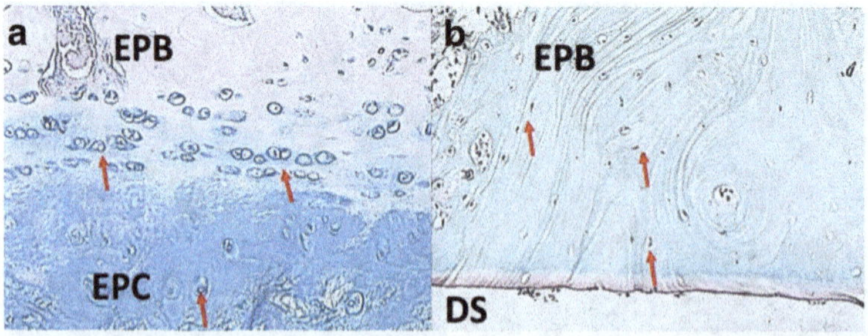

Fig. 5 Endplate bone Alcian blue stain (stains for proteoglycans). **a** Healthy disc ×8 magnification. The endplate cartilage (EPC) consists of chondrocytes (*red arrows*) embedded in a proteoglycan rich matrix (*blue stain on alcian blue*). The cartilage endplate borders to the endplate bone (EPB). **b** Discectomy disc ×4 magnification. The bony endplate with its cortical bone structure and osteoclasts (*red arrows*) borders directly to the disc space. There is no cartilage endplate in between

described as chondrocyte metaplasia (Fig. 6). All specimen showed no residual NP tissue in the disc space (Fig. 4b).

Both endplates were thinned and disrupted. The cartilage endplate completely disappeared (Fig. 7) and bony endplate (subchondral bone) displayed sclerotic changes (Fig. 4b). There was no new bone formation present on histological sections. The average degeneration grade according to the Bergknut classification was 19.4 out of 24 indicating terminal degenerative changes.

Discussion

Disc herniation is a common neurological condition in dogs, specifically in small and chondrodystrophoid breeds such as the beagle [23]. Discectomy procedures are commonly performed independently or in conjunction with a laminectomy or ventral slot approach for this condition.

They are also performed prophylactically as fenestration procedures. Due to their technical similarity, the term discectomy and fenestration can be used synonymously in this manuscript.

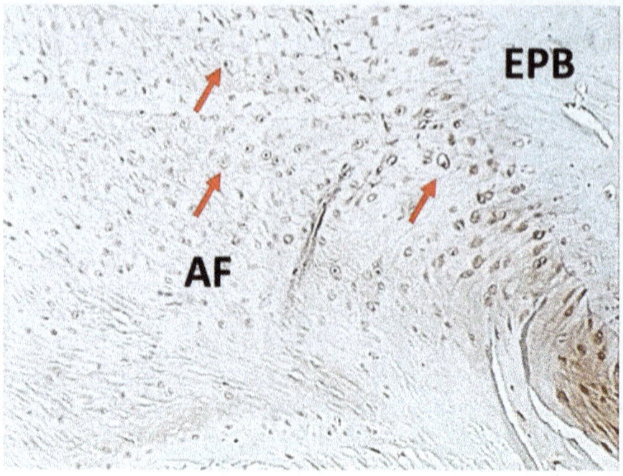

Fig. 6 Safranin-O stain of the Annulus Fibrosus which is attached to the endplate bone (EPB). Chondrocytes (*red arrows*) are infiltrating the annulus replacing fibroblasts, a degenerative process called chondrocytic metaplasia

The goal of this study was to evaluate the degenerative effects of discectomies in the canine spine.

We could show that IVDs undergoing discectomies displayed terminal signs of radiographic, and histological degeneration according to established grading scales. These alterations occurred relatively early after a 16 week follow up. Degeneration affected all three components of the IVD: the NP, AF and endplates.

NP changes

The NP plays a crucial role for segmental biomechanical functionality. It has a relatively high proteoglycan content leading to a high water binding capability [24]. The water content allows the NP to establish a hydrostatic pressure, which separates both endplates thereby maintaining disc height [24]. The relatively high water content is also responsible for the nuclear viscoelastic mechanical properties which facilitates its important damping quality [25].

According to MR based NP voxel count measurements, over 95% of the nucleus were removed from the discectomy procedure by week 16. The morphological appearance of "black discs" on T2 weighted images confirmed these quantitative assessments. Loss of NP T2 signal intensity represents loss of tissue hydration [26, 27]. It is a critical degenerative parameter according to the MR Pfirrmann grading, indicating terminal degenerative changes. Histological sections confirmed the almost complete loss of NP tissue, which is also a critical degenerative parameter [28].

AF changes

The AF, with its complex multilamellar fiber structure, is crucial for maintaining segmental stability by opposing axial rotation as well as lateral bending [29]. It works in tandem with the NP by opposing nuclear hydrostatic pressure facilitating maintenance of disc height.

Compared to the NP, there are less typical radiological signs for the AF to describe degenerative changes such

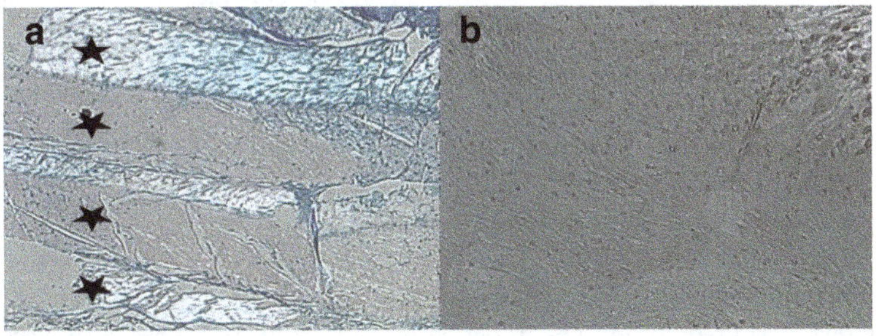

Fig. 7 Alcian *Blue* stained slides of the AF under polarized light (×4). **a** Healthy disc, the AF is organized in a multilamellar structure. The lamellae (*black star*) are composed of parallel aligned fibers and are therefore birefringent (bright) under polarized light. They alternate in their orientation resulting in alternating birefringence. **b** Dorsal annulus of a discectomy disc. Tissue lost its multilamellar organization. The Annular fibers lost their organization and parallel alignment indicated by lost in birefringent behavior under polarized light

as signal alterations. However, MR imaging showed bulging of the AF towards the spinal canal which is an important degenerative parameter according to canine specific Seiler MR grading [18]. Annular bulging most likely developed due to the loss of disc height and the resulting outwards displacement of annular fibers. Reduced disc height as well as reduced damping properties due to NP loss leads to redistribution of axial load and shear forces to the AF which results in structural changes [30, 31]. Histological sections of the AF in our study revealed early signs of these structural changes with cleft formation, reduced organization of lamellar structure and chondrocyte metaplasia.

Cartilage endplate

The cartilage endplate, with its high proteoglycan content, allows for high solute diffusivity that facilitates nutrition supply to the avascular NP [32, 33]. The endplate also has a mechanical function, as it absorbs hydrostatic pressure from the NP and works as a barrier to prevent bulging of the NP into the endplate [34].

Similar to the AF, there are no established radiographic signs to describe cartilage endplate degeneration. There are however indirect MR signs of endplate pathology. Modic changes, specifically type II, are described as increased T2 signal intensity in the vertebral body bone tissue adjacent to the endplate [34]. The histopathological correlate of type II Modic changes are disruption of the end plate with signs of an active inflammatory reaction [34]. Both increased endplate T2 signal intensity as well as disruption of the endplate on histological sections were seen in discectomized discs in our study. Modic changes have shown to correlate with back pain in humans [35]; a potential clinical relevance has so far not been studied in the canine spine. Endplate disruption can impact its physiological function. Disrupted endplates demonstrated an impaired ability to contain hydrostatic pressure from the NP which could result in disc height loss [36]. Endplate discontinuity has also shown to induce degenerative changes of IVDs, likely by impacting nutrient transport to nuclear cells [34, 37, 38].

It is unclear if endplate damage and thinning resulted from a post discectomy degenerative process or from the procedure itself. While it is possible this was the result of iatrogenic damage, it is unlikely since we took great care to not damage the endplates during discectomy procedures.

Comparison to literature

To our knowledge, this is the first in vivo study evaluating degenerative changes following ventral discectomy procedures performed with a standard surgical technique. Shores et al. studied degenerative changes of canine spinal segments after disc fenestration using a needle puncture technique with partial Nucleus Pulposus aspiration. Similar to our study, there was radiographic evidence of disc height narrowing 24 weeks post surgery. Histological sections showed no inflammation, dissolution or fibrotic changes on the residual NP. The only histological changes described were vascular and fibrous tissue invasion of the punctured AF [13]. Compared to our study, it appears that smaller puncture defects with retained NP tissue induce less degenerative changes than incising the AF with complete NP removal. However, similar studies in rabbit and rat demonstrated that puncture defects lead to terminal degenerative changes over time [16, 39]. They have also shown that the AF has a very low intrinsic healing capability [40, 41] and that residual NP tissue can herniate through annular needle puncture defects [16] over time.

While we did not evaluate mechanical alterations of discectomized discs, others have conducted mechanical studies on canine cervical cadavers undergoing C5/C6 discectomy procedure. They demonstrated a significant increase in flexion/extension range of motion post surgery indicating that these procedures may have a destabilizing effect of the involved segment [8, 12].

Clinical considerations

We could demonstrate that discectomy procedures as described are effective in completely removing NP tissue which makes herniations at prophylactically treated segments less likely to occur.

This corroborates studies showing a lower reherniation rate in animals treated with prophylactic fenestrations [42, 43].

However, discectomy procedures induced degenerative changes in a relatively short period of time. The most significant change was loss of disc height which led to a subsequent loss of neuroforaminal height. Reduced neuroforaminal height can lead to nerve root impingement which subsequently can cause radicular symptoms such as referred pain, muscle weakness or loss of sensation. Discectomy procedures also lead to protrusion of the AF into the spinal canal which could in certain cases cause symptomatic spinal cord compression. However, neither disc protrusion nor neuroforaminal stenosis led to significant impingement of neural structures after 16 weeks. There was also no deformity present on MR or radiographic imaging. It has to be kept in mind that 16 weeks is a short term follow up and that spinal degenerative changes such as spinal canal stenosis or deformity have a tendency to occur and progress over time.

Considering the degenerative effect demonstrated in our study, prophylactic discectomies in the form of fenestration procedures should be carefully considered specifically when they involve segments without significant preoperative radiographic signs of degeneration. Besides degenerative changes, fenestration procedures have further reported disadvantages such as longer surgery times, higher morbidity with increased postoperative pain and deficits as well as complications such as seroma formation or life threatening hemorrhages into the thorax cavity potentially leading to postoperative death [43].

Limitations

The main limitation of this study is the relative short term follow up. Degenerative changes described could progress over time. Another limitation is that healthy discs underwent discectomies whereas in clinical practice treated discs often already display signs of degeneration, which could alter histological appearance. Another limitation is that only one level underwent a discectomy. Prophylactic discectomies are often performed on several levels, which could worsen spinal malalignment.

Conclusion

Discectomies lead to significant degenerative changes of the affected discs according to histological, MR and radiographic assessments. Degenerative changes involved all three components of the IVD: the nucleus, Annulus Fibrosus and endplate. Therefore, discectomy procedures should be considered carefully especially when performed for prophylactic purposes.

Abbreviations

AF: Annulus Fibrosus; EPB: Endplate bone; EPC: Endplate cartilage; IM: Intramuscular; IV: Intravenous; IVD: Intervertebral disc; MRI: Magnetic resonance imaging; NP: Nucleus Pulposus; ROI: Region of Interest; T2-RT: T2 Relaxation time

Acknowledgments

We would like to thank Dr. Doty from the Hospital of Special Surgery for his help with preparing and interpreting histological slides used for this study.

Authors contribution

PG initiated the research project, performed surgical procedures, developed the hypothesis and design of the study, analyzed imaging and histology results. Wrote manuscript and submitted grants for funding. YM performed procedures and statistical analysis. BG helped to analyze data and evaluated it's relevance for veterinary neurosurgery. Edited manuscript. RR Performed anesthesia and postoperative care for animals undergoing surgery. Edited manuscript. LB helped to gather funding for this study, edited manuscript, helped with study design. RH helped to perform surgical procedures, worked on study design, gathered funding for the study. Edited manuscript. All authors have read and approved the final version of the manuscript.

Funding

This study was funded by the NIH (CTSC grant), the AO-spine and a New York State grant.

Competing interests

The authors declare that they have no competing interests.

Consent for publication

Not applicable.

Author details

[1]Department of Neurological Surgery, Weill Cornell Medicine, New York-Presbyterian Hospital, Weill Cornell Brain and Spine Institute|, 525 East 68th Street, Box 99, New York, NY 10065, USA. [2]Department of Neurological Surgery, Swedish Neuroscience Institute, Seattle, WA, USA. [3]Department of Orthopedics and Neurosurgery VCA-Animal Specialty, Yonkers, NY, USA. [4]Center of Comparative Medicine and Pathology, Memorial Sloan Kettering Cancer Center & Weill Cornell Medicine, New York City, NY, USA. [5]Department of Biomedical Engineering, Cornell University, Ithaca, NY, USA.

References

1. Hoerlein BF. Intervertebral disks. In: Hoerlein BF editors: Canine Neurology, 3rd ed. Philadelphia, WB Saunders; 1978. p. 470–560.
2. Shores A. The intervertebral disk syndrome in the dog: Part III. Thoracolumbar disk surgery. The Compendium on Continuing Education for the Practicing Veterinarian. 1982;4:24–31.
3. Nakama S, Taura Y, Tabaru H, Yasuda M. A retrospective study of ventral fenestration for disk diseases in dogs. J Vet Med Sci. 1993;55(5):781–4.
4. Brisson BA, Moffatt SL, Swayne SL, Parent JM. Recurrence of thoracolumbar intervertebral disk extrusion in chondrodystrophic dogs after surgical decompression with or without prophylactic fenestration. J Am Vet Med Assoc. 2004;224(11):1808–14.
5. Forterre F, Konar M, Spreng D, Jaggy A, Lang J. Influence of intervertebral disc fenestration at the herniation site in association with hemilaminectomy on recurrence in chondrodystrophic dogs with thoracolumbar disc disease: a prospective MRI study. Vet Surg. 2008;37(4):399–405.
6. Flo GL, Brinker WO. Lateral fenestration of thoracolumbar discs. JAAHA. 1975;11(5):619 26.

3. Nakama S, Taura Y, Tabaru H, Yasuda M. A retrospective study of ventral fenestration for disk diseases in dogs. J Vet Med Sci. 1993;55(5):781–4.
4. Brisson BA, Moffatt SL, Swayne SL, Parent JM. Recurrence of thoracolumbar intervertebral disk extrusion in chondrodystrophic dogs after surgical decompression with or without prophylactic fenestration. J Am Vet Med Assoc. 2004;224(11):1808–14.
5. Forterre F, Konar M, Spreng D, Jaggy A, Lang J. Influence of intervertebral disc fenestration at the herniation site in association with hemilaminectomy on recurrence in chondrodystrophic dogs with thoracolumbar disc disease: a prospective MRI study. Vet Surg. 2008;37(4):399–405.
6. Flo GL, Brinker WO. Lateral fenestration of thoracolumbar discs. JAAHA. 1975;11(5):619–26.
7. Knapp DW, Pope ER, Hewett JE, et al. A retrospective study of thoracolumbar disk fenestration in dogs using a ventral approach: 160 Cases (1976 TO 1986). JAAHA. 1990;26:543–9.
8. Macy NB, Les CM, Stover SM, Kass PH. Effect of disk fenestration on sagittal kinematics of the canine C5-C6 intervertebral space. Vet Surg. 1999;28(3):171–9.
9. Melrose J, Ghosh P, Taylor TK, Hall A, Osti OL, Vernon-Roberts B, et al. A longitudinal study of the matrix changes induced in the intervertebral disc by surgical damage to the annulus fibrosis. J Orthop Res. 1992;10:665–76.
10. Vasseur PB, Saunders G, Steinback C. Anatomy and function of the ligaments of the cervical spine in the dog. Am J Vet Res. 1981;42:1002–6.
11. Upadhyayula PS, Yue JK, Hoshide R, Curtis E, Ciacci JD. Elective Anterior Cervical Discectomy and Fusion vs Cervical Artificial Disc Replacement: A Comparison of Perioperative Morbidity and Early Outcomes. Neurosurgery. 2016;63(Suppl 1):201–2.
12. Fauber AE, Wade JA, Lipka AE, McCabe GP, Aper RL. Effect of width of disk fenestration and a ventral slot on biomechanics of the canine C5-C6 vertebral motion unit. Am J Vet Res. 2006;67(11):1844–8.
13. Shores A, Cechner PE, Cantwell HD, Wheaton LG, Carlton WW. Structural changes in thoracolumbar disks following lateral fenestration a study of the radiographic, histologic, and histochemical changes in the chondrodystrophoid dog. Vet Surg. 1985;14(2):117–23.
14. Fingeroth JM. Fenestration. Pros and cons. Probl Vet Med. 1989;1(3):445–66.
15. Harari J, Marks SL. Surgical treatments for intervertebral disc disease. Vet Clin North Am Small Anim Pract. 1992;22(4):899–915.
16. Grunert P, Gebhard HH, Bowles RD, James AR, Potter HG, Macielak M, et al. Tissue-engineered intervertebral discs: MRI results and histology in the rodent spine. J Neurosurg Spine. 2014;20(4):443–51.
17. Yu LP, Qian WW, Yin GY, Ren YX, Hu ZY. MRI assessment of lumbar intervertebral disc degeneration with lumbar degenerative disease using the Pfirrmann grading systems. PLoS One. 2012;7(12):e48074.
18. Seiler G, Häni H, Scheidegger J, Busato A, Lang J. Staging of lumbar intervertebral disc degeneration in nonchondrodystrophic dogs using low-field magnetic resonance imaging. Vet Radiol Ultrasound. 2003;44(2):179–84.
19. Grunert P, Hudson KD, Macielak MR, Aronowitz E, Borde BH, Alimi M, et al. Assessment of intervertebral disc degeneration based on quantitative magnetic resonance imaging analysis: an in vivo study. Spine (Phila Pa 1976). 2014;39(6):E369–78.
20. Bergknut N, Smolders LA, Grinwis GC, Hagman R, Lagerstedt AS, Hazewinkel HA, et al. Intervertebral disc degeneration in the dog. Part 1: Anatomy and physiology of the intervertebral disc and characteristics of intervertebral disc degeneration. Vet J. 2013;195(3):282–91.
21. Smolders LA, Bergknut N, Grinwis GC, Hagman R, Lagerstedt AS, Hazewinkel HA, et al. Intervertebral disc degeneration in the dog. Part 2: chondrodystrophic and non-chondrodystrophic breeds. Vet J. 2013;195(3):292–9.
22. Lu DS, Shono Y, Oda I, Abumi K, Keneda K. Effects of chondroitinase ABC and chymopapain on spinal motion segment biomechanics. An in vivo biomechanical, radiologic, and histologic canine study. Spine. 1997;22:1828–34.
23. Itoh H, Hara Y, Yoshimi N, Harada Y, Nezu Y, Yogo T, et al. A retrospective study of intervertebral disc herniation in dogs in Japan: 297 cases. J Vet Med Sci. 2008;70(7):701–6.
24. Iatridis JC, MacLean JJ, O'Brien M, Stokes IA. Measurements of proteoglycan and water content distribution in human lumbar intervertebral discs. Spine (Phila Pa 1976). 2007;32(14):1493–7.
25. Iatridis JC, Weidenbaum M, Setton LA, Mow VC. Is the nucleus pulposus a solid or a fluid? Mechanical behaviors of the nucleus pulposus of the human intervertebral disc. Spine (Phila Pa 1976). 1996;21(10):1174–84.
26. Detiger SE, Holewijn RM, Hoogendoorn RJ, van Royen BJ, Helder MN, Berger FH, et al. MRI T2* mapping correlates with biochemistry and histology in intervertebral disc degeneration in a large animal model. Eur Spine J. 2015;24(9):1935–43.
27. Marinelli NL, Haughton VM, Muñoz A, Anderson PA. T2 relaxation times of intervertebral disc tissue correlated with water content and proteoglycan content. Spine (Phila Pa 1976). 2009;34(5):520–4.
28. Rutges JP, Duit RA, Kummer JA, Bekkers JE, Oner FC, Castelein RM, et al. A validated new histological classification for intervertebral disc degeneration. Osteoarthr Cartil. 2013;21(12):2039–47.
29. Costi JJ, Stokes IA, Gardner-Morse M. Direct measurement of intervertebral disc maximum shear strain in six degrees of freedom: motions that place disc tissue at risk of injury. J Biomech. 2007;40(11):2457–66.
30. O'Connell GD, Vresilovic EJ, Elliott DM. Human intervertebral disc internal strain in compression: the effect of disc region, loading position, and degeneration. J Orthop Res. 2011;29(4):547–55.
31. Iatridis JC, MaClean JJ, Ryan DA. Mechanical damage to the intervertebral disc annulus fibrosus subjected to tensile loading. J Biomech. 2005;38(3):557–65.
32. Roberts S, Urban JP, Evans H, Eisenstein SM. Transport properties of the human cartilage endplate in relation to its composition and calcification. Spine. 1996;21:415–20.
33. Roberts S, Menage J, Urban JP. Biochemical and structural properties of the cartilage end-plate and its relation to the intervertebral disc. Spine (Phila Pa 1976). 1989;14(2):166–74.
34. Lotz JC, Fields AJ, Liebenberg EC. The role of the vertebral end plate in low back pain. Global Spine J. 2013;3(3):153–64.
35. Albert HB, Kjaer P, Jensen TS, Sorensen JS, Bendix T, Manniche C. Modic changes, possible causes and relation to low back pain. Med Hypotheses. 2008;70(2):361–8.
36. Moore RJ. The vertebral end-plate: what do we know? Eur Spine J. 2000;9:92–6.
37. Nachemson A, Lewin T, Maroudas A, Freeman MA. In vitro diffusion of dye through the end-plates and the annulus fibrosus of human lumbar intervertebral discs. Acta Orthop Scand. 1970;41(6):589–607.
38. Cinotti G, Della Rocca C, Romeo S, Vittur F, Toffanin R, Trasimeni G. Degenerative changes of porcine intervertebral disc induced by vertebral endplate injuries. Spine (Phila Pa 1976). 2005;30(2):174–80.
39. Masuda K, Aota Y, Muehleman C, Imai Y, Okuma M, Thonar EJ, et al. A novel rabbit model of mild, reproducible disc degeneration by an anulus needle puncture: correlation between the degree of disc injury and radiological and histological appearances of disc degeneration. Spine (Phila Pa 1976). 2005;30(1):5–14.
40. Hampton D, Laros G, McCarron R, Franks D. Healing potential of the anulus fibrosus. Spine (Phila Pa 1976). 1989;14(4):398–401.
41. Fazzalari NL, Costi JJ, Hearn TC, Fraser RD, Vernon-Roberts B, Hutchinson J. Mechanical and pathologic consequences of induced concentric anular tears in an ovine model. Spine (Phila Pa 1976). 2001;26(23):2575–8.
42. Brisson BA, Holmberg DL, Parent J, Sears WC, Wick SE. Comparison of the effect of single-site and multiple-site disk fenestration on the rate of recurrence of thoracolumbar intervertebral disk herniation in dogs. J Am Vet Med Assoc. 2011;238(12):1593–600.
43. Freeman P, Jeffery ND. Re-opening the window on fenestration as a treatment for acute thoracolumbar intervertebral disc herniation in dogs. J Small Anim Pract. 2017;58(4):199–204.

6

The effect of strontium ranelate on the healing of a fractured ulna with bone gap in rabbit

Mohd Rafiq Mohd Ibrahim[1], Simmrat Singh[1], Azhar Mahmood Merican[1], Hanumantha Rao Balaji Raghavendran[1], Malliga Raman Murali[1], Sangeetha Vasudevaraj Naveen[1] and Tunku Kamarul[1,2*]

Abstract

Background: Fracture healing in bone gap is one of the major challenges encountered in Orthopedic Surgery. At present, the treatment includes bone graft, employing either internal or external fixation which has a significant impact on the patient, family and even society. New drugs are emerging in the markets such as anabolic bone-forming agents including teriparatide and strontium ranelate to stimulate bone growth. Based on the mechanism of their actions, we embarked on a study on the healing of a fractured ulna with bone gap in a rabbit model. We segregated ten rabbits into two groups: five rabbits in the test group and five rabbits in the control group. We created a 5 mm bone gap in the ulna bone, removing the periosteum as well. Rabbits in the test group received 450 mg/kg of strontium ranelate via oral administration, daily, for six weeks. The x-rays, CT scans and blood tests were performed every two weeks. At the end of six weeks, the rabbits were sacrificed, and the radius and ulna bones harvested for histopathological examination.

Results: Based on the x-rays and CT scans, fracture healing or bone formation was observed to be faster in the control group. From the x-ray findings, 80 % of the fracture united and by CT scan, 60 % of the fracture united in the control group at the end of the six-week study. None of the fractures united in the test group. However, the histopathology report showed that a callus of different stages was being formed in both groups, consisting of 80 % of bone. The serum levels of osteocalcin and alkaline phosphatase initially remained similar up to three weeks and changed slightly at the end of six weeks.

Conclusions: We conclude that the strontium effect begins slowly, and while it may not interfere with bone cell proliferation it may interfere in the mineralization and delay the acute stage of fracture healing. We recommend that a larger sample size and a longer duration of the study period be implemented to confirm our finding.

Keywords: Fracture, Strontium, Ulna, Osteocalcin, Alkaline phosphatase

Background

The treatment of delayed unions, nonunions, malunions and bone loss pose great challenges for orthopedic surgeons [1]. Fracture healing disorders negatively affect the patient's quality of life and result in high healthcare costs, as a second surgery is necessitated to stabilize the fracture and stimulate bone biology. In most cases, successful union will be achieved by restoration of the alignment and stable fixation of the fracture. However, many cases call for adjunctive measures such as bone-grafting or bone transports to stimulate bone-healing and fill bone defects. The gold standard for bone defect repairs is autograft but their usage is affected by morbidity at the donor site and limited supply [2]. Limitations of the allograft include the immunogenic response by the host to the graft and the potential for disease transmission. To overcome these limitations an increasing number of new orthobiologic materials are being developed to aid in the management of bony defects. In future, advanced biotechnologies that accelerate fracture healing may be useful tools, which might also prevent the onset of these disorders [3]. The several options available for bone

* Correspondence: tkzrea22@gmail.com
[1]Tissue Engineering Group (TEG), National Orthopaedic Centre of Excellence in Research and Learning (NOCERAL), Department of Orthopaedic Surgery, Faculty of Medicine, University of Malaya, Kuala Lumpur, Malaysia
[2]Clinical Investigative Centre, Faculty of Medicine, University Malaya Medical Center, Kuala Lumpur, Malaysia

replacement are autologous bone or allogeneic cancellous or cortical bone, demineralized bone matrix, calcium phosphate-based bone-graft substitute or autologous bone marrow. The biology of each of these grafts varies but they perform one or several essential functions such as osteoconduction, osteoinduction, osteogenesis and structural support [4, 5].

Besides bone graft and bone graft substitutes, orthopedic surgeons at present use anabolic agents such as teriparatide and strontium ranelate to promote fracture healing and increase bone quality. An anabolic agent is one that raises the bone strength by increasing the bone mass due to an overall increase in bone remodeling combined with a positive bone balance [6]. Several case reports on strontium promoting fracture healing have been reported in the literature. Strontium ranelate accelerates filling of the bone defect and improves the properties of bone healing in rats [7]. Strontium nucleus is almost similar in size to that of calcium, the body easily absorbs it, incorporating it into the bones and tooth enamel instead of calcium [8]. Strontium ranelate acts via a dual action mode with its bone-forming and bone-resorbing properties, resulting in improved bone microarchitecture [9]. This agent is approved for the prevention of vertebral and hip fracture in postmenopausal osteoporosis. Preclinical studies have demonstrated enhanced fracture healing and osseo-integration with strontium ranelate, coupled with the improvement in bone microarchitecture [9]. Studies have also showed contradicting results in which 3 weeks of treatment with strotium increased the thickness of the healing mid-femoral cortical bone defects in rats, but did not influence volume, mechanical properties, periosteal callus volume, either 3 or 8 weeks. Furthermore, strontium had no effect on the microstructure and mechanical properties of the vertebral bodies [10, 11].

The ulna is found to have similar function, in both humans and four-footed animals. If the ulna breaks, it will most commonly occur at either the point where the radius and ulna form a joint or where the ulna forms a joint with the hand's carpal bones. Ulnar fractures cause severe pain, difficulty in moving the affected joint and even lead to deformity of the arm if the fracture is compound. So far reported studies have focused on the development of biocomposite materials or scaffold on different type of bone fractures and as well as ulna bone, while the effect of strontium ranelate has not been tested on ulna bone. The maximum period for spontaneous healing of the bone fracture is around 6 weeks, so we anticipated the treatment with strontium ranelate would trigger faster healing in rabbits compared with control [12].

Methods

Design and methodology

In this study, New Zealand white male rabbits (*Oryctolagus cuniculus;* $n = 5$) were used. Prior to this study, approval was obtained from the animal ethics committee of the Animal House of the University Malaya Medical Centre (UMMC). All the rabbits were maintained in accordance with the Institutional Animal Care & Use Committee approved protocol.

The rabbits selected for the study were all males, between 28 and 32 weeks of age, and within the weight range of 2.0–2.5 kg at the time of the surgery. All of the rabbits had free access to pellet food and water *ad libitum* and were housed in the animal experimental block of the UMMC at a constant temperature of 26–28 °C and a humidity of 60 %. The rabbits were caged individually in stainless steel cages measuring 9 cubic meters, employing a fenestrated flooring to allow the feces or droppings to fall into a collection pan.

Sterilization

All the instruments and gauze employed in the surgical procedure were sterilized by autoclaving in the Aesculap 420 laboratory and Eschmann SES 225B autoclave. The instruments were first washed under running water with disinfectant soap and sterilized at a pressure of 220 kPa and a temperature of 134 °C for approximately 15 min. Then they were automatically dried by the autoclaving machine and left for one hour to cool down.

All the surgical procedures were performed in the Animal Theater in the Animal House. Marking the ears of all the rabbits was done with a number assigned to them using a permanent marker for identification. All the cages were also labeled according to their respective numbers. The animals were weighed prior to the surgical procedure, and the amount of anesthesia (Ketamine 20 mg/kg IM) was calculated including the sedative and muscle relaxant, Xylazine (3 mg/kg). Then the antibiotic (Kombitrim 240, 1 ml/10 kg IM) was injected intramuscularly. The left fore-leg of the rabbit was shaved. All the rabbits gained 0.1–0.3 kg on average throughout the experiment.

Surgical techniques

After anesthesia had been achieved and the limb shaved, the rabbit then was placed on the operating table in the supine position. The left fore-leg was then cleaned with povidone and properly draped with disposable sterile drapes. The surgery was then performed using the aseptic technique taking adequate precautions all the time.

The center of the ulna bone at the diaphysis was identified and marked on the skin surface. Local anesthesia was administered to the rabbit at the planned incision site. Next, 1.5 cm long longitudinal incisions were made. The intramuscular septum was identified and the midshaft of the ulna was exposed. Soft tissues were gently dissected to expose the bone. A longitudinal incision 4 cm in length was made on the anteromedial surface of the left ulna at the cutaneous border, 2 cm proximal and

2 cm distal to the center of the diaphysis which had been marked prior. The fascia was then cut and the extensor muscles were identified and retracted to expose the ulna bone. Care was taken to split the muscular layer by blunt dissection to expose the ulnar bone. The planned site for the osteotomy was marked on the bone, and measured with a small stainless steel ruler. The osteotomy was then performed using an oscillating saw, carefully avoiding damage to the periosteum. Washing was done with some normal saline during the osteotomy. A 5 mm defect was created in each ulna. All the rabbits tolerated the surgery well and resumed their normal activity within a few days. No wound infection was observed. All the rabbits were freely ambulating one day post-surgery.

No neurological insults such as paralysis, convulsion, respiratory distress or signs of pain were observed.

Strontium treatment

Each rabbit was supplemented (orally) with 5 ml of strontium ranelate solution (2 grams of strontium ranelate mixed in 10 ml of distilled water) in the treatment group using a feeding tube for six weeks.

Macroscopic evaluation

After necropsy, the radius and ulna were harvested and the soft tissue removed. The bone defect site was observed macroscopically and photographs were also recorded.

X-ray and CT scan

The bone defect healing of all the rabbits was evaluated using the X-ray (DRX-Evolution, 50kVp, 2mAs Carestream, Malaysia) and CT scan. Scanning was done at weeks 1, 3 and 6 for each rabbit. They were scanned weekly for six weeks to determine the progress of defect healing in each group. While under general anesthesia, the rabbits were positioned accurately on the CT scan machine (Siemens Somatom Definition AS 128, Germany) in the right lateral position with the left fore-leg elevated on a sample holder. The long axes of the radius and ulna were aligned orthogonally to the axis of the x-ray beam. All the radius and ulnar bones were scanned using 35.5 μm isotropic resolutions at 80 kVp energy and 60 μA intensity in 150 ms integration time. Images had 0.6 mm slice thickness and resolution of 2048 × 2048 pixels. Images obtained from the scan were saved in DICOM (Digital Imaging and Communication in Medicine) format. The assessment such as calcification, appearance of callus, continuity of bone trabeculae was done by a Senior Orthopedic Surgeon who was blinded using the same score.

Qualitative bone growth evaluation

The radiographs were evaluated objectively and subjectively in collaboration with a consultant orthopedic surgeon. They were evaluated for initial and bridging callus formation. The 3D reconstruction images were obtained for better viewing and bone regeneration evaluation. For this study, we defined union based on the radiographic evaluations. Union was considered to have been achieved in the rabbit ulnar model if visible bridging callus was observed across the fracture on the radiographs, which was grade 4 and above on the Cheung (2000) criteria. Bridging callus needed to be visible in three cortices on two views on the x-ray. We could not do a clinical assessment for the fracture union because the radius was intact and the rabbits were able to weight-bear immediately post -surgery. The pattern and behavior of the bone growth in each group was also evaluated and analyzed from the radiographs enlisting the help of a radiologist.

Biochemical test

Serum levels of osteocalcin, ALP, calcium and phosphate at weeks 1, 3 and 6 were obtained via the ear vein and centrifuged at 10,000 x g for 10 min. The plasma was then analyzed for osteocalcin, ALP, calcium and phosphate concentrations using the corresponding kit according to the Standard Operating Procedure in the Tissue Engineering Group Laboratory in the National Orthopedic Center for Excellence and Learning (NORCERAL), University of Malaya. The results were measured with the respective optical densities for each parameter on a microplate reader.

Histopathology

At the culmination of the study after necropsy, the radius and ulnar bones were harvested and the specimens prepared for histopathological slides. Samples for histological evaluation were stored in 10 % neutral buffered formalin for four days and then decalcified for five days in 10 % formic acid. The samples thus processed were embedded in paraffin, sectioned longitudinally and stained with hematoxylin-eosin (Sigma USA). The sections were examined under a light microscope with magnification. The histopathological sections were examined by a single pathologist who was also blinded regarding the content of the current study. The progression of the fracture callus in each specimen was quantified based on the relative percentages of the lamellar bone, woven bone, cartilage, fibrous tissues, endochondral ossification and intramembranous ossification. The qualitative bone growth data were collected using x-ray and CT scan. Statistical analysis was done using the Fisher Exact Test.

Results

Radiographic examination of the radius-ulna of the strontium treated rabbits was performed at the end of study. None of the samples showed radiological union at the end of the six-week study (Fig. 1). However, excessive callus formation was observed in between the radius and ulna rather than in the fracture gap. From the findings mentioned above it was evident that the strontium treatment did not significantly improve fracture healing in rabbit ulna with bone gap. The union and nonunion rates using x-ray in the test and control groups were assessed by Cheung's method (Fig. 2a & b) and the *p*-value was calculated as 0.44 using Fisher Exact Test. There is no association of healing of the ulnar fracture with strontium.

An obvious increase in the union rate was recorded using Cheung's scoring method. However, the control group showed a better union rate on scoring method. All the rabbits were reviewed and the CT scans were taken within the first week post-surgery. No evidence of any callus formation was observed and the 0.5 cm gap was clearly seen. At around three weeks, evidence of minimal callus formation was seen. The callus began to form from the edges of the osteotomized bones. More calluses were noted in between the radius and ulna rather than within the bone gap. At six weeks, only two samples showed radiological union.

The CT scans of the rabbit fore-arm at the end of study in Group A (with strontium) and Group B (without Strontium) at the end of study (without strontium) are shown in Fig. 3. Post-surgery all the rabbits in both groups were reviewed and the CT scans were done within the first week of surgery. No evidence of any callus formation was initially found. At three weeks post-surgery, patchy calcifications were noted around the center of the defect and bone edges. The patchy calcifications moved towards the center of the bone defect. The callus in the center of the defect enlarged gradually and expanded proximally and distally. At around four weeks post-surgery, the proximal callus, which grew faster, met and united with the center callus. Then, it

	Rabbit on Strontium	**Rabbit Without Strontium**
1st. Week	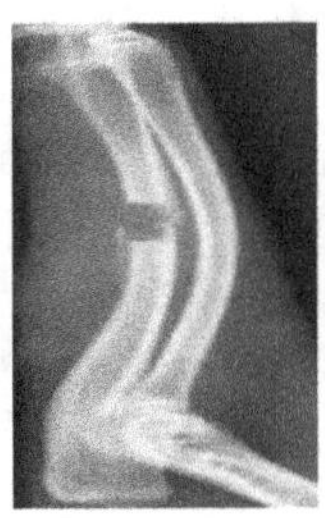	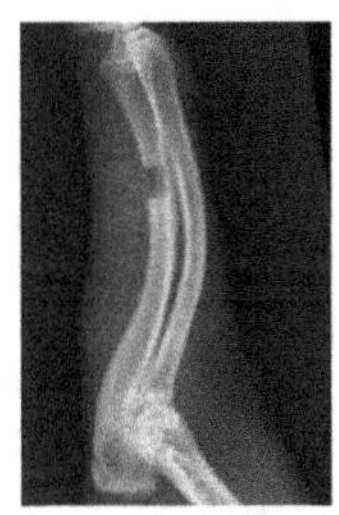
2nd. Week	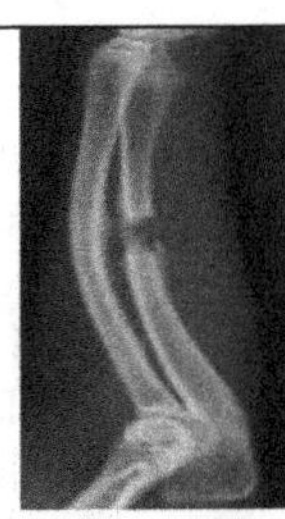	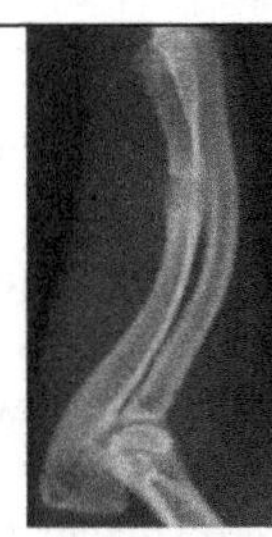
4th. Week	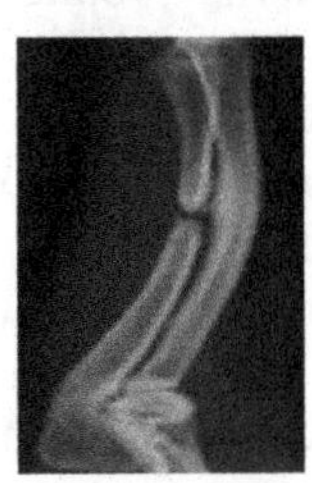	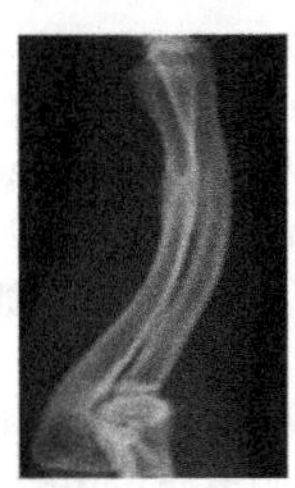

Fig. 1 Comparison of radius and ulna radiographs of rabbits with and without Strontium ranelate. The pattern of callus formation in the group treated with strontium or without strontium was observed using radiographs

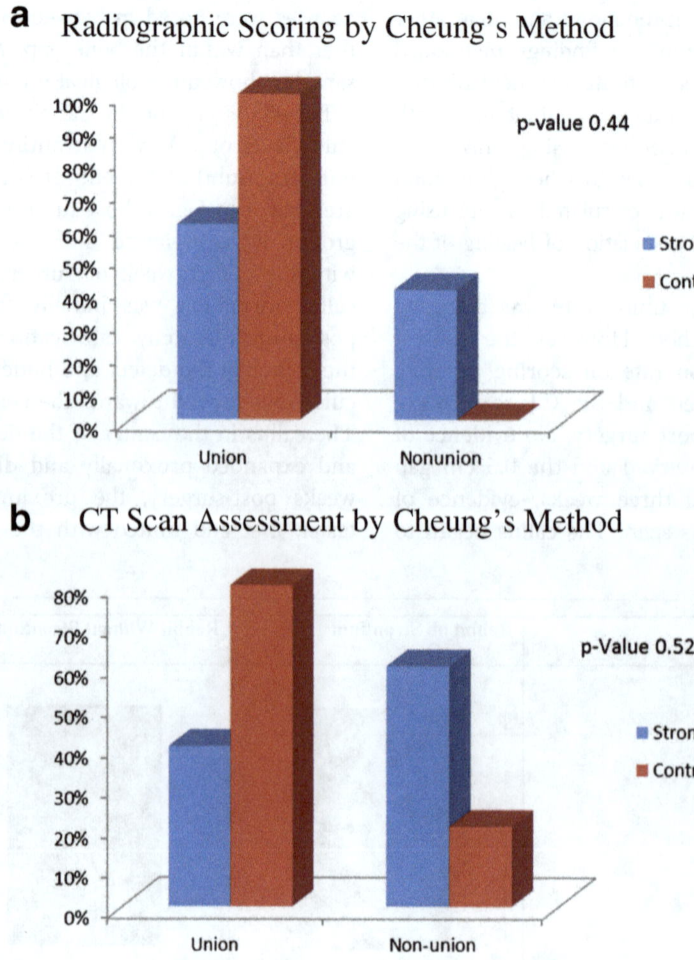

Fig. 2 a Radiographic scoring by Cheung's method and **b** CT Scan Assessment by Cheung's Method, Based on the radio graphical data X-Ray and CT scan the percentage of healing has been indicated

slowly grew distally and met the distal callus at around six weeks. At this point in time, no fracture gaps were observed. The bone growths were noted to fill up the whole osteotomy site. At six weeks, the fracture had united and there were continuity between the bone trabeculae but no remodeling noted. The diameter sizes of the newly formed bone were smaller than the actual defect. The p-value by Fisher Exact Test is 0.52. In the control group, the union rate is 100 % with x-ray and 80 % with the CT scan using Cheung's scoring methodology, which is almost two times higher than that of the test group. A comparison of the union rates from the x-rays and CT scans by Cheung's Method are shown in Fig. 4.

The biochemical markers including the levels of serum alkaline phosphatase, serum calcium, serum phosphate and serum osteocalcin were taken at weeks 1, 3 and 6 post surgery (Figs. 5a-d). The level serum markers were compared as the callus grew old. Serum levels of calcium and phosphate showed no change at weeks 1, 3 and 6. However, a significant statistical difference was observed in the serum levels of ALP and osteocalcin at week six, where the serum ALP was higher and osteocalcin was lower in the strontium treated group. Based on the histological examination, the grading and percentage of lamellar bone, woven bone, cartilage and fibrous tissue are shown in (Tables 1 & 2). The presence of lamellar bone in the specimen with radiological nonunion may have been contributed by the radius. However, no significant difference in the healing was observed between the strontium treated and untreated groups.

Discussion

Fracture healing in the presence of bone defect is a significant clinical issue. Non-union is a well-known complication of segmental loss in bone defect [10]. One of the main challenges in successful bone healing and new bone formation is the in-growth of soft tissue which may disturb the osteogenesis and cause non-union. Such defects greatly impact the patient's quality of life due to

	Rabbit on Strontium	Rabbit Without Strontium
1st. Week	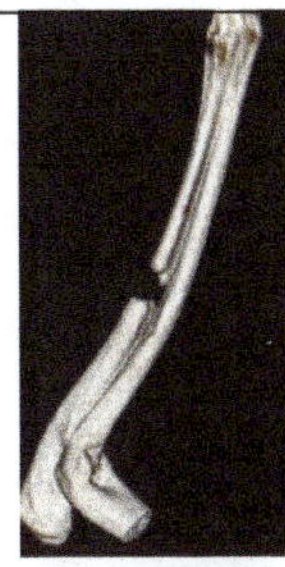	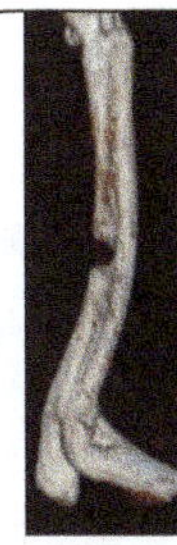
2nd. Week	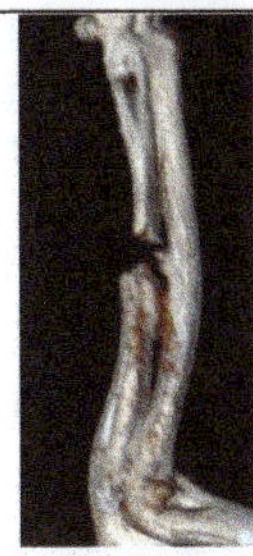	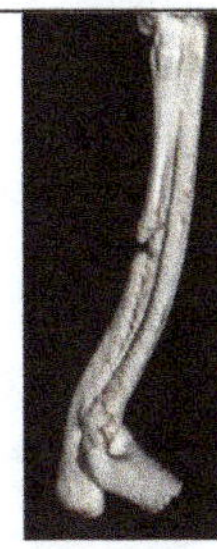
4th. Week	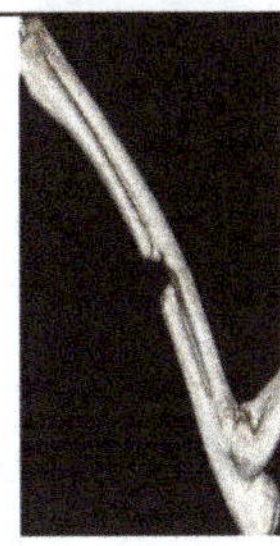	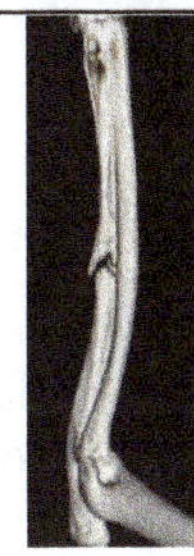

Fig. 3 Comparison of radius and ulna CT scans of rabbits with and without Strontium ranelate. The pattern of bone repair in the group treated with strontium or without strontium was observed using radiographs

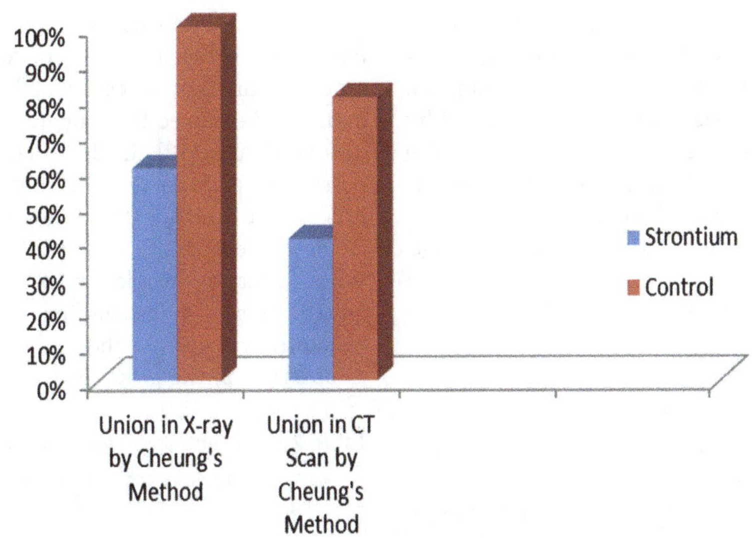

Fig. 4 Comparison showing X-ray and CT scan by Cheung's scoring system. The healing percentage has been indicated in scale based on the callus formation

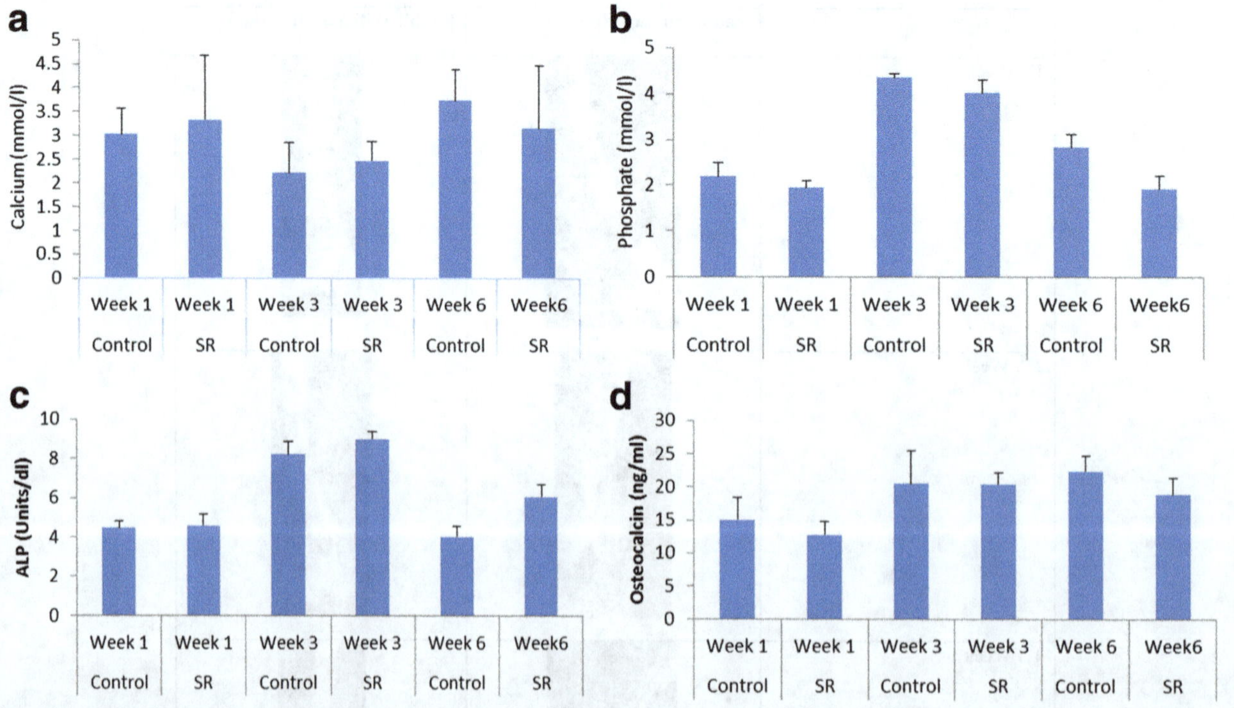

Fig. 5 a-d The levels of calcium, phosphate, ALP, and osteocalcin release in serum at variable time points. Serum separated from blood samples were examined using microtitre plate reader

limb length discrepancy and prolonged postoperative treatment. Furthermore, it will become an added financial load to the patient causing a socio-economic burden to the family as treatments for this condition are complicated. The current treatment option involves the use of the Ilizarov technique by distraction osteogenesis [11]. However, this treatment includes complications of its own; pin site infection, bulky implant, expensive cost, long hospital stay etc. Recently, anabolic bone-forming agents on fractures in animal models have been reported. The ulnar bone was selected in this study, as it is one of the common sites for fracture and segmental bone loss in humans, especially in trauma cases. Rabbit ulnar bone is easily accessible and the bone size is also appropriate to use. It is relatively easier to perform the surgical procedure in the ulnar bone as it is subcutaneous in location with less soft tissue coverage. Furthermore, it has a splinting effect from the radius and no implant is required.

Table 1 A six-point score to grade the radiographs

Grade	Radiographic description
Grade 1	Indicates no calcification at the fracture site.
Grade 2	Indicates patchy calcification
Grade 3	Indicates that the calcification takes on the appearance of the callus
Grade 4	Shows callus bridging across the fracture gap
Grade 5	Indicates continuity of bone trabeculae
Grade 6	Demonstrates remodeling to normal bone.

A 0.5 cm bone defect was created in this study as we desired to see the difference in the physiological repair process through the fracture gap between the group undergoing strontium ranelate treatment and the control group. The ulnar diameter on average was 6–8 mm, measured at the midshaft region. The 0.5 cm bone defects were made in the rabbits at the midshaft of the bone to assess the osteogenesis capacity of the rabbit ulna through the fracture gap. According to the earlier report, in the short experimental time, bone healing was partial and involved the immature bone and fibrous connective tissues [13]. Under such conditions, it became possible to evaluate the effect of an agent in the healing process and whether the healing would be satisfactory as far as tissue quantity and quality were concerned. The callus formation in relation to the repair period was required to assess the healing bone quantitatively and qualitatively; however, the treatment was not significant as observed in the group given strontium ranelate when

Table 2 Histopathological examination and statistical analysis

	Lamellar bone	Woven bone	Cartilage	Fibrous tissue
Control group	70 %	20 %	5 %	4 %
Test group	58 %	28 %	7 %	7 %
p-value	0.53	0.64	0.17	0.30

compared with the control group [14]. In fact, the best tissue quality should be achieved within the shortest time period, assuming that the bone will be remodelled during the animal's entire lifetime. In general, bone regeneration will be initiated from the periosteum (periosteal callus) and grow in a circumferential pattern from the outside into the centre of the defect. Bone regeneration without periosteum will occur from the primary response callus initially, later the medullary callus and follow a linear growth pattern of growth. The proximal bone edge callus will grow faster than the distal bone edge callus. In our study, the periosteum was removed in both the control group and test group which will exert a negative effect on bone healing. However, in the control group, the fracture unites even without the periosteum when compared with the test group, which received the bone stimulant, strontium ranelate. Therefore, we may conclude that strontium may not be effective if the periosteum is removed. Studies have previously demonstrated that periosteum is important for the acceleration of bone growth after stripping. The grown acceleration has been reported after transection of periosteal and resection [15–17]. Reports has also compared the different procedures head to head in the same mammalian model, transverse transection of the longitudinal periosteal fibers appears to be the most important aspect in accelerating growth [18–20].

From the X-ray findings, four of the five samples in the control group fulfilled the criteria for union using cheung's scoring method, all five samples from the control group and three samples from the strontium group showed bony union. At the end of the six-week study, four samples from the control group and two samples from the strontium group achieved radiological union from the CT scan findings using Cheung's method. The radiological findings revealed an association between the use of strontium ranelate and delayed unions or non-unions. Fibrous tissues (fibroblast) which grow faster than the bone (osteoblast) were observed to rapidly migrate and repopulate into the bone defect; however, no significant effect was observed after six weeks between the strontium ranelate treated group and the untreated group [21].

All the samples showed 80 % bone formation within the fracture gap created. The bones that formed were either lamellar bone or bone woven with the minimal fibrous tissue formation, between 5 and 10 %. We expected to see more fibrous tissues in the specimens from the radiological findings of the big bone gaps. Instead, we observed various stages of callus formation. The seven slides were prepared initially by cutting the radius and ulna longitudinally in the sagittal plane to facilitate the comparison of the callus and surrounding normal bones. When the results showed that 80 % of the bones in all the slides were in contrast to our imaging studies, we suspected a mixing of the callus with the surrounding normal bones. We removed the radius in the last three slides prepared, but we still observed the same results. These results demonstrated that the strontium ranelate treatment could interfere with the mineralization process, even though it did not inhibit callus formation. The results of the blood parameters showed no significant statistical difference in the serum levels of calcium and phosphate at weeks 1, 3 and 6. Statistical difference was noted in the serum alkaline phosphatase and osteocalcin at week six with the serum ALP being higher and serum osteocalcin dropping lower in the strontium treated group. This shows that strontium has slow action onset on the bone markers.

Reports have shown strontium ranelate has bone anabolic and anti-resorption effect which probably increase healing of bone defects [22–24]. In addition some reports have shown strontium ranelate seems to decrease bone resorption as well preserves or increases bone formation. Preclinical studies on fracture healing have shown that it has a positive effect on hard callus formation and bone strength [25, 26]. From our assessment using the radiographs and CT scans, strontium ranelate does not promote fracture healing within the first six weeks, especially a fracture with a bone gap, as none of the fractures were observed to unite in the treatment group. However, the HPE report revealed that the gap became filled with lamellar bone or woven bone of differing maturity. It may have initially delayed the fracture healing or impaired the mineralization process. However, changes in the serum levels of the bone markers such as osteocalcin and alkaline phosphatase showed that strontium has a slow onset of action on bone activity. We are, however, still unsure about the long-term effect of the strontium on fracture healing with bone gap. However, based on the x-ray and CT scan findings, strontium did not have a significant impact on fracture healing in the acute setting compared with the control group. One of the reasons why the callus was unable to bridge the gap could be the absence of the perisoteum. The surrounding soft tissue could have prolapsed and blocked the bone gap thus inhibiting the osteogenesis process. But, in specimens with the strontium supplement, the bone grew faster in any case. One of the possibilities is that the periosteum is essential for the strontium to act.

Conclusions

In conclusion, strontium ranelate is not found to promote bone healing and in fact may delay bone formation, especially during the early stages of fracture healing with bone gap, in rabbit. Further studies are warranted using bigger animal models to confirm the role of strontium ranelate.

Acknowledgment

The authors gratefully acknowledge the financial support received from the University of Malaya under the HIR-MoE Grant (Reference number – UM.C/625/1/HIR/MOHE/MED/32 Account number – H20001-E000071).

Authors' contributions

MRMI, SS, AM did animal work, MRM, SVN guided biochemical protocol, HBR, TK performed data analysis and drafted the article. All authors read and approved the final manuscript.

Competing interest

The authors declare that they have no competing interests.

Consent for publication

Not applicable.

References

1. Gómez-Barrena E, Rosset P, Lozano D, Stanovici J, Ermthaller C, Gerbhard F. Bone fracture healing: cell therapy in delayed unions and non-unions. Bone. 2015;70:93–101.
2. Amini AR, Laurencin CT, Nukavarapu SP. Bone tissue engineering: recent advances and challenges. Crit Rev Biomed Eng. 2012;40(5):363–408.
3. Giannotti S, Trombi L, Bottai V, Ghilardi M, D'Alessandro D, Danti S, et al. Use of autologous human mesenchymal stromal cell/fibrin clot constructs in upper limb non-unions: long-term assessment. PLoS One. 2013;8:1–9.
4. Nandi SK, Roy S, Mukherjee P, Kundu B, De DK, Basu D. Orthopaedic applications of bone graft & graft substitutes: a review. Indian J Med Res. 2010;132:15–30.
5. Puvaneswary S, Talebian S, Raghavendran HB, Murali MR, Mehrali M. Fabrication and in vitro biological activity of βTCP-Chitosan-Fucoidan composite for bone tissue engineering. Carbohyd Polym. 2015;134:799–807.
6. Brandi ML. Drugs for bone healing. Expert Opin Investig Drugs. 2012;21(8): 1169–76.
7. Zacchetti G, et al. Systemic Treatment with Strontium Ranelate Accelerates the Filling of a Bone Defect and Improves the Material Level Properties of the Healing Bone. BioMed Res Int. 2014;10:1–10.
8. Marie PJ. Effective doses for strontium ranelate. Osteoporos Int. 2008;19: 1813.
9. Fonseca JE, Brandi ML. Mechanism of action of strontium ranelate: What are the facts? Clin Cases Miner Bone Metab. 2010;7(1):17–8.
10. Fayaz HC, Giannoudis PV, Vrahas MS, Smith RM, Moran C, Pape HC, et al. The role of stem cells in fracture healing and nonunion. Int Orthop. 2011;35(11):1587–97.
11. Rahal SC, Volpi RS, Ciani RB, Vulcano LC. Use of the Ilizarov method of distraction osteogenesis for the treatment of radial hemimelia in a dog. J Am Vet Med Assoc. 2005;226(1):65–8. 52.
12. Terjesen T. Healing of rabbit tibial fractures using external fixation. Effects of removal of the fixation device. Acta Orthop Scand. 1984;55(2):192–6.
13. Passeri G, Cacchioli A, Ravanetti F, Galli C, Elezi E, Macaluso GM. Adhesion pattern and growth of primary human osteoblastic cells on five commercially available titanium surfaces. Clin Oral Implants Res. 2010;21(7):756–65.
14. Tarantino U, Celi M, Saturnino L, Scialdoni A, Cerocchi I. Strontium ranelate and bone healing: report of two cases. Clin Cases Miner Bone Metab. 2010;7 (1):65–8. doi:10.1186/s12917-016-0724-6.
15. Lorenzoni M, Pertl C, Polansky R, Wegscheider W. Guided bone regeneration with barrier membranes—a clinical and radiographic follow-up study after 24 months. Clin Oral Implants Res. 1999;10:16–23.
16. Bertone AL, Turner AS, Park RD. Periosteal transection and stripping for treatment of angular limb deformities in foals: clinical observations. J Am Vet Med Assoc. 1985;187:145–52.
17. Garces GL, Hernandez Hermoso JA. Bone growth after periosteal stripping in rats. Int Orthop. 1991;15:49–57.
18. Hernandez JA, Serrano S, Marinoso ML, Aubia J, Lloreta J, Marrugat J, Diez A. Bone growth and modeling changes induced by periosteal stripping in the rat. Clin Orthop Relat Res. 1995;320:211–9.
19. Dimitriou CG, Kapetanos GA, Symeonides PP. The effect of partial periosteal division on growth of the long bones. An experimental study in rabbits. Clin Orthop Relat Res. 1988;236:265–9.
20. Lynch MC, Taylor JF. Periosteal division and longitudinal growth in the tibia of the rat. J Bone Joint Surg (Br). 1987;69:812–6.
21. Read EK, Read MR, Townsend HG, Clark CR, Pharr JW, Wilson DG. Effect of hemi-circumferential periosteal transection and elevation in foals with experimentally induced angular limb deformities. J Am Vet Med Assoc. 2002;221:536–40.
22. Marie PJ. Strontium ranelate: a physiological approach for optimizing bone formation and resorption. Bone. 2006;38:S10–4.
23. Bonnelye E, Chabadel A, Saltel F, Jurdic P. Dual effect of strontium ranelate: stimulation of osteoblast differentiation and inhibition of osteoclast formation and resorption in vitro. Bone. 2008;42:129–38.
24. Stepan JJ. Strontium ranelate: in search for the mechanism of action. J Bone Miner Metab. 2013;31:606–12.
25. Vegger JB, Nielsen ES, Brüel A, Thomsen JS. Additive effect of PTH (1-34) and zoledronate in the prevention of disuse osteopenia in rats. Bone. 2014;66:287–95.
26. Brüel A, Olsen J, Birkedal H, et al. Strontium is incorporated into the fracture callus but does not influence the mechanical strength of healing rat fractures. Calcif Tissue Int. 2010;88:142–52.

7

Clinical monitoring of cardiac output assessed by transoesophageal echocardiography in anaesthetised dogs: a comparison with the thermodilution technique

Matheus M. Mantovani[1*], Denise T. Fantoni[2,4*], André M. Gimenes[1], Jacqueline R. de Castro[1], Patrícia B. Flor[2], Keila K. Ida[3] and Denise S. Schwartz[1]

Abstract

Background: Cardiac output (CO) is an important haemodynamic parameter to monitor in patients during surgery. However, the majority of the techniques for measuring CO have a limited application in veterinary practice due to their invasive approach and associated complexity and risks. Transoesophageal echocardiography (TEE) is a technique used to monitor cardiac function in human patients during surgical procedures and allows CO to be measured non-invasively. This prospective clinical study aimed to compare the transoesophageal echocardiography using a transgastric view of the left ventricular outflow tract (LVOT) and the thermodilution (TD) technique for the assessment of CO during mean arterial pressure of 65–80 mmHg (normotension) and <65 mmHg (hypotension) in dogs undergoing elective surgery. Eight dogs were pre-medicated with acepromazine (0.05 mg/kg, IM), tramadol (4 mg/kg, IM) and atropine (0.03 mg/kg, IM), followed by anaesthetic induction with propofol (3–5 mg/kg IV) and maintenance with isoflurane associated with a continuous infusion rate of fentanyl (bolus of 3 μg/kg followed by 0.3 μg/kg/min). The CO was measured by TEE (CO_{TEE}) and TD (CO_{TD}) at the end of expiration during normotension and hypotension (induced by isoflurane).

Results: There was a strong positive correlation between CO_{TEE} and CO_{TD} ($r = 0.925$; $P < 0.0001$). The bias between CO_{TD} and CO_{TEE} was 0.14 ± 0.29 L/min (limits of agreement, −0.44 to 0.72 L/min). The percentage error of CO measured by the two methods was 12.32%. In addition, a strong positive correlation was found between CO_{TEE} and CO_{TD} during normotension ($r = 0.995$; $P < 0.0001$) and hypotension ($r = 0.78$; $P = 0.0223$).

Conclusions: The results of this study indicated that the transgastric view of the LVOT by TEE was a minimally invasive alternative to clinically monitoring CO in dogs during anaesthesia. However, during hypotension, the CO obtained by TEE was less reliable, although still acceptable.

Keywords: Swan Ganz, Transgastric, Doppler, Aortic flow, Minimally invasive

* Correspondence: matheus2mvet@gmail.com; dfantoni@usp.br
[1]Departamento de Clínica Médica, Faculdade de Medicina Veterinária e Zootecnia, Universidade de São Paulo, São Paulo, Brazil
[2]Departamento de Cirurgia, Faculdade de Medicina Veterinária e Zootecnia, Universidade de São Paulo, São Paulo, Brazil
Full list of author information is available at the end of the article

Background

Cardiac output (CO) is an important haemodynamic parameter to monitor in patients during surgery. However, the majority of the techniques for measuring CO have a limited application in veterinary practice due to their invasive approach and associated complexity and risks [1].

The thermodilution technique (TD) is the gold standard for monitoring CO in veterinary medicine [2, 3]. It requires the insertion of a catheter into the pulmonary artery through the jugular vein, and the application of a cold solution to calculate the CO by temperature differences between the blood within the right atrium and the pulmonary artery [4]. Therefore, the TD technique is an invasive and sometimes limited method considering the risks associated with the development of arrhythmias, infection, thrombosis, and rupture of the pulmonary artery [5, 6].

Transoesophageal echocardiography (TEE) is a technique used to monitor cardiac function in human patients during surgical procedures [7, 8]. The Doppler technique allows CO to be measured non-invasively by multiplying the velocity-time integral (VTI) of blood flow through the transversal area of the vessel (CSA) with heart rate (HR) (CO = CSA x VTI × HR) [9].

A transgastric approach on TEE proposed for visualisation of the left ventricular outflow tract (LVOT), which has been allowed to quantify the aortic flow and, therefore, to calculate CO in human patients during surgery, has shown a good correlation with TD [7, 8, 10]. Although TEE is used for interventional procedures in veterinary patients [11, 12], no studies have described the transgastric approach of LVOT, the CO measured through this view, or the accuracy of the technique.

Therefore, the aim of this study was to compare the TEE transgastric view of the LVOT and the TD for measuring CO in anaesthetised dogs during surgery. The hypothesis is that CO can be accurately and non-invasively monitored using the TEE technique during clinical anaesthesia in dogs.

Methods

Animals

The study was authorized by written consent of the owners and the protocol (1936/2012) was approved by the university's ethical committee in the use of animals (CEUA). Eight dogs ASA 1 or 2, weighing 24.5 ± 2.1 kg, and undergoing surgery in the Veterinary Hospital of our institution were included in the study. The sample size for paired data was calculated using power analysis, indicating that a minimum of 8 dogs per group was required to have a 80% chance (with 5% risk) of detecting a difference of 0.78 L/min in the CO between groups and considering a standard deviation of 0.8 L/min.

Anaesthesia and monitoring

Food was withheld for 12 h and water for 4 h before anaesthesia. All animals were pre-medicated with acepromazine (0.05 mg/kg, IM; acepromazina, Syntec, Brazil), tramadol (4 mg/kg, IM; Tramadon, Cristália, São Paulo, Brazil), and atropine (0.03 mg/kg, IM; Plasmodex, Isofarma, Brazil). After 15 min, the cephalic vein was catheterised, and anaesthesia was induced with propofol to effect (3–5 mg/kg; Propovan, Cristália), administered through the catheter. After orotracheal intubation, anaesthesia was maintained with an initial end-tidal isoflurane concentration (ET_{ISO}) of 1.3% in 70% oxygen associated with fentanyl (bolus of 3 μg/kg followed by a constant rate infusion of 0.3 μg/kg/min; Fentanest, Cristália).

Neuromuscular blockade was instituted by rocuronium (0.6 mg/kg, IV; Esmeron, Organon, São Paulo, Brazil), and the mechanical ventilation (rebreathing circuit with a microprocessor-controlled anaesthesia ventilator; Shogun, Takaoka, São Paulo, Brazil) was then started using the pressure-controlled ventilation mode, with a peak inspiratory pressure of 10 cmH_2O, inspiratory-to-expiratory time ratio of 1:2, and a respiratory rate (RR) adjusted to maintain an end-tidal carbon dioxide concentration ($ETCO_2$) of 35–45 mmHg.

A 7F pulmonary artery catheter (Swan Ganz; Edwards Lifesciences, Irvine, CA, USA) was aseptically and percutaneously introduced into the right jugular vein using the Seldinger technique in dogs in dorsal recumbency. The distal sensor of the catheter was located in the pulmonary artery, which was confirmed by waveform analysis (DX2020; Dixtal, Brazil) and by transoesophageal echocardiographic imaging. Pressure transducers were connected to a multi-parametric data collection system for continuous monitoring of the pressures and waveforms (DX2020; Dixtal).

Heart rate (HR), RR and pulse oximetry (SpO_2) were monitored using a multiparametric monitor (DX2020; Dixtal). The end-tidal isoflurane concentration (ET_{ISO}) and $ETCO_2$ were assessed by using a gas analyser (PoetIQ2-8500Q; Criticare Systems, WI, USA). The invasive systolic, mean and diastolic pressures (SAP, MAP and DAP, respectively) were monitored by catheterisation of the dorsal podal artery. All cardiopulmonary data were monitored continuously and registered at the same time-points as the CO measurement. A continuous infusion of lactated Ringer's solution was delivered throughout (5 mL/kg/h).

Cardiac output measuring

The cardiac output assessed through the thermodilution technique (CO_{TD}) was measured at the end of expiration by administering 3 mL of 5% glucose at 5°C into the right atrium through the pulmonary artery catheter. The temperature change was detected by the thermosensitive

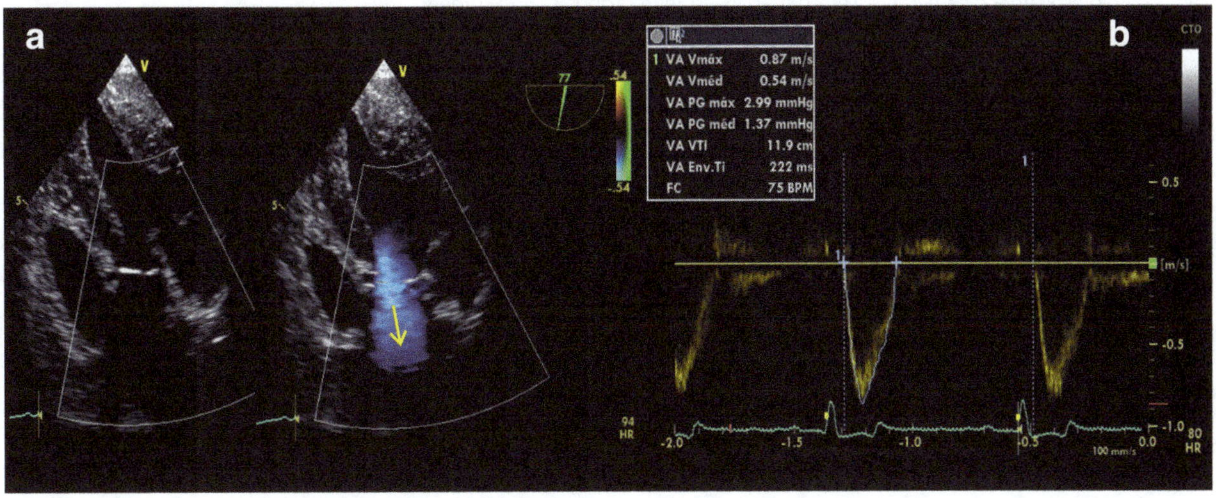

Fig. 1 Transgastric view of the left ventricular outflow tract assessed by transoesophageal echocardiography. **a** The almost parallel alignment between the volume sampled by the pulsate Doppler and the aortic blood flow (arrow) was obtained through this view. **b** The velocity-time integral (VTI) of aortic flow was calculated by the outline of the aortic blood flow

tip of the catheter located into the pulmonary artery, and the CO value was automatically calculated by the multiparametric monitor (DX 2020; Dixtal). The mean value of three measurements within ±10% was registered as CO_{TD}.

The cardiac output assessed through transoesophageal echocardiography (CO_{TEE}) was determined by using a multiplanar 2–5 MHz transoesophageal ultrasound transducer introduced into the mouth and passed into the oesophagus until visualisation of the aortic valve through the transverse caudal view. At this window, the planimetry of the aortic valve was performed to measure the transverse area of the aorta, as previously described by Boon [9]. Then, the transducer was inserted into the gastric cavity for visualisation of the short axis of the left ventricle at the level of the papillary muscles through the transverse transgastric view by ventroflexion movements of the transducer. At this level, the LVOT and the ascending portion of the aorta could be visualised by rotation of the ultrasonographic beam to approximately 90°-120° (Fig. 1a), allowing for a better alignment between the volume sampled by the pulsate Doppler and the aortic blood flow. The transgastric view of the LVOT could be improved by slight adjustments in the position of the transducer, which included the rotation or ventroflexion movements. From the transgastric view of the LVOT, the aortic blood flow was obtained via pulsate Doppler with the volume sampled immediately below the aortic valve. The velocity-time integral of aortic flow (VTI_{aortic}) was calculated by the outline of the aortic blood flow (Fig. 1b). The CO_{TEE} corresponded to the mean of three consecutive values calculated by the formula $CO_{TEE} = CSA \times VTI_{aortic} \times HR$ at three consecutive cardiac cycles, respectively.

The CO_{TD} and CO_{TEE} were always measured at the same time at expiration, and the values of CO_{TD} were not revealed to the echocardiographic examiner. Both techniques were applied after 20 min of anaesthetic stabilisation at a MAP of 65–80 mmHg (normotension) and then at an MAP <65 mmHg (hypotension) induced

Table 1 Breed, genre, bodyweight, surgery and ASA classification of the anaesthetic risk of 8 dogs undergoing cardiac output monitoring assessed by the transesophageal echocardiography and thermodilution techniques

Animal	Breed	Gender	Bodyweight (kg)	Surgery	ASA
1	Mixed-breed	F	17.2	Orthopaedic procedure	2
2	Mixed-breed	F	16.8	Laparotomy	2
3	Mixed-breed	M	24.3	Orthopaedic procedure	2
4	Boxer	M	29.5	Laparotomy	2
5	Pit bull	F	23	Orthopaedic procedure	2
6	Mixed-breed	F	26	Orthopaedic procedure	2
7	Mixed-breed	F	22.6	Laparotomy	2
8	Beagle	M	18.4	Ophthalmic procedure	1

ASA: *American Society of Anaeshesiologists* classification of physical status

Table 2 Cardiorespiratory parameters assessed in 8 anaesthetised dogs during surgery

Parameters	Normotension (MAP 65–80 mmHg)	Hypotension (MAP <65 mmHg)	*P*-value
HR (bpm)	97 (88–112)	96 (93–113)	0.9373
RR (mpm)	12 (10–14)	11 (10–15)	0.9572
SAP (mmHg)	105 ± 15	78 ± 12	0.0012
MAP (mmHg)	73 ± 5	56 ± 4	0.0027
DAP (mmHg)	60 ± 6	46 ± 3	0.0079
$ETCO_2$ (mmHg)	40 (37–43)	39 (36–42)	0.6913
ET_{ISO} (mmHg)	1.4 (1.00–1.82)	2.0 (1.57–2.47)	0.0340
SpO_2 (%)	98 (97–99)	97 (96–99)	0.9685

HR: heart rate; bpm: beats per minute; RR: respiratory rate; mpm: movements per minute; SAP: systolic arterial pressure; MAP: mean arterial pressure; DAP: diastolic arterial pressure; $ETCO_2$: end-tidal carbon dioxide concentration; ET_{ISO}: end-tidal isoflurane concentration; SpO_2: pulse oxymetry. Mean ± SD; paired Student t-test ($P < 0.05$). Median (interquartile interval); Wilcoxon test ($P < 0.05$)

by increasing the ET_{ISO} [18]. Arterial hypotension was treated immediately after measuring CO by reducing ET_{ISO} to baseline values. If necessary, hypotension was treated by further decreasing ET_{ISO} and by administering a bolus of crystalloids or colloids, and a bolus of 0.1 mg/kg of ephedrine until normalisation of MAP; these treatments, if any, were registered accordingly.

Statistical analysis

The distribution of all variables was analysed for normality using the Shapiro-Wilk test. The variables with a normal distribution were analysed using the paired Student t-test. The variables with a non-parametric distribution were analysed using the Wilcoxon matched-pairs signed rank test.

The Pearson coefficient, the intraclass correlation coefficient (ICC), and a model of linear regression (CO_{TEE} as the dependent variable and CO_{TD} as the independent variable) were calculated to assess the association between CO_{TEE} and CO_{TD}.

The agreement between CO_{TD} and CO_{TEE} was assessed by the Bland-Altman test [16]. The bias between the techniques was calculated as the mean of the differences between the CO measured by each technique. The limits of 95% agreement were calculated as the bias ± (2 × standard deviation). The ratio of the agreement limits for the CO value (percentage of the error; expressed as %) was calculated as 100 × (± 2 × standard deviation) ÷ CO (resulting from the overall mean of the two methods). A *P* -value <0.05 was considered statistically significant for all analysis.

Repeatability CO_{TEE} measurements was assessed using five animals. Each echocardiogram was evaluated three times in a given day by the same observer (intraobserver analysis) and by another independent observer (interobserver analysis). The VTI_{aortic} and CSA were measured three times in consecutive cardiac cycles in the same frame. The resulting mean values and standard deviations were used to determine the coefficients of variation. The echocardiogram analyses were performed offline.

Results

Animals included in the study are shown in Table 1. The haemodynamic and respiratory variables, and the CO of each animal included in the study are presented in Tables 2 and 3, respectively. The CO, SAP, MAP, and DAP had a normal distribution and were analysed using paired t-Student test. The HR, RR, $ETCO_2$, ET_{ISO}, and SpO_2 had a non-parametric distribution and were analysed using the Wilcoxon test.

The ET_{ISO} was 1.4% (1.00–1.82%) during normotension and 2.0% (1.57–2.47%) during hypotension (Table 2). No other treatments but decreasing ET_{ISO} was necessary to normalise MAP after isoflurane-induced hypotension.

A strong positive correlation was found between CO_{TEE} and CO_{TD} (r = 0.925; P < 0.0001). The ICC between CO_{TEE} and CO_{TD} was 0.920 (P < 0.0001) for isolate measurements and 0.958 (P < 0.0001) for the mean

Table 3 Cardiac output (L/min) of 8 dogs assessed by thermodilution technique (TD) and by transesophageal echocardiography (TEE) during a mean arterial pressure of 65–80 mmHg (normotension) and <65 mmHg (hypotension)

	Normotension		Hypotension	
Dog	TD	TEE	TD	TEE
1	2.35	2.26	1.69	1.9
2	4.79	4.78	1.76	2.12
3	3.24	3.24	2.64	3.27
4	2.85	2.79	1.88	2.45
5	2.77	2.77	3.05	2.63
6	3.17	3.14	1.96	2.66
7	2.88	2.95	3.01	3.23
8	2.89	3.02	1.82	1.77
Mean ± SD	3.11 ± 0.72	3.11 ± 0.73	2.22 ± 0.57	2.50 ± 0.56

of measurements. The linear regression analysis between CO_{TEE} and CO_{TD} was $r^2 = 0.855$ ($P < 0.0001$) and resulted in the following equation: $CO_{TEE} = 0.581 + 0.835 \times CO_{TD}$ (Fig. 2).

The agreement between CO_{TEE} and CO_{TD} showed a bias of 0.14 ± 0.29 L/min with a limit of agreement from −0.44 to 0.72 L/min (Fig. 3). A 12.32% error was found for the CO measured by both techniques.

There were no significant differences between CO_{TEE} and CO_{TD} during normotension ($P = 0.9612$) and hypotension ($P = 0.0761$) (Table 3; Fig. 4). A strong positive correlation was found between CO_{TEE} and CO_{TD} during normotension ($r = 0.995$; $P < 0.0001$) and hypotension ($r = 0.78$; $P = 0.0223$). The ICC between CO_{TEE} and CO_{TD} during normal arterial pressure was 0.995 ($P < 0.0001$) for isolate measurements and 0.998 ($P < 0.0001$) for the mean of the measurements. During arterial hypotension, the ICC between CO_{TEE} and CO_{TD} was 0.780 ($P < 0.007$) for isolate measurements and 0.876 ($P < 0.007$) for the mean of the measurements.

The linear regression analysis between CO_{TEE} and CO_{TD} resulted in a $r^2 = 0.991$ ($P < 0.0001$) and an equation of $CO_{TEE} = 0.044 + 0.985 \times CO_{TD}$ during normal blood pressure, and a $r^2 = 0.609$ ($P = 0.022$) and $CO_{TEE} = 0.221 + 0.801 \times CO_{TD}$ during hypotension.

The measurements bias for the condition of normotension and hypotension was 0.001 ± 0.07 L/min (limit of agreement: −0.13 to 0.14 L/min) and 0.27 ± 0.37 L/min (limit of agreement −0.46 to 1.01 L/min), respectively. A 2.55% error was found for the CO measured by both methods during normal arterial pressure and 15.26% during hypotension.

The coefficient of variation for the intraobserver and interobserver analysis for the CO_{TEE} measurements ranged from 0.47% to 7.77% and from 0.63% to 8.66%, respectively.

All dogs had ventricular arrhythmia during insertion of the pulmonary artery catheter that resolved spontaneously. With regard to the TEE, no complications were recorded.

Discussion

The study showed that the TEE transgastric approach of the LVOT has a clinically acceptable correlation and agreement with the gold standard thermodilution technique, and that it can be used for measuring CO in dogs during surgery.

Invasive CO monitoring during surgery is infrequently performed in dogs using the pulmonary artery catheter [3] due to many factors, including associated complications such as arrhythmias, thromboembolism or pulmonary artery rupture [5], the availability of equipment and costs. The high incidence of cardiac arrhythmia observed in the present study indicates that the risk-benefit ratio of the

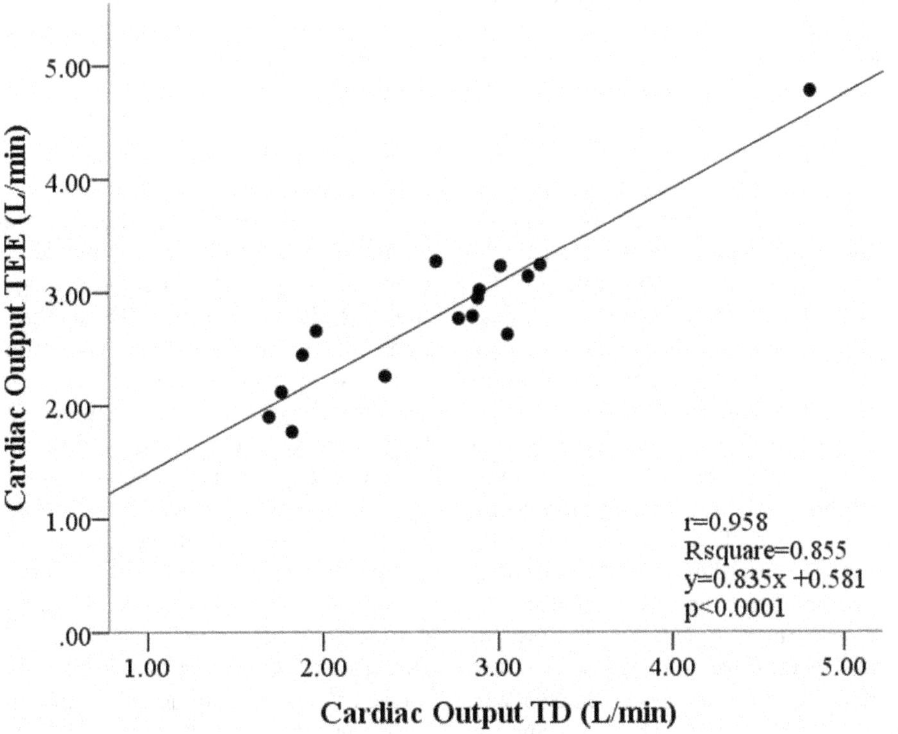

Fig. 2 Graphical dispersion of cardiac output (CO) values obtained by transoesophageal echocardiography (TEE) and the thermodilution technique (TD) in anaesthetised dogs undergoing surgery

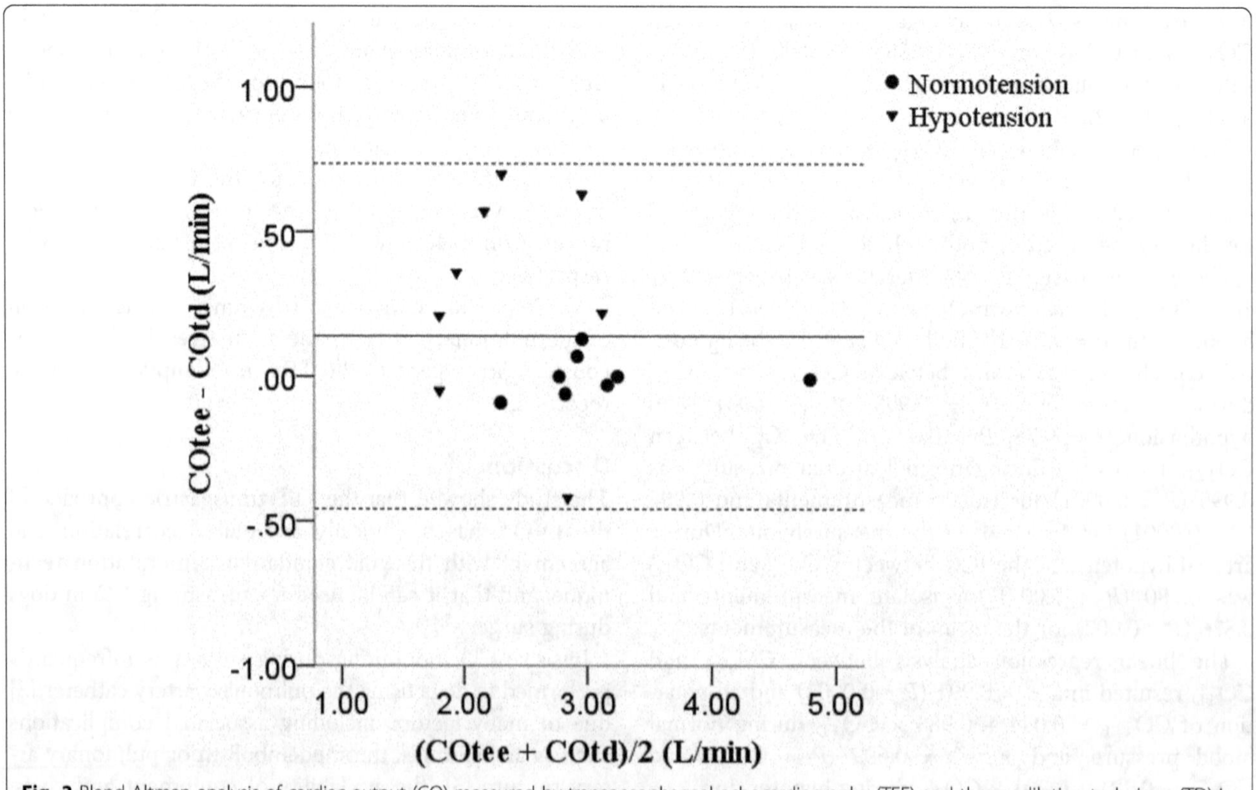

Fig. 3 Bland-Altman analysis of cardiac output (CO) measured by transoesophageal echocardiography (TEE) and thermodilution technique (TD) in eight dogs with a mean arterial pressure of 65–80 mmHg (normotension) and <65 mmHg (hypotension) arterial pressure. All comparisons were within the thresholds of agreement (dotted line)

right cardiac catheterisation should be considered according to the haemodynamic status of the patient. In contrast, the TEE was shown to be a less invasive technique with no cardiopulmonary complications and with an availability similar to that described in human patients for CO monitoring during surgery [7, 8].

Previous studies in veterinary patients have described the technique and the views obtained by the TEE [12, 13]. However, to the knowledge of the authors, this is the first clinical study to describe the application of the transgastric view of the LVOT for assessing CO in dogs during surgery. This echocardiographic window was obtained in all dogs of the study with an availability similar to that described for human patients [7, 8, 10].

The accuracy of the transthoracic echocardiography for measuring CO was demonstrated by other authors [14, 15], but the technique is often inappropriate for monitoring CO during surgery. TEE uses the same methodology as transthoracic echocardiography for calculating CO. Through this methodology, the CO is calculated by multiplying the SV with the HR [14]. To measure the stroke volume of the left ventricle, the cross-section area of the aorta is multiplied by the velocity-time integral aortic flow obtained by spectral Doppler [15]. By using the transgastric view of the LVOT, it was possible to obtain a parallel alignment between the volume sampled by the pulsate Doppler and the aortic blood flow and, therefore, to decrease bias when measuring the stroke volume [8].

A strong correlation was found between the techniques TEE and TD to obtain the CO, similar to that described in human patients [7, 8]. According to Bland & Altman [16], the correlation coefficient and regression analysis are not adequate statistical analyses for comparing two methods of measurement. The data analysis through the Bland-Altman technique is considered more adequate for assessing the agreement between the techniques, because it excludes the errors obtained from the use of the correlation coefficient, as it assesses the association of the measurements rather than the agreement between them. The agreement between techniques is considered satisfactory according to the Bland-Altman method, when the percentage error has a value lower than 30% [17]. In the present study, the error percentage between TEE and TD was 2.55% during normotension and 15.26% during hypotension, and there were no significant differences between CO calculated by TEE and TD in both arterial pressure conditions.

Coefficients of variation for intra- and interobserver measurement variability to the COTEE were lower than 10%, similar to that reported by other studies using transthoracic echocardiography [15, 17].

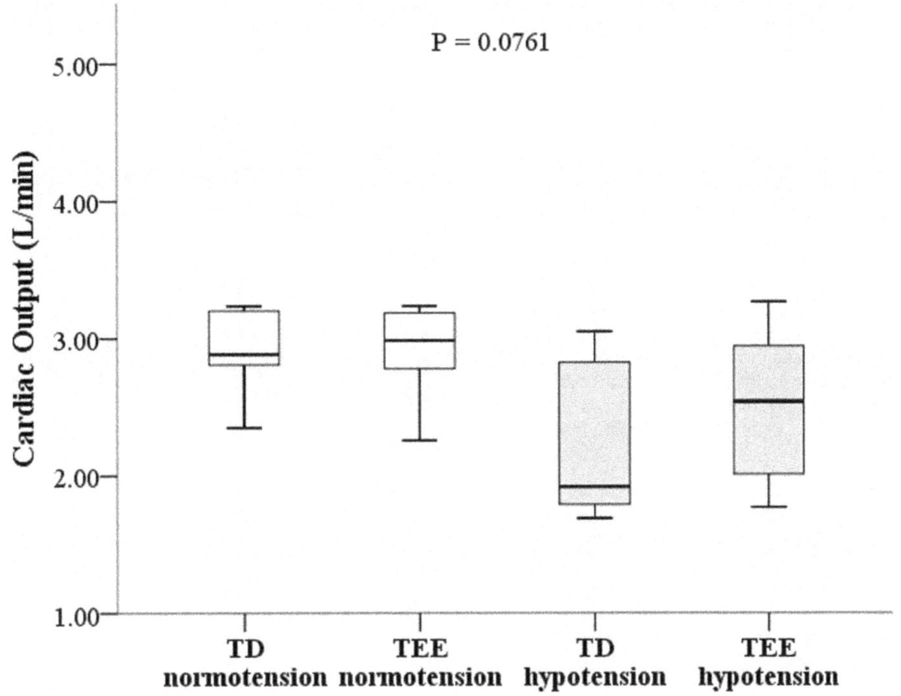

Fig. 4 Cardiac output measured in anaesthetised dogs with an adequate (normotension) and low (hypotension) arterial pressure during surgery. The line within the box indicates the median of the observations. The top and low parts of the box indicate the first and the third quartile, respectively. There were no significant differences between the cardiac output measured by the thermodilution technique (TD) and the transoesophageal echocardiography (TEE) during arterial normotension (P = 0.9612) and hypotension (P = 0.0761), according to the results obtained with the Student paired t-test

During the study, hypotension was induced in all animals during surgery and then reversed by reducing the isoflurane supply and/or administrating LR bolus. The decrease in arterial pressure was expected since isoflurane is an anaesthetic drug that reduces vascular resistance and that can be used as an inductor of hypotension in dogs undergoing experimental studies [18]. Despite an increase in HR expected during hypotension, this was not observed due to a decrease in the baroreflex induced by isoflurane and due to an increase in parasympathetic activity caused by fentanyl [19].

Some limitations of the study should be discussed. The TD technique can be relatively imprecise when measuring CO due to factors that can influence the accuracy of the measurement, such as dead space of the catheter, velocity of the administration and temperature of the solution [2]. However, this is still considered the gold standard for CO determination [3]. Despite the results of the present study having demonstrated that the TEE is an alternative technique to TD for measuring CO, in some situations, such as in surgeries of the oral, oesophageal or gastric areas, this technique cannot be applied.

Conclusion

The results of the study indicated that the transgastric view of the LVOT acquired by transoesophageal echocardiography is a minimally invasive alternative to TD for monitoring CO in anaesthetised dogs during surgery. However, during hypotension, the CO obtained by TEE was less reliable, although still acceptable.

Abbreviations

CO: Cardiac output; CO_{TD}: Cardiac output measured by thermodilution technique; CO_{TEE}: Cardiac output measured by transoesophageal echocardiography; DAP: Diastolic arterial pressure; $ETCO_2$: End-tidal carbon dioxide concentration; ET_{ISO}: End-tidal isoflurane concentration; HR: Heart rate; ICC: Intraclass correlation coefficient; LR: Lactated Ringer's solution; LVOT: Left ventricular outflow tract; MAP: Mean arterial pressure; SAP: Systolic arterial pressure; SpO_2: Oxyhaemoglobin saturation; TD: Thermodilution technique; TEE: Transoesophageal echocardiography; VTI: Velocity-time integral; VTI_{aortic}: Velocity-time integral of aortic flow

Acknowledgements

The authors gratefully acknowledge the veterinarians of the veterinary hospital of the Faculty of Veterinary Medicine and Animal Sciences of University of Sao Paulo for their contribution of cases. We thank all dog owners for their assistance and willingness to take part in this study.

Funding

This research received funding from FAPESP (Research Support Foundation of the State of São Paulo) and CNPq (National Council for Scientific and Technological Development).

Authors' contributions

DTF and DS designed the study, obtained the funding for the study, evaluated the data and revised the manuscript. MMM, AMG, JRC and PBF conducted the experiments, collected and analysed all of the data, and helped to write the manuscript. KKI analysed the data and helped to write, edit and review the manuscript. All authors read and approved the final manuscript.

Consent for publication
Not applicable.

Competing interests
The authors declare that they have no competing interests.

Author details
[1]Departamento de Clínica Médica, Faculdade de Medicina Veterinária e Zootecnia, Universidade de São Paulo, São Paulo, Brazil. [2]Departamento de Cirurgia, Faculdade de Medicina Veterinária e Zootecnia, Universidade de São Paulo, São Paulo, Brazil. [3]Laboratório de Investigação Médica 8, Anestesiologia, Faculdade de Medicina, Universidade de São Paulo, São Paulo, Brazil. [4]Faculdade de Medicina Veterinária e Zootecnia da Universidade Federal de São Paulo, Av. Prof Dr Orlando Marques de Paiva 87, São Paulo, SP 05508-270, Brazil.

References

1. Gonzalez J, Delafosse C, Fartoukh M, Capderou A, Straus C, Zelter M, Derenne JP, Similowski T. Comparison of bedside measurement of cardiac output with the thermodilution method and the Fick method in mechanically ventilated patients. Crit Care. 2003;7(2):171–8.
2. Levett JM, Replogle RL. Thermodilution cardiac output: a critical analysis and review of the literature. J Surg Res. 1979;27(6):392–404.
3. Shih A, Maisenbacher HW, Bandt C, Ricco C, Bailey J, Rivera J, Estrada A. Assessment of cardiac output measurement in dogs by transpulmonary pulse contour analysis. J Vet Emerg Crit Care. 2011;21(4):321–7.
4. Swan HJ, Ganz W, Forrester J, Marcus H, Diamond G, Chonette D. Catheterisation of the heart in man with use of a flow-directed balloon-tipped catheter. New Engl J Med. 1970;283(9):447–51.
5. Smart FW, Husserl FE. Complications of flow-directed balloon-tipped catheters. Chest. 1990;97(1):227–8.
6. Swain FR, Martinez F, Gripp M, Razdan R, Gagliardi J. Traumatic complications from placement of thoracic catheters and tubes. Emerg Radiol. 2005;12(1–2):11–8.
7. Stoddard MF, Prince CR, Ammash N, Goad JL, Vogel RL. Pulsed Doppler transoesophageal echocardiographic determination of cardiac output in human beings: comparison with thermodilution technique. Am Heart J. 1993;126(4):956–62.
8. Perrino AC Jr, Harris SN, Luther MA. Intraoperative determination of cardiac output using multiplane transoesophageal echocardiography: a comparison to thermodilution. Anesthesiol. 1998;89(2):350–7.
9. Boon JM. The M-mode and Doppler examination. In: boon JA, editor. Veterinary echocardiography. 2nd edn. Iowa, USA: Wiley-Blackwell. 2011:76–105.
10. Descorps-Declere A, Smail N, Vigue B, Duranteau J, Mimoz O, Edouard A, Samii K. Transgastric, pulsed Doppler echocardiographic determination of cardiac output. Intens Care Med. 1996;22(1):34–8.
11. Porciello F, Caivano D, Giorgi ME, Knafelz P, Rishniw M, Moise NS, Bufalari A, Fruganti A, Birettoni F. Transoesophageal echocardiography as the sole guidance for occlusion of patent ductus arteriosus using a canine ductal occluder in dogs. J Vet Intern Med. 2014;28(5):1504–12.
12. Domenech O, Oliveira P. Transoesophageal echocardiography in the dog. Vet J. 2013;198(2):329–38.
13. Loyer CT, Biplane WP. Transoesophageal echocardiography in the dog: technique, anatomy and imaging planes. Vet Radiol Ultrasound. 1995;36:212–6.
14. Lopes PC, Sousa MG, Camacho AA, Carareto R, Nishimori CT, Santos PS, Nunes N. Comparison between two methods for cardiac output measurement in propofol-anaesthetised dogs: thermodilution and Doppler. Vet Anaesth Analges. 2010;37(5):401–8.
15. Uemura K, Kawada T, Inagaki M, Sugimachi M. A minimally invasive monitoring system of cardiac output using aortic flow velocity and peripheral arterial pressure profile. Anaesthes Analges. 2013;116(5):1006–17.
16. Bland JM, Altman DG. Statistical methods for assessing agreement between two methods of clinical measurement. Lancet. 1986;1(8476):307–10.
17. Critchley LA, Critchley JA. A meta-analysis of studies using bias and precision statistics to compare cardiac output measurement techniques. J Clin Monitor Comput. 1999;15(2):85–91.
18. Morgaz J, Granados Mdel M, Munoz-Rascon P, Dominguez JM, Fernandez-Sarmiento JA, Gomez-Villamandos RJ, Navarrete R. Comparison of thermodilution, lithium dilution, and pulse contour analysis for the measurement of cardiac output in 3 different hemodynamic states in dogs. J Vet Emerg Crit Care. 2014;24(5):562–70.
19. Griffioen KJ, Venkatesan P, Huang ZG, Wang X, Bouairi E, Evans C, Gold A, Mendelowitz D. Fentanyl inhibits GABAergic neurotransmission to cardiac vagal neurons in the nucleus ambiguus. Brain Res. 2004;1007(1–2):109–5.

8

A retrospective analysis of the risk factors for surgical site infections and long-term follow-up after transpalpebral enucleation in horses

Tsjester Huppes*, Hanneke Hermans and Jos M. Ensink

Abstract

Background: Implants are often used to improve the cosmetic appearance of horses after enucleation of the eye. When surgical site infection (SSI) occurs, the implant will almost always be lost. The aim of this study is to collect data on the risk factors for SSIs and report long-term follow-up (cosmetic results and return to work) after transpalpebral enucleations. In this retrospective study, records of horses undergoing transpalpebral enucleation were reviewed (2007–2014) and telephone interviews were used to obtain long term follow-up. The potential risk factors for SSIs (indication for enucleation, use of an implant, standing procedures, duration of surgery, opening of the conjunctival sac and prolonged use of antimicrobials) were analysed for their association with the outcome measure 'SSI' vs 'no SSI' by multivariable binary logistic regression testing. Indications for enucleation were grouped as follows: Group 1 (clean) included equine recurrent uveitis, too small or too large globes, and intraocular tumours, Group 2 (non-clean) included corneal perforation/rupture and infected ulcers and Group 3 (tumour) included extraocular tumours.

Results: One hundred and seven cases of enucleation were evaluated. An implant was used in 49 horses. The overall number of SSIs was 8 (7.5%). Multivariable logistic regression testing showed implants (OR 7.5, $P = 0.04$) and standing procedures (OR 12.1; $P = 0.03$) were significantly associated with the percentage of SSIs and increased the risk of SSI. The eyes of horses in Groups 2 and 3 trended towards a larger risk for developing SSIs (OR 4.9; $P = 0.09$ and OR 5.9; $P = 0.1$, respectively). Prolonged use of antimicrobials, long surgery times and the opening of the conjunctival sac during dissection did not show significant associations with SSI risk.

Conclusions: The risk of SSI after enucleation is low in clean eyes and when no implant is used. Placing an implant or performing a standing enucleation significantly increases the risk of SSIs. Although implants can be used for eyes that fall into Groups 2 and 3, 17% of the horses in these two groups developed an SSI leading to loss of the implant.

Keywords: Horse, Transpalpebral, Enucleation, Risk factors, Surgical site infection

* Correspondence: t.huppes@uu.nl
Department of Equine Sciences, Faculty of Veterinary Medicine, Utrecht University, Yalelaan 114, 3584 CM Utrecht, Netherlands

Background

Enucleation is a commonly performed orbital surgery, in which the palpebral margins, nictitating membrane and its associated glands, conjunctiva and globe are removed. It is indicated in eyes that are painful and non-visual. It can also be indicated in eyes that still have visual function if they have a poor long term prognosis [1]. For simple enucleations, a transpalpebral or subconjunctival approach with primary closure of the eyelids can be used. Although preoperative flushing of the cornea and upper and lower fornices of the conjunctiva with povidone-iodine preparations significantly decrease the conjunctival flora [2, 3], in cases where sepsis or neoplasia involves the corneoconjunctival surface, the transpalpebral method is indicated because the closed conjunctival sac formed in this technique serves to prevent orbital contamination during surgery [4]. When performing a transpalpebral enucleation, care must be taken during dissection not to open the conjunctival sac as this may increase the risk of contamination. However, even with precise dissection, a miniscule opening in the conjunctival sac is always made in the medial canthus when the nasolacrimal system is transected. Therefore, based on the National Research Council's wound classification [5], enucleation can be considered a clean-contaminated procedure and perioperative antimicrobial prophylaxis is usually administered as a standard procedure.

Transpalpebral enucleation is often performed with the horse anaesthetized and in lateral recumbency, but a standing procedure has also been described [6, 7]. The standing procedure eliminates the expense and risk of general anaesthesia, but asepsis may be more difficult to maintain, which may increase the risk of surgical site infection.

Enucleation may lead to a deep indentation of the skin over the orbit, and implantation of an orbital prosthesis is a safe and inexpensive method in horses for improving cosmetic appearance after enucleation [8]. However, an implant serves as foreign material, which can be a nidus for infection and may allow biofilm formation [9, 10]. During clean-contaminated surgery, using an implant may increase the risk of surgical site infection (SSI). Unfortunately, in the advent of an SSI the implant will almost always be lost. In one study, a failure rate of 10.7% (3/28) is reported for silicone orbital implants after enucleation in the horse [8]. Therefore, the cosmetic advantage of an implant must be weighed against the disadvantage of an increased risk of SSI.

The aim of this retrospective study was to collect data on the risk factors for SSI and on long term follow-up (cosmetic results and return to work) following transpalpebral enucleation, to better inform clientele on the best surgical option for their horse.

Methods

Study design

Records of all horses undergoing transpalpebral enucleation at the Utrecht University's Equine Clinic between 1 May 2007 and 1 October 2014 were reviewed. Data retrieved from case records included indication for enucleation, which eye was enucleated, the position of the horse during surgery (recumbent or standing), the cosmetic approach used (use of an implant or no implant), surgical findings (opening of the conjunctival sac and surgery time) and postoperative findings (development of SSI and duration of antimicrobial use).

Follow-up information (no implant >30 days of follow up; implant >1 year of follow-up) from the owners' evaluation forms or a telephone interview with the owner was used to retrieve long-term information about the development of an SSI. A telephone interview (>1 year after surgery) was used to determine the pre- and post-operative use and the performance ability of the horse and to evaluate the owners' opinion about the final cosmetic appearance of the implant. Owners were asked to rate the cosmetic outcome as excellent, good or poor, with excellent for perfectly fitting implants (appearance identical to a closed contralateral eye; Figure 1), good for an implant showing minimal eyelid sinkage around the implant and poor for too large or too small implants.

Indications for enucleation were grouped into three groups. Group 1 (clean) included equine recurrent

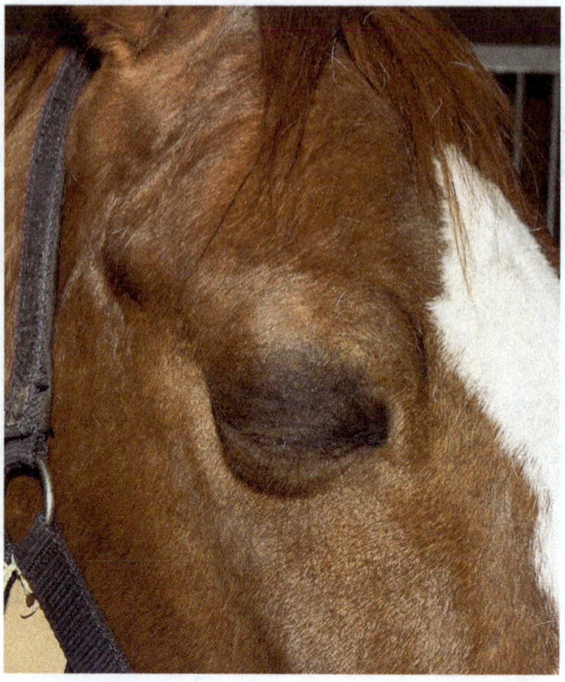

Fig. 1 Image of a horse several months after enucleation with implant and an excellent cosmetic appearance

uveitis (ERU), too small globes (phthisis bulbi, microphthalmia) or too large globes (glaucoma, buphthalmos), and intraocular tumours. Group 2 (non-clean) included corneal perforation and rupture and infected ulcers. Group 3 (tumour) included extraocular tumours (including squamous cell carcinoma).

Wounds were classified as 'infected' when persistent serohaemorrhagic or purulent drainage from the surgical wound was observed by the surgeon or owner. Based on the Centers for Disease Control and Prevention (CDC) definitions, a deep or superficial SSI must have an onset within thirty days after operation or within one year if the operation included placement of an implant [5]. Therefore, when no implant was used, infection within thirty days after operation was considered an SSI and, when an implant was used, an infection up to one year after surgery was considered an SSI. Wounds were classified as 'not infected' if there were either no wound complications or (sero)haemorrhagic exudation was only observed within 24 h postoperatively.

Surgical procedure of transpalpebral enucleation

Medical perioperative treatments were similar for all horses. Flunixin meglumine (1.1 mg/kg bwt, IV) was administered preoperatively. Prophylactic antibiotics (ampicillin (15 mg/kg bwt) or a combination of benzylpenicillin (40.000 IU/kg bwt) and gentamicin (6.6 mg/kg bwt)) were administered intravenously just before surgery, and all horses received a single intramuscular injection of procaine penicillin (22.000 IU/kg bwt) immediately after surgery. A longer, additional postoperative analgesic (meloxicam, 0,6 mg/kg bwt, PO) or antibiotic treatment was only provided to horses demonstrating signs of pain, postoperative swelling, or fever.

Surgeries were performed under general anaesthesia in lateral recumbency or standing with sedation and local analgesia. All horses received a retrobulbar block and, for horses undergoing a standing procedure, additional nerve blocks were performed as described in Pollock et al. [6]. A standard transpalpebral enucleation was performed [1] and the same surgical technique was used for the standing and the recumbent procedures. Preoperatively the surgical site was clipped and aseptically prepared, including flushing the lacrimal duct and the conjunctival sac with a mild disinfectant (0.1% povidone-iodine in saline). The eyelids were sutured together with a 2–0 non- absorbable monofilament suture in a continuous fashion. After closing the eyelids, the surgical site was again aseptically prepared and the transpalpebral enucleation was performed. Briefly, a full-thickness skin incision was created around the eyelid margins and a blunt and sharp subcutaneous dissection was performed posteriorly. After transecting the medial and lateral canthal ligaments, blunt dissection was continued along the sclera and the extraocular muscles and the optic nerve were transected. Before surgery the owners were always informed about the option of placing an orbital implant into the orbit to improve the cosmetic outcome. If preferred by the owner, after removal of the eye, a spherical silicone implant with a diameter dependent on the size of the orbit, was placed in the orbit (spherical silicone implants from Jardon eye prosthetics[1]). No preoperative or intraoperative measurements of the globe were performed to determine its size for selection of the implant. The optimal implant size was determined during surgery by fitting implants of different sizes into the orbit. The largest diameter size that could be fitted into the orbit without resistance - created by the size of the bony orbital rim - was chosen. Wounds were always closed completely, but the suture technique and material were at the surgeon's discretion. No sutures were placed over the orbital implant to secure it in the orbital rim. When an implant was used a two layered closure was performed over the implant. The subcutaneous tissues of upper and lower eyelids were apposed using polygalactin 910 (Vicryl; Ethicon) or poliglecaprone 25 (Monocryl; Ethicon) in a simple continuous pattern. The skin was apposed with monofilament suture material; a continuous intradermal suture pattern (poliglecaprone 25) was used or a perforating simple interrupted pattern (poliglecaprone 25 or nylon (Ethilon; Ethicon)) was used. When no implant was used subcutaneous tissues and skin were closed using a two layered method - as described above -, or an interrupted perforating pattern was used for concurrent closure of the skin and subcutis (interrupted vertical mattress and simple interrupted pattern) using poliglecaprone 25 or nylon. If non-absorbable sutures or perforating patterns were used suture removal was performed 10–12 days after surgery. After surgery, wounds were covered with an adhesive bandage for recovery. The adhesive bandage was removed within 24 h after recovery and no (stent) bandage was used to cover the wound after this period.

Data analysis

Variables analysed in this study are all categorical and are described in Table 1.

Univariable binary logistic regression was used to screen all variables for their association with the outcome measure 'SSI' vs 'no SSI'. Multivariable binary logistic regression testing was performed with all variables and a manual backward elimination procedure was performed to fit a multivariable model. Non-significant variables were eliminated if their elimination did not affect the log OR of the significant variables more than 15%. Odds ratios and confidence intervals were determined for all variables. Due to the small numbers of SSIs

Table 1 The statistical variables included in the study

Variables:	
Indication	Group 1 (clean)
	Group 2 (non-clean)
	Group 3 (tumour)
Position of the horse	Recumbent
	Standing
Implant use	No implant
	Implant
Antibiotic treatment	Short term (24 h)
	Long term (>24 h)
Duration of the surgery	<mean surgery time
	>mean surgery time
Conjunctival sac	Not opened
	Opened

no interaction between variables was tested. All statistical tests were performed using SPSS statistical software (SPSS 22). Statistical significance was set at $P \leq 0.05$.

Results

One hundred and seven cases of transpalpebral enucleation with primary closure and available follow-up about the development of an SSI were identified. Fifty-eight left eyes and 46 right eyes were removed. Eleven horses were operated on while standing and 96 horses were operated in lateral recumbency. Forty-nine horses had an implant used. The mean surgery time was 59 ± 22 min (range 23–123 min). No significant difference was found between the mean surgery time of recumbent (58 ± 21 min) and standing (72 ± 29 min) surgery (independent t-test $P = 0.1$). Enucleation was performed for a variety of reasons and, based on the previously described classification, 58 horses had a Group 1 indication (clean eye), 31 horses had a Group 2 indication (non-clean eye) and 18 horses had a Group 3 indication (tumour). Ninety-eight horses received a single dose of preoperative antibiotics (short term antibiotic treatment) and nine horses received prolonged antibiotic treatment (long term antibiotic treatment). Mean long term antibiotic treatment was 6.8 days (range, 3–18 days). Antibiotic treatment was prolonged for various reasons; in 2 cases antibiotic treatment was prolonged because perforation of the conjunctival sac occurred during surgery and increased contamination was considered likely. In 7 cases treatment was prolonged because of post-operative findings (postoperative swelling or fever) that might predispose to compromised wound healing. In two of these cases infection occurred (in one horse with an implant infection was presumed based on clinical signs, and in one horse without an implant infection was confirmed with culture), and an attempt was made to prevent implant loss by long-term antibiotic therapy. Neither infections resolved during antibiotic therapy and when clear signs of a sustained infection were apparent, antibiotic treatment was stopped and wounds were opened (with implant removal in the case with an implant) to allow sufficient drainage which resolved the infection quickly without negative consequences.

Surgical site infections

Based on our inclusion criteria of infection there were 8 SSIs, resulting in an overall infection rate of 7.5% (8/107). Three infections were noted within 10 days after surgery, 3 between 10 days and 1 month, and 2 infections were noted between 1 and 6 months. In 4 cases of SSI, samples for culture were taken and they were positive for *S. equi zooepidemicus* ($n = 2$), *S. aureus* ($n = 1$), and several anaerobes ($n = 1$). Two owners reported late postoperative infection with purulent drainage and loss of the implant (3 and 4 years after surgery). In one case a sample for culture was taken which was positive for *S. equi zooepidemicus*. Based on the CDC definitions, these cases were not rated as SSIs. Including these two cases, the overall long-term (1–8 years follow-up after surgery) loss of an implant due to infection was 14.3% (7/49).

The incidence of SSIs in the different patient categories and their univariable screening for their association with the outcome measure 'SSI' vs 'no SSI' are outlined in Table 2.

The following non-significant differences in percentages of SSI were found within the groups: horses with implants had a higher risk of SSI than those without implants (OR 2.1); horses in the non-clean eyes group (Group 2) and tumour group (group 3) had a higher risk of SSI than the horses in the clean eyes group (Group 1) (OR 2 (group 2) and 2.3 (group 3)); horses that underwent surgery in a standing position had a higher risk of SSI than those who were operated in a recumbent position (OR 3.3); horses that underwent prolonged antibiotic use had a higher risk of SSI than those that had short term antibiotic use (OR 4.4); horses with surgery time that was shorter than the mean surgery time had a higher risk of SSI than horses that had longer surgery times (OR 1.3); and finally, horses with surgeries in which the conjunctival sac was opened had a higher risk of SSI than horses that underwent surgeries in which the conjunctival sac remained closed during surgery (OR 1.4).

As shown in Table 3, horses in Group 1 had a significantly higher percentage of horses that received an implant compared with horses in the other groups (Fisher's Exact Test $P < 0.001$).

Therefore, multivariable logistic regression testing was performed with all variables in Table 2 to determine

Table 2 Percentage of SSIs for the different patient categories

	no SSI	SSI	Total	OR[a]	95% confidence interval[a]		Sig[a]
					Lower	Upper	
Indication							
Group 1: clean eye	55 (94.8%)	3 (5.2%)	58 (54.2%)	1			0.6[b]
Group 2: non-clean eye	28 (90.3%)	3 (9.7%)	31 (29%)	2	0.4	10.4	0.4
Group 3: tumour	16 (88.9%)	2 (11.1%)	18 (16.8%)	2.3	0.4	14.9	0.4
Total	99 (92.5%)	8 (7.5%)	107 (100%)				
Implant use							
No implant	55 (94.8%)	3 (5.2%)	58 (54.2%)	1			
Implant	44 (89.8%)	5 (10.2%)	49 (45.8%)	2.1	0.5	9.2	0.3
Total	99 (92.5%)	8 (7.5%)	107 (100%)				
Position of the horse							
Recumbent	90 (93.8%)	6 (6.3%)	96 (89.7%)	1			
Standing	9 (81.8%)	2 (18.2%)	11 (10.3%)	3.3	0.6	19	0.2
Total	99 (92.5%)	8 (7.5%)	107 (100%)				
Antibiotic treatment							
Short term	92 (93.9%)	6 (6.1%)	98 (91.6%)	1			
Long term	7 (77.8%)	2 (22.2%)	9 (8.4%)	4.4	0.7	25.9	0.1
Total	99 (92.5%)	8 (7.5%)	107 (100%)				
Surgery time							
< mean surgery time	55 (91.7%)	5 (8.3%)	60 (56.1%)	1.3	0.3	5.9	0.7
> mean surgery time	44 (93.6%)	3 (6.4%)	47 (43.9%)	1			
Total	99 (92.5%)	8 (7.5%)	107 (100%)				
Conjunctival sac							
Not opened	80 (93%)	6 (7%)	86 (80.4%)	1			
Opened	19 (90.5%)	2 (9.5%)	21 (19.6%)	1.4	0.3	7.5	0.7
Total	99 (92.5%)	8 (7.5%)	107 (100%)				

[a]Values are from the univariable logistic regression model
[b]Overall significance for indication

their association with the outcome measure 'SSI' vs 'no SSI' followed by a manual backward elimination procedure of nonsignificant variables. Table 4 presents the 3 variables found to be associated with SSI in the multivariable model ('indication' was a confounder and was kept in the model).

The use of an implant (OR 7.5; $P = 0.04$) and a standing surgical procedure (OR 12.1; $P = 0.03$) were significantly associated with the development of SSI. Horses in

Table 3 Distribution of implants over the groups (by indication)

	No implant	Implant	Total ($P < 0.001^*$)
Indication			
Group 1: clean eye	21 (36.2%)	37 (63.8%)	58 (54.2%)
Group 2: non-clean eye	22 (71%)	9 (29%)	31 (29%)
Group 3: tumour	15 (83.3%)	3 (16.7%)	18 (16.8%)
Total	58 (54.2%)	49 (45.8%)	107 (100%)

* *P*-value from Fisher's exact test

Table 4 Based on a multivariable logistic regression model, variables found to be associated with the likelihood of a horse having an SSI after enucleation

	OR	95% Confidence interval		Sig.
		Lower	Upper	
Indication				
Group 1: clean eye	1			0.1[a]
Group 2: non-clean eye	4.9	0.8	31.1	0.09
Group 3: tumour	5.9	0.7	49.4	0.1
Implant use				
No implant	1			
Implant	7.5	1.1	51.4	0.04
Position of the horse				
Recumbent	1			
Standing	12.1	1.3	112.9	0.03

[a]Overall significance for indication

Groups 2 and 3 trended towards being at a higher risk for developing an SSI (OR 4.9; P = 0.09 and OR 5.9; P = 0.1). Prolonged use of antimicrobials, the length of the surgery and whether the conjunctival sac was opened during dissection did not show a significant association with the risk of developing an SSI.

Final cosmetic appearance of the implant

Long term follow-up on the final cosmetic appearance of the implant was obtained for 40 horses (in 4 horses long term follow-up about cosmetic appearance was not available and 5 horses lost their implant within 1 year after surgery because of a surgical site infection). Thirty-eight (95%) owners reported excellent to good cosmetic results. Two owners (5%) reported poor cosmetic outcome. Overall 97.5% (39/40) of the owners reported that in a similar case they would again opt for an implant.

Return to work after unilateral enucleation

Long term follow-up information about pre- and post-operative use of 95 horses was available for evaluation. Based on pre-surgical discipline, the number of horses returning to their previous use was evaluated and the results are shown in Table 5.

Ninety-eight percent (84/86) of the horses returned to their pre-operative performance after enucleation. Two owners reported that their horses were not able to return to their preoperative use due to behavioural changes related to monocular vision; one horse did not return to work as a sport horse (harness), and one did not return to work as a pleasure horse. Nine horses were already retired at the time of the surgery so it was not possible to qualify their postoperative performance ability, but the owners reported that these horses had no difficulties in adapting to their life after enucleation.

Discussion

The prevention of SSIs is a major goal during surgery, and proper surgical technique such as effective hemostasis, eradication of dead space and minimalizing wound contamination can reduce the risk of infection [11]. In this respect, some challenges are encountered during transpalpebral enucleation. Maintaining strict aseptic techniques is impaired because a small opening in the conjunctival sac is always made in the medial canthus when the nasolacrimal system is transected. Complete and effective haemostasis or eradication of dead space is not achievable during enucleation; although transecting the extraocular muscles at their tendinous insertions minimizes haemorrhage [1], removal of the eye - without subsequent placement of an orbital implant - always leaves a dead space that inevitably fills with blood. In this respect, dead space is reduced by placing an implant which might confound its predisposing factor for infection. The surgical site can be closed in three layers, and the orbital septum can be closed to secure the implant and to assist with haemostasis [1]. Although one can argue that this technique can help to reduce dead space, in the cases evaluated in this retrospective study no attempt was made to do so. These predisposing factors related to the technique of enucleation might have contributed to an overall infection rate of 7.5% in this study. Compared to Group 1, horses in Groups 2 or 3 (non-clean or tumour) had a considerably higher percentage of SSIs (9.7% and 11.1%, respectively). In Group 2, although the eyelids were sutured together before final aseptic preparation of the surgical site, minimal leakage from the conjunctival sac might have occurred during surgery causing an elevated concentration of microorganisms per gram tissue and increasing the risk of SSI. In Group 3, the intention to remove a tumour completely might have necessitated more extensive dissection, causing more tissue trauma, an increased inflammatory response and a larger dead space, which may explain the increased risk of SSIs.

Preoperatively, owners were always informed about the option of placing an orbital implant into the orbit to improve the cosmetic outcome, but they were

Table 5 Return to work after unilateral enucleation, grouped on preoperative discipline

		Performance		Total
		Return	No return	
Discipline	Recreational/pleasure–/trail riding	52 (98%)	1 (2%)	53 (56%)
	Sport horse (dressage)	14 (100%)	0 (0%)	14 (15%)
	Sport horse (jumping)	4 (100%)	0 (0%)	4 (4%)
	Sport horse (harness)	4 (80%)	1 (20%)	5 (5%)
	Harness horse (pleasure)	5 (100%)	0 (0%)	5 (5%)
	Riding school horse (group lessons)	3 (100%)	0 (0%)	3 (3%)
	Broodmare	2 (100%)	0 (0%)	2 (2%)
	Retired	9 (100%)	0 (0%)	9 (10%)
Total		93 (97.9%)	2 (2.1%)	95 (100%)

discouraged from placing an orbital implant when there was evidence of neoplasia or infection (horses in Groups 2 and 3) [12]. The final decision about implant use was based on the owner's preference, but as a result of our pre-operative advice, in Group 1, a significantly higher percentage of horses received an implant than in both of the other groups, which influenced the overall infection rate in Group 1. In Group 1, where no implant was used, no SSIs developed (0/21). In Group 1, horses that received implants 8.1% (3/37) developed an SSI.

Because transpalpebral enucleation is considered a clean-contaminated surgery, a small degree of contamination can be expected. In surgical wounds a number of microorganisms greater than 10^5 per gram of tissue increases the risk of SSIs [13]. In the presence of foreign material the amount of contamination necessary for infection is markedly reduced [14]. Horses in groups 2 and 3 trended towards an increased risk of SSIs. Although implants can be used for horses that fall into one of these two groups, 17.6% (3/12) of the horses that did have implants used developed an SSI with loss of the implant.

The number of standing enucleations is small (n = 11) so no firm conclusions can be drawn. In the study of Pollock et al. (2008) evaluating 40 standing enucleations, 1 out of 32 horses (3.1%) with long term follow-up had serosanguinous discharge from the incision for 3 days [6]. In their study, an implant was used after standing enucleation in 4 out of 40 horses, but eight horses were lost to long-term follow-up and it was not further specified how many of them had an implant. Compared to this study we found a considerably higher infection rate of 18.2% for standing enucleation. In our study, the significant increase of SSIs in the standing enucleations compared to enucleations performed under general anaesthesia, may be explained by the difficulty in preventing contamination if the horse moves its head. It suggests that when implant placement is intended, an enucleation under general anaesthesia is preferable. Out of 11 standing enucleations performed in our study, in only one case was an implant used and in this case, the horse developed an SSI.

In one horse enucleation was started as a standing procedure, but due to continuous non-cooperative behaviour of the horse during closure of the eyelids - even after additional sedation and local analgesia - the procedure was eventually performed under general anaesthesia. This implies that character of the horse can also influence the final decision about performing enucleation with the horse standing or under general anaesthesia. One study about complications associated with anaesthesia for ocular surgery found that these horses were at greater risk of unsatisfactory recoveries [15]. In this respect, the advantage of avoiding the expenses and risks of general anaesthesia when performing a standing enucleation should also be taken into account.

The effect of accidentally opening the conjunctival sac on the percentage of SSIs is limited (OR 1.4) and shows that even when the conjunctival sac is opened an implant can be used. Eleven percent (1/9) of the horse in which the conjunctival sac was opened and an implant was used, developed an SSI. Eight percent (1/12) of the horses in which the conjunctival sac was opened developed an SSI when no implant was used. Surgeries were all performed after thorough flushing of the conjunctival sac and nasolacrimal duct with a mild disinfectant and with peri-operative antimicrobial prophylaxis. In two cases the post-operative antibiotic treatment was preventively prolonged after the conjunctival sac had been opened. These actions might have contributed to the limited deleterious effect of inadvertently opening the conjunctival sac during surgery.

A higher rate of SSI was found in horses that received prolonged antibiotic treatment, but this probably reflects the fact that prolonged antibiotic treatment was used in cases where infection was more likely. In 2 cases antibiotic treatment was prolonged because perforation of the conjunctival sac occurred during surgery and increased contamination was considered likely. In 7 cases treatment was prolonged because of post-operative findings (postoperative swelling or fever) lead us to anticipate possible compromised wound healing.

Apart from the 8 SSIs classified in this study, two late infections (after 3 and 4 years, respectively) were reported in the group with implants. Out of all horses with their implants in place after one year (no SSI; n = 44), in two horses (4.5%) late infection and loss/removal of the implant occurred. In both cases acute swelling of the orbital region occurred, followed by purulent drainage. According to the Centers for Disease Control and Prevention (CDC) definitions, an SSI must have an onset within one year if the operation included placement of an implant [5]. For the infections that occurred after 3 and 4 years, it is hard to imagine that the infection was there all that time in a subclinical form and these cases do not meet the criteria of an SSI. The surface of the implant may be a site of lower resistance where haematogenic bacteria have a better chance of producing an infection at a later stage. An infection of the implant might also be acquired through neighbouring tissue, after local trauma of the skin covering a slightly bulging implant at the nonvisual side. In the follow-up of horses that underwent enucleation without an implant, no late infection was reported.

Thirty-eight (95%) owners reported excellent to good cosmetic results. In our study, cosmetic outcome was reviewed by the owner and no objective postoperative measurement or standardized evaluation by the veterinary surgeon was performed. Although this would have been a more accurate way to rate cosmesis, achieving owner satisfaction about the cosmetic result is the most important goal in cosmetic procedures. In a study comparing enucleation with and without the use of a suture meshwork implant, 68% of the owners rated the cosmetic appearance after the use of an implant as 'bad', with a marked or deep sunk-in appearance [16]. In our study, only 2 owners reported poor cosmetic outcome because of the suboptimal size of the implants. One owner reported that the implant was too large and that the protruding implant led to frequent trauma of the skin (the horse showed late infection with loss of the implant 4 years postoperatively). The second owner reported that the implant was too small. In this case the spherical implant did not occupy the complete orbital volume and during the healing process, sinkage of the eyelids occurred and the implant within an orbital delineation was clearly visible under the skin. Due to the favourable cosmetic outcome of the spherical implants, it is advised to place this implant after transpalpebral enucleation if cosmetic appearance is important to the owner. If the owner is primarily concerned with the welfare of the horse, no implant should be used because cosmetic appearance is not of interest for the horse and increases the risk of SSI.

Since no preoperative or intraoperative measurements of the globe were performed to determine the size of the implant, fitting implants of different sizes into the orbit during surgery was needed to determine the optimal implant size. In our experience and based on high owner satisfaction about the cosmetic outcome, this is an effective method to determine the optimal size.

Two percent (2/86) of the horses failed to return to their pre-operative performance after enucleation due to behavioural changes related to monocular vision. A study reviewing 34 horses of different breeds and a variety of pre-surgical occupations, reported that 12% failed to return to work following unilateral enucleation for reasons related to monocular vision [17]. A large percentage of the population in that study were racing horses (10/34) and 20% of them were not returned to work. The population of horses in our study included no racing horses and this can be an explanation for the differences found. Independent of the differences in populations, our results confirm the conclusion that horses are able to return to a variety of occupations after unilateral enucleation.

Because this study was retrospective, several limitations were encountered. Since in some horses clinical signs did occur after the hospitalization period we lack samples for culture in 4/8 cases. Therefore, the classification of infection was limited to persistent serohaemorrhagic or purulent drainage. In 4/8 cases a sample for culture was taken and all samples confirmed infection. In 4/8 cases no culture or cytology was performed and in these cases non-infectious wound discharge and dehiscence or implant rejection can't be excluded. As a consequence of how we did define infection some of the cases reported herein as infected, may not have been infected. This might have overrated the actual overall infection rate. Because of the single-centred nature of this study a relatively small number of horses were evaluated, but consequently no potential interhospital variations were applicable. Between 2007 and 2014 no temporal changes in the approach to patients or clients occurred in our hospital that we are aware of. Because we only started using the standing technique in 2011, the standing and recumbent surgeries are not equally distributed over time. In our clinic a standardized approach is employed by the veterinary technicians regarding aseptic preparation of the surgical patient and surgical instrumentation. These protocols are identical for all patients and were applied during the entire study period. Although all surgeons follow standardized guidelines regarding aseptic techniques employed, limitations such as the lack of complete similarity in surgical aseptic preparation (e.g. gloving technique) between surgeons were encountered. Between 2007 and 2014 a large variety of surgeons (n = 14) did perform the surgeries and none of the surgeons did the majority of the cases. Therefore, the results were not controlled for different surgeons and aseptic techniques employed. Even with these limitations valuable information to better inform the owners was obtained.

Conclusion

Based upon this report the risk of SSI after enucleation is low in clean eyes and when no implant is used. Placing an implant and performing a standing enucleation significantly increases the risk of SSI. Enucleations performed in non-clean eyes and eyes with an extraocular tumour show a trend towards increased risk of SSI. Although implants can be used in these groups, 17% developed an SSI with loss of the implant. Owners should be informed about these risks so that they can make an informed decision about the choice of technique. If owners prioritize quick, uncomplicated healing above the final cosmetic outcome, an implant should not be placed. If final cosmetic outcome with implant placement is important to the owner, then an enucleation under general anaesthesia may be preferable.

Placing a silicone implant during enucleation is a simple and affordable technique to improve cosmesis and a high owner satisfaction about the cosmetic outcome is achieved.

Horses are able to return to a variety of occupations after unilateral enucleation.

Endnotes

[1]Jardon Eye Prosthetics, Inc. Southfield, USA

Abbreviations

CDC: Centers for Disease Control and Prevention; SSI: Surgical site infection

Acknowledgements

The authors wish to thank Dr. J.C.M. Vernooij (Utrecht University) for his assistance with the statistical analyses.

Funding

No sources of funding to report for this submission.

Authors' contributions

TH was involved in the experimental study design, study execution, data analysis and interpretation, and final preparation of the manuscript. HH assisted in gathering data and in the preparation of the manuscript. JE contributed to gathering and analysis of the data and writing of the manuscript, and provided assistance in designing the study. All the authors assisted in the reviewing of this manuscript during the writing process. All authors read and approved the final version of the manuscript and have significantly contributed to writing the draft manuscript.

Competing interests

None of the authors of this paper has a financial or personal relationship with other people or organizations that could inappropriately influence or bias the content of the paper.

Consent for publication

Not applicable.

References

1. Pierce KE, Townsend WM. Surgery of the globe and orbit. In: Auer JA, Stick JA, editors. Equine surgery. 4th ed. St. Louis: Saunders; 2012. p. 737–8.
2. Apt L, Isenberg S, Yoshimori R, Paez JH. Chemical preparation of the eye in ophthalmic surgery: III. Effect of povidone-iodine on the conjunctiva. Arch Ophthalmol. 1984;102(5):728–9.
3. Binder CA. Miño de Kaspar H, Klauss V, Kampik a. Preoperative infection prophylaxis with 1% polyvidon-iodine solution based on the example of conjunctival staphylococci. Ophthalmologe. 1999;96(10):663–7.
4. Herring IP. Enucleation and Orbital Exenteration. In: Bojrab MJ, Waldron DR, Tooms JP, editors. Current Techniques in Small Animal Surgery. 5th ed. Jackson: Teton NewMedia; 2014. p. 165.
5. Mangram AJ, Horan TC, Pearson ML, Silver LC, Jarvis WR. Guideline for prevention of surgical site infection, 1999. Center for Disease Control and Prevention (CDC) hospital infection Control practices advisory committee. Infect Control Hosp Epidemiol. 1999;20(4):250–78.
6. Pollock PJ, Russell T, Hughes TK, Archer MR, Perkins JD. Transpalpebral eye Enucleation in 40 standing horses. Vet Surg. 2008;37(3):306–9.
7. Hewes C, Keoughan GC, Gutierrez NS. Standing enucleation in the horse: a report of 5 cases. Can Vet J. 2007;48(5):512–4.
8. Hamor RE. Use of orbital implants after enucleation in dogs, horses, and cats: 161 cases (1980-1990). J Am Vet Med Assoc. 1993;203(5):701–6.
9. Freeman K, Woods E, Welsby S, Percival SL, Cochrane CA. Biofilm evidence and the microbial diversity of horse wounds. Can J Microbiol. 2009;55(2): 197–202.
10. Costerton JW, Montanaro L, Arciola CR. Biofilm in implant infections: its production and regulation. The International journal of Artificial Organs. 2005;28(11):1062–8.
11. Santschi EM. Prevention of Postoperative Infections in Horses. Vet Clin North Am Equine Pract. 2006;22(2):323–34.
12. Michau TM, Gilger BC. Cosmetic globe surgery in the horse. Vet Clin N Am Equine Pract. 2004;20(2):467–84.
13. Raahave D, Friis-Moller A, Bjerre-Jepsen K, Thiis-Knudsen J, Rasmussen LB. The infective dose of aerobic and anaerobic bacteria in postoperative wound sepsis. Arch Surg. 1986;121(8):924–9.
14. Merritt K, Hitchins VM, Neale AR. Tissue colonization from implantable biomaterials with low numbers of bacteria. J Biomed Mater Res. 1999;44(3): 261–5.
15. Parviainen AKJ, Trim CM. Complications associated with anaesthesia for ocular surgery: a retrospective study 1989?1996. Equine Vet J. 2000;32(6): 555–9.
16. Maninchedda U, Nottrott K, Gangl M. Enucleation in equids with and without the use of an orbital suture meshwork implant: a retrospective study of 37 cases. Vet Rec. 2015;177(14):367.
17. Utter ME, Wotman KL, Covert KR. Return to work following unilateral enucleation in 34 horses (2000-2008). Equine Vet J. 2010;42(2):156–60.

9

Quantitative evaluation of canine urinary bladder transitional cell carcinoma using contrast-enhanced ultrasonography

Francesco Macrì, Simona Di Pietro, Cyndi Mangano, Michela Pugliese*, Giuseppe Mazzullo, Nicola M. Iannelli, Vito Angileri, Simona Morabito and Massimo De Majo

Abstract

Background: In veterinary medicine, contrast-enhanced ultrasonography allowed the accurate quantification of liver, splenic and kidney vascularization in healthy dogs and the differentiation between malignant and benign hepatic, renal, and splenic nodules in dogs and cats based on perfusion patterns. The utility of contrast-enhanced ultrasonography in other applications is still under study.

The aim of this study was to develop diagnostic criteria by contrast-enhanced ultrasonography in 8 client-owned adult dogs affected by urinary bladder transitional cell carcinoma with definitive diagnosis made by cytopathologic evaluation after suction biopsy. The contrast enhancement pattern and the quantification of blood flow parameters of this tumor were reported.

Results: Examinations with B-mode, Doppler ultrasonography and contrast-enhanced ultrasonography were performed in all not sedated dogs. Assessments of bladder masses and bladder wall infiltration were performed. Each dog received 2 bolus injections of sulfur hexafluoride during the contrast-enhanced ultrasonography. Quantitative analysis of the contrast-enhanced ultrasonography images were performed. For each dog, one region of interest was manually drawn around the entire tumor. Software analysis of contrast-enhanced time-intensity curves was used to identify peak enhancement, time to peak enhancement, regional blood volume, regional blood flow, and mean transit time.

Contrast-enhanced ultrasonography showed an avid enhancement of the tumour tissue, with a heterogeneous or homogeneous pattern. The exam also showed the loss of planes between the lesion and the muscular layer. The presence of vascularized tissue through the bladder wall confirms the infiltrative feature of the tumour. Post-processing quantitative analysis showed a time-intensity curve with a rapid wash-in, a low level of signal intensity and a slow wash-out.

Conclusions: Contrast-enhanced ultrasonography provided useful clinical information and defined a vascular enhancement patterns and calculated parameters associated with TCC. It may be a useful, noninvasive and reproducible tool for detecting these tumors in dogs.

Keywords: Dog, Contrast-enhanced ultrasonography, Diagnostic ultrasound, Urinary bladder, Sonovue, Qontrast

* Correspondence: mpugliese@unime.it
Department of Veterinary Sciences, University of Messina, Polo Universitario Annunziata, 98168 Messina, Italy

Background

Contrast-enhanced ultrasound is a technique that involves the use of ultrasound contrast agents to improve the traditional ultrasonography both in human and veterinary medicine [1, 2].

Contrast agents used in CEUS are composed of gas-filled microbubbles, which are injected into the bloodstream. When the power of the ultrasound beam is low enough, microbubbles resonate, rapidly contracting and expanding in response to the pressure changes of the sound wave. Multiple harmonic signals are produced that can be recorded [3].

Following injection, the bubbles greatly increase the amplitude of the scattered signals not only from large vessels but also from the microvasculature, providing real-time assessment of vascular perfusion of target organs and/or lesions [4]. Contrast media are safe products and are well tolerated by dogs and cats [5].

In veterinary medicine, CEUS allowed the accurate quantification of liver, splenic and kidney vascularization in healthy dogs [6–8] and the differentiation between malignant and benign hepatic, renal, and splenic nodules in dogs and cats based on perfusion patterns [9–13].

The utility of CEUS in other applications is still under study. Recently, the use of CEUS has been extended to imaging of the urinary bladder in humans, improving the differential diagnosis between urinary bladder intraluminal masses and clots and allowing the differentiation between enhancing and nonenhancing lesions [14, 15].

Some Authors also demonstrated that it is possible to predict the human bladder neoplasm grading by the pattern of CEUS time–intensity curves [16, 17].

Contrast-enhanced ultrasound also resulted to be superior to grayscale ultrasound in assessing infiltration of the muscle wall-layer [3].

In veterinary medicine, urinary bladder tumors affects commonly dogs and the most common cancer of the canine urinary bladder is the invasive TCC of intermediate to high grade.

A study reported ultrasonographic findings such as wall involvement, heterogeneous mass and trigone location could be reliable prognostic indicators in canine TCC [18].

To our knowledge, there are no published reports using CEUS in the diagnosis of urinary bladder diseases in dogs.

In this study we describe the application of qualitative and quantitative CEUS in eight dogs affected by bladder TCC, reporting the contrast enhancement pattern and the quantification of blood flow parameters of this tumor, in order to provide a useful diagnostic tool for a more complete evaluation of the canine bladder TCC.

We hypothesized that CEUS would improve the detection of the infiltrative feature of this tumor by observing the abnormal intramural perfusion pattern.

Methods

Study population

To test our hypothesis, over a year's time (October 2015, November 2016) we recruited 8 consecutive dogs with cytopathologic diagnosis of TCC based on suction biopsy as "gold standard".

The cytological examination, reviewed by a veterinary pathologist (GM), showed scarce basophilic background, sometimes strongly hematic. Cells were represented by two types of epithelial elements. A first type consisted of single or small groups of epithelial elements in dysplastic squamous features. The second type was represented by more or less large epithelial aggregates with basophilic, vacuolated cytoplasm and rounded margins. Nuclei were single, sometimes multiple, often bulky, irregularly shaped, with angled profile or indented and abundant chromatin disposed in granules or large clusters. Anisocytosis, anisokaryosis and pleomorphism were evident. N/C ratio > 1 and the mitotic index was moderate. The findings were strongly suggestive of a cytological diagnosis of transitional cell carcinoma.

There were 3 spayed female, 2 entire female, 3 entire males. There was 1 each Saint-Bernard, Spinone Italiano dog, Cocker, Collie, Beagle and 3 mixed breed. The mean (± SD) age of the eight enrolled dogs was 6.8 (± 2.6) years (range: 3 to 10 y).

Dogs were excluded, if they had evidence of cardiac disease or a history of anaphylactic reactions to vaccines or other medications, to avoid adverse reactions due to the microbubble contrast agent. Dogs were also excluded if their complete blood count and serum biochemistry were not within normal range.

B-mode and color Doppler ultrasonography

Examinations with B-mode, Doppler ultrasonography and CEUS were performed on all dogs.

Informed owners' consents were obtained. All treatments, housing, and animal care were in compliance with EU Directive 2010/63/EU on the protection of animals used for scientific purposes and with Department's Animal Ethics Council approval (no. 13/2017).

The conventional ultrasonography and the CEUS examinations were performed by the same investigator, using a scanner[1] equipped with contrast-tuned imaging technology[2] in not sedated dogs in dorsal recumbency. Hairs over the ventral portion of the abdomen were clipped. Alcohol and coupling gel were applied to the skin.

B-mode and Color Doppler ultrasonography of bladder was performed with microconvex (5.0 to 8.0-MHz) and linear (10 to 12-MHz) transducers. Transverse and longitudinal planes were used to fully assess the bladder.

Ultrasonographic assessments of bladder masses included: size and shape (pedunculated or nonpedunculated), echo pattern (homogeneous or heterogeneous), location (apex, body, trigone or all sites), and involvement of the bladder wall. Bladder masses having uniform echogenicity or mixed echogenicity with hyperechoic and hypoechoic interior areas were recorded as "homogeneous" or "heterogeneous", respectively.

The main diagnostic criterion used to diagnose tumor infiltration of the bladder wall was the interruption of hyperechoic (submucosal) and hypoechoic (muscular) layers of the bladder wall in the site of the lesion, as described in previous reports [18].

Contrast-enhanced ultrasonography

CEUS examination was performed immediately following B-mode ultrasonography, using a linear (5.0-7.5-MHz) transducer with contrast agent capability. The mechanical index was set from 0.08 to 0.09; only 1 focal zone was used, which was placed immediately below the urinary bladder.

The contrast agent was a sulphur hexafluoride signal enhancer[3] and it was prepared in accordance with the manufacturer's recommendations. Each vial of contrast agent (which contained 25 mg of freeze-dried powder) was reconstituted by injection of 5 mL of 0.9% sodium chloride; vials then were shaken vigorously for 20 s. An aliquot (0.05 mL/kg of body weight) of the contrast medium was rapidly injected via a 3-way valve and 18-20 G catheter inserted in the cephalic vein. The contrast injection was immediately followed by a 5 mL saline flush, as previously reported [13].

Each dog received 2 bolus injections of contrast agent; the second injection of ultrasound contrast agent was 10 min later the first. The activation of a timer was performed simultaneously with the contrast agent dose inoculation.

All CEUS examinations were performed by two operators. The first operator injected the contrast medium through the catheterized vein, while the second performed the US scans of the urinary bladder.

Raw data (good-quality video clips) obtained during CEUS were stored digitally on a hard disk and subsequently they were analysed by two co-authors.

Post processing quantitative analysis of video-clips was performed by use of image-analysis software.[4] For each dog, one region of interest (ROI) was manually drawn around the entire tumor. During ROI selection adjacent portions of the bladder wall that appeared unaffected were excluded.

Contrast-enhanced TICs were generated for each ROI. Analysis of tissue perfusion was based on video SI changes over time using CEUS.

The SI of a white band in the gray scale bar (8 bit) was defined as maximal (100%) SI. Other pixels in the image were then assigned SI values based on this reference.

Within the selected ROI, during the period of enhancement, the following parameters were computed: peak enhancement, TTP perfusion, MTT, RBV and RBF. Peak enhancement (%) is defined as the percentage increase in SI - from 0 to 100 as maximal intensity - reached during transit of the contrast agent at a specific time point. The TTP (seconds) is defined as the interval until maximum SI of the contrast agent. The MTT is defined as the circulation time of the contrast agent in the examined tissue. The RBV is defined as the integral of the video SI (%) changes during the extrapolated transition time without recirculation. The RBF is defined as the ratio between regional blood volume and MTT.

A three-dimensional color map was reconstructed to visually assess regional blood flow of the corresponding bladder tumor.

Descriptive statistical analysis of quantitative CEUS-derived data included Shapiro-Wilk test, assessing the normal distribution of variables. Obtained data are expressed as mean ± standard deviation.

Results

Trans-abdominal grey-scale ultrasonography, performed on dog 1, revealed the presence of a large non pedunculated cauliflower shaped mass (40 × 40 mm), located at the level of the entire dorsal wall of the bladder and protruding into the lumen. Furthermore, it had jagged margins. The echo pattern of the mass was heterogeneous. Colour Doppler showed an abundant vascularization with more than one vascular pole (Fig. 1a and b).

In all other dogs pedunculated round shaped masses of variable size from 10 to 30 mm, located at the level of the trigone (4 cases) and apex (3 case) of the urinary bladder, protruding into the lumen were observed. Conventional B-mode and Doppler ultrasonography showed different patterns of tumors (Figs. 2a, b, 3a, b).

In all cases, the normal bladder wall was identified by ultrasound as two hyperechoic parallel thin layers and a hypoechoic layer that corresponds to the muscular layer, placed between the two previous ones. The portion of bladder wall located at base of tumor showed the loss of normal layering, that induced the suspicion of an intramural neoplastic invasion.

Contrast-enhanced ultrasound images showed in the arterial phase, at 8-9 s after the contrast injection, an avid enhancement of the tumour tissue in all dogs, with a heterogeneous enhancement in dog no. 1 and no. 3 (Figs. 1c and 3c) for the presence of several small non-enhancing areas into the contest lesion consistent with necrotic lesions, and with a homogeneous enhancement of masses in all other dogs (Fig. 2c).

Contrast-enhanced ultrasound images also showed the loss of planes between the lesion and the bladder wall layers, with disappeared hyperenhancing submucosal layer and hypoenhancing muscular layer, due to the presence of the hyperenhancing tumor tissue. The disruption of the

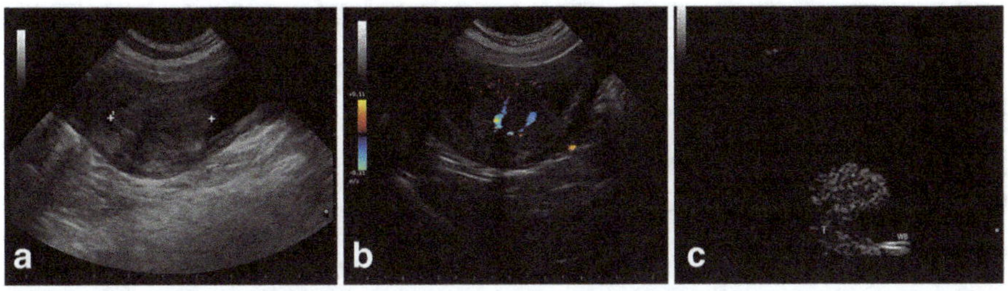

Fig. 1 6 year-old entire male Spinone Italiano dog with pedunculated round shaped mass, located at the level of the bladder apex, staged with gray-scale ultrasound and CEUS. **a**- Conventional B-mode sonography shows the bladder mass with homogeneous echo pattern and interruption of hyperechoic bladder wall by less echogenic tumor tissue. **b** – Colour Doppler shows the presence of discrete vascular poles within the mass. **c** - CEUS image shows the avid homogenous enhancement of tumour tissue and the loss of bladder wall hypoenhancing muscular layer at base of tumor due to the appearance of hyperenhancing tumor tissue (T). In the normal wall bladder (WB) adjacent to the tumour the submucosal and serous hyperenhancing lines and the hypoenhancing muscular layer were preserved

bladder wall muscular layer by enhancing tumor tissue confirms the infiltrative feature of tumour (Figs. 1c, 2c and 3c).

In the venous phase there was a slow and progressive reduction of enhancement in the tumour tissue.

Enhancement of the normal wall bladder adjacent to the tumour is almost imperceptible, throughout the arterial and venous phases. During the initial arterial phase, the bladder mural vascularization was characterized by the first appearance of the external layer, followed by small vessels perpendicular to the axis of the wall, into the hypoenhancing muscular layer, that appeared approximately 11 s after the contrast agent injection. About 22 s from the contrast dose, the submucosal layer became progressively enhanced. In the normal portions of the wall bladder the submucosal and serous hyperecoic lines were preserved (Figs. 1c, 2c, 3c).

Post-processing quantitative analysis showed a time intensity curve characterized by a rapid wash-in, a low level of SI and a slow wash-out (Fig. 4).

The three-dimensional images of regional blood flow underlined a homogeneous perfusion patterns of the tumor tissue, as well as observed during the qualitative analysis, providing a more intuitive reconstruction of vascular features that characterized the urinary bladder TCC (Fig. 5).

Descriptive statistical analysis of the quantitative CEUS-derived parameters revealed a normal distribution for each value of its mean and standard deviation, provided below: peak enhancement was 22,05 ± 1,73%; TTP was 30,38 ± 4,78 s; RBV was 1064.15 ± 184,39 L/min; RBF was 25,17 ± 3.29 L/min; MTT was 42,19 ± 3,81 s.

In all cases the contrast micro-bubbles were well tolerated by dogs and no side effects were noted.

Discussion

Transitional Cell Carcinoma is the most common malignancy of the urinary bladder in dogs (50-75%), generally invasive and often metastatic to the lung, regional lymph nodes or liver [19, 20]. Multiple risk factors for the development of canine TCC are involved, including both genetic and environmental factors. A breed predisposition (Scottish Terrier, Shetland Sheepdog, Collie, Airedale and Beagle) and a major incidence of TCC in older females were reported [19]. The most common

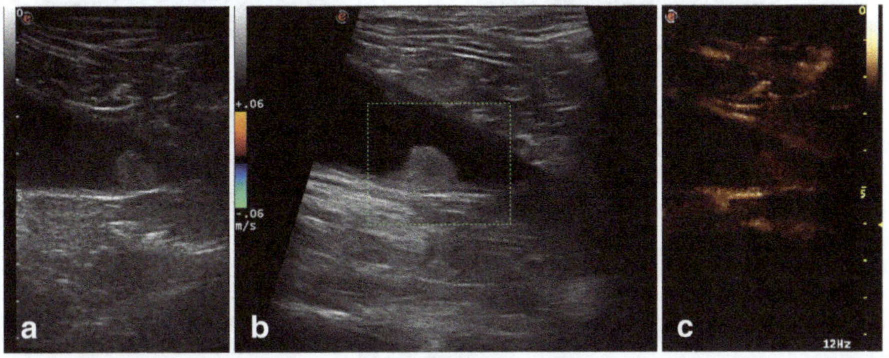

Fig. 2 9 year-old entire female mixed breed dog with nonpedunculated round shaped mass, located at the level of the bladder trigone. B-mode ultrasonography shows the bladder mass with homogeneous echo pattern and interruption of hyperechoic bladder wall by less echogenic tumor tissue (**a**), without evidence of vascular signal (**b**). CEUS image shows the avid homogenous enhancement of tumour tissue and the loss of bladder wall hypoenhancing muscular layer at base of tumor (**c**)

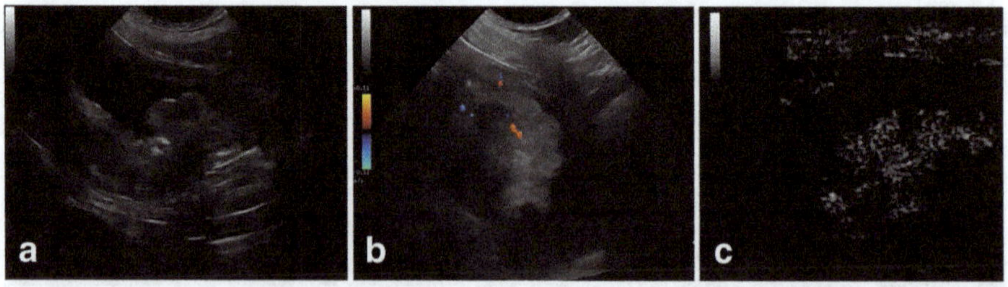

Fig. 3 3 year-old entire male Saint-Bernard dog with nonpedunculated cauliflower shaped mass, located at the level of the bladder body. **a**- Conventional B-mode sonography shows the bladder mass with heterogeneous echo pattern and interruption of hyperechoic bladder wall by less echogenic tumor tissue. **b** – Colour Doppler shows the presence of discrete vascular poles within the mass. **c** - CEUS image shows a heterogeneous enhancement of tumour tissue and the loss of bladder wall hypoenhancing muscular layer at base of tumor due to the appearance of hyperenhancing tumor tissue

clinical sign in dogs is dysuria, including haematuria, abnormally frequent and painful excretion of drop by drop urine, and it can be present for weeks to months prior to definitive diagnosis [21]. This tumor is frequently located in the trigon region of the canine urinary bladder [22–24]; sometimes an urethral involvement, that can lead to dysuria and partial or complete obstruction of the urinary tract, may be seen [25].

It is associated with short-survival time [19, 21]. Due to the progressive nature of this disease, the treatment, including the surgical excision and the combination chemotherapy, is palliative.

Diagnostic methods to detection the TCC include radiography (double contrast cystography) and ultrasound examination. Definitive diagnosis can be achieved through histopathologic examination of a tissue sample obtained by cystotomy, cystoscopy, or a catheter biopsy [22, 24].

In the present study, the diagnostic criteria of the canine TCC were based on a cytopathologic evaluation of a sample of cancerous cells obtained through an ultrasound-guided suction biopsy and smeared on slides and then stained with May-Grümwald Giemsa.

An accurate evaluation of tissue layers of the urinary bladder wall is required for diagnosing and predicting prognosis in transitional cell carcinoma, so that it can be differentiated from other benign lesions [18].

Ultrasonography is commonly used as the first-line imaging modality in order to diagnose a bladder cancer, because it is not invasive, widely available and does not require anesthesia [26]. Furthermore, the detection of tumoral angiogenesis using an imaging technique is very important to achieve a diagnosis of malignant cancers. So, imaging techniques performed with the injection of intravascular contrast agents become the gold standard to fully study an invasive bladder tumors in humans as well as in animals.

Various studies demonstrated that high-field magnetic resonance imaging and computed tomography using iodinate contrast media could be valuable for evaluation of wall involvement in human and canine bladder cancer [20, 27, 28].

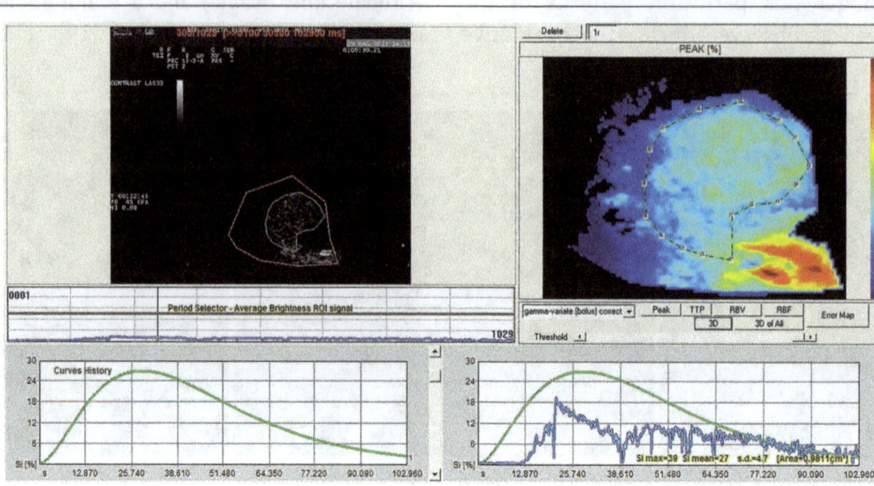

Fig. 4 Quantitative analyses performed after injection of contrast agent with dedicated perfusion software. Time-intensity curve was created from the ROI positioned in the tumor tissue of a representative dog with urinary bladder TCC. The jagged gray line was generated from actual data, whereas the curved black line was generated from data fitted by use of a corrected γ function

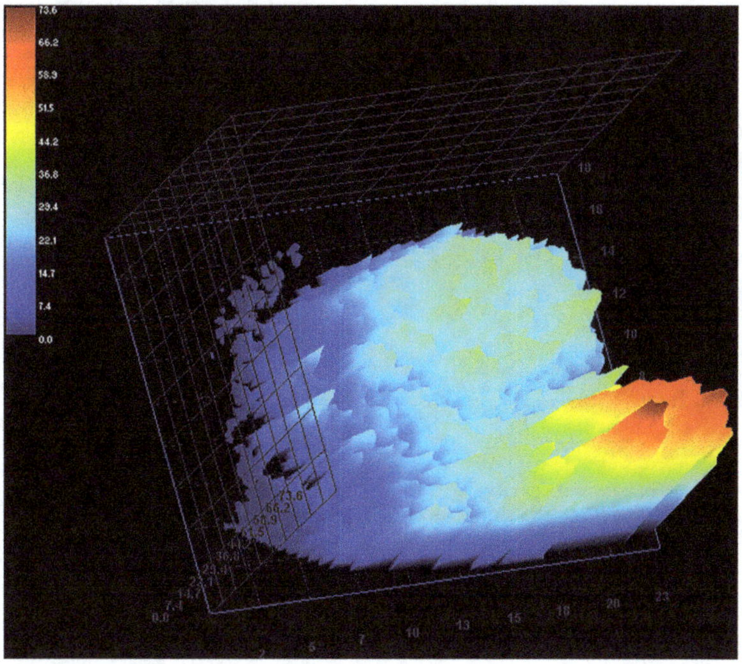

Fig. 5 Three-dimensional CEUS reconstruction demonstrating regional blood flow of the tumor tissue during the wash-in phase in a dog with urinary bladder TCC, expressed in arbitrary units of signal intensity. Note the homogeneous perfusion pattern of the tumor tissue

However, in clinical practice computed tomography and magnetic resonance imaging scan require anesthesia, are very expensive and therefore not widely available and sometimes unsafe because of adverse reactions associated with the use of iodine as a contrast medium.

So, CEUS may play a role in urinary bladder diagnostic field, being helpful in differentiating pathological entities, as clots or surgical wall changes, from bladder cancer, detecting bladder tumour neovascularisation enhancement [14].

In human medicine, qualitative contrast ultrasound has been used to identify bladder tumors and to evaluate enhancement patterns [14, 29].

Some Authors showed that CEUS had a very high sensitivity for the presence of human bladder cancer and that it is very sensitive in revealing tumor microvascularisation [14].

In veterinary medicine, some Authors reported that in canine urinary bladder lesions wall involvement, as revealed by B-mode ultrasound, was significantly ($P =$ 0.00005) associated with histological muscular layer involvement with a sensitivity of 93% and specificity of 92%, showing that this ultrasonographic finding could be reliable indicator of prognosis in canine transitional cell carcinoma [18].

A recent study was carried out to evaluate the feasibility of using contrast-enhanced cadence contrast pulse sequencing ultrasound estimates of microvascular density to predict clinical and angiogenic response to treatment in dogs affected by bladder tumors undergoing to chemotherapy [30].

In our study, using a contrast-tuned imaging technology, CEUS provided useful clinical information and defined a vascular enhancement patterns and calculated parameters associated with TCC.

The purely intravascular contrast agent provide detailed viewing of the microvascular pattern of the tumor lesion and a more accurate reading of ultrasound images.

The qualitative analysis showed a hyperechoic CEUS pattern of the tissue tumor. Previously hypoperfused muscle layer under the mass became hyperenhanced, suggesting that the tumor had infiltrated the bladder wall.

These findings support the use of detailed evaluation of the bladder wall by CEUS for prediction of prognosis in canine TCC, although further studies could be advisable for targeting differential diagnosis among TCC and other proliferative lesions of the canine urinary bladder.

The quantification of blood flow parameters was also reported, although the qualitative analysis of perfusion pattern is more reliable in arriving to a definitive diagnosis. In fact, the ultrasound enhancement measurements may be influenced by several patient-related (i.e. cardiac output, blood pressure, respiratory rate and interactions with the contrast medium) and technical variables related factors (i.e. scanner setting, gain setting, type, preparation and injection protocol of the contrast medium), all of which are potential source of variability.

Conclusions

In conclusion, our results must be interpreted in light of the relatively small number of dogs enrolled. We believe that this finding should be included in contrast ultrasonography of the canine TCC. CEUS exam may be a useful, noninvasive and reproducible tool for detecting tumors that infiltrate the muscle layer of the bladder wall.

Endnotes

[1]Mylab 40/Vet, Esaote, Genova, Italy.
[2]CnTI, Esaote, Genova, Italy.
[3]SonoVue®, Bracco Imaging, Milan, Italy.
[4]Qontrast™, Bracco, Milan, Italy.

Abbreviations

CEUS: Contrast-enhanced ultrasonography; MTT: Mean transit time; RBF: Regional blood flow; RBV: Regional blood volume; ROI: Region of interest; SI: Signal intensity; TCC: Transitional cell carcinoma; TIC: Time-intensity curve; TTP: Time to peak

Acknowledgments

No third-party funding or support was received in connection with this study or the writing or publication of the manuscript.

Authors' contribution

FM, MDM and SDP conceived the study. FM, MDM, CM performed the diagnostic examinations. FM, SDP and MDM performed the CEUS off-line quantification analysis, statistical analysis and wrote the manuscript. MP managed the patients and contrast media during the ultrasounds and contributed to reviewing the manuscript. SM, NMI and VA analyzed the data and assisted to drafting the manuscript. GM performed the cytological examinations of the urinary bladder catheter biopsies and assisted in drafting the manuscript. All authors read and approved the final manuscript.

Funding

None.

Consent for publication

Not applicable.

Competing interests

The authors declare that they have no competing interests.

References

1. Piscaglia F, Nolsoe C, Dietrisch DO, Cosgrove DO, Gilja OH, et al. The EFSUMB guidelines and recommendations on the clinical practice of contrast enhanced ultrasound (CEUS): update 2011 on non-hepatic applications. Ultraschall Med. 2012;33:33–59.
2. Ohlerth S, O'Brien RT. Contrast ultrasound: general principles and veterinary clinical applications. Vet J. 2007;174:501–12.
3. Caruso G, Salvaggio G, Campisi A, Melloni D, Midiri M, Bertolotto M, Lagalla R. Bladder tumor staging: comparison of contrast-enhanced ultrasound and gray-scale. AJR Am J Roentgenol. 2010;194:151–6.
4. Tang MX, Mulvana H, Gauthier T, Lim AKP, Cosgrove DO, Eckersley RJE, Stride E. Quantitative contrast-enhanced ultrasound imaging: a review of sources of variability. Interface Focus. 2011;1:520 39.
5. Seiler GS, Brown JC, Reetz JA, Taeymans O, Bucknoff M, Rossi F, et al. Safety of contrast-enhanced ultrasonography in dogs and cats: 488 cases (2002–2011). J Am Vet Med Ass. 2013;242:1255–9.
6. Ziegler LE, O'Brien RT, Waller KR, Zagzebsky JA. Quantitative contrast harmonic ultrasound imaging of normal canine liver. Vet Radiol Ultrasound. 2003;44:451–4.
7. Nyman HT, Kristensen AT, Kjelgaard-Hansen M, Mc Evoy F. Contrast-enhanced ultrasonography in normal canine liver. Evaluation of imaging and safety parameters. Vet Radiol Ultrasound. 2005;46:243–50.
8. Nakamura K, Sasaki N, Yoshikawa M, Ohta H, Hwang SJ, Mimura T, Yamasaki M, Takiguchi M. Quantitative contrast-enhanced ultrasonography of canine spleen. Vet Radiol Ultrasound. 2009;50:104–8.
9. O'Brien RT, Lani M, Matheson J, Delaney F, Young K. Contrast harmonic ultrasound of spontaneous liver nodules in 32 dogs. Vet Radiol Ultrasound. 2004;45:547–53.
10. Webster N, Holloway A. Use of contrast ultrasonography in the diagnosis of metastatic feline visceral haemangiosarcoma. J Feline Med Surg. 2008;10: 388–94.
11. Kanemoto H, Ohno K, Nakashima K, Takahashi M, Fujino Y, Nishimura R, Tsujimoto H. Characterization of canine focal liver lesions with contrast-enhanced ultrasound using a novel contrast agent—Sonazoid. Vet Radiol Ultrasound. 2009;50:188–94.
12. Haers H, Vignoli M, Paes G, Rossi F, Taeymans O, Daminet S, Saunders JH. Contrast harmonic ultrasonographic appearance of focal space-occupying renal lesions. Vet Radiol Ultrasound. 2010;51:516–22.
13. Macrì F, Di Pietro S, Liotta L, Palumbo Piccionello A, Pugliese M, De Majo M. Effects of size and location of regions of interest examined by use of contrast-enhanced ultrasonography on renal perfusion variables of dogs. Am J Vet Res. 2016;77(8):869–76.
14. Nicolau C, Bunesch L, Peri L, Salvador R, Corral JM, Mallofre C, Sebastia C. Accuracy of contrast-enhanced ultrasound in the detection of bladder cancer. Br J Radiol. 2011;84:1091–9.
15. Drudi FM, Di Leo N, Maghella F, Malpassini F, Iera J, Rubini A, Orsogna N, D' Ambrosio F. CEUS in the study of bladder, method, administration and evaluation, in technical notes. J Ultrasound. 2013;17:57–63.
16. Drudi FM, Cantisani V, Liberatore M, Iori F, Erturk SM, Cristini C, Di Pierro G, D'Ambrosio U, Malpassini F, De Felice C, Di Leo N. Role of low mechanical index CEUS in the differentiation between low and high grade bladder carcinoma: a pilot study. Ultraschall Med. 2010;31:589–95.
17. Li QY, Tang J, He EH, Li YM, Zhou Y, Zhang X, Chen G. Clinical utility of three-dimensional contrast-enhanced ultrasound in the differentiation between noninvasive and invasive neoplasms of urinary bladder. Eur J Radiol. 2012;81:2936–42.
18. Hanazono K, Fukumoto S, Endo Y, Ueno H, Kadosawa T, Uchide T. Ultrasonographic findings related to prognosis in canine transitional cell carcinoma. Vet Radiol Ultrasound. 2013;55:79–84.
19. Knapp DW, Ramos-Vara JA, Moore GE, Dhawan D, Bonney PL, Young KE. Urinary bladder cancer in dogs, a naturally occurring model for cancer biology and drug development. ILAR J. 2014;55:100–18.
20. Lee K, Choi S, Choi S, Lee Y. Clinical experience of MRI in two dogs with muscle-invasive transitional cell carcinoma of the urinary bladder. J Vet Med Sci. 2016;78:1351–4.
21. Knapp DW, McMillan SK. Tumors of the urinary system. In: Withrow SJ, Vail D, Page R, editors. Withrow & MacEwen's small animal clinical oncology. St. Louis: Elsevier -Saunders; 2013. p. 572–82.
22. Caswell M. Transitional cell carcinoma of the urinary bladder in a 14-year-old dog. Can Vet J. 2011;52:673–5.
23. Henry CJ. Management of transitional cell carcinoma. Vet Clin North Am Small Anim Pract. 2003;33:597–613.
24. Mutsaers AJ, Widmer WR, Knapp DW. Canine transitional cell carcinoma. J Vet Intern Med. 2003;17:136–44.
25. Budreckis DM, Byrne BA, Pollard RE, Rebhun RB. Rodriguez CO Jr, Skorupski KA. Bacterial urinary tract infections associated with transitional cell carcinoma in dogs. J Vet Intern Med. 2015;29:828–33.
26. Nicolau C, Bunesch L, Sebastia C, Salvador R. Diagnosis of bladder cancer: contrast-enhanced ultrasound. Abdom Imaging. 2010;35:494–503.
27. Babjuk M, Oosterlinck W, Sylvester R, Kaasinen E, Böhle A, Palou-Redorta J. European Association of Urology (EAU). EAU guidelines on non-muscle invasive urothelial carcinoma of the bladder. Eur Urol. 2008;54:303–14.
28. Razavi SA, Sadigh G, Kelly AM, Cronin P. Comparative effectiveness of imaging modalities for the diagnosis of upper and lower urinary tract malignancy: a critically appraised topic. Acad Radiol. 2012;19:1134–40.

29. Wang X, Xu P, Wang Y, Grant EG. Contrast-enhanced ultrasonographic findings of different histopathologic types of breast cancer. Acta Radiol. 2011;52:248–55.
30. Pollard RE, Watson KD, Hu X, Ingham E, Ferrara KW. Feasibility of quantitative contrast ultrasound imaging of bladder tumors in dogs. Can Vet J. 2017;58:70–2.

10

Canine atlantoaxial optimal safe implantation corridors – description and validation of a novel 3D presurgical planning method using OsiriX™

Guillaume Leblond[1], Luis Gaitero[1*], Noel M. Moens[1], Alex zur Linden[1], Fiona M. K. James[1], Gabrielle Monteith[1] and John Runciman[2]

Abstract

Background: Canine ventral atlantoaxial (AA) stabilization is most commonly performed in very small dogs and is technically challenging due to extremely narrow bone corridors. Multiple implantation sites have been suggested but detailed anatomical studies investigating these sites are lacking and therefore current surgical guidelines are based upon approximate anatomical landmarks. In order to study AA optimal safe implantation corridors (OSICs), we developed a method based on computed tomography (CT) and semi-automated three-dimensional (3D) mathematical modelling using OsiriX™ and Microsoft®Excel software. The objectives of this study were 1- to provide a detailed description of the bone corridor analysis method and 2- to assess the reproducibility of the method. CT images of the craniocervical junction were prospectively obtained in 27 dogs and our method of OSIC analysis was applied in all dogs. For each dog, 13 optimal implant sites were simulated via geometrical simplification of the bone corridors. Each implant 3D position was then defined with respect to anatomical axes using 2 projected angles (ProjA). The safety margins around each implant were also estimated with angles (SafA) measured in 4 orthogonal directions. A sample of 12 simulated implants was randomly selected and each mathematically calculated angle was compared to direct measurements obtained within OsiriX™ from 2 observers repeated twice. The landmarks simulating anatomical axes were also positioned 4 times to determine their effect on ProjA reproducibility.

Results: OsiriX could be used successfully to simulate optimal implant positions in all cases. There was excellent agreement between the calculated and measured values for both ProjA ($\rho_c = 0.9986$) and SafA ($\rho_c = 0.9996$). Absolute differences between calculated and measured values were respectively [ProjA = 0.44 ± 0.53°; SafA = 0.27 ± 0.25°] and [ProjA = 0.26 ± 0.21°; SafA = 0.18 ± 0.18°] for each observer. The 95 % tolerance interval comparing ProjA obtained with 4 different sets of anatomical axis landmarks was [−1.62°, 1.61°] which was considered appropriate for clinical use.

Conclusions: A new method for determination of optimal implant placement is provided. Semi-automated calculation of optimal implant 3D positions could be further developed to facilitate preoperative planning and to generate large descriptive anatomical datasets.

Keywords: Canine, Atlantoaxial joint, Atlantoaxial surgery, Computed tomography, Three-dimensional, Neurosurgical methods

(Continued on next page)

* Correspondence: lgaitero@uoguelph.ca
[1]Department of Clinical Studies, Ontario Veterinary College, University of Guelph, Guelph, ON N1G 2W1, Canada
Full list of author information is available at the end of the article

(Continued from previous page)

Abbreviations: 3D, Three-dimensional; AA, Atlantoaxial; AAI, Atlantoaxial instability; C1, Atlas; C2, Axis; CT, Computed tomography; DICOM, Digital imaging and communication in medicine; MPR, Multi-planar reconstruction; OSIC(s), Optimal safe implantation corridor(s); ProjA, Projected angle; ROI(s), Region(s) of interest; SafA, Safety angle; TSF, Transarticular screw fixation; VR, Volume rendering

Background

Canine AA instability (AAI) has been treated via surgical stabilization for almost 50 years [1]. Methods of stabilization have evolved from simple dorsal AA sutures to ventral transarticular screw fixation (TSF) and more complex constructs composed of multiple ventral implants embedded in polymethylmethacrylate cement [2–6]. Despite overall satisfactory outcomes obtained with modern procedures [6–8], ventral AA stabilization remains technically challenging and is associated with relatively high mortality rates (5 %) [8].

The small size of affected dogs and extremely narrow bone corridors used to position stabilizing implants are often considered major technical limitations of these procedures [9, 10]. These technical difficulties have led neurosurgeons to develop novel techniques to either improve accuracy of implant placement or to multiply the number of implants to better distribute the load applied on the stabilizing construct [2–6, 9, 10]. Complications directly resulting from such narrow bone corridors include iatrogenic bone fracture and violation of the vertebral canal by the stabilizing implants. Both of these complications can have disastrous consequences for the patient either by compromising the stability of the construct or by causing iatrogenic spinal cord injury. Although the incidence of either complication in canine AA stabilization is unknown, experimental studies on ventral placement of pedicular and monocortical implants in other cervical vertebrae have demonstrated that vertebral canal violation is common [11, 12]. It can be hypothesized that vertebral canal violation in AA stabilization is likely as common and underestimated by clinicians given that radiographs have a low sensitivity to detect vertebral canal violation and that postoperative CT is not commonly performed in veterinary medicine [13].

In human medicine, extensive precautions are taken to avoid both vertebral canal violation and vertebral artery injury when performing cervical and AA stabilization. Routine stabilization procedures rely on readily available anatomical data defining OSICs, preoperative planning using advanced imaging and various imaging-based intraoperative guidance techniques [14–19]. In veterinary spinal surgery, preoperative planning is often limited and intraoperative neuronavigation is not routinely available, leaving neurosurgeons with the descriptive data provided by the literature to guide implant placement.

Traditionally, vertebral OSICs have been characterized using radiographic and CT images. This has been achieved by identifying a theoretical plane within which the optimal implant is to be positioned. Using such a predefined plane allows simplification of a complex 3D problem into a bidimensional description. This method has been applied successfully along most of the vertebral column because stabilizing implants are typically positioned within the transverse plane of each vertebra [20–23]. However, most of the reported atlas (C1) and axis (C2) implantation sites have an oblique direction precluding the use of these traditional methods. As a result, AA implant sites have been subjectively defined without detailed anatomical description. The only OSIC that has been more precisely studied in dogs is the corridor used for TSF fixation [5, 9]. However, available studies have used different subjective definitions of the optimal implant position and therefore obtained slightly different results. Overall, precise objective surgical guidelines are currently lacking for AA ventral stabilization.

Our initial objective was to provide data to the veterinary community describing as precisely as possible optimized methods of AA stabilization. As we began to work on the description of optimal implant positioning, we realized that a new method of analysis of bone corridors would be necessary to precisely depict the complex 3D interrelationships between anatomical structures and implants. Therefore, we planned to develop a novel approach for the analysis of CT 3D data, using the Digital Imaging and Communication in Medicine (DICOM) software OsiriX™. In order to apply this method in a time-efficient manner, a mathematical model was also developed to semi-automatize the process.

In the present study, our objective was to describe and validate this new method of bone corridor analysis. We hypothesized 1- that mathematical calculations would have high concordance when compared to manual measures, and 2- that predefined anatomical landmarks could be used reliably to calculate 3D implant coordinates.

Methods

Preliminary review of the literature

An extensive online literature search was conducted prior to the study in order to identify available descriptions of canine AA anatomy as well as bone corridors previously used for ventral AA stabilization. Both

PubMed and Google scholar search engines were used to identify pertinent publications with the search terms "ventral atlantoaxial dog", "atlantoaxial instability dog" or "atlantoaxial subluxation dog". When using Google scholar, only the first 250 references were assessed for relevance. Articles written in a language other than English were excluded. All identified journal articles and textbook chapters describing AA anatomy or ventral AA stabilization techniques were reviewed in detail, including identification of pertinent cited references which were also reviewed.

Study population and CT image acquisition

Between October 2012 and December 2013, dogs were prospectively recruited in order to obtain a CT scan of their craniocervical region. The objective was to recruit approximately 10 dogs affected with AAI and 20 dogs with a normal AA joint (including 10 Toy breed dogs and 10 Beagle dogs). Toy breed dogs were defined as dogs with a body weight less than 5 kg. A minimal age of 6 months was subjectively selected to avoid excessive anatomical variations due to growth stage. The CT scans obtained from dogs with a normal AA joint were either obtained from cadavers or client owned animals anesthetized at the Ontario Veterinary College Health Sciences Centre for clinical reasons unrelated to this study after owner consent was obtained. For AAI dogs, obtaining a CT scan of the AA region is standard-of-care practice for diagnostic workup and/or pre-surgical planning in our institution. A diagnosis of AAI was reached if dens separation, agenesis, or hypoplasia was identified in conjunction with clinical signs consistent with a cranial cervical myelopathy or if unequivocal AA subluxation was visible in the CT study.

CT images of the craniocervical junction were obtained using a 16 slice detector GE Brightspeed CT scanner.[1] The raw data was acquired with a standardized protocol in helical mode, 1.0 s rotation time, 0.562:1 pitch, 120 kV and 250mAs, 25 cm collimation, 512x512 matrix size, 0.488 mm in plane resolution, 0.625 mm through plane resolution using both standard and bone algorithms. Both algorithms were reviewed but only the images captured in a bone algorithm were used for OSIC analysis. The images were subsequently imported into the free version of OsiriX™ DICOM viewer[2] using an Apple® computer.[3] The images were reviewed using the window width and level preset in OsiriX™ for bone CT images in the 2D viewer, 3D multi-planar reconstruction (MPR) and 3D volume rendering (VR) modes.

3D optimal implant simulation using OsiriX™

In order to define objective optimal implant placements for each available bone corridor, we developed a method based on geometrical simplification of the bone corridors. The purpose of this simplification was to obtain 3D geometrical shapes with well-defined centered axes, that could then be used to define optimal implant placements. To be surgically applicable, the insertion point for each implant had to be located on the ventral surface of C1 or C2. The geometrical shapes simulating the bone corridors were delineated in OsiriX™ by placing region of interest (ROI) points either in 3D-MPR mode or 3D-VR mode. These ROI points were subsequently used as landmarks in 3D-MPR mode to determine centered axes of the bone corridors using various geometrical methods (Fig. 1). Each optimal implant placement could then be simulated by placing 2 ROI points along the centered axis representing the insertion and exit points of the implant. Further details on how each specific bone corridor was geometrically simplified and each optimal implant placement was obtained is provided in additional files (see Additional file 1).

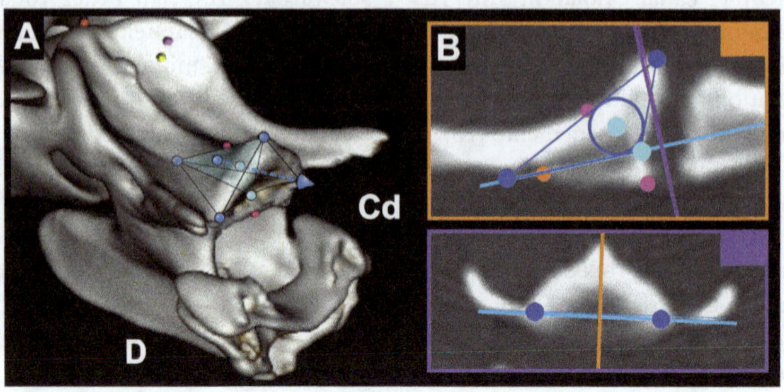

Fig. 1 Principles of determination of optimal implant placement using the geometrically centered method. **a** Example of simplification of a bone corridor into a pyramidal shape (*theoretical black lines*) using ROI points (*in blue*) placed in 3D-VR mode. An optimal implant can be positioned using an axis centered within the pyramid (blue dashed line). **b** This centered axis is determined in 3D-MPR mode using ROI points (*in blue*) as landmarks and geometrical shapes (*dark blue lines*) [see Additional file 1 for more details]. D: dorsal; Cd: caudal. ROI points in other colors correspond to different implant sites

Determination of optimal implant 3D coordinates by manual measurements

Each implant direction was defined using 2 ProjA on anatomical planes, which were used as 3D coordinates (Fig. 2a). It is important to note that projections onto anatomical planes are not identical between C1 and C2 because of the significant range of motion existing between these vertebrae. In this study, a projection on C1 anatomical planes was operated for C1 implants and respectively for C2 implants. Transarticular implants involving C1 and C2 were defined using C1 projections. OsiriX™ allowed determination of the ProjA by aligning 3D-MPR planes with anatomical planes. This was achieved by identifying 1 anatomical plane and 1 anatomical axis. For both C1 and C2, the sagittal plane was defined as the plane of symmetry of the vertebra which was determined in 3D-MPR mode. Then, an anatomical axis was identified in the sagittal plane to complete the alignment of all 3 planes. For C1, the ventrodorsal axis was defined as the sagittal cranial border of C1 dorsal and ventral arches. For C2, the craniocaudal axis was defined as the sagittal ventral border of the C2 vertebral foramen (Fig. 2b). Once anatomical alignment was obtained in 3D-MPR mode, ProjA could be measured manually by centering the intersection of the 3 planes on the insertion point followed by shifting the plane of interest until the exit point was visualized (Fig. 2c).

Estimation of the safety margins of each OSIC by manual measurements

In order to provide an estimation of the safety margins associated with each implant site, we developed a new method considering both the bone margins and the diameter of the implant used. The general principle of the method was to study the bone corridor associated with each optimal implant site in 2 subjectively defined orthogonal planes using OsiriX™ 3D-MPR mode. In each of these planes, 2 safety margins were determined by rotating the central axis of the implant away from the optimal position around the insertion point until the implant position became considered unsafe (either due to inappropriate bone purchase or violation of vital structures). Bone purchase was considered inappropriate when the virtual implant central axis reached a line tangent to the inner surface of the near (cis) vertebral cortex. Vital structures included the spinal cord, nerve roots or blood vessels passing through or in between C1 and C2. These structures were delineated in CT images by the vertebral, lateral, alar, transverse and intervertebral foramen. The first point encountered along each rotation of the implant that was causing it to become unsafe was identified by placing an ROI point representing a safety margin of the bone corridor. For sagittal implants directed toward the vertebral canal, 75 % of the corridor length was used to position safety margin points. This method allowed identification of 4 safety margin points for each bone corridor. SafA could then be determined using the optimal implant ROI points, the safety margin ROI points and circles simulating the implant diameter as demonstrated in Fig. 3.

Mathematical determination of optimal implant 3D coordinates and OSIC safety margins

The methods of determination of ProjA and SafA described above were considered excessively time consuming to apply on a large sample size and to be used

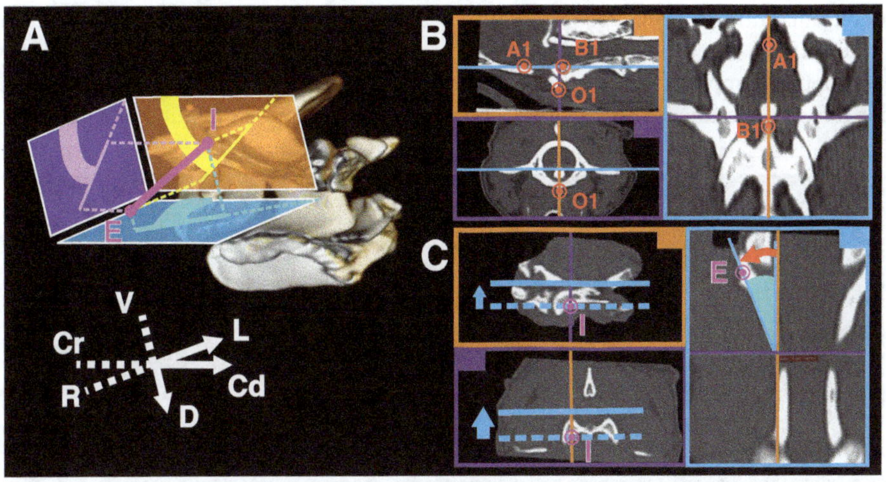

Fig. 2 Manual measurement of ProjA using OsiriX™. **a** Sagittal, transverse and dorsal ProjA can be used as the implant 3D coordinates. **b** To determine ProjA using OsiriX™ 3D-MPR mode, the 3 planes are first aligned with the anatomical planes (points OAB are used as landmarks – see Fig. 4). **c** ProjA measurement is obtained by shifting the plane of projection from the insertion point (I) to the exit point (E) of the studied implant (this is an example of dorsal ProjA). V: ventral; D: dorsal; R: right; L: left; Cr: cranial; Cd: caudal

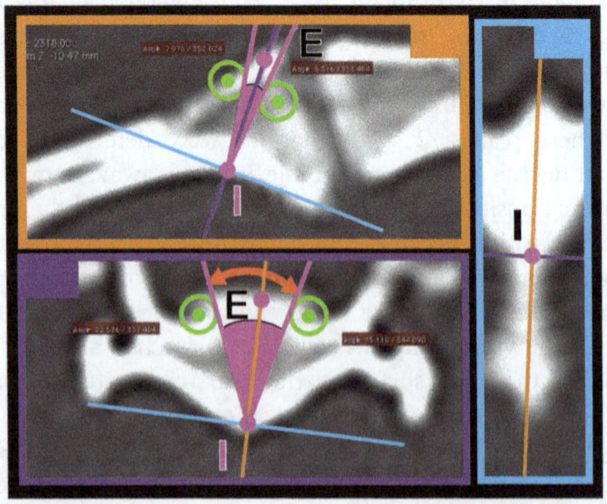

Fig. 3 Manual method of determination of SafA using OsiriX™ 3D-MPR mode. First, 2 orthogonal planes containing the safety margin points (*green points*) are identified. The intersection of these 2 planes simulates the implant site (IE). Then, circles of the same diameter as the simulated implant are positioned around the safety point (*green circles*). Tangent lines to each circle passing through the insertion point are used to measure SafA (*red arrows*)

routinely in the clinical setting. Given that we intended to study multiple implant sites in approximately 30 dogs, we elected to develop a method of mathematical calculation of these angles that would be more time efficient. All mathematical calculations were performed using Microsoft® Excel software.[4] The calculations were based on the CT 3D coordinates of the ROI points simulating the optimal implants and their respective safety margins. An open-source OsiriX™ plugin[5] allowing exportation of 3D coordinates into Microsoft® Excel was used to optimize the process and limit the risk of error while transferring the 3D data.

Mathematical determination of ProjA required advanced vectorial calculations (see Additional file 2 for details). Briefly, each optimal implant was considered as a vector oriented from its insertion to exit point. The coordinates of these points provided by the CT scan could not be directly utilized for ProjA calculations. Instead, a change of coordinate system (also called change of basis) was performed to provide vector coordinates defined with respect to the anatomical axes. This was achieved by defining anatomical coordinate systems for C1 and C2 using 3 ROI points strategically selected in the sagittal plane of each vertebra (Fig. 4a). Once the coordinates of the vector were determined with respect to the anatomical axes, the ProjA could easily be calculated using standard trigonometric equations (Fig. 4b). Each step of the calculations was then entered into a Microsoft® Excel sheet semi-automating the process.

Mathematical equations for calculation of the SafA could be established through trigonometry as depicted in Fig. 5a. The CT coordinates of the safety margins ROI points could be used without any change of basis, as these angles are defined with respect to the axis of the optimal implant. The diameter of the implant used had to be known to calculate SafA. The same safety margin ROI points could also be used to estimate the width of the bone corridor in both orthogonal planes as depicted in Fig. 5b. An example of the spreadsheet with all pre-entered equations for all 13 implant sites is provided as an additional file (see Additional file 3).

Mathematical model validation and estimation of angle measurement errors

In order to validate our semi-automated method of determination of ProjA and SafA, a complete OSIC simulation was performed by 1 author (GL) including simulation of 13 optimal implants (2 ROIs/implant), safety margins (4 ROIs/implant) and C1/C2 anatomical axes (6 ROIs/dog) in all dogs. A sample of 12 dogs was then randomly selected within the recruited population and 1 implant was randomly selected for each dog using random numbers generated with SAS OnlineDoc® software.[6] Prior to any angle measurements and calculation, the ROI points simulating the selected optimal implant

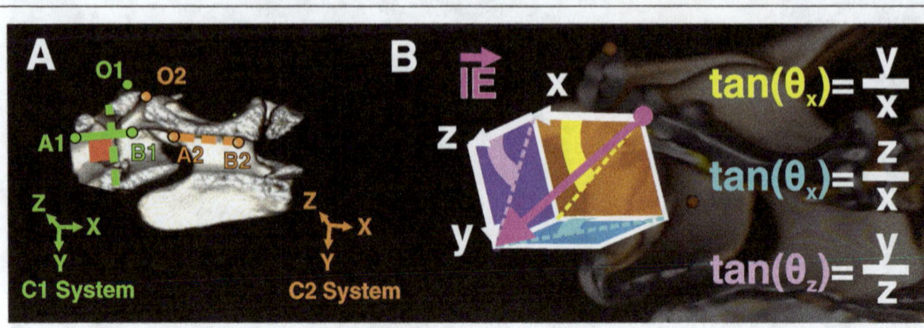

Fig. 4 Trigonometric equations used for ProjA calculations based on anatomical coordinates. **a** Anatomical coordinate systems were defined for C1 and C2 by positioning 3 points (O, A, B) in the sagittal plane of each vertebra. The point O represents the origin of the coordinate system, while (AB) represents the craniocaudal axis (X). **b** Geometrical demonstration of sagittal (*yellow*), dorsal (*blue*) and transverse (*purple*) ProjA (Θ) calculation based on anatomical coordinates (x, y, z) of a vector ($\overrightarrow{IE}$)

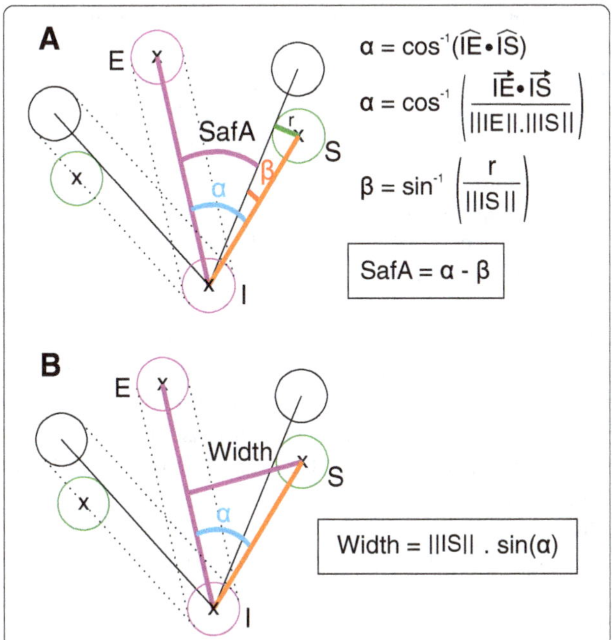

Fig. 5 Geometrical demonstration of SafA and OSIC width calculations. **a** Method of SafA calculation; (**b**) Method of OSIC width calculation. In the schematics, the IE segment represents the optimal implant position (*in pink*) and the S point is the safety margin identified on CT images by rotating the axis of the implant around its insertion point until the position is considered unsafe. The insertion point (I), exit point (E), safety margin (S), and radius of the implant (r) are all known entities

and its associated anatomical coordinate system and safety margins were imported in OsiriX™ for each dog. These ROI points were then used to determine 2 ProjA and 4 SafA mathematically and compared to measures obtained manually for each of the 12 selected implants. The manual measures were obtained by 2 observers (AZ and GL) and repeated after a 1-week interval. For determination of SafA, implant diameter was subjectively set at 1.5 mm. Agreements between the calculated values and manual measures and 95 % tolerance limit intervals were determined to validate the mathematical model.

In order to estimate the error generated by the operator when measuring ProjA and SafA manually, calculated values were considered as gold standard. The measurement error was determined for each observer by calculating the absolute difference between the manually measured and calculated values.

In order to estimate the error on ProjA measurements generated by the operator when identifying the anatomical axes, 6 ROI points representing the anatomical coordinate systems of C1 (O_1, A_1, B_1) and C2 (O_2, A_2, B_2) were positioned by 2 observers (AZ and GL) with 2 repeats in all 12 dogs. This provided 4 sets of 6 ROIs per dog, each representing the same anatomical axes with a slight variation due to operator variability. To estimate the effect of this variability on ProjA values, all previously determined ROI points representing all of the studied implant sites (13/dog) were imported into OsiriX™ for all 12 dogs. For each implant site, 2 ProjA were calculated 4 times based on the 4 coordinate systems obtained by the 2 observers. Because the exact position of the anatomical axes cannot be objectively determined, the mean of the 4 repeats of each ProjA values was used as gold standard for that part of the study. Agreements and absolute error between each of the 4 obtained values and the gold standard as well as 95 % tolerance limit intervals were determined to estimate the ProjA calculation error. Agreements and 95 % tolerance limit intervals were also determined between observers, between repeats and within subsamples (specific coordinate systems or specific projection planes) in order to identify the most significant sources of error.

Statistical analysis

Agreements between different methods of angle determination (automatically calculated vs manual) and between repeated measures were obtained using the Bland-Altman method and concordance correlation. This method also allowed calculation of 95 % tolerance intervals, representing the range of values that would theoretically be obtained for a single measure with 95 % probability. These values estimated the reproducibility of the method which is defined as the degree to which repeated measurements provide similar results [24]. Statistical analysis of the data was performed using statistical software SAS OnlineDoc®. Statistical significance was set at a maximum p value of 0.05.

Results

Sampled population and CT images acquisition

Over the recruitment period, 27 dogs were recruited to participate in this study. The recruited population differed slightly from the initial objective and included 9 mature Beagle dog cadavers, 13 Toy breed dogs with a normal AA joint and 5 Toy breed dogs affected with AAI. One unaffected Toy breed dog was 3 weeks younger than our inclusion criteria but was not excluded given the CT images revealed complete fusion of the vertebral growth plates suggesting the AA region had reached adult stage. CT images of the craniocervical junction were successfully obtained in 25 dogs using the pre-established protocol. In 2 AAI dogs, the slice thickness was set at 1.25 mm instead of 0.625 mm due to a protocol error.

Definition of AA OSICs and simulation of optimal implant 3D positions

The online search of the literature identified 32 pertinent references [4–7, 9, 10, 22, 25–49]. Upon review of these references, 9 safe bone corridors were defined corresponding to anatomical parts of the AA vertebrae. These bone corridors included the lateral masses (C1, bilateral), ventral arch (C1, sagittal), cranial articular surfaces (C2, bilateral), cranial vertebral body (C2, sagittal), pedicles (C2, bilateral) and caudal vertebral body (C2, sagittal). Each corridor was simplified into a geometrical shape, including pyramids, prisms and hemi-ellipsoids (Fig. 6). The general principle used to simulate optimal implants was to identify well-defined centered axes of the geometrical shapes (see Additional file 1). In addition, a transarticular optimal implant position was defined (C1-C2, bilateral) using the lateral mass corridors to define its axis and the ventral surface of C2 to position its insertion point. For the caudal vertebral body corridor, 3 different centered implant positions could be defined. Therefore in total, 13 optimal implant sites could be objectively defined (Fig. 6). For implants located in the sagittal plane, a traditional method was used by identifying 1 point of the optimal axis within the sagittal plane which was then used in 3D-MPR mode to center the implant axis (see Additional file 1).

The method of OSIC analysis was used successfully in all 27 cases although some limitations were observed while positioning ROI points. Even though OsiriX™ 3D modes generated continuous 3D space, ROI points placed in 3D-MPR or 3D-VR modes remained associated to specific slices. In other words, the space located between each slice could not be represented using ROI points. Another seemingly random difficulty encountered in 3D-VR mode was an occasional software glitch when placing ROI points. Instead of positioning the point on the visible bone surface, the point would be placed on the opposite side of the vertebra. This malfunction could be overcome by positioning the vertebra so that the bone surface of interest was tangent to the operator view.

Validation of the mathematical model and estimation of measurement errors

The raw data of manually measured and calculated values from the 2 observers is presented in Table 1. The 2 CT studies that had 1.25 mm slice thickness (instead of 0.625 mm) were excluded from the random sampling process. Sagittal implants were also excluded due to only 1 projected angle value defining them.

Excellent agreement was observed between the calculated and measured values for both ProjA ($\rho_c = 0.9986$) and SafA ($\rho_c = 0.9996$). The 95 % tolerance intervals obtained by concordance analysis to estimate operator-induced error for manual angle measurements by comparison to semi-automated calculations (gold standard) were respectively, [−1.23°,1.20°] and [−0.65°,0.70°] for ProjA and SafA. Absolute errors were, respectively, [ProjA = 0.44 ± 0.53°; SafA = 0.27 ± 0.25°] and [ProjA = 0.26 ± 0.21°; SafA = 0.18 ± 0.18°], for each observer. Results from this concordance analysis and measurement errors are summarized in Tables 2 and 3, and graphically represented in Fig. 7. These results implied that our mathematical model was in agreement with manual measures and that manual measurement of these angles was very reproducible with minimal operator-induced error.

Validation of the anatomical axes simulation and estimation of the error induced by landmark placements

The raw data of ProjA values calculated based on 4 sets of anatomical landmarks representing C1 and C2 coordinate systems is presented in the additional files (see Additional file 4). Agreements between each value and the gold standard (mean of 4 values) revealed to be excellent ($\rho_c = 0.9985$) with an overall low 95 % tolerance interval [−1.62°, 1.61°]. The absolute error (mean ± SD) was determined by comparing the gold standard to each individual value (0.58 ± 0.54°), to the mean of 2 values from the same observer (0.42 ± 0.39°) and to the mean

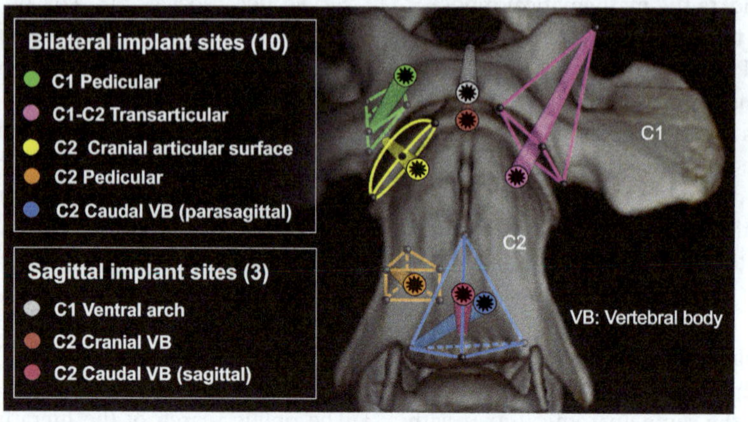

Fig. 6 Simulation of 13 optimal implants using geometrical simplification of AA bone corridors (*ventral view*)

Table 1 Mathematically calculated and manually measured values of ProjA and SafA

Case	Implant	Observer	Repeat	ProjA1 (°)	ProjA2 (°)	SafA1 (°)	SafA2 (°)	SafA3 (°)	SafA4 (°)
7	8	1	1	35.67	20.60	16.33	11.54	17.52	5.60
		1	2	34.59	22.66	15.9	11.9	17.42	5.65
		2	1	34.72	21.36	16.48	11.29	17.46	5.41
		2	2	34.39	21.43	16.59	11.16	17.44	5.51
		Gold standard		**34.51**	**21.42**	**16.50**	**11.25**	**17.38**	**5.51**
3	3	1	1	35.78	33.80	13.38	10.29	4.02	4.58
		1	2	35.69	34.34	13.01	9.99	4.51	4.49
		2	1	35.21	33.77	13.02	10.51	4.19	4.46
		2	2	35.60	34.52	13.45	10.27	4.23	4.39
		Gold standard		**35.61**	**34.30**	**13.20**	**10.19**	**4.15**	**4.44**
22	1	1	1	25.67	23.66	44.28	12.71	7.68	9.30
		1	2	25.63	24.04	44.54	13.38	7.75	9.31
		2	1	25.39	24.06	44.23	13.34	7.35	9.34
		2	2	25.28	23.96	44.76	13.50	7.37	9.42
		Gold standard		**25.61**	**24.10**	**44.38**	**13.21**	**7.55**	**9.29**
18	4	1	1	41.14	37.39	24.12	21.55	40.16	15.95
		1	2	43.13	37.12	23.38	21.88	41.39	14.61
		2	1	43.29	38.21	23.72	21.56	40.87	15.69
		2	2	42.97	37.94	24.39	20.94	40.52	15.74
		Gold standard		**42.81**	**38.27**	**23.54**	**21.63**	**40.65**	**15.83**
15	0	1	1	30.03	16.73	44.61	11.91	16.48	6.62
		1	2	30.3	19.61	45.86	10.82	16.29	6.25
		2	1	30.32	19.99	45.61	10.72	16.29	5.63
		2	2	30.00	19.42	45.57	10.69	16.46	6.04
		Gold standard		**29.83**	**19.68**	**45.64**	**10.72**	**16.17**	**6.30**
25	8	1	1	26.09	14.03	17.62	19.69	13.60	3.29
		1	2	26.13	15.66	17.17	19.51	13.69	3.71
		2	1	26.09	15.36	16.83	19.86	13.88	3.53
		2	2	25.93	15.26	17.88	19.72	13.91	3.40
		Gold standard		**26.08**	**14.93**	**17.35**	**19.85**	**13.81**	**3.41**
14	7	1	1	7.22	31.70	31.87	15.80	28.14	19.85
		1	2	8.18	31.95	31.35	15.5	27.73	19.16
		2	1	6.99	32.51	31.19	15.04	27.42	18.81
		2	2	6.90	31.16	31.37	15.46	26.99	19.56
		Gold standard		**7.30**	**31.62**	**31.21**	**15.56**	**27.51**	**19.21**
16	2	1	1	32.00	35.50	11.11	17.58	13.84	3.58
		1	2	31.94	35.41	11.27	17.18	13.49	3.51
		2	1	31.33	35.88	11.17	17.17	13.77	3.34
		2	2	31.32	35.22	11.07	17.03	13.76	3.40
		Gold standard		**31.33**	**35.34**	**11.21**	**17.09**	**13.74**	**3.41**
20	2	1	1	25.62	22.77	14.24	22.02	9.19	2.45
		1	2	25.82	22.91	14.15	21.81	8.81	2.31
		2	1	25.65	23.38	14.28	21.86	9.08	2.08
		2	2	25.69	23.27	14.14	21.73	8.87	2.25

Table 1 Mathematically calculated and manually measured values of ProjA and SafA *(Continued)*

		Gold standard		**25.61**	**23.13**	**14.23**	**21.81**	**9.08**	**2.17**
5	8	1	1	39.27	11.33	9.48	8.74	18.57	0.74
		1	2	39.25	10.63	9.12	8.79	18.57	0.45
		2	1	38.73	11.71	9.35	8.39	18.74	0.47
		2	2	39.00	11.41	9.04	8.55	18.89	0.43
		Gold standard		**38.98**	**11.06**	**9.22**	**8.60**	**18.80**	**0.38**
24	7	1	1	2.96	22.15	34.91	26.15	29.58	27.10
		1	2	2.34	22.61	33.99	26.9	30	26.41
		2	1	1.59	22.94	33.46	25.97	29.66	26.49
		2	2	2.19	22.25	34.04	26.72	29.27	27.36
		Gold standard		**2.45**	**22.71**	**33.96**	**26.54**	**29.32**	**26.95**
2	0	1	1	15.71	20.17	45.65	11.82	11.85	11.69
		1	2	15.32	20.35	46.05	12.23	12	12.35
		2	1	15.63	20.10	45.29	11.81	11.34	11.61
		2	2	15.30	19.58	45.54	12.22	11.92	11.21
		Gold standard		**15.49**	**20.00**	**45.66**	**12.04**	**11.97**	**11.48**

Implants were numbered as follows: C1 pedicular (0–1); C1-C2 transarticular (2–3); C2 cranial articular surface (4–5); C2 pedicular (6–7); C2 parasagittal caudal vertebral body (8–9); Right side (even #); Left side (odd #); Bold font: Mathematically calculated values (gold standard)

of 2 values from different observers (0.30 ± 0.25°). Agreement analysis within subsamples including coordinate system (C1 or C2) and the plane of projection used (Sagittal/Transverse/Dorsal) was conducted between observers and between repeats. This revealed that the widest 95 % tolerance interval was obtained when comparing inter-observer values calculated in C1 coordinate system [−3.58°, 3.72°]. Results from this concordance analysis and calculated errors are summarized in Tables 4 and 5, and graphically represented in Fig. 8. These results suggest that the simulation of anatomical axes in OsiriX™ using the previously defined OAB points is very reproducible. The largest predicted error on an individual ProjA value was estimated at 3.7° (with 95 % probability).

Discussion

This study provides a detailed description of a new method of AA OSIC analysis using OsiriX™. This method overcame the problem of subjective optimal implant placement definitions. Three-dimensional simplification of bone corridors into geometrical shapes not only permitted the description of corridors of complex / oblique distribution, but also to objectively localize the optimal implant position in space. For the transarticular OSIC, the geometrical determination of the corridor centered axis was based on the C1 lateral masses while the insertion point was located on the C2 cranial articular surface. Some occasional issues were encountered when placing ROI points in 3D-VR mode in some cases but they did not preclude successful OSIC simulation in any case. This step was the most time consuming and could not be automatized. Improvement in 3D surgical planning software would be necessary to allow such automation.

For the determination of numerical values describing 3D optimal implant placements and bone corridor

Table 2 Concordance analyses validating our mathematical method and estimating error generated by manual measures

Angle	Value 1	Value 2	n	R^2	ρ_c	Low TL	Up TL	Low CI	Up CI	Bias (°)	*P*-value
ProjA	**GS**	**Single value**	96	0.9972	**0.9986**	**−1.23**	**1.20**	−0.13	0.09	−0.019	0.726
	Rep1	Rep2	48	0.9944	0.9971	−1.94	1.75	−0.32	0.13	−0.092	0.415
	Obs1	Obs2	48	0.9937	0.9968	−1.99	1.92	−0.27	0.20	−0.033	0.779
SafA	**GS**	**Single value**	192	0.9992	**0.9996**	**−0.65**	**0.70**	−0.02	0.07	0.027	0.239
	Rep1	Rep2	96	0.9984	0.9992	−1.04	1.00	−0.11	0.07	−0.020	0.677
	Obs1	Obs2	96	0.9983	0.9991	−0.94	1.17	0.02	0.21	0.116[a]	0.019

[a]statistically significant bias (considered clinically non-significant); Bold font: agreement between GS and manually measured values
n: number of measures compared, R^2 correlation coefficient, ρ_c concordance coefficient, *TL* 95 % tolerance interval limit (in degrees), *CI* 95 % confidence interval limits (in degrees), *GS* gold standard (mathematically calculated values), *Obs* observer, *Rep* repeat

Table 3 Absolute errors determined by comparison between manual and mathematical values

Angle	Repeats	Observer 1	Observer 2
ProjA	1	0.55 ± 0.65	0.31 ± 0.25
	2	0.34 ± 0.35	0.21 ± 0.14
	Both	0.44 ± 0.53	0.26 ± 0.21
Saf A	1	0.29 ± 0.26	0.18 ± 0.18
	2	0.24 ± 0.25	0.17 ± 0.18
	Both	0.27 ± 0.25	0.18 ± 0.18

Values (in degrees) reported as Mean ± Standard deviation

characteristics, we developed a semi-automated procedure relying on the 3D coordinates of pre-identified ROI points. This study demonstrated excellent concordance between the semi-automated mathematical calculations and manually measured values which validated our first hypothesis. Our data also implied that SafA and ProjA could be accurately obtained using OsiriX™ measurement tools, although this would be more time consuming compared to the semi-automated method. Similar concordance analysis revealed that positioning of the landmarks used for anatomical space modeling induced

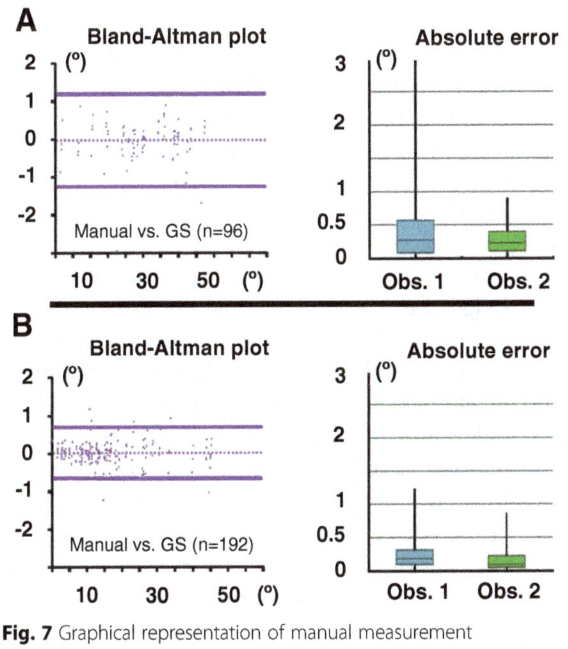

Fig. 7 Graphical representation of manual measurement reproducibility and absolute operator-induced error. **a** Bland-Altman and 4 quartiles box plots of absolute errors on ProjA values. **b** Bland-Altman and 4 quartiles box plots of absolute errors on SafA values. Bland-Altman plots are used to represent the difference between each measurement and the gold standard (GS) on the y axis. If perfect agreement between the 2 compared methods was present, all the points would be located on the 0 line. The 2 lines parallel to the 0 line represent the 95 % tolerance limits which is the expected error on a single measurement with respect to the gold standard with 95 % probablity

low errors (overall 1.6°, up to 3.7° for some subsamples with 95 % probability). It should be emphasized that this source of error is inherent to the use of ProjA values as 3D coordinates. Similar limitations are encountered when using neuronavigation based on fiducial markers [50]. Based on our results, landmark induced error can be significantly reduced if 2 observers position the ROI points successively and the mean of the 2 obtained ProjA values is used instead of an individual value. Regardless, the observed range of error of only a few degrees was considered small given that a minimum 15–20° bone corridor angular width would likely be necessary to recognize a corridor as acceptably safe. A theoretical error in any ROI positioning was expected of up to half the CT study slice thickness (0.3125 mm) which would also have a low impact on most of the OSIC calculated values. This type of error could have been minimized by reformatting all CT studies to 0.1 mm slice thickness.

Overall, these results validated our second hypothesis, allowing us to conclude that the use of OsiriX™ with implementation of mathematical equations on exported 3D coordinates was an efficient and reproducible tool which could be applied on a larger scale to describe AA OSICs. The major advantage of the described method is it can generate 3D data defined with respect to anatomical coordinates. Such data could be used for applications beyond OSIC descriptions. For instance, 3D data can be used to study the biomechanics of complex motions between vertebral motion units or to characterize pathological range of motion such as observed in AAI. Another possible application of this type of analysis would be to develop software able to automatically reduce AA subluxation at the planning stage. This type of 3D anatomical realignment would be extremely helpful to optimize implant positioning for each individual patient and compare different stabilization constructs such as plating systems or other customized implants in virtual 3D space.

These clinical applications all heavily rely on the definition of anatomical coordinate systems. Consequently, a good understanding of these definitions and how angle projections are made is essential. Identification of the sagittal plane is the most intuitive step to define a ProjA as it is also the plane of symmetry of the vertebra. An anatomical axis is then needed within that plane to define a proper coordinate system. In a previous report, the craniocaudal axis for C2 was defined as the ventral border of the vertebral foramen, which is what was also used in our study [9]. To our knowledge, a similar axis had not yet been described for C1. Therefore, we subjectively defined the cranial border of the dorsal and ventral arches as representing the ventrodorsal axis. The implicit assumption was that these C1 and C2 anatomical

Table 4 Concordance analyses estimating the reproducibility and error generated by OAB landmark placements

Angle	Value 1	Value 2	n	R^2	ρ_c	Low TL	Up TL	Low CI	Up CI	Bias (°)	*P*-value
ProjA	**GS**	**Single value**	1104	0.9970	**0.9985**	**−1.62**	**1.61**	−0.05	0.04	−0.006	0.801
	GS	**Mean 2 Obs**	552	0.9992	**0.9996**	**−0.83**	**0.83**	−0.04	0.03	−0.003	0.861
	Obs1	Obs2	552	0.9912	0.9956	−2.85	2.79	−0.15	0.08	−0.032	0.579
	Obs1-Sag	**Obs2-Sag**	264	0.9909	**0.9955**	**−3.37**	**3.25**	−0.25	0.13	−0.060	0.533
	Obs1-Tr	Obs2-Tr	144	0.9815	0.9905	−2.02	2.27	−0.04	0.29	0.123	0.135
	Obs1-Dors	Obs2-Dors	144	0.9844	0.9921	−2.96	2.69	−0.35	0.08	−0.137	0.207
	Obs1-C1	**Obs2-C1**	192	0.9621	**0.9808**	**−3.58**	**3.72**	−0.17	0.32	0.074	0.549
	Obs1-C2	Obs2-C2	360	0.5493	0.9976	−2.48	2.31	−0.21	0.03	−0.089	0.142
	GS	**Mean 2 Rep**	552	0.9984	**0.9992**	**−1.18**	**1.18**	−0.05	0.05	−0.001	0.957
	Rep1	Rep2	552	0.9943	0.9971	−2.33	2.20	−0.16	0.03	−0.065	0.163
	Rep1-Sag	Rep2-Sag	264	0.9941	0.9970	−2.77	2.58	−0.25	0.06	−0.098	0.211
	Rep1-Tr	Rep2-Tr	144	0.9846	0.9922	−1.97	1.95	−0.16	0.14	−0.008	0.916
	Rep1-Dors	Rep2-Dors	144	0.9918	0.9959	−2.11	1.98	−0.22	0.09	−0.063	0.421
	Rep1-C1	Rep2-C1	192	0.9795	0.9890	−2.92	2.56	−0.36	0.00	−0.179	0.054
	Rep1-C2	Rep2-C2	360	0.9965	0.9983	−2.06	2.05	−0.11	0.10	0.930[a]	−0.005

Bold font: most clinically relevant concordance analyses including comparisons with GS and widest tolerance limit intervals
n number of measures compared, R^2 correlation coefficient, ρ_c concordance coefficient, *TL* 95 % tolerance interval limit (in degrees), *CI* 95 % confidence interval limits (in degrees), *GS* gold standard (mean of 4 values), *Obs* observer, *Rep* repeat, *Sag* sagittal ProjA, *Tr* transverse ProjA, *Dors* dorsal ProjA, *C1* angle projected in C1 system, *C2* angle projected in C2 system
[a]statistically significant bias (considered clinically non-significant)

axes would have good alignment when the AA joint is placed in neutral position. Further investigation on the neutral position of the AA joint would be necessary to assess the accuracy of that assumption. Misalignment of the anatomical axes could result in clinically significant consequences when placing C1 implants. Indeed, only a very small portion of C1 can be visualized intraoperatively which means that estimation of C1 implant 3D position in surgery is mostly based on landmarks present on the ventral surface of C2. Fortunately, this type of misalignment would have limited impact on the risk of vertebral canal violation (except for a C1 ventral arch implant) as it would only affect the implant direction along the sagittal plane, not lateromedially.

One significant limitation in our study was the small number of recruited dog suffering from AAI, the population of clinical interest. However, most implant positions were simulated using the exact same protocol in all 3 groups. One notable difference in methodology in the AAI group was the fact that the insertion point of transarticular implants normally placed on C2 ventral surface had to be approximated due to AA misalignment. In contrast AA misalignment did not affect transarticular implant directions nor their ProjA values as they were solely defined using C1 landmarks (independently from C2 position). Overall, the low number of AAI cases could affect certain descriptive values such as the estimated length of transarticular implants but was not expected to have any significant impact on the optimal implant direction nor the reproducibility of our method.

Neuronavigation can be defined as a group of techniques designed to target neuroanatomical structures intraoperatively using 3D data obtained via advanced imaging. These methods include frame-based systems where the 3D space is defined with respect to a rigid frame, and frameless systems which require more advanced intraoperative 3D calculations, but allow for greater freedom of movement for the surgeon [50]. In veterinary medicine, neuronavigation represents a promising technical advancement in surgical accuracy, even though it remains cost-prohibitive for most clinical practices. The main alternative to neuronavigation is precise pre-surgical planning. The free open-source DICOM

Table 5 Absolute errors determined by comparison between the gold standard and individual values or the mean of 2 values

Angle	Repeats	Observer 1	Observer 2	Mean 2 Observers
ProjA	1	0.63 ± 0.59	0.54 ± 0.60	0.30 ± 0.25
	2	0.60 ± 0.50	0.56 ± 0.44	
	Mean 2 Repeats	0.42 ± 0.39		Overall single values 0.58 ± 0.54

Values (in degrees) reported as Mean ± Standard deviation

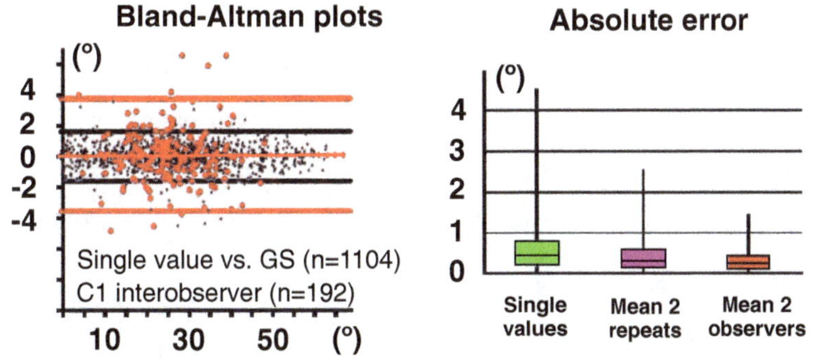

Fig. 8 Graphical representation of OAB landmarks reproducibility and absolute operator-induced error on ProjA calculations. Two Bland-Altman plots are superimposed including the overall comparison between the gold standard (GS) and single ProjA calculated values (*in black*) and the widest observed 95 % tolerance limit interval comparing values from 2 different observers in C1 system subsample (*in red*)

software OsiriX™ was initially developed by a human radiologist to improve multidimensional navigation and display of large datasets generated by advanced imaging modalities such as PET-CT or Cardiac CT [51]. The accuracy and reliability of the software have been validated experimentally and compared to other image analysis programs [52–54]. Good accuracy and low measurement error of the software have been demonstrated which is critical for surgical planning of implant placement with narrow safety margins. OsiriX™ rapidly became a successful 3D navigation tool due to its extremely fast and optimized 3D graphics. More recently, several publications in human medicine have reported its use for fast pre-surgical planning, notably in emergency situations where advanced neuronavigation planning is considered excessively time consuming [53, 55]. In our study, OsiriX™ proved relatively intuitive, and overall easy to use. The method presented here is currently relatively cumbersome due to the necessity to export 3D data in a separate software. However, OsiriX could be complemented with pre-surgical planning tools through the development of plugins incorporating mathematical equations similar to those we used in our study. This would allow generating optimal implant placement definitions considering individual morphological variations of the patient. Precise calculations of such coordinates may improve surgical accuracy; however, this would require the development of intraoperative guiding systems able to use these values to position implants in vivo.

Without such guiding system the precise coordinate values provided by our method would remain difficult to apply to actual patients as intraoperative implant positioning would still rely on the surgeon's ability to reproduce these values in vivo. Current neuronavigation techniques are difficult to use in the AA region of Toy breed dogs due to the small operation field and limited space available for fiducial markers. Therefore, our group has developed a 3D drill guide device using ProjA values to help the surgeon estimate optimal implant position intraoperatively, although investigation of the accuracy of the device will be necessary. In any case, we expect that the method of determination of OSICs presented here may improve accuracy of implant positioning.

Conclusion

Individual anatomical variations are becoming more commonly recognized in the canine population, and therefore the need for individualized pre-surgical planning will likely be increasing. Neuronavigation is an appealing solution to this problem, but such advanced technology remains currently inaccessible to most veterinary practices. This study described a novel semi-automated method of OSIC analysis using OsiriX™ DICOM viewer software. Geometrical simplification of bone corridors could be applied in the most commonly reported implant sites used for ventral AA stabilization. The method of calculation of ProjA and SafA was successfully validated by comparing the results to manually measured values. The principles described in our method could be further developed as an interactive pre-operative/intraoperative planning tool for individualized surgical planning of spinal fixation.

Endnotes

[1]GE Brightspeed CT scanner, GE Healthcare, Milwaukee, WI, USA.

[2]OsiriX™ versions 5.8–6.0, Pixmeo SARL, Bernex, Switzerland.

[3]Apple® computer Mac mini, Apple Inc., Cupertino, CA, USA.

[4]Microsoft® Excel software version 2011, Microsoft Corp., Redmond, WA, USA.

[5]ExportROIs version 1.3.1.

[6]SAS OnlineDoc® version 9.2, 2007, SAS Institute Inc. Cary, NC, USA.

Additional files

Additional file 1: Detailed optimal safe implantation corridor method of analysis. Step by step method of geometrical simplification of all studied bone corridors and simulation of associated optimal implant placements.

Additional file 2: Cartesian vectorial calculations used to determine projected angles of optimal implants. Step by step demonstration of the mathematical equations used for semi-automation of the method.

Additional file 3: Calculation sheet used to analyze the 3D data extracted from ROI points. Equations demonstrated in Additional file 2 are pre-entered in this calculation sheet to automate the calculation process.

Additional file 4: Raw data of projected angle values calculated based on 4 different sets of anatomical landmarks. This data was used to determine the reproducibility of projected angle calculations considering the variability caused by anatomical axes simulation.

Acknowledgements
The authors would like to thank Sue Kinsella (AHT) and Alexandra Gillan (BScH, DVM) for their help with case recruitment, Carolyn Bennett (AHT, BSc) and Sheila Currie (RVT) for their technical expertise in collecting CT images, and the members of the Ontario Veterinary College Health Sciences Centre Anesthesia Service for their excellent standard of care.

Funding
This project was funded by the Ontario Veterinary College Pet Trust Fund. Once approval of the study design was obtained, the funding body was not involved in the collection, analysis, and interpretation of data and was also not involved in writing the manuscript.

Authors' contributions
All authors were involved in the study design, grant submission, data interpretation and writing of the manuscript. LG, NM and GL provided the original ideas from which the study was designed. GL and AZ collected the CT studies and performed all OSIC simulations and manual measurements. GL and JR set up the vectorial calculations used to automatize the method. GM performed statistical analysis of the data. All authors read and approved the final manuscript.

Authors' information
The data from this manuscript is extracted from a thesis submitted by GL to the University of Guelph's Department of Clinical Studies as partial fulfillment of the requirements for a Doctorate in Veterinary Science (DVSc). The results were partially presented as a poster at the annual American College of Veterinary Internal Medicine Forum (Indianapolis, IN, June 2015). LG and NM are both Associate Professors at the University of Guelph who were co-advisors on the DVSc advisory committee. AZ, JR and FJ were members of the advisory committee.

Competing interests
The authors declare that they have no competing interests.

Consent for publication
Not applicable.

Author details
[1]Department of Clinical Studies, Ontario Veterinary College, University of Guelph, Guelph, ON N1G 2W1, Canada. [2]School of Engineering, University of Guelph, Guelph, ON N1G 2W1, Canada.

References

1. Geary JC, Oliver JE, Hoerlein BF. Atlanto axial subluxation in the canine. J Small Anim Pract. 1967;8:577–82.
2. Kishigami M. Application of an atlanto-axial retractor for atlanto-axial subluxation in the cat and dog. J Am Anim Hosp Assoc. 1984;20:413–9.
3. LeCouteur RA, McKeown D, Johnson J, Eger CE. Stabilization of atlantoaxial subluxation in the dog, using the nuchal ligament. J Am Vet Med Assoc. 1980;177:1011–7.
4. Schulz KS, Waldron DR, Fahie M. Application of ventral pins and polymethylmethacrylate for the management of atlantoaxial instability: results in nine dogs. Vet Surg. 1997;26:317–25.
5. Sorjonen DC, Shires PK. Atlanto-axial Instability - a ventral surgical technique for decompression, fixation, and fusion. Vet Surg. 1981;10:22–9.
6. Aikawa T, Shibata M, Fujita H. Modified ventral stabilization using positively threaded profile pins and polymethylmethacrylate for atlantoaxial instability in 49 dogs. Vet Surg. 2013;42:683–92.
7. Beaver DP, Ellison GW, Lewis DD, Goring RL, Kubilis PS, Barchard C. Risk factors affecting the outcome of surgery for atlantoaxial subluxation in dogs: 46 cases (1978-1998). J Am Vet Med Assoc. 2000;216:1104–9.
8. Slanina MC. Atlantoaxial Instability. Vet Clin North Am Small Anim Pract. 2016;46:265–75.
9. Vizcaino Reves N, Stahl C, Stoffel M, Bali M, Forterre F. CT scan based determination of optimal bone corridor for atlantoaxial ventral screw fixation in miniature breed dogs. Vet Surg. 2013;42:819–24.
10. Platt SR, Chambers JN, Cross A. A modified ventral fixation for surgical management of atlantoaxial subluxation in 19 dogs. Vet Surg. 2004;33:349–54.
11. Hettlich BF, Allen MJ, Pascetta D, Fosgate GT, Litsky AS. Biomechanical comparison between bicortical pin and monocortical screw/polymethylmethacrylate constructs in the cadaveric canine cervical vertebral column. Vet Surg. 2013;42:693–700.
12. Hicks DG, Pitts MJ, Bagley RS, Vasavada A, Chen AV, Wininger FA, et al. In vitro biomechanical evaluations of screw-bar-polymethylmethacrylate and pin-polymethylmethacrylate internal fixation implants used to stabilize the vertebral motion unit of the fourth and fifth cervical vertebrae in vertebral column specimens from dogs. Am J Vet Res. 2009;70:719–26.
13. Hettlich BF, Fosgate GT, Levine JM, Young BD, Kerwin SC, Walker M, et al. Accuracy of conventional radiography and computed tomography in predicting implant position in relation to the vertebral canal in dogs. Vet Surg. 2010;39:680–7.
14. Kazan S, Yildirim F, Sindel M, Tuncer R. Anatomical evaluation of the groove for the vertebral artery in the axis vertebrae for atlanto-axial transarticular screw fixation technique. Clin Anat. 2000;13:237–43.
15. Kamimura M, Ebara S, Itoh H, Tateiwa Y, Kinoshita T, Takaoka K. Cervical pedicle screw insertion: assessment of safety and accuracy with computer-assisted image guidance. J Spinal Disord. 2000;13:218–24.
16. Ludwig SC, Kramer DL, Balderston RA, Vaccaro AR, Foley KF, Albert TJ. Placement of pedicle screws in the human cadaveric cervical spine: comparative accuracy of three techniques. Spine. 2000;25:1655–67.
17. Igarashi T, Kikuchi S, Sato K, Kayama S, Otani K. Anatomic study of the axis for surgical planning of transarticular screw fixation. Clin Orthop Relat Res. 2003;408:162–6.
18. Chung SS, Lee CS, Chung HW, Kang CS. CT analysis of the axis for transarticular screw fixation of rheumatoid atlantoaxial instability. Skeletal Radiol. 2006;35:679–83.
19. Fu M, Lin L, Kong X, Zhao W, Tang L, Li J, et al. Construction and accuracy assessment of patient-specific biocompatible drill template for cervical anterior transpedicular screw (ATPS) insertion: an in vitro study. PLoS One. 2013;8:e53580.
20. Corlazzoli D. Bicortical implant insertion in caudal cervical spondylomyelopathy: a computed tomography simulation in affected Doberman Pinschers. Vet Surg. 2008;37:178–85.
21. Knell SC, Kircher P, Dennler M, Montavon PM, Voss K, Hurter K. Angle of insertion and confirmation of angles measured after in vitro implantation during laminar vertebral stabilization in vertebral columns obtained from canine cadavers. Am J Vet Res. 2011;72:1674–80.
22. Watine S, Cabassu JP, Catheland S, Brochier L, Ivanoff S. Computed tomography study of implantation corridors in canine vertebrae. J Small Anim Pract. 2006;47:651–7.
23. Vallefuoco R, Bedu AS, Manassero M, Viateau V, Niebauer G, Moissonnier P. Computed tomographic study of the optimal safe implantation corridors in feline thoraco-lumbar vertebrae. Vet Comp Orthop Traumatol. 2013;26:372–8.
24. de Vet HC, Terwee CB, Knol DL, Bouter LM. When to use agreement versus reliability measures. J Clin Epidemiol. 2006;59:1033–9.
25. Cerda-Gonzalez S, Dewey CW. Congenital diseases of the craniocervical junction in the dog. Vet Clin North Am Small Anim Pract. 2010;40:121–41.

26. Denny HR, Gibbs C, Waterman A. Atlanto-axial subluxation in the dog: a review of 30 Cases and an evaluation of treatment by lag screw fixation. J Small Anim Pract. 1988;29:37–47.
27. Dewey C, Marino D, Loughin C. Craniocervical junction abnormalities in dogs. N Z Vet J. 2013;61:202–11.
28. Dewey CW. A practical guide to canine & feline neurology. 2nd ed. Danvers: Blackwell Publishing; 2008.
29. Dewey CW. Surgery of the cervical spine. In: Fossum TW, Dewey CW, Horn CV, Johnson AI, MacPhail CM, Radlinsky MG, Schulz KS, Willard MD, editors. Small Animal Surgery Textbook. St. Louis: Elsevier Mosby; 2013. p. 1467–507.
30. Dickomeit M, Alves L, Pekarkova M, Gorgas D, Forterre F. Use of a 1.5 mm butterfly locking plate for stabilization of atlantoaxial pathology in three toy breed dogs. Vet Comp Orthop Traumatol. 2011;24:246–51.
31. Evans HE, de Lahunta A. Miller's anatomy of the dog. 4th ed. St. Louis: Elsevier/Saunders; 2012.
32. Forterre F, Vizcaino Reves N, Stahl C, Rupp S, Gendron K. Atlantoaxial synovial cyst associated with instability in a Chihuahua. Case Rep Vet Med. 2012. doi:10.1155/2012/898241.
33. Galban EM, Gilley RS, Long SN. Surgical stabilization of an occipitoatlantoaxial malformation in an adult dog. Vet Surg. 2010;39:1001–4.
34. Jeserevics J, Srenk P, Beranek J, Jaggy A, Touru S, Cizinauskas S. Stabilisation of atlantoaxial subluxation in the dog through ventral arthrodesis. Schweiz Arch Tierheilkd. 2008;150:69–76.
35. Johnson SG, Hulse DA. Odontoid dysplasia with atlanto-axial instability in a dog. J Am Anim Hosp Assoc. 1989;25:400–4.
36. Kent M, Eagleson JS, Neravanda D, Schatzberg SJ, Gruenenfelder FI, Platt SR. Intraaxial spinal cord hemorrhage secondary to atlantoaxial subluxation in a dog. J Am Anim Hosp Assoc. 2010;46:132–7.
37. Knipe MF, Sturges BK, Vernau KM, Berry WL, Dickinson PJ, Anor S, et al. Atlantoaxial instability in 17 dogs. J Vet Intern Med. 2002;16:368.
38. McCarthy RJ, Lewis DD, Hosgood G. Atlantoaxial subluxation in dogs. Comp Cont Educ Pract. 1995;17:215–27.
39. Parry AT, Upjohn MM, Schlegl K, Kneissl S, Lamb CR. Computed tomography variations in morphology of the canine atlas in dogs with and without atlantoaxial subluxation. Vet Radiol Ultrasound. 2010;51:596–600.
40. Sanders SG, Bagley RS, Silver GM, Moore M, Tucker RL. Outcomes and complications associated with ventral screws, pins, and polymethyl methacrylate for atlantoaxial instability in 12 dogs. J Am Anim Hosp Assoc. 2004;40:204–10.
41. Sharp NJH, Wheeler SJ. Small animal spinal disorders: diagnosis and surgery. 2nd ed. Philadelphia: Elsevier Mosby; 2005.
42. Stead AC, Anderson AA, Coughlan A. Bone plating to stabilize atlantoaxial subluxation in 4 dogs. J Small Anim Pract. 1993;34:462–5.
43. Thomas WB, Sorjonen DC, Simpson ST. Surgical management of atlantoaxial subluxation in 23 dogs. Vet Surg. 1991;20:409–12.
44. Voss K, Steffen F, Montavon PM. Use of the ComPact UniLock System for ventral stabilization procedures of the cervical spine - A retrospective study. Vet Comp Orthop Traumatol. 2006;19:21–8.
45. Warren-Smith CM, Kneissl S, Benigni L, Kenny PJ, Lamb CR. Incomplete ossification of the atlas in dogs with cervical signs. Vet Radiol Ultrasound. 2009;50:635–8.
46. Watson AG, de Lahunta A, Evans HE. Morphology and embryological interpretation of a congenital occipito-atlanto-axial malformation in a dog. Teratology. 1988;38:451–9.
47. Watson AG, Evans HE, de Lahunta A. Ossification of the atlas-axis complex in the dog. Anat Histol Embryol. 1986;15:122–38.
48. Westworth DR, Sturges BK. Congenital spinal malformations in small animals. Vet Clin North Am Small Anim Pract. 2010;40:951–81.
49. Wheeler SJ. Atlantoaxial subluxation with absence of the dens in a rottweiler. J Small Anim Pract. 1992;33:90–3.
50. Wininger F. Neuronavigation in small animals: development, techniques, and applications. Vet Clin North Am Small Anim Pract. 2014;44:1235–48.
51. Rosset A, Spadola L, Ratib O. OsiriX: an open-source software for navigating in multidimensional DICOM images. J Digit Imaging. 2004;17:205–16.
52. Kim G, Jung HJ, Lee HJ, Lee JS, Koo S, Chang SH. Accuracy and reliability of length measurements on three-dimensional computed tomography using open-source OsiriX software. J Digit Imaging. 2012;25:486–91.
53. Fortin M, Battie MC. Quantitative paraspinal muscle measurements: inter-software reliability and agreement using OsiriX and ImageJ. Phys Ther. 2012;92:853–64.
54. Yamauchi T, Yamazaki M, Okawa A, Furuya T, Hayashi K, Sakuma T, et al. Efficacy and reliability of highly functional open source DICOM software (OsiriX) in spine surgery. J Clin Neurosci. 2010;17:756–9.
55. Jaimovich SG, Guevara M, Pampin S, Jaimovich R, Gardella JL. Neurosurgical planning using Osirix software [in Spanish]. Surg Neurol Int. 2014;5:S267–71.

11

The effect of surgery (Ovariohysterectomy) on the plasma disposition of meloxicam following intravenous administration in dogs

Umit Karademir[1], Dilek Aksit[2], Cavit Kum[1], Hasan Erdogan[3], Eyup Hakan Ucar[4], Cevdet Peker[4] and Cengiz Gokbulut[5*]

Abstract

Background: Meloxicam (MLX) is a nonsteroidal anti-inflammatory drug used in the relief of postoperative pain for human and veterinary medicine. This study was designed to investigate the effect of surgery on the plasma disposition of MLX in dogs undergoing ovariohysterectomy following a single intravenous injection at a dose of 0.2 mg/kg bodyweight. Eight crossbred bitches were used in the study. A two-phase experimental design with a 10-day washout period was used. Pre-operative MLX was administered intravenously to 8 bitches about 10 days before surgery (Phase I, control) at a dose of 0.2 mg/kg bodyweight and peri-operative MLX was administered intravenously after anaesthesia and 15 min before the start of surgery (Phase II). Blood samples were collected from all animals at various times between 1 and 96 h after the drug administrations in both phases. The drug concentrations were analysed using high performance liquid chromatography.

Results: The volume of plasma MLX distribution at steady-state (Vd_{ss}) of the control group (Vd_{ss}: 263.0 ml/kg) was significantly greater ($P < 0.05$) compared to that of the surgery group (Vd_{ss}: 149.3 ml/kg). The AUC values were higher (29.5 vs. 23.0 μg.h^2/ml) and the CL values were lower (7.7 vs. 10.5 ml.h/kg) in the surgery group compared to the control group, respectively, but differences were not significant.

Conclusions: The results of the present study indicated that surgery could alter the plasma disposition of MLX and thus the drug efficacy and side effects such as gastrointestinal ulceration, unusual bleeding and loss of kidney function/failure when repeated doses are used.

Keywords: Dog, Meloxicam, Pharmacokinetics, Surgery

Background

Analgesic drugs including nonsteroidal anti-inflammatory drugs (NSAIDs), opioids and local anaesthetic agents are used in dogs as peri- and post-surgery pain relievers. NSAIDs are used in veterinary medicine for treating especially musculo-skeletal and abdominal pain [7]. These drugs have antipyretic, anti-inflammatory and analgesic properties. The common mechanism of action for this class of drugs can be attributed to a blockade of the biosynthesis of prostaglandins, resulting from the inhibitionof enzyme cyclooxygenase (COX) [3, 21].

Meloxicam (MLX), belongs to the enolic acid class of NSAIDs and is also effective as antipyretic, analgesic or anti-inflammatory agent [20]. It preferentially inhibits COX-2, which is induced by inflammatory stimuli in pathophysiological conditions [9]. MLX is about 12 times more potent at inhibiting COX-2 than COX-1 activity [17].

Surgery is a duration when there are some major stresses associated with pain, cardiovascular and possibly major haemodynamic changes peri- and post-operation, especially if there is a significant blood loss [1]. In general,

* Correspondence: cengizgokbulut@yahoo.com
[5]Department of Medical Pharmacology, Faculty of Medicine, Balikesir University, Balikesir, Turkey
Full list of author information is available at the end of the article

the pharmacokinetics of drugs in most species have been characterized in healthy animals. However, the plasma disposition of the active compound and its metabolites may be markedly altered in diseased animals or during peri- or post-operative period.

The pharmacokinetics data are available for some NSAIDs in dogs undergoing surgery and can be compared with other published data [6, 7, 11, 27]. However, to the best of our knowledge, this is the first study in which the pharmacokinetic disposition of an NSAID in dogs has been evaluated in the same animal with and without surgery. Our hypothesis was that surgery alters the plasma disposition of certain drugs including analgesics and anaesthetics administered pre- or peri-operatively. Therefore, this study was designed to investigate the effects of surgery on the plasma disposition of MLX in dogs undergoing ovariohysterectomy following a single intravenous injection at 0.2 mg/kg bodyweight.

Results

Clinically no adverse effects were observed during and after the MLX administration in dogs. The pre-operative biochemical and haematological parameters were within the normal ranges. Mean age, bodyweight, duration of surgery and the selected surgical variables during anaesthesia are shown in Table 1. The heart rate, respiratory rate and end tidal CO_2 values were 122.17 ± 10.6 beats/min, 8.5 ± 0.9 breaths/min and 42.06 ± 7.3 mmHg during anaesthesia, respectively. The albumin levels of each dog in the control group were similar to its own post-surgery plasma albumin concentration. In addition, the mean albumin concentration in the control group (2.43 ± 0.32 g/dl) was not significantly different (P: 0.719) compared with that observed in the surgery group (2.50 ± 0.23 g/dl).

The analysis yielded linear regression lines ranging from 0.025 to 10 μg/ml of MLX with a correlation coefficient of 0.999. The limits of detection and quantification of the MLX assay were 0.005 μg/ml and 0.02 μg/ml, respectively. The mean recovery was 98.32 % (inter assay CV = 2.09 %) and the accuracy ranged from 96 % to 103 %.

Table 1 Mean (±SD) values of general characteristics and selected surgical variables during anaesthesia of eight dogs undergoing ovariohysterectomy

Characteristic	Mean ± SD
Operation time (min)	29 ± 7.9
Age (year)	1.4 ± 0.4
Bodyweight (kg)	18.25 ± 4.4
Time from MLX injection to start of surgery (min)	15 ± 0.0
Heart rate (per min)	122.17 ± 10.6
Respiration rate (per min)	8.5 ± 0.9
End tidal CO2 (mmHg)	42.06 ± 7.3
Oxyhaemoglobin (%)	>98

Pharmacokinetic parameters of MLX following intravenous administration (0.2 mg/kg) are given in Table 2. Semi logarithmic plot of the mean plasma concentration *vs.* time curves are shown in Fig 1. In additions, the scatter plots of the pharmacokinetic parameters (Vd_{ss}, $T_{1/2}$, Cl and AUC) in control *vs.* surgery group are presented in Fig. 2.

The differences in most pharmacokinetic parameters between the control and surgery groups were not significant, however, variability was high for each phase. Nevertheless, the terminal half-life ($T_{1/2\lambda z}$) and total body clearance (Cl_B) values were longer and higher, but the area under the curve (AUC) value was smaller in the control group ($T_{1/2\lambda z}$: 17.21 h, Cl_B: 10.50 ml.h/kg and AUC: 23.00 μg.h/ml) compared to the surgery group ($T_{1/2\lambda z}$: 12.77 h, Cl_B: 7.70 ml.h/kg and AUC: 29.50 μg.h/ml), respectively. The volume of MLX distribution at steady-state (Vd_{ss}) of the control group (Vd_{ss}: 263.00 ml/kg) was significantly larger ($P < 0.05$) compared to that of the surgery group (Vd_{ss}: 149.30 ml/kg). The Vd_{ss} value of each individual animal decreased in phase I compared with that of the same animals in phase II. Moreover, $T_{1/2\lambda z}$, AUC and MRT values in 7 out of 8 dogs were altered in the post-surgery group compared to the control group.

Discussion

The plasma concentration of MLX in dogs following intravenous administration exhibits slight fluctuations, especially in the early hours of the administration in both phases of the present study. Similar observations were also reported by studies performed recently in

Table 2 Median pharmacokinetic parameters with lower and upper confidence intervals of meloxicam in control and surgery groups following intravenous (0.2 mg/kg) administration to bitches ($n = 8$)

Parameters	Control group	Surgery group	*P* values
$T_{1/2\lambda z}$ (h)	17.21 (12.8–40.1)	12.77 (9.8–24.3)	0.289
C_0 (μg/ml)	1.05 (0.7–9.92)	5.3 (1.9–14.2)	0.298
AUC_{last} (μg.h/ml)	21.2 (10.8–30.8)	28.5 (18.7–45.6)	0.176
$AUC_{0\to\infty}$ (μg.h/ml)	23.0 (12.4–41.0)	29.5 (19.4–51.5)	0.322
$AUMC_{0\to\infty}$ (μg.h²/ml)	698 (378–2815)	588 (329–2150)	0.959
Cl_B (ml.h/kg)	10.5 (6.0–20.6)	7.7 (4.9–11.35)	0.191
Vd_{ss} (ml/kg)	263.0 (211–470)	149.3 (122.4–172.7)	0.016*
$MRT_{0\to\infty}$ (h)	28.1 (19.5–56.0)	20.7 (14.4–34.3)	0.303

C_0: plasma concentration at time 0, $AUC_{0\to\infty}$: area under the (zero moment) curve from time 0 to infinity, $T_{1/2\lambda z}$: terminal half-life, $AUMC_{0\to\infty}$: area under the moment curve from time 0 to infinity; Cl_B: total body clearance of drug; Vd_{ss}: volume of distribution at steady-state; $MRT_{0\to\infty}$: mean residence time
*The kinetic parameters in control group are significantly different ($P < 0.05$) from the surgery group

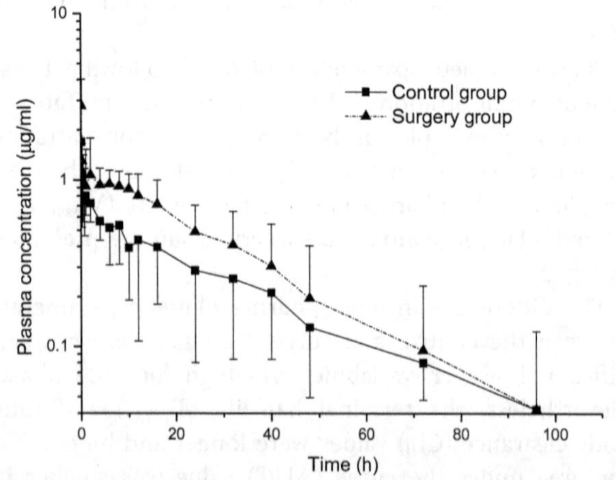

Fig 1 Semi log plot of mean (±SD) plasma concentrations *vs.* time curves of meloxicam in control and surgery groups following intravenous (0.2 mg/kg) administration to bitches ($n = 8$)

dogs, cats and horses subjected to ketorolac treatment [7, 11, 27]. The reason of such characteristics in plasma concentrations is not clear and probably not associated with the anaesthetic agents and surgical procedures employed in the experiments, since similar fluctuations were observed in the animals of the control group.

There is a reasonable body of literature evaluating peri- or post-operative analgesic effects and plasma dispositions of some NSAIDs in dogs undergoing surgery [4, 7, 8, 12, 24]. However, to our knowledge this is the first study in which the pharmacokinetics of an NSAID in dogs have been evaluated in the same animal with and without surgery. Although, all animals under surgery receive at least 1 drug during the operation for pre-anesthetic medication, anesthesia or analgesia in the surgery unit, there is no information available on the alterations in drug disposition following surgery in veterinary medicine. During the surgery, many hemodynamic and metabolic alterations such as fluctuating hemodynamics, alteration of protein catabolism and anabolism may occur.

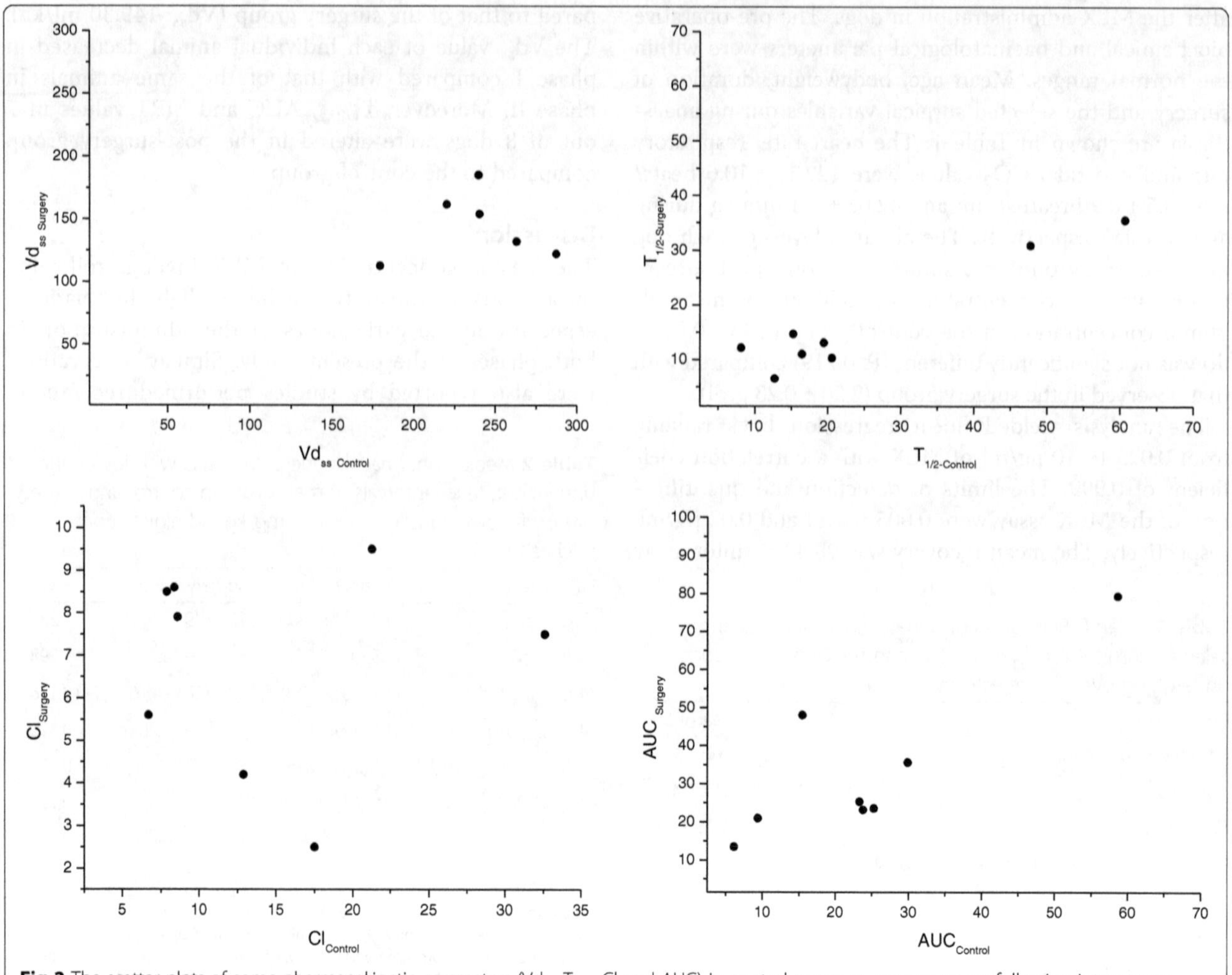

Fig 2 The scatter plots of some pharmacokinetic parameters (Vd_{ss}, $T_{1/2}$, Cl and AUC) in control group *vs.* surgery group following intravenous (0.2 mg/kg) administration of meloxicam to dogs ($n = 8$)

The changes in circulation, blood volume, extracellular fluid and blood protein levels, such as α1-acid glycoprotein and albumin may affect the distribution of drugs used during the peri- and post-operative periods [18].

The kinetic parameters of MLX observed from the control group in the present study exhibits a low apparent volume of distribution (263.00 ml/kg) and a long plasma half-life (17.21 h) and residence time (28.10 h) in dogs following the intravenous administration. These findings are in agreement with the results of a previous study [5], regarding the values of V_{ss} (320 ml/kg), $T_{1/2}$ (24.0 h), MRT (34.8 h) and AUC (21.5 μg.h/kg) in healthy dogs.

The differences in most pharmacokinetic parameters between the control and surgery groups were not significant, however, variability was high for each phase. The dogs in the control group were demonstrated to have a prolonged half-life (17.21 h *vs* 12.77 h), smaller AUC (23.00 μg.h/ml *vs* 29.50 μg.h/ml) and greater body clearance (Cl_B) (10.50 ml.h/kg *vs* 7.70 ml.h/kg) when compared to themselves in the surgery group. Moreover, the volume of MLX distribution at steady-state in the control group (Vd_{ss}: 263.00 ml/kg) was significantly greater than that of the surgery group (Vd_{ss}: 149.30 ml/kg). Volume of distribution (Vd_{ss}) is one of the most important parameters for the evaluation of the pharmacokinetic characteristics of the drugs and depends on many factors, including the physicochemical properties of the drug, binding strength of plasma proteins, binding capacity to the other tissues. The reason for low levels of Vd_{ss} measured in surgery group is probably associated with major haemodynamic changes during the surgery and/or drug-drug interaction. The hepatic activity increases during the post-operative period. Serum albumin turnover elevates, drug-albumin binding characteristics alter and the level of serum proteins, including albumin decreases dramatically for a period following surgery [18]. In addition, it has been reported that the serum albumin level was significantly reduced in dogs with inflammation compared with the healthy dogs [2]. Besides, high plasma albumin binding of MLX could be altered by the anaesthetic drugs, since it has been reported that the plasma proteins (albumin, globulin) decreases in under isoflurane anaesthesia in flying fox [15]. Both the duration and the intensity of drug action with the free drug concentration being the active compound are affected by the level of protein binding [26]. In these circumstances, the protein binding is influenced, particularly for the drugs which have more than 90 % protein bound [18]. The protein binding ratio of MLX in dogs was reported as 97 % [5] and MLX exhibits a high degree of binding to albumin [16]. Generally, the reduction of plasma protein leads the increase of distribution volume and clearance of drugs via the decrease in the plasma protein bindings. However, the mean albumin concentration in the control group (2.46 g/dl) was not significantly different (P: 0.719) compared with that observed in the surgery group (2.48 g/dl) in the present study. Consequently, the difference on Vd_{ss} of MLX is probably not related to the different plasma albumin level between the control and surgery groups. The reason for lower Vd_{ss} in the surgery group was however unclear. It is probably related to the other factors such as drug-drug interaction which may have changed the drug-protein binding capacity in the surgery group since atropine sulphate, propofol and isoflurane were combinely used for premedication and as anaesthesia. Also ovariohysterectomy may have affected reproductive hormones and thus the disposition of the drugs. In addition, the reason for lower Vd_{ss} in the surgery group could be, at least in part, due to smaller Cl_B and MRT as $Vd_{ss} = Cl_B \times MRT$. Moreover, there was a limitation since the control and surgery phases (I and II) were arranged in a sequence, but not in a crossover fashion. This experimental design may potentially induce a period effect. However, this is judged to be unlikely as a 10-day washout period was considered to be sufficiently long [22].

In the present study, the effect of surgical operation on the plasma disposition of MLX was investigated in only crossbred and female dogs. However, the plasma disposition of MLX may be different in pure-bred and between male and female dogs. The elimination half-life of naproxen in beagles ($T_{1/2}$: 35 h) was much shorter [25], compared with that of observed in mongrels ($T_{1/2}$: 74 h) [13]. This difference probably reflects a breed difference, since it is known that beagles metabolise drugs more rapidly than other breeds [14]. Besides, it has been reported that, female dogs showed lower AUC and elimination $T_{1/2}$ values of MLX, compared with male dogs [5].

Conclusions

Vd_{ss} of MLX in the control group is significantly greater compared to that of the surgery group. Generally limited or lowered distribution may decrease the drug exposure into tissues. However, the consequent reduction in volume of distribution leads to higher plasma concentrations of MLX. Besides, higher plasma concentration of the increased unbound MLX fraction in plasma may increase risk of side effects such as gastrointestinal ulceration, unusual bleeding and loss of kidney function/failure when repeated doses are used. The change in the disposition of some drugs pre-, peri- and post-operatively administered for pre-medication, anaesthesia or prevention of post-operative infections may result in changing efficacy and/or increasing side effects or toxicity.

Methods

Experimental animals

A total of 8 client-owned, cross-bred bitches, 2–4 years old and weighing 18.25 ± 4.4 kg were used in the study. Animals were judged to be healthy on the basis of physical examinations and haematological and biochemical blood tests. All animals were housed in single boxes and each dog was identified by natural markings. Water was supplied *ad libitum* and animals were fed a standard commercial diet twice daily with an appropriate quantity of feed during the experimental period. The animals were acclimated for 5 days before the study and food was withdrawn 12 h before the drug administrations in pre- and peri- surgery.

The study was designed as a two-phase trial with a 10-day washout period as this time duration was reported to be adequate for ensuring the clearance of the drug in dogs [22]. A bolus of MLX was administered intravenously to each dog about 10 days before the surgery (Phase I, control) at a dose of 0.2 mg/kg bodyweight and peri-operative MLX was administered intravenously after the anaesthesia and 15 min before the start of the surgery (ovariohysterectomy) (Phase II) at the same dose 0.2 mg/kg bodyweight. MLX administration and blood sampling were performed through the different cephalic veins of each dog. All animals were enrolled after written consent of the owners. The experimenters were blinded to the pharmacological treatment, while processing data and making exclusion decisions. All procedures were carried out under a protocol approved by the Animal Ethics Committee of Adnan Menderes University (Reference number: 64583101/2014/170). All sections of this paper adheres to the ARRIVE Guidelines for reporting animal research [19].

Pre-surgical and surgical procedures

All dogs in phase II were administered to the following anaesthetic protocol: premedication by subcutaneous atropine sulphate (0.045 mg/kg bwt, Teknovet Atropine; Teknovet, Turkey), induction by intravenous bolus of propofol (4 mg/kg bwt, Propofol 1 %; Fresenius, Fresenius Kabi) administered for inducing the anaesthesia. After intubation, the anaesthesia was maintained with isoflurane (Isoflurane USP; Adeka, Turkey). Different levels of isoflurane were used during anaesthesia, to maintain an appropriate depth of anaesthesia based on clinical assessment; heart rate (HR), invasive blood pressure (IBP), muscle relaxation, the degree of nystagmus and response to the surgery were monitored.

MLX (Bavet Meloxicam; Bavet, Istanbul-Turkey) was administered intravenously as a bolus at a dose of 0.2 mg/kg bodyweight after intubation and 15 min before the start of the surgery.

After the dog was anesthetized, a standard aseptic preparation was performed, which was followed by elective ovariohysterectomy via a routine ventral midline approach. Same surgeon performed all ovariohysterectomy operations. Respiration rate, HR, IBP, $EtCO_2$, oxyhaemoglobin saturation, electrocardiography (lead II), and body temperature were recorded every 5 min during the operation period using an Utech monitor (VS2000V Vital Signs Monitor; Utech Co. Ltd., China).

Sample collection

Heparinized blood samples (3 ml) were collected by cephalic venepuncture using a 20 G catheter (B&D Medical Systems; Istanbul, Turkey) prior to drug administration (0 h), 5, 15, 30, 45 min and 1, 2, 4, 6, 8, 10, 12, 16, 24, 32, 40, 48, 72 and 96 h after the administration of MLX. Blood samples were centrifuged at 3000 g for 20 min and plasma was transferred to plastic tubes (5 ml). Heparinized drug-free blood samples for analytical method development and validation process were collected from other dogs not included in the study. All the plasma samples were stored at −20 °C until the estimations of drug concentrations.

Analytical procedures

The parent compounds of MLX in dog plasma were analysed using validated high performance liquid chromatography (HPLC) following a liquid-liquid phase extraction procedure. Plasma concentrations of MLX were measured by minor modifications of the methods described by Eniko et al. [10].

Stock solution (100 µg/ml) of pure standard of MLX (Dr. Reddy's Laboratory, India) was first prepared using acetonitrile: water (20:80) as solvent. The resulting stock was then further diluted to produce 0.05, 0.5, 1, 2.5, 5 and 10 µg/ml solutions for calibration as standard curves and to add to the drug-free plasma samples to determine the recovery.

The mobile phase consisted of acetonitrile : 1 % aqueous glacial acetic acid (40:60, v/v) and was delivered (Agilent 1260 Series binary pump; Waldron, Germany) at a flow rate of 1.2 ml/min. An analytical column (Zorbax CN, 5 µm, 4.6 mm x 250 mm; Agilent Technologies, Wilmington, DE) was used for the analysis of MLX. The eluate was continuously monitored using a photodiode array detector (Agilent 1260 Series Technologies; Waldron, Germany) at a wavelength of 360 nm.

The method for MLX analysis in plasma was validated before the start of the analysis of the study samples. The chromatographic peak of MLX was identified with the retention times of its analytical standard. Recovery of the molecule was determined by comparison of the peak areas from the spiked plasma samples with the areas resulting from direct injections of the analytical reference standard.

The inter- and intra-assay precisions of the extraction and chromatography procedures were evaluated by processing replicate aliquots of drug-free dog plasma samples containing known amounts of the drug on different days. Calibration graphs were prepared (linear range 0.025-10 µg/ml). The slope of the lines between peak areas and drug concentration was determined by least squares linear regression and showed a correlation coefficient between 0.9987 and 0.9999. The detection limit of the molecule was established with HPLC analysis of blank plasma spiked with the analytical standard and measuring the baseline noise at the peak retention time. The limit of detection (LOD) and limit of quantification (LOQ) were determined for the HPLC method. The limits were determined based on the standard deviation amongst response and slope of the curve at the lowest concentrations.

Plasma albumin concentrations of all samples of each animal were determined by autoanalyser (Sinnowa D280, China), using bromocresol green (Archem A2011, İstanbul, Turkey) as described by Lolekha and Charoenpol [23].

Pharmacokinetics and statistical analysis of data

The plasma concentration *vs.* time curve obtained after the treatment was fitted with the WinNonlin software program (version 5.2, Pharsight Corp., Mountain View, California, US). The pharmacokinetics parameters for each animal were estimated using non-compartmental model analysis. The trapezoidal rule was used to calculate the area under the plasma concentration time curve (AUC).

The pharmacokinetic parameters are reported as median with lower and upper confidence intervals. The characteristics of dogs (Table 1), the plasma albumin concentrations (Table 2) and the plasma concentrations *vs.* time curves of MLX (Fig. 1) were expressed as mean ± SD. The pharmacokinetic parameters and plasma albumin concentrations were statistically compared with a Wilcoxon's signed rank test a nonparametric approach for paired data. All statistical analyses were performed by using MINITAB for Windows (release 12.1, Minitab Inc., State College, PA, USA). Mean values were considered significantly different at $P < 0.05$.

Abbreviations

$AUC_{0\to\infty}$: area under the (zero moment) curve from time 0 to infinity; $AUMC_{0\to\infty}$: area under the moment curve from time 0 to infinity; C_0: plasma concentration at time 0; Cl_B: total body clearance of drug; COX: cyclooxygenase; MLX: meloxicam; $MRT_{0\to\infty}$: mean residence time; NSAIDs: nonsteroidal anti-inflammatory drugs; $T_{1/2\lambda z}$: terminal half-life; Vd_{ss}: volume of distribution at steady-state.

Competing interests

The authors declare that they have no competing interests.

Authors' contributions

All authors have made substantial contributions to all of the following: the conception and design of the study (UK, CG), the animal phase of the experiments (UK, CK, HE, EHU, CP), the analytical phase of the study (CG, DA), drafting the article (CG, UK). All authors have read and approved the final manuscript.

Acknowledgements

The authors would like to thank Prof Hayrettin Cetin for his expert advice with the experimental procedures carried out during the study and Prof. Mehmet Bilgen for proof reading and commenting on the work.

Author details

[1]Department of Pharmacology and Toxicology, Faculty of Veterinary Medicine, University of Adnan Menderes, Isikli Koyu, Aydin, Turkey. [2]Department of Pharmacology and Toxicology, Faculty of Veterinary Medicine, Balikesir University, Balikesir, Turkey. [3]Department of Internal Medicine, Faculty of Veterinary Medicine, University of Adnan Menderes, Isikli Koyu, Aydin, Turkey. [4]Department of Obstetrics and Gynecology, Faculty of Veterinary Medicine, University of Adnan Menderes, Isikli Koyu, Aydin, Turkey. [5]Department of Medical Pharmacology, Faculty of Medicine, Balikesir University, Balikesir, Turkey.

References

1. Barker SJ, Gamel DM, Tremper KK. Cardiovascular effects of anaesthesia and operation. Crit Care Clin. 1987;3:251–68.
2. Belpaire FM, De Rick A, Dello C, Fraeyman N, Bogaert MG. Alpha 1-acid glycoprotein and serum binding of drugs in healthy and diseased dogs. J Vet Pharm Ther. 1984;10:43–8.
3. Botting RM. Cyclooxygenase: Past, present and future. A tribute to John R. Vane (1927–2004). J Therm Biol. 2006;31:208–19.
4. Budsberg SC, Cross AR, Quandt JE, Pablo LS, Runk AR. Evaluation of intravenous administration of meloxicam for perioperative pain management following stifle joint surgery in dogs. Am J Vet Res. 2002;63:1557–63.
5. Busch U, Schmid J, Heinze G, Schmaus H, Baier J, Huber C, et al. Pharmacokinetics of meloxicam in animals and the relevance to humans. Drug Metab Dispos. 1998;26:576–84.
6. Cagnardi P, Zonca A, Gallo M, Villa R, Carli S, Beccaglia M, et al. Pharmacokinetics and perioperative efficacy of intravenous ketorolac in dogs. J Vet Pharm Ther. 2013;36:603–8.
7. Cagnardi P, Ferraresi C, Zonca A, Pecile A, Ravasio G, Zani DD, et al. Clinical pharmacokinetics of tramadol and main metabolites in horses undergoing orchiectomy. Vet Quar. 2014;34:143–51.
8. Caulkett N, Read M, Fowler D, Waldner C. A comparison of the analgesic effects of butorphanol with those of meloxicam after elective ovariohysterectomy in dogs. Can Vet J. 2003;44:565–70.
9. Engelhardt G, Homma D, Schlegel K, Utzmann R, Schnitzler C. Meloxicam: a potent inhibitor of adjuvant arthritis in the Lewis rat. Inf Res. 1995;44:548–55.
10. Eniko C, Ibolya F, Daniela-Lucia M. Development of a HPLC-UV method for determination of meloxicam in human plasma and pharmaceutical dosage forms. Acta Med. 2014;60:142–5.
11. Ferraresi C, Villa R, Ravasio G, Zonca A, Carli S, Pecile A, et al. Pharmacokinetics of IV Ketorolac in Horses Undergoing Orchiectomy. J Equine Vet Sci. 2014;34:870–5.
12. Fowler D, Isakow K, Caulkett N, Waldner C. An evaluation of the analgesic effects of meloxicam in addition to epidural morphine/mepivacaine in dogs undergoing cranial cruciate ligament repair. Can Vet J. 2003;44:643–8.
13. Frey HH, Rieh B. Pharmacokinetics of naproxen in the dog. Am J Vet Res. 1981;42:1615–7.
14. Frey HH, Loscher W. Pharmacokinetics of antiepileptic drugs in the dog: A review. J Vet Pharm Ther. 1985;8:219–33.
15. Heard DJ, Huft VJ. The effect of short term physical restraint and isoflurane anaesthesia on haematology and plasma biochemistry in the island flying fox (Pteropus hypomelanus). J Zoo Wild An. 1998;29:14–7.
16. Jolliet P, Simon N, Brée F, Urien S, Pagliara A, Carrupt PA, et al. Blood-to-brain transfer of various oxicams: effects of plasma binding on their brain delivery. Pharm Res. 1997;14:650–6.
17. Kay-Mugford P, Benn SJ, Lamarre J, Conlon P. In vitro effects of nonsteroidal anti-inflammatory drugs on cyclooxygenase activity in dogs. Am J Vet Res. 2000;61:802–10.
18. Kennedy JM, Riji AM. Effects of surgery on the pharmacokinetic parameters of drugs. Clin Pharm. 1998;35:293–312.
19. Kilkenny C, Browne WJ, Cuthill IC, Emerson M, Altman DG. Improving bioscience research reporting: the arrive guidelines for reporting animal research. Plos Biology. 2010;8:1–5.

20. Kum C, Voyvoda H, Sekkin S, Karademir U, Tarimcilar T. Effect of carprofen and meloxicam on C-reactive protein, ceruloplasmin and fibrinogen concentrations in dogs undergoing ovariohysterectomy. Am J Vet Res. 2013; 74:1267–73.
21. Lees P, Giraudel J, Landoni MF, Toutain PL. PK-PD integration and PK-PD modelling of nonsteroidal anti-inflammatory drugs: principles and applications in veterinary pharmacology. J Vet Pharm Ther. 2004;27:491–502.
22. Lees P, Landoni MF, Giraudel J, Toutain PL. Pharmacodynamics and pharmacokinetics of nonsteroidal anti-inflammatory drugs in species of veterinary interest. J Vet Pharm Ther. 2004;27:479–90.
23. Lolekha PH, Charoenpol W. Improved automated method for determining serum albumin with bromcresol green. Clin Chem. 1974;20:617–9.
24. Mathews KA, Pettifer G, Foster R, Mcdonell W. Safety and efficacy of preoperative administration of meloxicam, compared with that of ketoprofen and butorphanol in dogs undergoing abdominal surgery. Am J Vet Res. 2001;62:882–8.
25. Runkel R, Forchielli E, Boosz G, Chaplin M, Hill R, Sevelius H, et al. Naproxen metabolism, excretion and comparative pharmacokinetics. Scan J Rheum. 1973;2:24–36.
26. Van Dalen R, Vree TB. Pharmacokinetics of antibiotics in critically ill patients. Intens Care Med. 1990;16:235–8.
27. Villa R, Ravasio G, Ferraresi C, Zonca A, Carli S, Borghi L, et al. Pharmacokinetics of intravenous ketorolac in cats undergoing gonadectomy. N Z Vet J. 2015;63:162–6.

12

A preliminary study evaluating cardiac output measurement using Pressure Recording Analytical Method (PRAM) in anaesthetized dogs

Angela Briganti[1], Flavia Evangelista[1], Paola Centonze[2], Annaliso Rizzo[2], Francesco Bentivegna[2], Antonio Crovace[2] and Francesco Staffieri[2*]

Abstract

Background: Haemodynamic variations normally occur in anaesthetized animals, in relation to the animal status, administered drugs, sympathetic and parasympathetic tone, fluid therapy and surgical stimulus. The possibility to measure some cardiovascular parameters, such as cardiac output (CO), during anaesthesia would be beneficial for both the anaesthesia management and its outcome. New techniques for the monitoring of CO are aimed at finding methods which are non invasive, accurate and with good trending ability, which can be used in a clinical setting. The aim of this study was to compare the Pressure Recording Analytical Method (PRAM) with the pulmonary artery thermodilution (TD) for the measurement of cardiac output in 6 anaesthetized critically ill dogs.

Results: Fifty-four pairs of CO measurements were obtained with a median (range) of 3.33 L/min (0.81–7.21) for PRAM-CO and 3.48 L/min (1.41–6.56) for TD-CO. The Bland-Altman analysis showed a mean bias of 0.17 L/min with limits of agreement (LoA) of – 0.46 to 0.81 L/min. The percentage error resulted 18.2%. The 4-quadrant plot analysis showed an acceptable concordance (93%) between the 2 methods. The polar plot showed a good trending ability with the mean angular bias of 3.9° and radial LoA ± 12.1°.

Conclusions: The PRAM resulted in good precision, acceptable concordance and good trending ability for the measure of CO in the anaesthetized dog, representing a promising alternative to thermodilution for the measurement of CO. Among all the pulse contour methods available on the market it is the only one that does not require any calibration or adjustment of the measurement. Further studies are required to verify the ability of this method to accurately measure cardiac output even during unstable hemodynamic conditions.

Keywords: Pressure recording analytical method, Cardiac output, Pulse contour, Dog, Anaesthesia

Background

Haemodynamic monitoring represents a support tool for the assessment of the clinical status of patients, guidance of therapeutic decisions and evaluation of response to intervention, both in human and veterinary patients [1–3].

Cardiac output (CO) is a macrocirculatory measure of total body blood flow, defined as the volume of blood pumped by the heart in 1 min, and is a major determinant of DO_2 [4]. Since most organs rely on flow rather than pressure for optimal function, measurement of CO is a pivotal component of the haemodynamic evaluation of high risk human patients, providing an indirect indication of global tissue perfusion [5]. The need to monitor this parameter in the perioperative period has led to the development of various devices and techniques. Thermodilution, through the use of pulmonary artery catheters (PAC-TD), based on the Stewart-Hamilton principle, is considered as the clinical standard method for the measurement of cardiac output in human medicine and it is often considered the reference method when other

* Correspondence: francesco.staffieri@uniba.it
[2]Dipartimento delle Emergenze e Trapianti di Organo, Università degli Studi di Bari "Aldo Moro," Sezione di Cliniche Veterinarie e P.A, Bari, Italy
Full list of author information is available at the end of the article

devices or measuring techniques are compared [5, 6]. However, the use of PAC-TD in clinical practice is limited, mainly because of additional costs and risks associated with pulmonary artery catheterization [7]. For this reason, in the last years less invasive procedures, such as pulse contour monitors, are under evaluation in order to find new techniques that can be used for the CO evaluation. Recent veterinary studies concluded that results obtained from the evaluated pulse contour methods [8–11] are not reliable for the CO evaluation in dogs in the clinical setting.

Pressure Recording Analytical Method (PRAM) is a pulse contour method, which estimates stroke volume and other hemodynamic parameters from the analysis of the arterial pulse waveform [12]. It is based on the principle for which the arterial blood pressure waveform results from the interaction between the systolic ejection volume and the physical characteristics of the systemic vascular system (vascular compliance, aortic impedance and peripheral arterial resistance). Stroke volume is estimated from the area under the systolic portion of an arterial pressure curve and a variable called Z. This variable indicates the dynamic impedance of the cardiovascular system, representing all the factors which oppose to the propagation of the pressure wave on the arterial tree. The variable Z is computed from the pressure curve through a proprietary algorithm on each beat [12–14]. The monitor allows a beat-by-beat assessment of CO from the arterial pressure wave, it is minimally invasive because it only needs the insertion of a regular, non-dedicated arterial catheter and doesn't need calibration prior to clinical use. In addition to the CO, heart rate, systolic, diastolic and mean arterial pressures, pulse pressure, systolic pressure, pulse pressure variation (PPV), stroke volume (SV) and stroke volume variation (SVV) are also continuously provided by the monitor [13, 14].

PRAM has been validated for the measurement of CO in a swine model under different haemodynamic states [15, 16] and in human patients undergoing cardiac surgery [17], patients supported with a left ventricular assist device [18] and in patients supported with aortic counterpulsation after cardiac surgery [19].

The objective of this study was to evaluate the performances of the PRAM technology integrated in the MostCare® monitor compared to PAC-TD for the measurement of CO in selected cases in which dogs received a Swan-Ganz catheter for their clinical management. We hypothesized that CO measurement obtained by PRAM would be in agreement with those obtained by thermodilution.

Methods

The study was conducted at the Section of Veterinary Clinics and Animal Production, DETO, University of Bari, Italy after the approval of the Ethical Committee (Prot. n. 48/16-DETO) and written owner consent was obtained before enrolling the dogs in the study.

Animals

Six female dogs, affected by early stage sepsis, anesthetised for major abdominal surgical procedures, were enrolled for this study. In all dogs a Swan-Ganz catheter was placed for the monitoring of the cardiac output during anaesthesia and thereafter in the intensive care unit, based on the judgment of the clinician in charge. Patients that required administration of inotropic and/or vasoactive drugs and/or with cardiac arrhythmias were not included in the study.

Before anaesthesia all the animals were submitted to clinical and laboratory exams in order to evaluate the clinical conditions and assign the ASA Physical Status.

Breed, age, weight, ASA Physical Status and the main pathological reasons for surgery are reported in Table 1.

Anaesthetic protocol

Dogs were premedicated with methadone[1] 0.3 mg/kg intramuscularly and were induced with propofol[2] to effect to obtain orotracheal intubation at 30 min after the premedication. Anaesthesia was maintained with isoflurane[3] in oxygen with an oxygen inspired fraction (FiO_2) > 0.8. The end tidal concentration of isoflurane was maintained at 1–1.3% during all the procedure according to the patients' requirements. During the procedure all the animals were mechanically ventilated in a volume controlled mode with a tidal volume of 10 mL/kg, a respiratory rate of 12 breaths per minute and an inspiration-expiration ratio of 1:2; the ventilator setting was modified in order to maintain the carbon dioxide end tidal ($EtCO_2$) values between 35 and 45 mmHg.[4] Surgery started at the completion of the placement of the monitoring and the surgical scrubbing. Ringer Lactate solution[5] was administrated at a minimum of 10 mL/kg/h IV and its rate was adjusted based on the specific requirements of the patients. At the end of surgery anaesthetic drugs administration was discontinued and patients were recovered in the intensive care unit (ICU) with the appropriate support. Before surgery and in the postoperative period dogs were treated with 22 mg/kg IV of ampicillin[6] every 8 h and enrofloxacin[7] 10 mg/kg IV every 24 h. Moreover, methadone (0.2 mg/kg IV) was administered every 4 h. Fluid therapy, pain management, cardiovascular support, sedation and any additional treatment were based on the judgment of the clinician in charge of the case. The Swan-Ganz and arterial catheters were left in place up to a maximum of 48 h.

Cardiac output measurements

After induction of anaesthesia patients were positioned in dorsal recumbency. A 6F 12 cm introducer was

Table 1 Breed, age, weight, type of surgery and ASA status of the dogs included in the study

Case n.	Breed	Age (years)	Weight (kg)	Surgery	ASA Status
1	Golden Retriever	1	17	Pyometra	III
2	Mixed Breed	2	15	Septic peritonitis for intestinal rupture (foreign body)	IV
3	Beagle	3	17	Septic peritonitis for a rupture of an hepatic abscess	III - IV
4	German Shepherd	2	23	Pyometra	IV
5	Mixed Breed	2	14	Pyometra	III - IV
6	Mixed Breed	1	14	Septic peritonitis for anastomotic dehiscence	IV

transcutaneoulsy placed in the right external jugular vein by means of the Seldinger technique, and through it a 5F Swan-Ganz pulmonary arterial catheter[8] was advanced to the lumen of the pulmonary artery to obtain the cardiac output measurements with the thermodilution technique (TD) using a dedicated monitor.[9] The catheter's position was confirmed by observation of characteristic pulmonary arterial pressure waves. The computation constant for the computer was adjusted for a 5F Swan-Ganz catheter, injection volume of 5 mL, and an injectate temperature of 0–5 °C, which was measured at the injection site. Each measurement was taken with the administration of 5 mL of cold (0–3 °C) 0.9% sodium chloride[10] over less than 3 s, the measurement was repeated for three times with 1 min intervals between each determination. Injections were done manually always by the same person, and the mean of three measurements within 10% was used. A 18 gauge × 25 mm catheter[11] was transcutaneously positioned in the femoral artery and connected to the PRAM monitor[12] for the evaluation of the CO.

Both the Swan-Ganz and the arterial catheters were connected to a transducer[13] with a dedicated saline-filled line included in the kit and zeroed at the right atrial level. The accuracy of the signal was verified by a square wave test, before starting data collection.

The CO values obtained with PRAM (PRAM-CO) were recorded and stored automatically every 30 s on a personal computer. At each time of determination of CO with TD, a marker was stored on the PRAM monitor in order to detect that specific determination, a posteriori, on the PRAM data sheet. The corresponding PRAM determination was considered as the value registered at the time of the marker. The average of the values recorded for the three consecutive determinations at each time point of the study was taken as the representative result for PRAM-CO. The CO measurements were done after the placement of the catheters (T0) and thereafter every 10–15 min up to 8 measurements (T1, T2, T3, T4, T5, T6, T7, T8) for a total of 9 time points.

Monitoring

During the procedure heart rate (HR, beats/min), systolic, diastolic, mean arterial pressures (SAP, DAP and MAP, mmHg)[12], end-tidal carbon dioxide tension ($EtCO_2$, mmHg), peripheral capillary oxygen saturation (SpO_2, %), respiratory rate (RR, breaths/min) and oesophageal temperature (T, °C) were monitored with a multiparameter monitor[14] and recorded every 5 min on a data sheet. Moreover, central venous pressure (CVP, mmHg), cardiac output (CO, L/min) were measured and systemic vascular resistances (SVR, dyn·s/cm^{-5}) were calculated.

Statistics

Data were analysed for normal distribution with a Kolmogorov Smirnov test and expressed as mean and standard deviation. A one-way ANOVA for repeated measures was used to compare the clinical parameters for each recorded time; if significant, Tukey's test was applied for post hoc comparison between the different conditions. A Spearman correlation test was used to evaluate the correlation between pairs of values (TD-CO vs PRAM-CO) and a coefficient of determination (r^2) was calculated. P values < 0.05 were considered significant.

The agreement between TD-CO and PRAM-CO measurements was assessed using the Bland Altman method for multiple observations per individual [20, 21]. Mean bias (mean difference between measurements), standard deviation (SD), percentage bias (mean of 100 x [bias/(TD-CO + PRAM-CO)/2]), 95% limits of agreement (LoA; mean bias ±1.96 SD) and percentage error (100 × 1.96 SD/mean CO of both methods) were calculated. A percentage error not exceeding 30% was considered acceptable to indicate clinical reliability [22]. Precision of method (POM) of each series of triplicate CO measurements was calculated as 2 times the coefficient of error (CE) and CE was obtained dividing the coefficient of variation by the square root of number of replicates [11, 23]. The obtained POMs were used to calculate the precision of agreement (POA) [23].

Ability of the PRAM to track changes towards the TD method was evaluated by 4-quadrant plot and polar plot analysis. Sequential percentage changes in PRAM-CO were plotted on the y axis and corresponding changes in the TD-CO were visualized on x axis. The graph was then divided in 4-quadrants by the intersection of lines originated from zero in both axes. Delta CO measurements < 10% were excluded according to the bibliography

[24]. The concordance was calculated as the numbers of points in the upper right and lower left quadrants, divided by the total number of points and considered as a percentage as following: > 95% good concordance, between 95% and 90% acceptable or marginal and < 90% poor concordance.

The delta CO (ΔCO) changes were then calculated as arithmetic mean of ΔCO of the tested (PRAM-CO) and reference (TD-CO) method. The polar angle was calculated as the angle of divergence of the ΔCO from the line of identity (45°) [25]. As recommended by Critchley et al. (2011) good trending ability based on polar plot analysis was defined by the mean angular bias ≤ `5° with radial LoA ≤ `30°.

For statistical test and graphic presentation different specific softwares[15,16,17] were used.

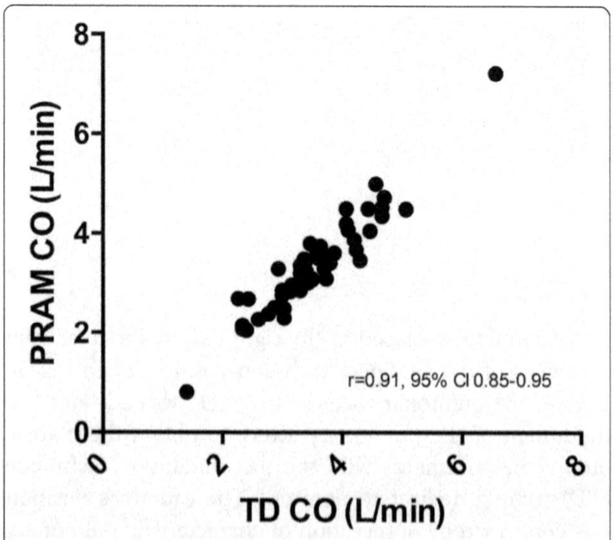

Fig. 1 Plot of PRAM-CO values (y axis) and TD-CO values (x axis) with Spearman correlation test results

Results

All the enrolled animals survived to the surgical procedure and the anaesthesia. The median (range) duration of surgery and anaesthesia was 153 min (125–185) and 195 min (156–215) respectively. No complications related to the Swan-Ganz arterial catheters were reported in the records of the dogs.

No differences were detected between each recorded time for clinical parameters (Table 2).

Fifty-four pairs of CO measurements were obtained (Fig. 1).

The median and range of the CO values were 3.33 L/min (0.81–7.21) for the PRAM and 3.48 L/min (1.42–6.56) for the TD. The Bland-Altman analysis showed a mean bias of 0.17 L/min with LoA of – 0.46 to 0.81 L/min. The percentage error resulted 18.2% (Table 3). A Bland-Altman plot is shown in Fig. 2. The POM of the TD-CO was 9.2% and POM of PRAM-CO was 8.8%. POA expected if the reference technique was compared to itself (POA $_{REFxREF}$) resulted 13%; POA of test versus reference technique (POA $_{TESTxREF}$) resulted 12.7%.

The 4-quadrant plot analysis (Fig. 3) showed an acceptable concordance (92%) between the 2 methods (Table 4). The polar plot showed a good trending ability

Table 2 Mean values and standard deviation of measured physiological parameters of dogs for 9 time points corresponding to CO measurements

	T0	T1	T 2	T 3	T 4	T 5	T 6	T 7	T 8
HR (beats/min)	84 ± 17	78 ± 29	81 ± 24	79 ± 16	70 ± 19.	65 ± 13	72 ± 18	75 ± 21	80 ± 17
SAP (mmHg)	105 ± 16	111 ± 19	115 ± 14	118 ± 17	145 ± 31	123 ± 23	115 ± 14	114 ± 17	111 ± 18
MAP (mmHg)	74 ± 12	79 ± 16	83 ± 12	88 ± 16	114 ± 26	90 ± 25	86 ± 14	84 ± 16	81 ± 18
DAP (mmHg)	58 ± 9	64 ± 14	67 ± 11	73 ± 15	98 ± 24	79 ± 17	70 ± 13	68 ± 15	66 ± 17
CVP (mmHg)	5 ± 1	7 ± 3	6 ± 2.4	7 ± 1	8 ± 2	8 ± 2	7 ± 2	7 ± 2	6 ± 2
PRAM –CO (L/min)	2.8 ± 0.5	3.0 ± 0.5	3.4 ± 0.5	3.4 ± 0.7	3.9 ± 0.5	3.0 ± 1.2	4.1 ± 1.6	3.1 ± 0.8	3.2 ± 0.9
TD-CO (L/min)	2.8 ± 0.5	3.3 ± 0.6	3.6 ± 0.4	3.5 ± 0.9	4.1 ± 0.3	3.1 ± 0.9	4.1 ± 1.3	3.4 ± 07	3.5 ± 0.6
SV_{PRAM} (mL)	33 ± 11	46 ± 21	45 ± 16	42 ± 10	66 ± 24	42 ± 19	48 ± 16	43 ± 13	40 ± 12
SV_{TD} (mL)	33 ± 7	48 ± 22	48 ± 17	45 ± 11	63 ± 18	49 ± 17	58 ± 13	48 ± 15	45 ± 9
$ETCO_2$ (mmHg)	43 ± 4	42 ± 3	43 ± 3	40 ± 6	38 ± 6	44 ± 6	45 ± 6	43 ± 5	44 ± 5
SPO_2 (%)	95 ± 1	95 ± 2	96 ± 1	95 ± 1	97 ± 1	97 ± 1	96 ± 1	96 ± 1	97 ± 1
T (°C)	36.9 ± 0.6	36.6 ± 0.7	36.4 ± 0.9	36.4 ± 0.9	35.9 ± 0.6	35.7 ± 0.4	35.4 ± 0.5	35.6 ± 0.4	35.5 ± 0.5
RR (breaths/min)	14 ± 3	14 ± 3	14 ± 3	14. ± 2	15 ± 3	16 ± 2	16 ± 2	16 ± 2	16 ± 2

HR heart rate, *SAP* systolic arterial pressure, *MAP* mean arterial pressure, *DAP* diastolic arterial pressure, *CVP* central venous pressure, *PRAM-CO* cardiac output measurements obtained by PRAM, *TD-CO* cardiac output measurements obtained by pulmonary artery thermodilution, SV_{PRAM} stroke volume measurements obtained by PRAM, SV_{TD} stroke volume measurements obtained by pulmonary artery thermodilution, $EtCO_2$ end-tidal carbon dioxide tension, SpO_2 peripheral capillary oxygen saturation, *T* temperature, *RR* respiratory rate

Table 3 Results of Bland Altman Analysis for 54 pairs of CO measurements

	TD-CO vs PRAM-CO
mean bias (L min^{-1})	0.17
SD of bias (L min^{-1})	0.32
mean percentage bias (%)	6.38
upper LOA (L min^{-1})	0.81
lower LOA (L min^{-1})	−0.46
percentage error (%)	18.2

with the mean angular bias of 3.9° with radial LoA ± 12.1° (Table 3 and Fig. 4).

Discussion

This is the first study in which the PRAM technology is compared to the thermodilution method in the canine species. These preliminary findings showed a close agreement between thermodilution and PRAM. The PRAM method tends to underestimate CO compared to thermodilution measurements with a mean bias of 0.17 L/min (and a mean percentage bias of 6.38%). The percentage error is a statistical measure of agreement between the two methods [24]. A limit of 30% of the percentage error value has been recommended as an objective criterion to define clinical acceptability of a new method compared to the reference method [22]. The percentage error in this study, calculated from the Bland-Altman plot, resulted 18%, largely acceptable for the aforementioned limit of percentage error. This value is consistent to percentage errors found in other validation studies of CO measuring methods, and even better performing than other studies involving the validation of PRAM in man [12, 18, 19, 26]. The limitation to the commonly utilization of the 30% cut-off value for the percentage error is due to the fact that precision of thermodilution technique can vary and, in case of rigorously applied techniques, or when CO is derived from more than 1 measurement, a low PE of the reference method can compensate for higher PE of the tested technique. For this reason the most recent studies, evaluating new techniques for the cardiac output comparison, put in evidence the necessity to calculate the specific precision of each used method [27]: both the one considered the reference method (POM_{REF}) and the new one studied (POM_{TEST}). With this calculation it was possible to evaluate the precision of each method (POM) employed in the present study, both for the reference (TD-CO: 9,2%) and the tested method (PRAM-CO: 8,8%). POM itself can not be used to compare the two techniques because it describes the similarity of a method's repeated measurements for one and the same true value [27]. The main problem in using a POM in CO studies is that the CO itself is not a constant true value, but it can rapidly change over time depending on several factors such as heart rate, stroke volume and mean arterial pressure. For simplicity, in this kind of studies, it is assumed that for each time point cardiac output is fairly constant during the multiple measurements obtained by both techniques [11]. POM_{REF} and POM_{TEST} can be used to calculate the POA, which describes the variability in the agreement or disagreement between methods [27]. Usually POA between the studied technique and the reference technique ($POA_{TESTxREF}$) is compared to the POA that would be expected if the reference technique was compared to itself. $POA_{REFxREF}$, defined as estimation of the POA when the reference technique is compared to itself, is an artificial POA, but can be used to define the acceptable percentage error of a specific study. In the present study the $POA_{REFxREF}$ resulted 13% and $POA_{TESTxREF}$ resulted 12.7%. In case of the POM of the studied technique and the reference technique were the

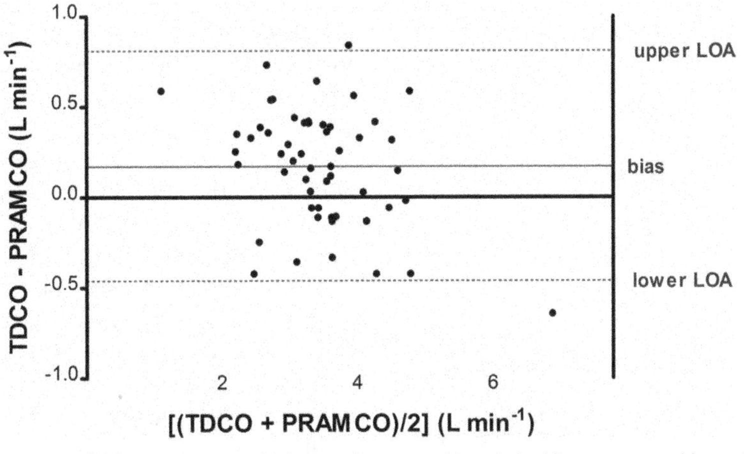

Fig. 2 Bland Altman plot for 54 pairs of CO measurements. Light grey line: mean bias; dashed lines: upper and lower limits of agreement

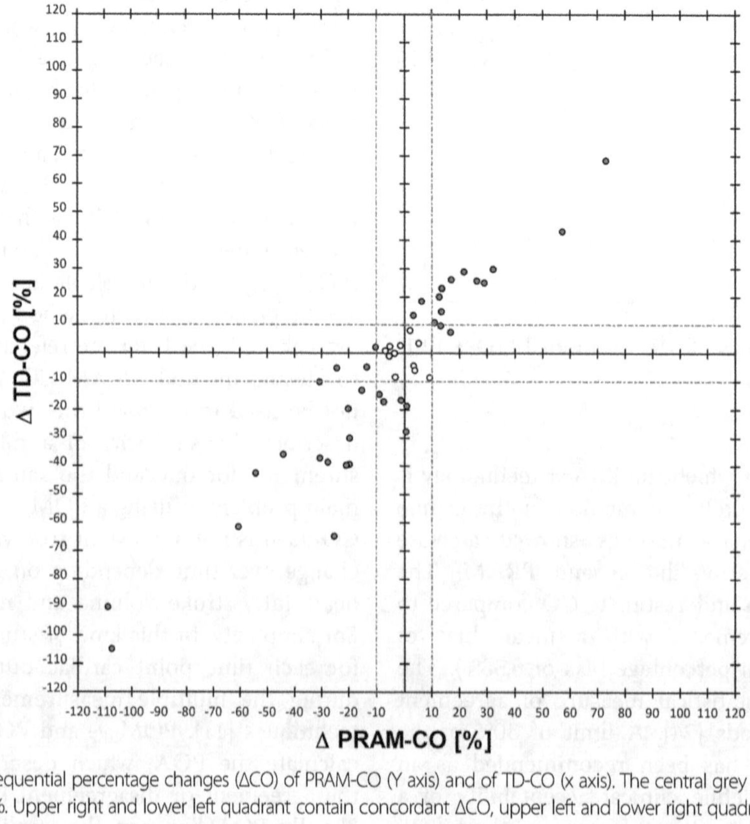

Fig. 3 Four-quadrant plot. Sequential percentage changes (ΔCO) of PRAM-CO (Y axis) and of TD-CO (x axis). The central grey zone represents the exclusion area that contains ΔCO < 10%. Upper right and lower left quadrant contain concordant ΔCO, upper left and lower right quadrant contain discordant ΔCO

same also the $POA_{REFxREF}$ and $POA_{TESTxREF}$ would be the same [27] and the tested technique would be accepted as in our case. It is fundamental to keep in mind that POM only describes deviations among repeated measurements of a true value, while the trueness describes the overall deviation of these measurements from that value, that in case of cardiac output measurement it is impossible to acquire [27].

In the validation process of a new technique, Bland-Altman analysis is the main instrument to assess if the new method agrees with the reference method and to which extent [28]. However it is important to point out that this statistical tool only addresses agreement and doesn't provide information about how reliably the new method detects changes in the measured values in time (trending ability); thus Bland-Altman analysis alone is not sufficient to determine if a new technique is clinically acceptable in comparison to a reference technique [28, 29]. To overcome this issue, other statistical tools are available. Trending ability analysis with concordance rate calculation and four quadrant plots [25, 28] and polar plots, with the calculation of the polar angle and radial limits of agreement [25, 29], can be used to assess the trending ability of the technique to be validated. In this study both the 4-quadrant analysis and the polar plot have been done in order to assess the concordance and the trending ability of the PRAM technique. The concordance resulted acceptable (92%) and the trending ability good (mean radial angle of 3.9° and radial LoA ± 12.1°).

Both for the 4 quadrant plot and for the polar plot, a central exclusion zone with data points ≤ 10% was identified and data inside it were excluded. Those data were considered to increase the signal-to-noise ratio, [24, 25] adding no information to the assessment of trending ability of the technique and representing very little clinical impact.

Table 4 Results of 4-quadrant plot and polar plot

	TDCO vs PRAMCO
Measurements < 10% (n)	11
Measurements > 10% in the right quadrants (n)	34
Measurements > 10% in the wrong quadrants (n)	3
Total measurements > 10% (n)	37
Concordance rate (%)	92
Mean angular bias (°)	3.9
Radial limits of agreement (°)	± 12.1

Concordance rate was calculated as: 100 × (data points in correct quadrant and > 10% CO)/data points > 10% CO. Concordance rates are considered to be good when above 95%, acceptable when between 90 and 95% and poor when below 90%. In the polar plot a mean angle with the horizontal axis < 5° and radial limits of agreement RLOA (= 95% confidence interval) < 30° are considered to indicate good trending ability

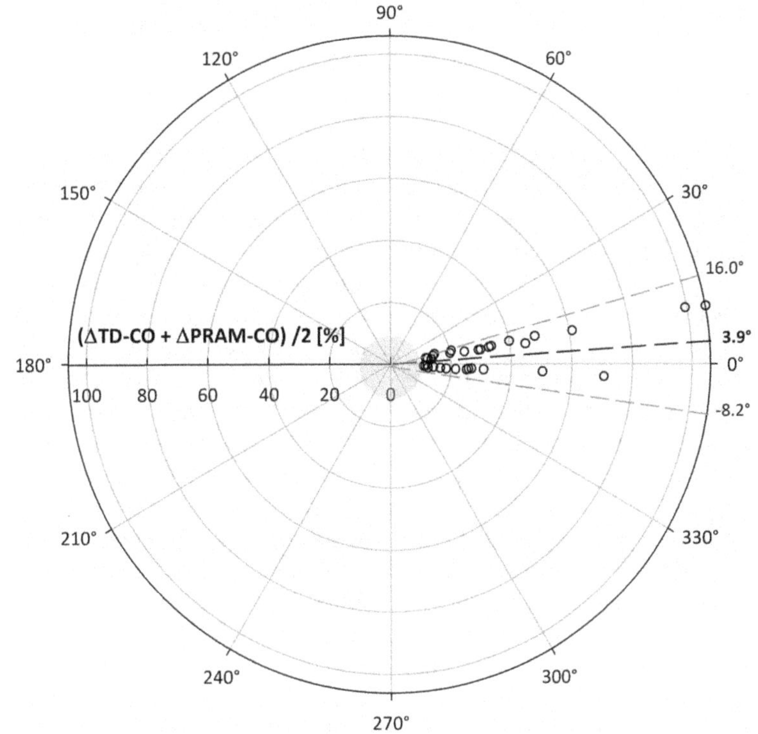

Fig. 4 Polar plot of ΔCO expressed as polar coordinates (radius and polar angle). The central grey circle represents the exclusion zone (mean ΔCO < 10%). The black dashed line represents the mean polar angle of 3.9° (mean angular bias), light gray dashed lines represent the radial LoA (± 12.1°). Sixteen data points were excluded from analysis because they fell in the exclusion zone

A recent evaluation of pulse contour methods in dogs has been published [8]. The authors evaluated PiCCO and PulseCO (both externally calibrated pulse contour methods, respectively with transpulmonary thermodilution and with pulmonary artery thermodilution), as well as transpulmonary thermodilution, all compared to pulmonary artery thermodilution. Since the assessment of agreement and of trending ability with the same statistical tools allows the comparison of different studies [28] we can compare our results to those obtained by Kutter and colleagues. They show a poor trending ability of PiCCO and PulseCO compared to pulmonary artery thermodilution with low concordance rates (respectively 77% and 74%), and an unacceptable percentage error (respectively 47% and 42%), far above the 30% criterion defined by Critchley (2010) for acceptability. In our study the concordance and the trending ability of PRAM resulted superior to all the techniques evaluated by Kutter and colleagues with a mean radial angle lower than 5° and all the measurements under ±30°.

Another recent study [28] evaluated the use a calibrated pulse contour analysis, PiCCO (calibrated with transpulmonary thermodilution) during pharmacological interventions on vascular tone (intravenous phenylephrine and nitroprusside) in dogs. The authors concluded that the use of PiCCO is limited in dogs when abrupt changes in peripheral vascular resistances occur, reporting low concordance (63%) and poor trending ability (mean radial angle 38°) compared to pulmonary artery thermodilution.

The Flotrac/Vigileo system, a pulse contour method, which needs an input of demographic data for calibration, has been evaluated in dogs in comparison to pulmonary artery thermodilution [9]. In light of a very high percentage bias between the two techniques (110%) and a high percentage error, far beyond the limits of acceptance (162%), the authors conclude that the use of this monitor is not recommended for measuring CO in dogs [9]. Moreover authors did a post-hoc trending ability analysis and poor trending ability with a concordance rate of 86% was found together with a mean polar angle of 9° as well as inadequately wide radial limits of agreement of ±48° (Kutter and Bektas, personal communication). The algorithm which underlies the functioning of FloTrac/Vigileo takes into account human demographic data which might not apply correctly to the cardiovascular system of dogs [9].

Pulmonary artery thermodilution is a technique which requires some time to obtain one single measurement. In this time frame the true value of CO can experience variations and therefore for each single measurement there is an intrinsic error, which can be reduced by averaging a certain number of single measurements. For

TD-CO determination it has been recommended to obtain the mean of three consecutive measurements of CO, which results in a precision of 6% within the true value with a 95% confidence interval, and allows a reliable detection in CO changes [30, 31].

For this reason a monitor which can rapidly detect changes in CO might be more suitable for use in critical and surgical patients, or in goal directed therapy, contexts in which it is crucial to detect fast hemodynamic changes. Pulse contour methods estimate SV from the arterial wave line and can perform a beat-to-beat estimation of CO.

If our results will be confirmed by more standardized and controlled studies, the PRAM technology could represent a promising alternative to thermodilution for the measurement of CO in dogs, both for clinical and research purposes. The PRAM method only needs a pressure waveform signal detected by an arterial catheter in a peripheral artery connected to a dedicated monitor, and among all the pulse contour methods available on the market it is the only one that does not require any calibration or adjustment of the measurement according to pre-obtained data [14]. The issue of calibration is overcome by PRAM, which obtains information about the arterial system elastic and mechanical properties in vivo, directly from the arterial waveform, for every beat [13]. Indeed pulse contour methods calculate SV from the ratio of the area under the arterial pressure curve and a variable called Z, which denotes the relationship between pressure and flow. Z takes into account physical properties of the cardiovascular system, which are closely interrelated, such as arterial impedance, arterial compliance and the peripheral arterial tree resistance. All these physical properties need to be evaluated simultaneously for a correct estimation of SV from the pressure wave [13]. In calibrated pulse contour methods, Z is computed starting from already existing data (Vigileo) or it is obtained from an external calibration method (PiCCO, PulseCO) and its value is applied over several SV estimations, even if the mechanical and elastic properties of the arterial system may change with time. PRAM, instead, directly estimates Z from the curve at every pulsation, considering both the systolic and diastolic contributions of the curve to the estimation of SV [13, 32]. Therefore the way that the variable Z is obtained may be the key difference between pulse contour methods that explains why PRAM has a superior performance in dogs, showing a good agreement and trending ability when compared to pulmonary artery thermodilution.

On the other side, PRAM has some limitations related to the need to detect dicrotic notch at every beat. If the monitor fails to correctly detect the dicrotic notch at each beat, the calculations are incorrect and CO measures might be artifactual. In our study the femoral artery has been catheterised, whereas other locations most commonly used in clinical patients, as dorsal pedal or dorsal metatarsal arteries, could be more influenced for the vascular elasticity and the dicrotic notch could not be as clear as in our results. The occurrence of arrhythmia or bradycardia is a typical scenario in which the monitor can mis-detect the notch and therefore return erroneous readings. However, the position of the dicrotic notch is highlighted on the screen at every beat, and the clinician can modify the settings on the PRAM monitor to adjust the dicrotic notch position if the quality of the detection is evaluated to be poor. Another issue is the necessity to have a correct damping of the arterial line: assessment of the damping is important since an over- or under-damped signal can generate an artefact which modifies the area under the curve and therefore affects the estimation of SV [32].

There is no information about the use of PRAM during acute changes in vascular resistance in dogs. Garofalo and colleagues (2016) report that when nitroprusside was infused intravenously in dogs, the dicrotic notch of the arterial waveform was blunted and difficult to detect by PiCCO; while the dicrotic notch was always detectable during a phenylephrine intravenous infusion. This is probably due to the dispersion of energy in the vascular tree during a vasodilated state, which decreases the magnitude of reflected backward waves from the peripheral arterial system to the heart, a phenomenon that could lead to failure of the device to detect the end of the systolic portion of the wave and to overestimate SV, artifactually increasing the area under the curve of the systolic portion [11].

The number of the cases is an important limitation of this study. Moreover, animals that required administration of vasoactive and/or inotropic drugs were excluded in order to avoid additional biases that could not have been controlled in a clinical setting. Accordingly, our observations were limited to more stable cardiovascular conditions. In the light of these encouraging results, further experimental and clinical studies are needed to determine whether PRAM has a good agreement and trending ability during cardiovascular instability and under the influence of drugs that alter the peripheral vessel tone, thus confirming the clinical reliability of this technique.

Conclusion

PRAM resulted in good precision, acceptable concordance and good trending ability for the measure of CO in the anaesthetized dog with a clinically stable hemodynamic status. As a minimally-invasive pulse contour method it seems to be very promising. Further studies are needed to assess the capacity of this method to be accurate even during instable hemodynamic conditions.

Endnotes

[1]Semfortan 10 mg/mL, Dechra S.r.l
[2]Propovet 10 mg/mL' Zooetis
[3]Vetflurane, 1000 mg/g, Virbac Animal Health
[4]Servo 900D, Siemens Elma, Sweden
[5]B.Broun Vet Care 500 ml
[6]Vetamplius 10 g 50 mL, Fatro Spa
[7]Baytril 10%, Bayer Spa
[8]Swan-Ganz, Edwards Lifesciences, Irvine, Calif
[9]Vigilance®, Edward Lifescience Corporation
[10]B.Broun Vet Care 500 ml
[11]Neo Delta Ven®, Delta Med, Medical Services
[12]Most Care®, Vytech, Padova, Italy
[13]Transpac®, IV Monitoring Kit, Icu Medical
[14]Siemens, SC 6002XL Patient Monitor
[15]GraphPad Prism 6.1, GraphPad Software, Inc.
[16]Microsoft ® Office Excel 2003, Microsoft Corporation
[17]SigmaPlot for Windows, Version 14.0, Systat Software, Inc.

Abbreviations

PAC: With pulmonary artery catheter; TD: Thermodilution; CE: Coefficient of error; CO: Cardiac output; CVP: Central venous pressure; DO_2: Systemic oxygen delivery; $EtCO_2$: Carbon dioxide end tidal; FiO_2: Oxygen inspired fraction; HR: Heart rate; LoA: Limit of agreement; PE: Percentage error; POA: Precision of agreement; POM: Precision of method; PRAM: Pressure Recording Analytical Method; RR: Respiratory rate; SAP, DAP, MAP: Systolic, diastolic, mean arterial pressure; SD: Standard deviation; SpO_2: Peripheral capillary oxygen saturation; SV: Stroke volume; SVR: Systemic vascular resistances; TD: Thermodilution; VO_2: Oxygen consumption; ΔCO: Delta cardiac output

Acknowledgements

The authors wish to thank Vygon Health (Padua, Italy) for kindly providing the MostCare device.

Funding

The study has been supported by an internal grant of the Department of Emergency and Organ Transplantation.

Authors' contributions

FS, AC designed the study. AB, FE, PC, FB, AR collected and analysed data, FS, AB and FE wrote the manuscript and made the figures. PC, AR, FB, AC supported with data acquisition. FS, FE, AB, AC helped with editing the manuscript. All authors read and approved the final manuscript.

Consent for publication

Not applicable

Competing interests

The authors declare that they have no competing interests.

Author details

[1]Department of Veterinary Sciences, University of Pisa, Pisa, Italy.
[2]Dipartimento delle Emergenze e Trapianti di Organo, Università degli Studi di Bari "Aldo Moro," Sezione di Cliniche Veterinarie e P.A, Bari, Italy.

References

1. Conti-Patara A, de Araújo Caldeira J, De Mattos-junior E, de Carvalho Hda S, Reinoldes A, Pedron BG, Patara M, Francisco Talib MS, Faustino M, de Oliveira CM, Cortopassi SR. Changes in tissue perfusion parameters in dogs with severe sepsis/septic shock in response to goal-directed hemodynamic optimization at admission to ICU and the relation to outcome. J Vet Emerg Crit Care. 2012;22(4):409–18.
2. Vallet B, Blanloeil Y, Cholley B, Orliaguet G, Pierre S, Tavernier B. Société française d'anesthésie et de réanimation. Guidelines for perioperative haemodynamic optimization. Ann Fr Anesth Reanim. 2013;32(10):e151–8.
3. Vincent JL, Pelosi P, Pearse R, Payen D, Perel A, Hoeft A, Romagnoli S, Ranieri VM, Ichai C, Forget P, Della Rocca G, Rhodes A. Perioperative cardiovascular monitoring of high-risk patients: a consensus of 12. Crit Care. 2015;8(19):224.
4. Peterson NW, Moses L. Oxygen delivery. Compend Contin Educ Vet. 2011; 33(1):E5.
5. Funk DJ, Moretti EW, Gan TJ. Minimally invasive cardiac output monitoring in the perioperative setting. Anesth Analg. 2009;108(3):887–97.
6. Alhashemi JA, Cecconi M, Hofer CK. Cardiac output monitoring: an integrative perspective. Crit Care. 2011;15(2):214.
7. Pinsky MR, Vincent JL. Let us use the pulmonary artery catheter correctly and only when we need it. Crit Care Med. 2005;33(5):1119–22.
8. Kutter AP, Bettschart-Wolfensberger R, Romagnoli N, Bektas RN. Evaluation of agreement and trending ability between transpulmonary thermodilution and calibrated pulse contour and pulse power cardiac output monitoring methods against pulmonary artery thermodilution in anesthetized dogs. J Vet Emerg Crit Care. 2016;26(4):531–40.
9. Bektas RN, Kutter AP, Hartnack S, Jud RS, Schnyder M, Matos JM, Bettschart-Wolfensberger R. Evaluation of a minimally invasive non-calibrated pulse contour cardiac output monitor (FloTrac/Vigileo) in anaesthetized dogs. Vet Anaesth Analg. 2012;39(5):464–71.
10. Canfrán S, Cediel R, Sández I, Caro-Vadillo A, Gómez de Segura IA. Evaluation of an oesophageal Doppler device for monitoring cardiac output in anaesthetised healthy normotensive dogs. J Small Anim Pract. 2015;56:450–5.
11. Garofalo NA, Teixeira-Neto FJ, Rodrigues JC, Cerejo SA, Aguiar AJ, Becerra-Velásquez DR. Comparison of Transpulmonary Thermodilution and calibrated pulse contour analysis with pulmonary artery Thermodilution cardiac output measurements in anesthetized dogs. J Vet Intern Med. 2016;30(4):941–50.
12. Romagnoli S, Bevilacqua S, Lazzeri C, Ciappi F, Dini D, Pratesi C, Gensini GF, Romano SM. Most care®: a minimally invasive system for hemodynamic monitoring powered by the pressure recording analytical method (PRAM). HSR Proc Intensive Care Cardiovasc Anesth. 2009;1(2):20–7.
13. Romano SM, Pistolesi M. Assessment of cardiac output from systemic arterial pressure in humans. Crit Care Med. 2002;30(8):1834–41.
14. Romagnoli S, Romano SM. Estimation of hemodynamic parameters by arterial waveform: available technologies. Anesth Analg. 2010;110(1):257–8.
15. Scolletta S, Romano SM, Biagioli B, Capannini G, Giomarelli P. Pressure recording analytical method (PRAM) for measurement of cardiac output during various haemodynamic states. Br J Anaesth. 2005;95(2):159–65.
16. Romagnoli S, Romano SM, Bevilacqua S, Ciappi F, Lazzeri C, Peris A, Dini D, Gelsomino S. Cardiac output by arterial pulse contour: reliability under hemodynamic derangements. Interact Cardiovasc Thorac Surg. 2009;8(6):642–6.
17. Giomarelli P, Biagioli B, Scolletta S. Cardiac output monitoring by pressure recording analytical method in cardiac surgery. Eur J Cardiothorac Surg. 2004;26(3):515–20.
18. Scolletta S, Franchi F, Taccone FS, Donadello K, Biagioli B, Vincent JL. An uncalibrated pulse contour method to measure cardiac output during aortic counterpulsation. Anesth Analg. 2011;113(6):1389–95.
19. Scolletta S, Miraldi F, Romano SM, Muzzi L. Continuous cardiac output monitoring with an uncalibrated pulse contour method in patients supported with mechanical pulsatile assist device. Interact Cardiovasc Thorac Surg. 2011;13(1):52–6.
20. Bland JM, Altman DG. Agreement between methods of measurement with multiple observations per individual. J Biopharm Stat. 2007;17(4):571–82.
21. Critchley LA. Validation of the MostCare pulse contour cardiac output monitor: beyond the bland and Altman plot. Anesth Analg. 2011;113(6): 1292–4.
22. Critchley LA, Critchley JA. A meta-analysis of studies using bias and precision statistics to compare cardiac output measurement techniques. J Clin Monit Comput. 1999;15(2):85–91.
23. Cecconi M, Rhodes A, Poloniecki J, Della Rocca G, Grounds RM. Bench-to-bedside review: the importance of the precision of the reference technique in method comparison studies with specific reference to the measurement of cardiac output. Crit Care. 2009;13:201.

24. Critchley LA, Yang XX, Lee A. Assessment of trending ability of cardiac output monitors by polar plot methodology. J Cardiothorac Vasc Anesth. 2011;25(3):536–46.
25. Saugel B, Grothe O, Wagner JY. Tracking changes in cardiac output: statistical considerations on the 4-quadrant plot and the polar plot methodology. Anesth Analg. 2015;121(2):514–24.
26. Romagnoli S, Ricci Z, Romano SM, Dimizio F, Bonicolini E, Quattrone D, De Gaudio R. FloTrac/Vigileo(TM) (third generation) and MostCare(®)/PRAM versus echocardiography for cardiac output estimation in vascular surgery. J Cardiothorac Vasc Anesth. 2013;27(6):1114–21.
27. Hapfelmeier A, Cecconi M, Sauge B. Cardiac output method comparison studies: the relation of the precision of agreement and the precision of method. J Clin Monit Comput. 2016;30:149–55.
28. Critchley LA, Lee A, Ho AM. A critical review of the ability of continuous cardiac output monitors to measure trends in cardiac output. Anesth Analg. 2010;111(5):1180–92.
29. Giavarina D. Understanding bland Altman analysis. Biochem Med (Zagreb). 2015;25(2):141–51.
30. Stetz CW, Miller RG, Kelly GE, Raffin TA. Reliability of the thermodilution method in the determination of cardiac output in clinical practice. Am Rev Respir Dis. 1982;126(6):1001–14.
31. Nilsson LB, Nilsson JC, Skovgaard LT, Berthelsen PG. Thermodilution cardiac output - are three injections enough? Acta Anaesthesiol Scand. 2004;48(10): 1322–7.
32. Romagnoli S, Franchi F, Ricci Z, Scolletta S, Payen D. The pressure recording analytical method (PRAM): technical concepts and literature review. J Cardiothorac Vasc Anesth. 2017;31(4):1460–70.

Comparison of contrast-enhanced multidetector computed tomography angiography and splenoportography for the evaluation of portosystemic-shunt occlusion after cellophane banding in dogs

Sebastian Schaub[1*], Antje Hartmann[2], Tobias Schwarz[3], Karsten Kemper[1], Kerstin H. Pueckler[1] and Matthias A. Schneider[1]

Abstract

Background: Many patients with a congenital extrahepatic portosystemic shunt (PSS) do not tolerate an immediate shunt closure. Therefore, slow progressive techniques were developed. To evaluate the success of shunt closure diagnostic imaging is essential to identify possible residual blood flow through the shunt vessel. There is a lack of information about the reliability of computed tomography angiography (CTA) for evaluating residual flow through a PSS after treatment. The purpose of this prospective study was to compare the results of CTA with splenoportography. Three months after cellophane banding CTA and splenoportography were performed in 20 dogs and reviewed by three independent examiners, respectively. In both imaging modalities the presences of a residual shunt was judged as present or absent and the extent of visibility of portal vasculature was recorded.

Results: Based on the evaluation of the splenoportography residual flow through shunt was present in 6 dogs. The classification of residual shunt present or absent showed a substantial to perfect agreement ($\kappa = 0.65–1.00$) between the observers in splenoportography and a slight to moderate agreement ($\kappa = 0.11–0.51$) for CTA. Sensitivity and specificity varied between 0.50 and 1.00 and 0.57–0.85, respectively. Significant correlation between CTA and splenoportography for the classification of residual shunt was present only in one observer but not in the other two.

Conclusion: More studies were classified as residual shunt positive with CTA compared to splenoportography. It remains unclear which methods do reflect reality better and thus which method is superior. The greater inter-rater agreement for splenoportography suggests a greater reliability of this technique.

Keywords: Computed tomography, Splenoportography, Angiography, Extrahepatic portosystemic shunt

Background

Portosystemic shunts describe anomalous vessels connecting the portal venous system to the systemic venous system and subsequently allow blood to bypass the liver. They can be classified as intrahepatic or extrahepatic [1, 2]. As a consequence of blood bypassing the liver there is a lack in hepatotrophic substances, especially insulin, and subsequent hepatic atrophy [3, 4]. Toxins from the intestines, such as ammonia or aromatic amino acids, in the systemic circulation are accounted for the clinical signs [2]. Blood work only allows for the suspicion of the presence of a portosystemic shunt (PSS). Diagnostic imaging modalities are used to prove vascular anomalies of the portal system. Portography is the gold-standard for the visualization of the portal system and diagnosis of PSS in veterinary medicine [1, 5–8]. However, portography is replaced by other, less invasive imaging modalities like ultrasonography,

* Correspondence: Sebast.schaub@gmail.com
[1]Department of Veterinary Clinical Sciences, Small Animal Clinic, Justus-Liebig-University Giessen, 35392 Giessen, Germany
Full list of author information is available at the end of the article

computed tomography angiography (CTA) and magnetic resonance imaging [5, 9–12].

Long-term prognosis is better in animals undergoing complete shunt occlusion compared to animals showing a residual flow through the shunt vessel [13]. Therefore, the main objective of surgical or interventional therapy is a complete occlusion of the PSS to establish normal liver function. An immediate complete occlusion is not possible in most animals due to the risk of fatal portal hypertension [13, 14]. Extravascular surgical techniques leading to slow occlusion include the use of an ameroid constrictor or cellophane bands [15–18]. Gradual occlusion of the PSS by cellophane banding occurs as a result of inflammation and thrombosis [18]. After cellophane banding, continued shunting can occur, either due to incomplete occlusion or due to the development of multiple acquired shunts [19].

One case report demonstrates the use of CTA in the evaluation of shunt closure after cellophane banding [20]. However, there is a lack of information in the literature concerning the reliability of CTA to assess the shunt closure after surgical treatment of PSS by cellophane banding. The objective of this prospective study was to compare CTA with splenoportography in the assessment of residual blood flow through the shunt vessel 3 months after cellophane banding.

Methods

Animals

All investigations were conducted in strict compliance with the restrictions of the German Animal Protection Law. The study was conducted prospectively and was approved by the Committee on the Ethics of Animal Experiments of the Justus Liebig University and local Hessian government (reference number GI 18/17 Nr. A 43/2012).

Twenty client owned dogs with a single congenital extrahepatic portosystemic shunt were included in this study. The owners of the dogs gave permission for their animals to be used in this study. The dogs were treated 3 months previously by cellophane banding without intraoperative attenuation as described previously [21]. A ventral midline laparotomy was performed and the shunt vessel was visualized. The cellophane band was placed around the shunt vessel and for fixation of the cellophane band a non-metal hemoclip (Hem-o-lok®, Teleflex Medical, Kernen, Germany) was used. No other inclusion criteria were applied. The dogs underwent a physical examination as well as a complete hematology and serum chemistry prior to anesthesia. An intravenous (IV) catheter was placed in a cephalic vein. Anaesthesia was induced with acepromazin (Vetranquil®, CEVA GmbH, Düsseldorf, Germany) and l-polamidon (L-Polamivet®, Intervet, Unterschleissheim, Germany) and maintained using isoflurane (IsoFlo®, Ecuphar GmbH, Greifswald, Germany). Each patient was placed in sternal recumbency. Ventilator aided hyperventilation and breath-hold techniques were used to eliminate motion during scanning.

Computed tomography

All images were obtained using a 16-slice CT scanner (Brilliance 16, Philips Healthcare, Best, Netherlands). Patients were positioned in sternal recumbency on the patient table of the CT scanner. Plain transverse images of the abdomen were acquired in helical mode using the following scanning parameters: 2 mm slice thickness, pitch of 1, tube current of 313 mA, tube voltage of 120 kVp and 0.75 s rotation time. Transverse images were reconstructed using a medium-frequency, non-enhancing filter with a 512x512 matrix. Scan direction was from caudal to cranial. To determine the scan delay for optimal contrast enhancement of the portal vein a dynamic CT scan was performed caudal to the porta hepatis.

For the dynamic CT scan a single slice was imaged sequentially to evaluate contrast enhancement of the portal vein over time. A low dose (150 mg Iodine/kg body weight) of contrast medium (Xenetix® 300, Guerbet, Sulzbach, Germany) was administered IV using a power injector (Injektron CT2, MEDTRON, Saarbruecken, Germany). The injection rate was 3 ml/s. Every 2 s one transverse image was acquired until twenty images were recorded. Scanning parameters for the dynamic scan were, 6 mm slice thickness, tube current of 40 mA, tube voltage of 120 kVp and 0.75 s rotation time. In the resulting image series a region of interest was positioned over the portal vein. A time attenuation curve was generated from which the time to peak enhancement was determined. The optimal time to start the CTA was calculated by subtracting the time the scanner needed to reach the position of the dynamic CT scan from the time to peak enhancement. For the CTA contrast medium was administered at a dose of 600 mg Iodine/kg body weight and an injection rate of 3 ml/s. The scan was started after the determined delay. Scan parameters were identical to the precontrast scan. A second scan was performed subsequently to the portal phase in cranial to caudal direction.

Splenoportography

For splenoportography the patient was placed in dorsal recumbency on the table of a biplane fluoroscopy system (Bicor HS, Siemens Healthcare, Erlangen, Germany). Under ultrasonographic guidance a 20 gauge venous catheter was inserted percutaneously into the splenic parenchyma. Contrast medium (Xenetix® 300, Guerbet, Sulzbach, Germany) was administered manually into the spleen (300 mg Iodine/kg body weight), at a flow rate of approximately 2 ml/s. During breath-hold lateral and dorsoventral angiographic cineloops were acquired simultaneously at a frame rate of 12.5 images/s. Fluoroscopic acquisition started immediately before contrast injection and lasted for 10 s. One cineloop was recorded, no follow up sequences were acquired.

Image analysis

Images were anonymized, patient information was removed from the image by deleting it from the DICOM information and an arbitrary number was assigned for the CT images and the digital cineloops of the splenoportography. Hence, reviewers assessing CTA images and splenoportography cineloops were blinded to which studies belonged to the same patient. To minimize image recognition review of splenoportography and CTA images was performed 6 months after the last set of images was acquired.

CTA images were reviewed in a soft tissue window by two board certified radiologists (AH and TS) and a radiology resident (SS). Original pre- and post-contrast transverse as well as multiplanar reformatted images were available for review. Reviewers could modify image orientation and windowing individually to optimize the images according to personal preference. Residual flow was judged as "absent" if there was no connection visible between the shunt vessel and the systemic vein (Fig. 1). Residual flow was classified as "present" if contrast was visible in the shunt vessel entering the systemic vein (Fig. 2). In addition, the branching pattern of the portal vein within the liver was graded using a simplification of a previously published angiographic grading system [22]: grade 1 (no intrahepatic portal vasculature visible), grade 2 (portal vessel stump visible within the liver parenchyma) or grade 3 (good portal vessel branching within the liver parenchyma).

Digital cineloops of the splenoportography were assessed by one board certified cardiologist (MS), one board certified radiologist (AH) and one radiology resident (SS). Also in splenoportography presence of a residual shunt was graded based on the visibility of flow of contrast medium to the systemic vein. The branching pattern of the portal vein in the liver was graded using the same modified grading system as for the CTA.

Statistical analysis

Statistical analysis was performed using commercially available statistics software (SPSS® Statistics 22, IBM Corporation, Armonk NY, USA). Inter-rater agreement for residual shunt judgement was measured by Cohen's kappa coefficient in splenoportography and CTA, separately.

The splenoportography evaluation of the examiner (MS) with the greatest experience in angiography of portosystemic shunts, based on long standing clinical practice in this technique, was used as reference for further analysis to which the results of splenoportography and CTA of the other reviewers were compared to.

Fisher's exact was used for comparison of residual shunt classification between the results of our reference (most experienced observer, MS) for splenoportography and the three different CTA analyses. Sensitivity and specificity were calculated for each observer of the CTA separately. Cramer's V correlation analysis was used for comparison of portal vein branching between CTA, assessed by the three different observers, and the results of splenoportography of our set reference (MS). Significance level was set at $p \leq 0.05$.

Results

Dogs included in this study were five mix-breed dogs, four Pug dogs, two Yorkshire terriers, two Miniature Pinschers and one Chihuahua, Bolognese, Maltese, Parson Russell terrier, Shi Tzu and Shetland sheepdog, respectively. There were ten female and ten male dogs. The median age of the patients was 15.5 months (range 6–68 month). The median body weight was 4.63 kg (range 2.0–9.7 kg). Based on intraoperative angiography ten dogs had a portocaval

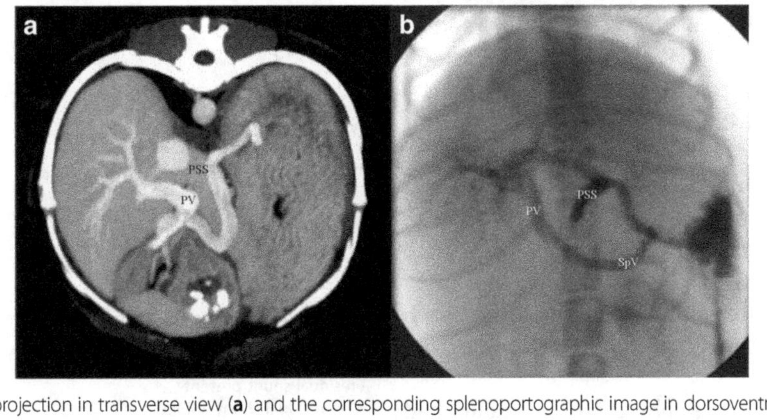

Fig. 1 Maximum intensity projection in transverse view (**a**) and the corresponding splenoportographic image in dorsoventral view (**b**) demonstrating a shunt vessel of a gastroduodenal-caval shunt which was graded as "closed" in splenoportography and CTA. Note the portal vein (PV), splenic vein (SpV) and the former shunt vessel (PSS)

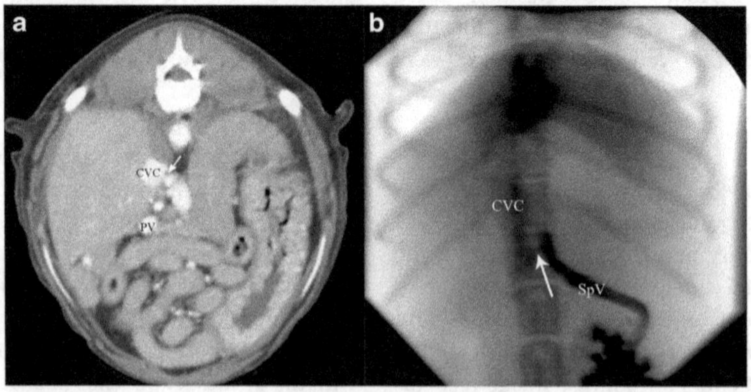

Fig. 2 Maximum intensity projection in transverse view (**a**) and the corresponding splenoportographic image in dorsoventral view (**b**) demonstrating a gastrospleno-caval shunt which was graded as "open" in splenoportography and CTA. Note the portal vein (PV), splenic vein (SpV) and the shunt vessel. There is still a fine hyperattenuating band (*arrow*) visible between the splenic vein and the caudal vena cava (CVC)

shunt arising from the gastroduodenal vein, ten dogs had shunt arising from the gastrosplenic vein entering the caudal vena cava ($n = 6$), the azygos vein ($n = 2$) or the phrenic vein ($n = 2$) (Table 1).

Residual shunting was found in splenoportography in 6/20 (30%) dogs by the most experienced observer.

Eight to eleven dogs (40–55%) showed a residual shunt in CTA for the three examiners of the CTA.

The results of splenoportography and CTA including the respective shunt type are summarized in Table 1.

All CTA studies showed a subjective good contrast enhancement of the portal vasculature. Inter-rater agreement for splenoportography was perfect for one observer ($\kappa = 1.0$) (comparison of MS with SS) and for two observers substantial ($\kappa = 0.66$) (comparison of AH with MS and AH with SS). Inter-rater agreement for CTA was slight to moderate for all observers ($\kappa = 0.12$; 0.38; 0.52) (comparison of AH with TS; AH with SS; TS with SS).

Between splenoportography and CTA significant association was found for one observer ($p = 0.001$), first author of this paper (SS), but not for the other two observers ($p = 0.16$ (TS); 0.64 (AH)). Compared to the results of the splenoportography the sensitivity of CTA for residual shunt detection was 50% (AH); 83% (TS); 100% (SS), respectively. The specificity of CTA was 57% (TS); 64% (AH); 86% (SS), respectively.

In splenoportography the most experienced observer (MS) classified the portal vein branching as grade 1 in three dogs and grade 3 in 17 dogs. Three observers classified the portal vein branching in CTA as grade 2 in none (AH), two (TS) and three dogs (SS); all remaining dogs were classified with grade 3. The results for each observer in relation to the type of shunt are summarized in Table 1.

Compared to splenoportography the CTA results had a fair correlation (Cramers-V = 0.21 (SS); 0.33 (TS)) in two observers for the assessment of the branching of the

Table 1 Shunt type, residual shunting and intrahepatic portal vein branching classified in splenoportography and computed tomography angiography by different observers (MS, TS, AH, SS)

Patient	Type of shunt	Residual shunting				Portal vein branching			
	Origin – End	SP (MS)	CTA (TS)	CTA (AH)	CTA (SS)	SP (MS)	CTA (TS)	CTA (AH)	CTA (SS)
1	GdV – CVC	-	+	+	+	3	3	3	3
2	GsV – CVC	-	-	-	-	3	3	3	3
3	GdV – CVC	-	+	+	+	3	3	3	2
4	GsV – CVC	-	-	-	-	3	3	3	3
5	GdV – CVC	+	+	-	+	1	2	3	2
6	GsV – PhV	+	+	-	+	3	3	3	3
7	GsV – CVC	+	+	+	+	1	3	3	3
8	GdV – CVC	-	-	+	-	3	3	3	3
9	GsV – AzV	-	-	-	-	3	3	3	3
10	GdV – CVC	-	+	-	-	3	3	3	3
11	GdV – CVC	-	-	-	-	3	3	3	3
12	GsV – CVC	+	-	+	+	3	3	3	3
13	GdV – CVC	-	+	+	-	3	2	3	3
14	GdV – CVC	-	-	+	-	3	3	3	3
15	GdV – CVC	-	+	-	-	3	3	3	3
16	GsV – PhV	-	-	-	-	3	3	3	3
17	GsV – CVC	+	+	+	+	1	3	3	3
18	GsV– CVC	-	-	-	-	3	3	3	3
19	GdV– CVC	-	+	-	-	3	3	3	3
20	GsV – AzV	+	+	-	+	3	3	3	2

SP splenoportography, *CTA* computed tomography angiography, *GdV* gastroduodenal vein, *GsV* gastrosplenic vein, *CVC* caudal vena cava, *PhV* phrenico vein, *AzV* azygos vein
- residual shunt present
+ no residual shunt visible
1 no intrahepatic portal vasculature visible
2 portal vessel stump visible
3 good portal vessel branching

portal vein. In the third observer (AH) no correlation could be calculated because all dogs classified as grade 3 in CTA.

Discussion

Currently portography is considered the gold-standard for the assessment of a portosystemic shunt [1, 5, 6, 8]. However, sensitivity or specificity values are not reported for splenoportography [23]. CTA has proven to be a reliable imaging modality for diagnosing an extrahepatic PSS in dogs [5, 12, 24–26]. Sensitivity and specificity for detection of an extrahepatic PSS using CTA are reported to be 96 and 89%, respectively [27]. However, studies assessing the value of imaging techniques in the detection of residual flow through a PSS after treatment are lacking.

The study was performed 3-month post-surgery. This is the standard interim for the re-check after cellophane banding in our clinic. An earlier re-check would have most likely lead to an increased number of patients showing a residual flow, which would have been beneficial for the statistical evaluation in our study. It is reported that 2–6 month post-surgery 85% of dogs show a normal liver function, however no imaging was performed for shunt evaluation [15]. Others report that it takes more than 6 months for shunt occlusion to occur depending on the size of the shunting vessel [21]. Therefore, we did not expect that most patients show complete shunt attenuation after 3-month.

Inter-rater agreement was only slight to moderate ($\kappa = 0.12$ to 0.52) for CTA, whereas for splenoportography it was substantial to perfect ($\kappa = 0.66$ to 1.0). We found a varying sensitivity (50 to 100%) and specificity (57 to 85%) for the assessment of residual blood flow through the shunt vessel three months after cellophane banding using CTA.

During a consensus review of the CTA images, which was performed during preparation of the paper after statistical analysis, in order to identify possible causes for the wide variation in sensitivity and specificity and the poor inter-rater agreement between the different observers a fine hyperattenuating band between the portal vein and the systemic vein visible on some CTA images, showing no detectable flow during splenoportography (Fig. 3) was identified. This band has been assessed as a sign of residual flow through the shunt by some observers (residual flow present), whereas others interpreted it as contrast enhancing inflammatory reaction without residual blood flow encapsulating the previous shunting vessel. It remains unclear if this band represents a residual flow through the shunt vessel or not. Further assessment of this finding would have required surgical exploration and for example dye injection (e.g., methylene blue) in the previous shunt vessel (stump) or removal with histopathological examination of the tissue. All dogs were clinically unremarkable, therefore another surgery was not an option. Another possibility for the future might be the comparison between functional shunt closure accessed by laboratory tests and both imaging techniques.

CT has a possible submillimeter spatial resolution, modern fluoroscopy systems can only discriminate 2.5 to 3 line pairs per millimeter [28–30]. In addition, CT offers superior contrast resolution, allowing for a better distinction of structures with only minor differences in x-ray attenuation [31]. Therefore, splenoportography may under diagnose residual flow. Minimal flow through a small residual lumen of a shunt might not be visible on the fluoroscopy screen due to a lower spatial and contrast resolution compared to CT.

The small number of patients further enhances the wide variation in sensitivity and specificity between the different observers. It would be interesting if a dynamic scan over the shunt vessel can help to discriminate between inflammatory reaction and residual flow. For example, by assessing the time of arrival of the contrast medium in the area of shunt attenuation.

Contrast medium injection in splenoportography was done via injection into the splenic parenchyma under ultrasound guidance. Laceration of the spleen is a possible complication using this technique. However, ultrasonographic identification and puncturing of the spleen does help to minimize the risk of laceration of the spleen. Nevertheless, it requires the radiologist to be present in the examination room during image acquisition. Scatter radiation during splenoportography and subsequent exposure to radiation is a major downside of this procedure [1, 32].

Application of contrast media for a CTA is done by intravenous injection. Thus, allowing for the usage of a high power injector with a defined injection rate. Using a power injector allow for the personal to stay outside the scanner room during injection and image acquisition, avoiding radiation exposure to personal. Application of contrast medium for CTA of the portal system was done using a cephalic vein. Contrast medium applied by a saphenous vein can lead to beam hardening artifacts and a retrograde filling of the hepatic veins with contrast medium [26]. Injection into the splenic parenchyma as in splenoportography is also described [33]. This would require the presence of a person in the scanner room if images should be acquired during the portal phase. For radiation safety reasons this is not allowed in our country and a possible benefit of this technique should be critically questioned in countries where the presence of person in the room during radiation is legally allowed.

CTA was planned on the basis of a dynamic CT scan as it has been recommended in a previous study [12]. Other options would have been the use of bolus tracking

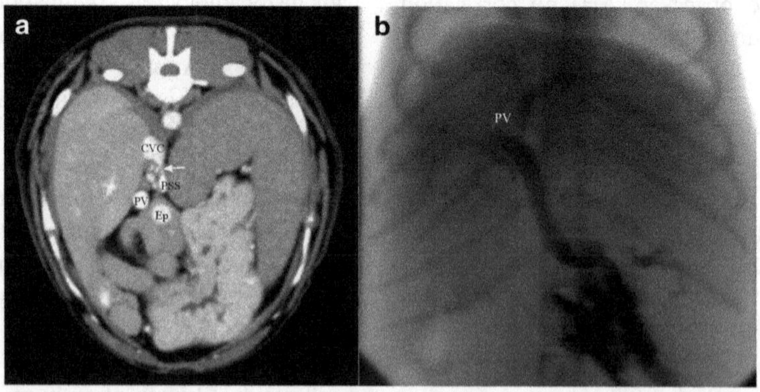

Fig. 3 Maximum intensity projection in transverse plane (**a**) and dorsoventral view projection in splenoportography (**b**) of a dog with gastroduodenal-caval shunt, which was graded as "open" in CTA and "closed" in splenoportography. In CTA there is a fine hyperattenuating connection (*arrow*) visible between the former shunt vessel (PSS) and the caudal vena cava (CVC). Note the portal vein (PV) ventral to the caudal vena cava and medial to the dilated epigastric vein (Ep) in CTA images. In splenoportography there was no flow of contrast medium into the caudal vena cava visible. All intrahepatic portal branches (PV) can be clearly seen in splenoportography with a fine arborization within the liver parenchyma

or a body weight dependent delay [5, 33, 34]. Using the bolus tracking technique, a region of interest is placed over the vessel which is going to be evaluated and the scan starts automatically when a given threshold value is reached. Respiration can cause artifacts leading to an inadvertent too early or late start of the CTA by moving the tracked vessel out of the region of interest [33, 34]. Using a published body weight dependent delay for the starting of the CT angiography proofed not practical in our clinic. The published values differ between 1.41 to 4.12 s per kg body weight, leading to wide range of possible starting points varying more than 100% for a given weight category [5].

For injection we used a constant injection rate of 3 ml/s. We performed a test injection to calculate the optimal timing for scanning. Therefore, we encountered no problems in acquiring images during peak enhancement. In patients with an insufficient attenuation of the shunt vessel no contrast enhancement of the entire intrahepatic portal vasculature could be visualized in the splenoportography. However, in CTA it was always possible, in this study, to visualize the complete intrahepatic portal vasculature even if the shunt vessel was still partially open. In splenoportography only minimal hemodilution of the contrast medium from the splenic blood pool occurs, therefore one would expect a distinct contrast enhancement of the portal vasculature also within the liver parenchyma [35].

In CTA hemodilution of contrast medium is much greater as in splenoportography owing to the peripheral injection technique. Nevertheless, we encountered a greater contrast enhancement and visibility of portal vasculature in CTA. One reason most likely contributing to the lack of visibility of the intrahepatic portal vessels in splenoportography is the location of contrast injection in relation to the shunt location. All three patients in which no contrast enhancement of the entire intrahepatic portal vasculature could be observed using splenoportography had a shunt type which involves mainly (spleno to caval shunt; $n = 2$) or partially (right gastric with left gastric to caval, $n = 1$) the splenic vein leading to a large proportion of the injected contrast medium flowing through the incompletely occluded shunt and not into intrahepatic portal vein branching. For these shunt forms it may have been better to inject the contrast medium directly into the portal vein. However, this problem has not been described previously and was only encountered during consensus review of all splenoportographies after statistical analysis, during manuscript preparation. Future studies may profit from this finding and use a different approach for contrast injection in PSS involving the splenic vein.

Another explanation contributing to the lack of visibility of the intrahepatic portal vessels in splenoportography is that the contrast resolution of the fluoroscopic images from splenoportography is too low to show blood that contains only a small amount of contrast medium entering the intrahepatic portal vasculature. Computed tomography is known to have a better contrast resolution compared to fluoroscopy [31]. With CT, minimal differences in attenuation can be detected, which go undetected with fluoroscopy. So, a faint contrast filling of the intraparenchymal liver vasculature can be depicted with CT but not with fluoroscopy. Based on the findings of CTA we consider this explanation the most likely cause for the inability to see the intrahepatic portal vasculature using splenoportography in patients with incomplete shunt occlusion. It seems unlikely that an insufficient contrast medium dose is the cause for the lack of visualization of the intrahepatic portal vasculature. Even considering that some contrast medium remained within the splenic parenchyma and therefore did not contribute to the blood pool good enhancement of the splenic vein draining the contrast medium from the spleen was present in all cases.

Thus the amount of contrast medium injected was considered sufficient and good opacification of the intrahepatic portal vasculature would have been expected. In addition pooling of contrast medium within the splenic parenchyma occurred in all patients, also in patients in which the intrahepatic vasculature was visible in splenoportography. Although quantification of how much contrast medium remained in the splenic parenchyma was not possible, we assume the percentage was similar in all patients thus the effect on the visibility of the intrahepatic portal vasculature was assumed to be similar between patients with visible and invisible intrahepatic portal vasculature.

A limitation of this study is the small number of observers for both modalities; in addition not every observer assessed each imaging modality further decreasing the number of observers per imaging modality. We decided for this experimental set up for multiple reasons. First, the observers which did only review images of one image modality had no experience in the other imaging technique, thus we expected a poor performance which would have led to skewing of our results. The second reason was to avoid subconscious influence by the knowledge of the result of the other imaging modality in at least some of our observers. To assess the unbiased potential of CT we therefore decided that the most experienced observers should only read the CT images. The observers reading images of both modalities had a low to medium experience in reading splenoportographic and CTA images, thus unwanted bias of the results based on a lack of experience with one imaging technique was not expected. This study was meant as a pilot study evaluating CTA for assessing residual shunting after partial shunt closure, we therefore considered a total of four observers sufficient. However, overall a larger number of observers would have been ideal.

Another limitation might be some degree of image recognition for the first author as all CTA studies were performed by him. We tried to minimize this risk by anonymizing the images and having a time gap of at least 6 months between image acquisition and analysis. The overall better performance of the first author of this paper might be the result of SS being trained by MS for splenoportography analysis, leading to a stronger correlation between the two.

Another limitation of our study is the relatively low number of dogs included (twenty animals).

Further studies evaluating the value of CT to assess the presence of residual shunting are necessary.

Conclusion

In summary, the results for CTA are heterogeneous compared to splenoportography for the evaluation of a possible residual flow through the shunt vessel. More studies were classified as residual shunt positive with the CTA compared to the splenoportography. However, it remains unclear which methods do reflect reality better. The better spatial and contrast resolution of CT might be superior to splenoportography in detecting residual blood flow through a shunt vessel, which remains invisible on splenoportography. Further studies are necessary to judge which imaging modality is correct. However, the substantial to perfect inter-rater agreement for splenoportography and only slight to moderate inter-rater agreement for CTA suggests a greater reliability of splenoportography due to less observer related effects on the results.

In any case, CTA is advantageous for the anatomic assessment of the portal vasculature.

Abbreviations

CT: Computed tomography; CTA: Computed tomography angiography; DICOM: Digital imaging and communications in medicine; IV: Intravenously; Kg: Kilogram; kVp: Peak kilovoltage; mA: Milliampere; mg: Milligram; ml: Milliliter; mm: Millimeter; PSS: Portosystemic shunt; S: Second

Acknowledgements

The technical assistance of Ella Wenz is gratefully acknowledged.

Funding

No funding was received for this study.

Authors' contributions

SS, AH, TS, KK, KP, MS contributed to the development and writing of the paper. SS performed the CT angiography in all dogs. MS performed the splenoportography in all dogs. SS, TS, MS, AH performed the measurements. All authors read and critically revised and approved the final manuscript.

Competing interests

The authors declare that they have no competing interests.

Consent for publication

Not applicable.

Author details

[1]Department of Veterinary Clinical Sciences, Small Animal Clinic, Justus-Liebig-University Giessen, 35392 Giessen, Germany. [2]Department of Clinical Veterinary Medicine, Vetsuisse Faculty, University of Bern, 3012 Bern, Switzerland. [3]Royal (Dick) School of Veterinary Studies, The University of Edinburgh, Roslin, Midlothian EH25 9RG, UK.

References

1. Haers H, Paepe D, Vermote K, Saunders JH, Daminet S, Risselada M. Portosystemic shunts in dogs and cats: imaging portosystemic shunts in small animals – hepatics vascular anatomy, shunt morphology, radiography. Vlaams Diergeneeskd Tijdschr. 2007;76(5):315–21.
2. van Steenbeek FG, van den Bossche L, Leegwater PA, Rothuizen J. Inherited liver shunts in dogs elucidate pathways regulating embryonic development and clinical disorders of the portal vein. Mamm Genome. 2012;23(1–2):76–84.
3. Baade S, Aupperle H, Grevel V, Schoon HA. Histopathological and immunohistochemical investigation of hepatic lesions associated with congenital portosystemic shunt in dogs. J Comp Pathol. 2006;134(1):80–90.
4. Rozga J, Jeppsson B, Bengmark S. Hepatotrophic factors in liver growth and atrophy. Br J Exp Pathol. 1985;66(6):669–78.

5. Frank P, Mahaffey M, Egger C, Cornell KK. Helical computed tomographic portography in ten normal dogs and ten dogs with a portosystemic shunt. Vet Radiol Ultrasound. 2003;44(4):392–400.
6. Lamb CR, Daniel GB. Diagnostic imaging of dogs with suspected portosystemic shunting. Compend Contin Educ Pract Vet. 2002;24(8):626–35.
7. Suter PF. Portal vein anomalies in the dog: their angiographic diagnosis. Vet Radiol. 1975;16(3):84–97.
8. Tillson DM, Winkler JT. Diagnosis and treatment of portosystemic shunts in the cat. Vet Clin North Am Small Anim Pract. 2002;32(4):881–99.
9. Brühschwein A, Foltin I, Flatz K, Zöllner M, Matis U. Contrast-enhanced magnetic resonance angiography for diagnosis of portosystemic shunts in 10 dogs. Vet Radiol Ultrasound. 2010;51(2):116–21.
10. d'Anjou MA. The sonographic search for portosystemic shunts. Clin Tech Small Anim Pract. 2007;22(3):104–14.
11. Szatmári V, Rothuizen J, Voorhout G. Standard planes for ultrasonographic examination of the portal system in dogs. J Am Vet Assoc. 2004;224(5):713–6.
12. Zwingenberger AL, Schwarz T. Dual-phase CT angiography of the normal canine portal and hepatic vasculature. Vet Radiol Ultrasound. 2004;45(2): 117–24.
13. Hunt GB, Hughes J. Outcomes after extrahepatic portosystemic shunt ligation in 49 dogs. Aust Vet J. 1999;77(5):303–7.
14. Hottinger HA, Walshaw R, Hauptman JG. Long-term results of complete and partial ligation of congenital portosystemic shunts in dogs. Vet Surg. 1995; 24(4):331–6.
15. Hunt GB, Kummeling A, Tisdall PL, Marchevsky AM, Liptak JM, Youmans KR, Goldsmid SE, Beck JA. Outcomes of cellophane banding for congenital portosystemic shunts in 106 dogs and 5 cats. Vet Surg. 2004;33(1):25–31.
16. Hunt GB, Culp WTN, Mayhew KN, Mayhew P, Steffey MA, Zwingenberger A. Evaluation of in vivo behavior of ameroid ring constrictors in dogs with congenital extrahepatic portosystemic shunts using computed tomography. Vet Surg. 2014;43(7):834–42.
17. Vogt JC, Krahwinkel DJ, Bright RM, Daniel GB, Toal RL, Rohrbach B. Gradual occlusion of extrahepatic portosystemic shunts in dogs and cats using the ameroid constrictor. Vet Surg. 1996;25(6):495–502.
18. Youmans KR, Hunt GB. Cellophane banding for the gradual attenuation of single extrahepatic portosystemic shunts in eleven dogs. Aust Vet J. 1998; 76(8):531–7.
19. Landon BP, Abraham LA, Charles JA. Use of transcolonic portal scintigraphy to evaluate efficacy of cellophane banding of congenital extrahepatic portosystemic shunts in 16 dogs. Aust Vet J. 2008;86(5):169–79.
20. Yoon H, Choi Y, Kim S, Kim K, Jeong S. Contrast-enhanced computed tomography angiography and volume-rendered imaging for evaluation of cellophane banding in a dog with extrahepatic portosystemic shunt. J S Afr Vet Assoc. 2011;82(2):125–8.
21. Frankel D, Seim H, MacPhail C, Monnet E. Evaluation of cellophane banding with and without intraoperative attenuation for treatment of congenital extrahepatic portosystemic shunts in dogs. J Am Vet Med Assoc. 2006; 228(9):1355–60.
22. White RN, Burton CA, McEvoy FJ. Surgical treatment of intrahepatic portosystemic shunts in 45 dogs. Vet Rec. 1998;142:358–65.
23. Scrivani PV, Yeaher AE, Dykes NL, Scarlett JM. Influence of patient positioning on sensitivity of mesenteric portography for detecting an anomalous portosystemic blood vessel in dogs: 34 cases (1997–2000). J Am Vet Med Assoc. 2001;219(9):1251–3.
24. Nelson NC, Nelson LL. Anatomy of extrahepatic portosystemic shunts in dogs as determined by computed tomography angiography. Vet Radiol Ultrasound. 2011;52(5):498–506.
25. Zwingenberger AL. CT diagnosis of portosystemic shunts. Vet Clin North Am Small Anim Pract. 2009;39(4):783–92.
26. Zwingenberger AL, Schwarz T, Saunders HM. Helical computed tomographic angiography of canine portosystemic shunts. Vet Radiol Ultrasound. 2005;46(1): 27–32.
27. Kim EK, Giglio RF, Reese DJ, Reese SL, Bacon NJ, Ellison GW. Comparison of computed tomographic angiography and ultrasonography for the detection and characterization of portosystemic shunts in dogs. Vet Radiol Ultrasound. 2013;54(6):569–74.
28. Bertolini G, Prokop M. Multidetector-row computed tomography: technical basics and preliminary clinical applications in small animals. Vet J. 2011; 189(1):15–26.
29. Flohr TG, Schaller S, Stierstorfer K, Bruder H, Ohnesorge BM, Schoepf UJ. Multi-detector row CT systems and image-reconstruction techniques. Radiology. 2005;235(3):756–73.
30. Sikkink CJJM, Reijnen MMPJ, Zeebregts CJ. The creation of the optimal dedicated endovascular suite. Eur J Vasc Endovasc Surg. 2008;35(2):198–204.
31. Ohlerth S, Scharf G. Computed tomography in small animals – Basic principles and state of the art applications. Vet J. 2007;173(2):254–71.
32. Haers H, Paepe D, Vermote K, Saunders JH, Daminet S, Risselada M. Portosystemic shunts in dogs and cats: imaging portosystemic shunts in small animals – ultrasonography, scinitgraphy, computed tomography, magnetic resonance imaging. Vlaams Diergeneeskd Tijdschr. 2007;76(5):322–30.
33. Echandi RL, Morandi F, Daniel WT, Paquette JL, Daniel GB. Comparison of transplenic multidetector ct portography to multidetector ct- angiography in normal dogs. Vet Radiol Ultrasound. 2007;48(1):38–44.
34. Bertolini G, Rolla EC, Zotti A, Caldin M. Three-Dimensional multislice helical computed tomography techniques for canine extra-hepatic portosysemic shunt assessment. Vet Radiol Ultrasound. 2006;47(5):439–43.
35. Moon ML. Diagnostic imaging of portosystemic shunts. Semin Vet Med Surg (Small Anim). 1990;5(2):120–6.

14

Has intravenous lidocaine improved the outcome in horses following surgical management of small intestinal lesions in a UK hospital population?

Shebl E. Salem[1,2], Chris J. Proudman[3] and Debra C. Archer[1,4*]

Abstract

Background: Perioperative lidocaine treatment is commonly used in horses that undergo surgical treatment of colic, to prevent or treat postoperative ileus and reduce the effects of intestinal ischaemia-reperfusion injury. However, its clinical efficacy has not been evaluated in a large population of horses undergoing small intestinal surgery. The aim of the current study was to evaluate whether systemic lidocaine administration reduced the prevalence, volume and duration of postoperative reflux and improved rates of survival following surgical treatment of small intestinal lesions. Data were collected as a part of two prospective studies investigating postoperative survival of surgical colic patients admitted to a UK equine referral hospital during the periods 2004–2006 and 2012–2014. Kaplan-Meier plots of cumulative probability of survival and the log-rank test were used to compare survival between horses that did or did not receive lidocaine. The Wilcoxon rank-sum test was used to compare the total reflux volume and duration of reflux between the groups. A multivariable Cox proportional hazards model was used to identify pre- and intraoperative risk factors for non-survival.

Results: Data from 318 horses were included in the final analysis. The overall prevalence of postoperative reflux was 24.5 %. This was significantly higher (34.8 %) in horses admitted in 2012–2014 compared to the 2004–2006 cohort (16.7). Perioperative lidocaine treatment had no effect on total reflux volume, duration of reflux or rates of postoperative survival nor was it a risk factor associated with altered postoperative survival. Variables identified to be associated with increased risk of postoperative mortality included packed cell volume on admission (hazard ratio [HR] 1.03 95 %, 95 % confidence interval [CI] 1.004–1.06, $p = 0.024$), heart rate on admission (HR 1.014, 95 % CI 1. 004–1.024, $p = 0.008$) and duration of surgery (HR 1.007, 95 % CI 1.002–1.01, $p = 0.008$).

Conclusions: Lidocaine therapy had no effect on the prevalence of postoperative reflux, total reflux volume and duration of reflux nor did it have any effect on postoperative survival in horses undergoing surgical management of small intestinal disease for treatment of colic. There is a need for a well-designed multicentre, prospective randomised controlled trial to fully investigate the efficacy of lidocaine across different hospital populations.

Keywords: Horse, Colic, Small intestine, Laparotomy, Lidocaine, Postoperative reflux, Postoperative ileus

* Correspondence: darcher@liverpool.ac.uk
[1]Institute of Infection and Global Health, Department of Epidemiology and Population Health, University of Liverpool, Wirral CH64 7TE, UK
[4]Philip Leverhulme Equine Hospital, School of Veterinary Science, University of Liverpool, Wirral CH64 7TE, UK
Full list of author information is available at the end of the article

Background

Postoperative ileus (POI) is a frequent complication in horses that have undergone small intestinal surgery for management of colic and it increases the risk of postoperative mortality [1–4]. In horses at high risk of POI or where POI develops postoperatively, prokinetic drugs are frequently used. Lidocaine, erythromycin, metoclopramide, cisapride, mosapride, and bethanechol are agents that have been evaluated as prokinetic drugs in horses through clinical [5–11] or experimental (both in vitro and in vivo) studies [12–16].

Lidocaine is a local anaesthetic agent, which has antiarrhythmic, analgesic and prokinetic properties when administered systemically in humans [17–19]. Several studies have also evaluated its effects in horses using in vitro and in vivo models. Systemically administered lidocaine has been found to have anti-inflammatory properties such as reduction of mucosal COX-2 expression and neutrophil count in ischaemic-injured equine intestine or amelioration of the negative effects of flunixin meglumine on recovery of injured mucosa [14, 15]. Lidocaine therapy has been proposed as a treatment option for horses with inflammatory conditions of the gastrointestinal tract including POI and recovery from ischaemic injury [20] and the authors of the latter study highlighted the need for further trials to evaluate its clinical effectiveness.

Studies that have investigated the prokinetic properties of lidocaine have reported conflicting results. A study that compared the effects of mosapride, cisapride, metoclopramide and lidocaine on jejunal motility in adult Thoroughbred horses found improved jejunal motility in response to cisapride, mosapride and metoclopramide but not with lidocaine treatment [16]. Additionally, lidocaine administration in normal horses that underwent laparotomy did not result in increased jejunal motility [13] and in a separate study was also associated with prolonged faecal transit time and reduced faecal output in normal horses [21]. More recent in vitro studies [22–24] reported positive effects of lidocaine on the contractility of smooth muscle isolated from equine jejunum in ischaemia and reperfusion injury models. The effect was found not to be specific to lidocaine and smooth muscle contractility was induced with other agents including mexiletine, bupivacaine, tetracaine and procaine [23]. Overall, limited evidence has been found to support the use of perioperative lidocaine as a therapy for POI [25]. Despite this, lidocaine therapy is frequently used in horses undergoing surgical treatment of colic. A recent survey of European Equine Internal Medicine and Surgery Diplomates reported that lidocaine was used intraoperatively in 50 % of cases and postoperatively in 67 % to prevent POI and was the drug of choice for 79 % of respondents in the management of POI in horses [26].

In the authors' hospital, intravenous lidocaine has become more frequently used in the perioperative management of horses undergoing surgical management of small intestinal lesions for treatment of colic, and in particular horses at increased risk of POI. The aim of the current study was to investigate whether routine use of lidocaine in this population of horses has had any effect on the prevalence, duration of postoperative reflux and total reflux volume in horses, and to determine whether it has altered rates of postoperative survival or is a risk factor for altered postoperative survival.

Methods

Study population

The study population consisted of two cohorts of horses that underwent surgical treatment of colic related to a primary small intestinal lesion at a UK equine hospital. Horses were recruited onto the study if they underwent exploratory laparotomy for treatment of colic, were diagnosed with a small intestinal lesion at surgery, and stood in the recovery box following general anaesthesia. The first cohort were horses admitted in October 2004–November 2006, when lidocaine was only used intermittently in colic patients, and the second cohort was admitted in October 2012–November 2014 after lidocaine use had become implemented more routinely in horses undergoing small intestinal surgery for treatment of colic based on studies published between the two time periods advocating its use [3, 11, 20]. Routine surgical and postoperative management of colic patients during this time remained otherwise unchanged. Briefly, this consisted of intravenous flunixin meglumine administration for a minimum of 72 h (1.1 mg/kg bwt q. 12 h), and antimicrobial therapy with procaine penicillin (12 mg/kg bwt i.m. q. 12 h) or procaine penicillin and gentamicin (6.6 mg/kg bwt i.v. q. 24 h) for 3–5 days based on the surgical procedure performed (e.g. enterotomy, resection and anastomosis) and clinician preference. In this group of horses that had primary small intestinal lesions, all received intravenous fluid therapy (lactated Ringer's solution) for at least the first 24 h postoperatively (unless they were able to tolerate oral fluids prior to this), and until oral fluid therapy could be initiated. Intravenous fluids were administered according to maintenance requirements (2 ml/kg bwt/h) together with additional fluid losses (e.g. net reflux volume) and were supplemented with calcium and potassium where required. Nasogastric intubation was performed at 2–4 hourly intervals once postoperative reflux developed. This continued until reflux ceased and oral water and feed were then gradually reintroduced over 3–4 days. Where reflux persisted, repeat laparotomy was undertaken or horses were euthanased based on lack of response to treatment and/or owner finances. Monitoring of small intestinal motility and diameter was performed ultrasonographically in some horses. Lidocaine therapy was usually administered during anaesthesia and immediately following placement in the stable following recovery from anaesthesia for most horses in the 2012–14 cohort unless clinician preference or lack of client finances dictated otherwise.

Data collection and follow-up

Preoperative data were collected in a specifically designed colic admission form, which included questions about signalment, use, current management practices and any recent management changes, and results of clinical and clinicopathological examinations (Additional file 1). Postoperatively, clinical parameters including the net volume of reflux obtained and medications administered were recorded in specifically designed hospital forms. For both cohorts, survival was monitored following hospital discharge by telephone questionnaires administered with the horse owner/carer. This was performed every 3 months following discharge for the first 12 months and then at 6 monthly intervals. The questionnaires were administered as a part of two separate prospective studies investigating postoperative survival following colic surgery [27] and Salem et al. (unpublished data). All data were entered onto a Microsoft access or a Microsoft SQL Server database for the 2004–2006 and 2012–2014 cohorts respectively.

Administration of lidocaine intra- or postoperatively was recorded based on examination of the anaesthetic and postoperative monitoring sheets. The standard dose used at the hospital was a 1.3 mg/kg bolus given intravenously over 15 min followed by a 0.05 mg/kg bwt/min intravenous continuous rate infusion (CRI). Due to the fact that it is difficult to confirm true POI and to differentiate it from other causes of small intestinal obstruction e.g. mechanical obstruction that may occur postoperatively [28, 29], the term postoperative reflux (POR) [30, 31] was used in the current study. This was defined as a net nasogastric reflux of ≥2 l on at least two consecutive occasions within 24 h postoperatively [32]. Due to the fact that pain was not assessed using a single, consistent scoring system, we could not assess the effect of lidocaine on postoperative pain and this was not one of the aims of the current study.

Data analysis

Descriptive data analysis

Survival time was calculated as a continuous variable starting from the date of surgery until the date of death or censoring. Horses were censored if they were lost to follow-up or were alive at the last interview date. Survival time was used to construct Kaplan-Meier plots of cumulative probability of survival and the log-rank test was used to compare survival between different surgical diagnosis categories, and between horses that did or did not receive lidocaine CRI intra- or postoperatively. A chi-square test of independence was used to compare frequencies of common surgical diagnosis categories and surgical procedures performed such as intestinal resection and anastomosis or types of anastomosis performed, use of prokinetic therapy and prevalence of POR between the two cohorts. The Wilcoxon rank-sum test was used to compare number of days that the horses were classified as having POR and total reflux volume between horses that received or did not receive lidocaine CRI intra- or postoperatively. Horses diagnosed with equine grass sickness (EGS) were excluded from statistical analyses [33].

Univariable analysis

Explanatory variables were screened for univariable association with time to death or censoring using univariable Cox proportional hazards models. Variables that had a likelihood ratio test (LRT) p value <0.25 were considered for inclusion into a multivariable model. Variables containing ≥30 % missing data were initially excluded from the analysis and categorical variables with few observations in some categories were re-categorised into fewer, biologically plausible categories. Pearson's correlation coefficient was used to test for collinearity between explanatory variables. If variables were highly correlated ($r \geq 0.7$) [34] or were considered to be measuring the same exposure, the variable that resulted in a greater reduction in residual deviance was selected [35]. The functional form of the relationships between continuous predictor variables and survival time was explored using penalized regression models [36]. The results from these models were examined graphically and variables that demonstrated a significant non-linear association with survival were fitted as P-spline smoothers, otherwise a linear fit was chosen. Data pre-processing and re-categorisation were performed using Epi Info7[1] software. Survival analysis was performed using the 'survival' statistical package (version 2.38.1) [37] in R software environment version 3.2.2 [38]. Critical probability was set at 0.05 for all analyses.

Multivariable analysis

A multivariable Cox proportional hazards model considering only variables measured pre- and intraoperatively was built using a forward stepwise selection procedure. Variables were added sequentially into the model and were retained if they significantly improved model fit. This was indicated by a LRT p value <0.05 and a reduction in Akaike information criterion by at least 2 (ΔAIC >2) when nested models were compared.

Eliminated variables were then forced back into the final model to assess for confounding and two-way interactions between variables remaining in this model were evaluated for statistical significance. The proportional hazard (PH) assumption was evaluated by plotting complementary log-log survival curves and scaled Schoenfeld residuals for variables remaining in the model. This was also assessed statistically using the Therneau-Grambsch non-proportionality test [39] as implemented by the 'survival::cox.zph' function in R. Scaled changes in regression coefficients associated with the exclusion of individual data points (delta-betas) were plotted in order to identify influential observations. The model was re-run following removal of any influential data point (−0.4 < delta-betas > 0.4) to evaluate their leverage on parameter estimates. Poorly fitted data points were also evaluated in a deviance residual plot. A data point was considered outlying if the corresponding deviance residual value is outside the range of (−2.5–2.5) [40]. The effect of surgeon and of anaesthetist on the probability of survival was tested in the final model by including each of these variables as a frailty term (random effect) in the final model.

Results

Of 342 horses that underwent laparotomy for treatment of a primary small intestinal lesion, 318 were recruited onto the study (24 horses were excluded due to a diagnosis of EGS). The follow-up periods were the same for both study cohorts and all interviews were concluded approximately 3 months following the last recruitment date. This resulted in 272.6 horse years of recorded survival time. The number of horses in each study cohort and the frequencies of the most common surgical diagnosis categories and anastomoses types if small intestinal resection was performed are shown in Table 1. There was a significant increase in number of horses diagnosed with idiopathic focal eosinophilic enteritis (IFEE) lesions in the 2012–2014 cohort compared to the 2004–2006 cohort (19.7 vs 7.2 %). Surgical management of these lesions also varied: 78.6 % (11/14) of horses diagnosed with IFEE lesions in 2004–2006 admission years had intestinal resection and anastomosis during surgery compared with none in 2012–2014 admission years. There was a significant reduction in the frequency of horses in which intestinal resection and anastomosis was performed, particularly the frequency of side-to-side jejunocaecal anastomosis in recent admission years.

Table 1 Results of descriptive data analyses comparing the two study cohorts

Diagnosis/types of small intestinal anastomosis/prokinetic drugs/postoperative reflux	2004–2006 admission years	2012–2014 admission years	χ2 *p* value	Total
Horses diagnosed with small intestinal lesions	195 (60.6)	147 (55.7)	0.23	342 (58.4)
Common diagnosis categories				
Pedunculated lipoma obstruction	52 (25.7)	39 (26.5)	0.98	91 (26.6)
Idiopathic focal eosinophilic enteritis	14 (7.2)	29 (19.7)	0.001	43 (12.6)
Epiploic foramen entrapment	29 (14.9)	14 (9.52)	0.14	43 (12.6)
Ileal impaction	11(3.2)	13 (3.8)	0.7	24 (7)
Equine grass sickness (EGS)	15 (7.7)	9 (6.1)	0.6	24 (7)
Horses undergoing intestinal resection and anastomosis (EGS cases excluded)	115 (63.9)	56 (41.8)	<0.001	171 (54.5)
Side-to-side jejunocaecal anastomosis	42 (24.3)	12 (9)	0.001	54 (17.2)
Side-to-side ileocecal anastomosis	3 (1.7)	0 (0.0)	-	3 (0.96)
Side-to-side jejunojejunal anastomosis	4 (2.2)	0 (0.0)	-	4 (1.3)
End-to-end jejunoileal anastomosis	9 (5)	15 (11.2)	0.04	24 (7.6)
End-to-end jejunojejunal anastomosis	57 (31.7)	29 (21.6)	0.049	86 (27.4)
Prokinetic drugs used (EGS cases excluded)				
Lidocaine CRI intraoperatively	25 (16.1)	86 (62.3)	<0.001	111 (37.9)
Lidocaine CRI postoperatively	7 (4)	102 (73.9)	<0.001	109 (34.8)
Metoclopramide	1 (0.6)	9 (6.5)	-	10 (3.2)
Erythromycin	0 (0.0)	7 (5.07)	-	7 (2.2)
Lidocaine CRI plus Metoclopramide	0 (0.0)	8 (5.8)	-	8 (2.5)
Postoperative reflux (EGS cases excluded)	30 (16.7)	48 (34.8)	<0.001	78 (24.5)

Results of descriptive data analyses comparing frequencies of small intestinal lesions, common diagnosis categories, types of small intestinal anastomosis performed, prokinetic drugs administered intra- or postoperatively, and postoperative reflux between the two study cohorts. Chi-square (χ2) test *p* values comparing these frequencies and total frequencies are shown. Descriptive data are presented as numbers (%)

Cumulative probabilities of survival of horses in the five most frequent diagnosis categories are shown in Fig. 1a. IFEE and ileal impaction cases had a fairly stable survival at around 0.8 throughout the study period. This was in contrast to epiploic foramen entrapment (EFE) cases, which demonstrated a rapid decline in postoperative survival resulting in a median survival time of 370 days. The log-rank test of the probability of survival between these small intestinal lesions was significant at $p = 0.038$. Cumulative probability of survival did not differ significantly between horses in the two study cohorts (log-rank test $p = 0.79$) (Fig. 1b).

Effect of lidocaine therapy

The prevalence of POR in all horses recruited onto the study was 24.5 %. This was significantly higher in horses admitted in 2012–2014 (34.8 %) compared to 16.7 % in horses admitted in 2004–2006 (Table 1). POR resulted in a significant reduction in the long-term probability of survival and this effect was evident throughout the follow-up period (Fig. 2a). There was no statistical evidence that intraoperative lidocaine administration had any effect on long-term postoperative survival (log-rank test $p = 0.72$) (Fig. 2b). Because postoperative lidocaine treatment was not assigned randomly and horses were administered this medication if they were considered to be at high risk of developing POR or occasionally once horses had developed POR, the data were stratified and the effect of lidocaine CRI on probability of survival was compared in horses that did or did not develop POR separately. Such comparison did not reveal any significant improvement in the probability of survival in lidocaine-treated horses (Fig. 2c and d). The median duration of POR and of total reflux volume did not

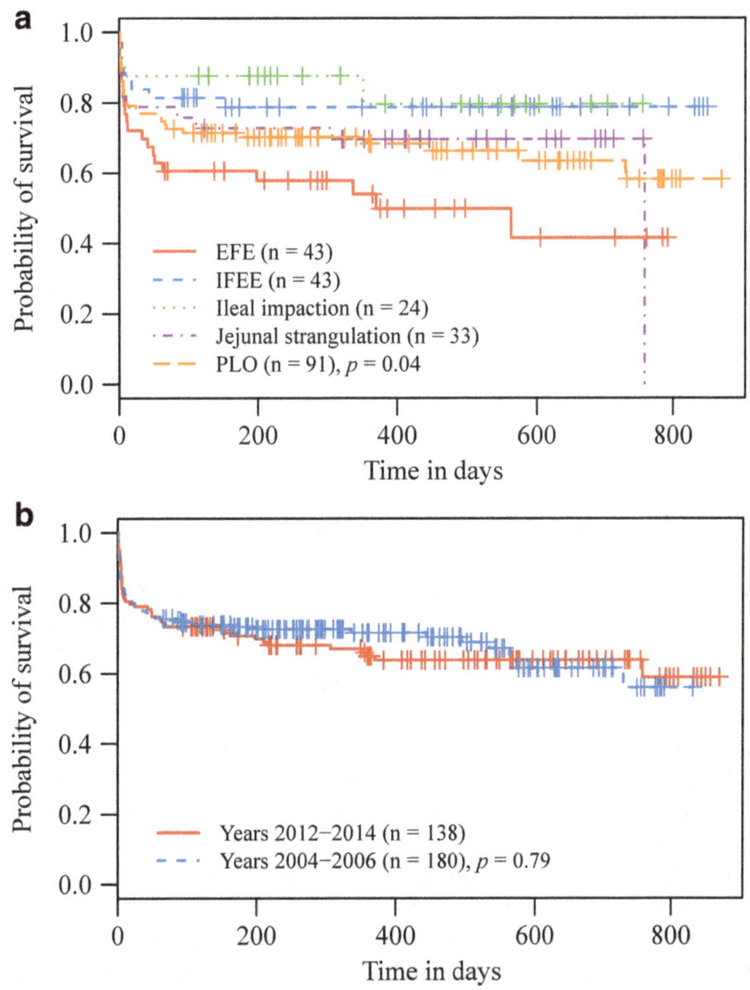

Fig. 1 Kaplan-Meier plots comparing commonly identified small intestinal lesions (**a**) and the study cohorts (**b**). Kaplan-Meier plots of cumulative probability of survival and the log-rank test were used to compare survival between the five most frequent surgical diagnosis categories and between horses that belong to each of the admission periods (2004–2006 and 2012–2014 admission years). Vertical lines on the curves represent censoring times. The log-rank test p values and number of horses in each category are shown. EFE = epiploic foramen entrapment, IFEE = idiopathic focal eosinophilic enteritis, PLO = pedunculated lipoma obstruction

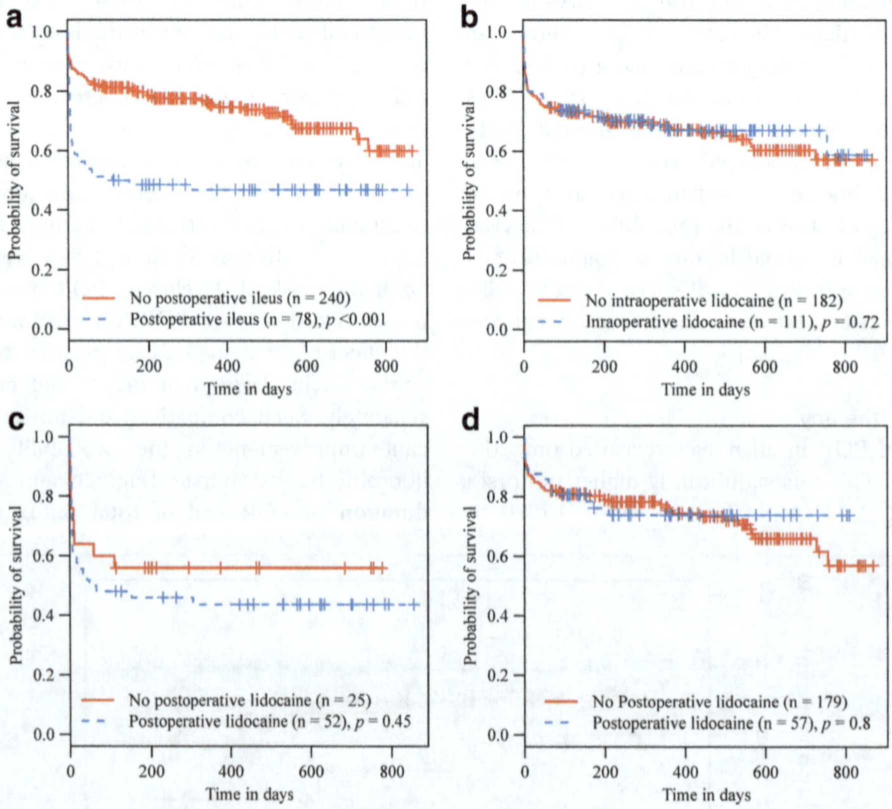

Fig. 2 Kaplan-Meier plots illustrating the effect of POR and of lidocaine therapy on postoperative survival. Kaplan-Meier plots of cumulative probability of survival and the log-rank test were used to compare survival between horses that developed or did not develop postoperative reflux (**a**), horses that received or did not receive lidocaine CRI intraoperatively (**b**). Following stratifying the data by postoperative reflux, the effect of postoperative lidocaine therapy was assessed in horses that developed (**c**) or did not develop postoperative reflux (**d**). The number of horses in each category and the log-rank test *p* values are shown

differ significantly between horses that were or were not administered intraoperative (Wilcoxon rank-sum $p = 0.75$ and 0.86 respectively) or postoperative lidocaine therapy (Wilcoxon rank-sum $p = 0.15$ and 0.14 respectively) (Fig. 3).

Risk factors for postoperative survival

Results of univariable analysis of continuous and categorical variables are available in Additional files 2 and 3. The functional form of the relationships examined by penalized regression models was non-linear for the variable heart rate on admission and therefore, this variable was evaluated as a penalized smoothed term in the multivariable model (Fig. 4). A final multivariable proportional hazards model is shown in Table 2. Variables identified to be associated with increased risk of postoperative mortality included packed cell volume on admission, heart rate on admission and duration of surgery. There was a significant multiplicative interaction between duration of surgery and EFE (hazard ratio 1.013, 95 % confidence interval 1.002–1.03, $p = 0.027$), meaning that the hazard ratio comparing horses with or without EFE depends on the duration of surgery. The random effects of surgeon and of anaesthetist tested in the final model were not significant ($p = 0.98$).

The proportional hazards assumption was satisfied in the final multivariable model (global p value from the Therneau-Grambsch non-proportionality test = 0.94). A single influential data point was identified for variable PCV on admission (Additional file 4). The observations had a censored survival time, yet it was from a horse that had a PCV of 74 % on admission. Removal of this influential observation and re-running the model resulted in 33 % increase in the regression coefficient of this variable. The observation was found to be accurately recorded, so it was retained in the model. Four poorly fitting data points were identified on a deviance residual plot (Additional file 5). They had deviance residual values of >2.5 and the values were positive which meant observed death happened before the model was able to predict it. These observations were from horses that had PCV on admission of ≤40 % and surgery duration of ≤105 min, yet they had a survival time of 1 day.

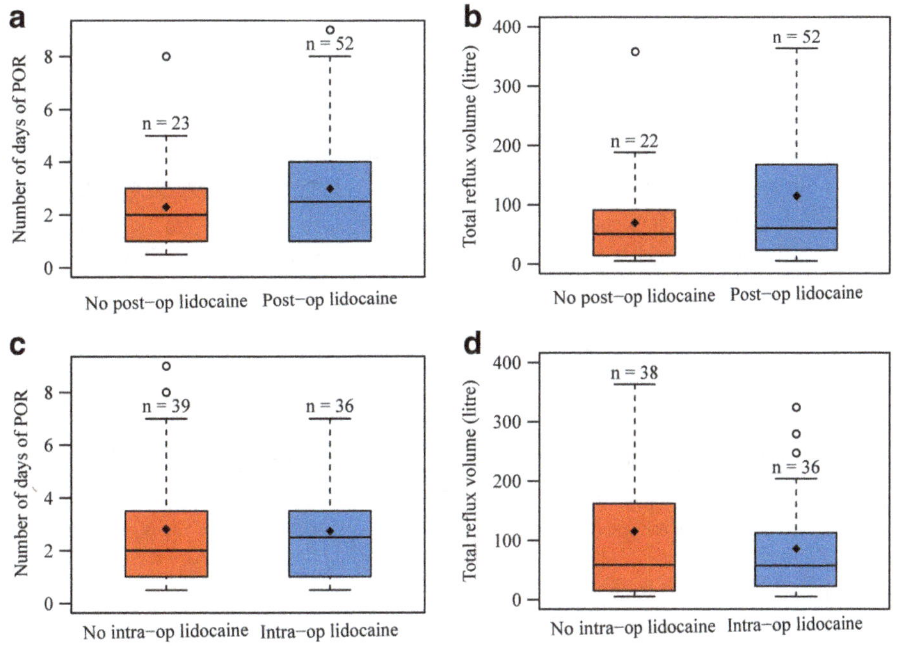

Fig. 3 Boxplots demonstrating the effects of lidocaine therapy on duration of POR and total reflux volume. Duration of postoperative reflux (POR) and total reflux volume were compared between horses that were administered lidocaine continuous rate infusion postoperatively (**a** and **b**) or intraoperatively (**c** and **d**). The box represents the 25th and 75th percentiles of the data, the horizontal line across the middle of the box represents the median and the *dot* is the mean. Post-op = postoperatively, Intra-op = intraoperatively

Discussion

The current study found no significant effect of intra- or postoperative lidocaine therapy on the duration of POR or total reflux volume in horses that underwent laparotomy for treatment of small intestinal lesions. Lidocaine administration also had no significant effect on postoperative survival, consistent with the findings of *Malone* et al. [11]. Lidocaine is currently commonly administered postoperatively in horses that have undergone surgical management of colic based on its perceived prokinetic properties [26]. These findings are important and demonstrate the need for further evaluation of the efficacy of lidocaine treatment in horses undergoing surgical management of colic related to small intestinal disease, particularly in horses at high risk of or that have developed POR, in a randomised controlled trial.

The prevalence of POR in the current study is comparable to previously reported rates of 9–33 % [3, 41–43]. The frequency of intra- or postoperative lidocaine treatment was significantly greater in horses that underwent surgical treatment of small intestinal lesions in 2012–2014 cohort, but the prevalence of POR doubled compared with the 2004–2006 admission years (34.8 vs 16.7 %), which was unexpected. The frequency of horses that were recovered from surgery that had undergone intestinal resection and anastomosis, particularly side-to-side jejunocaecal anastomoses was also significantly reduced in the 2012–2014 admission group. This is likely to be due to awareness of the effects of intestinal resection and anastomosis and of side-to-side jejunocaecal anastomosis on reduced postoperative survival, leading to some owners choosing to have horses euthanased on the operating table rather than continue with treatment or in equivocal cases, surgeons choosing not to resect potentially viable small intestine [27, 44–46]. It is not possible to determine why the prevalence of POR was increased in the 2012–2014 surgical cohort who routinely received perioperative lidocaine therapy, nor to attribute it directly to lidocaine use as this was not a randomised study. However, surgeons being more likely to leave small intestine that would undergo ischaemia-reperfusion injury may have resulted in increased prevalence of POR in the 2012–2014 cohort. The prevalence of IFEE lesions did differ between the two study periods which could have resulted in bias. Further exploration of the data using univariable and multivariable models with POR as the outcome demonstrated that the variable IFEE was not significantly associated with POR ($p = 0.58$) and inclusion of IFEE cases were therefore considered unlikely to have a significant impact on the study. In addition, whether resection was performed or not in IFEE cases was considered unlikely to alter the likelihood of postoperative mechanical obstruction occurring (and subsequent development of POR) as these are thickened lesions that cause acute colic due to simple obstruction at the site, and any physical thickening of

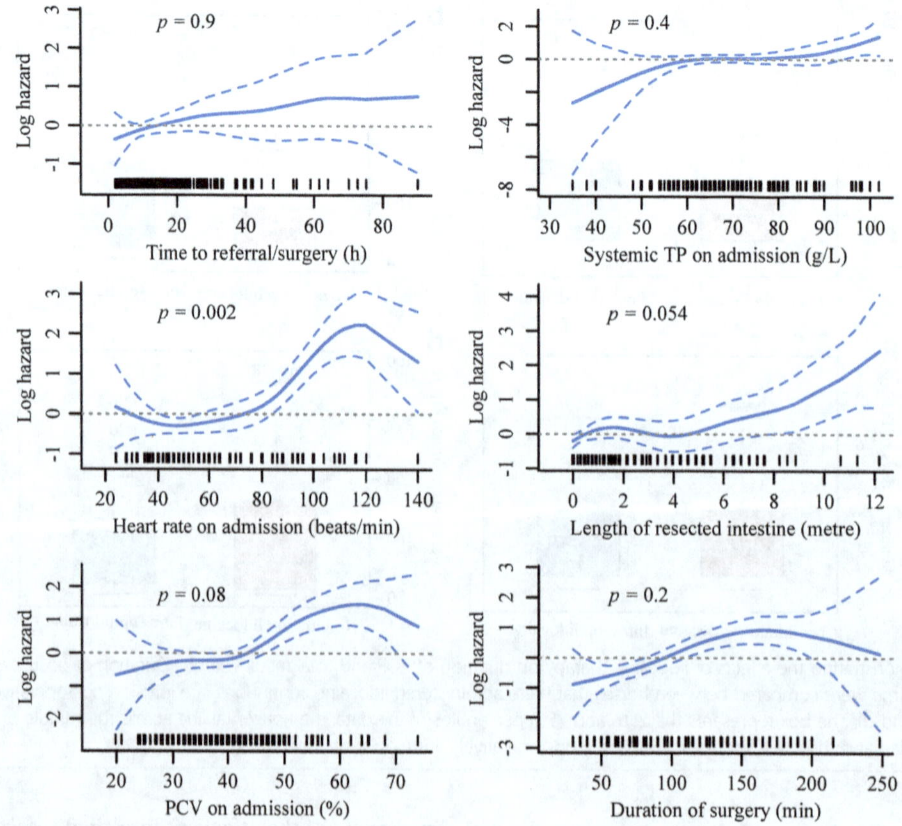

Fig. 4 Plots of P-spline smoothers of continuous pre- and intraoperative variables. Penalised regression models were used to investigate the functional form of the relationships between the log hazard of postoperative death and continuous variables measured pre and intraoperatively. The plots show the fitted curves with 95 % confidence intervals (*dashed lines*) and the rug plots along the x-axes represent the number of data points. *Dotted horizontal lines* are at log hazard of zero. The *p* values are from chi square tests for non-linearity where a significant *p* value ($p > 0.05$) indicates a non-linear association

intestine at the site of IFEE lesions left in situ (i.e. not resected) is comparable to that of an anastomosis.

In humans, systematic reviews and meta-analysis of randomised clinical trials have investigated the prokinetic and analgesic properties of lidocaine. Following open abdominal or laparoscopic surgery in adult humans, lidocaine has been found to be associated with significant reductions in postoperative pain scores [17, 47, 48]. However, the evidence for prokinetic efficacy is variable. Evidence of reduced time to first flatus, time to first bowel movement or likelihood of POI was found to be of low quality [17]. Comparison of the efficacy of 15 systemically acting prokinetic drugs for treatment of POI versus placebo in another systematic review reported that only lidocaine and neostigmine have an effect on gastrointestinal recovery in the form of reduction of time to first flatus and to first bowel movement [19]. Lidocaine treatment was also reported to be associated with reduced duration of hospital stay and of ileus following abdominal surgery in another systematic review [49].

The prokinetic properties of lidocaine have been evaluated previously in equine surgical colic patients in two separate randomised clinical trials [10, 11]. In one of these trials most of the horses were diagnosed with large intestinal lesions at surgery (20/28) and only two horses developed POI (one control, one treatment), and therefore the prokinetic properties of lidocaine could not be assessed [10]. In the study by *Malone* et al. [11], lidocaine administration to horses that developed nasogastric reflux resulted in significant reduction in number of horses refluxing at 30 h post-treatment and in duration of hospital stay compared to saline group. The study, however, did not report any differences in survival to hospital discharge or in the level of postoperative pain between groups. Limitations of the latter study include the fact that the study was performed on a small number of horses and included horses diagnosed with proximal duodenitis-jejunitis (DPJ) treated medically (8 DPJ and 24 POI horses), which are lesions with different pathobiology and relevance when considering lidocaine use in horses that have undergone small intestinal surgery [25]. A prophylactic effect of lidocaine in horses with POI was reported in a study by *Torfs* et al. [3]. In the latter study, lidocaine was frequently administered concurrently with

Table 2 Multivariable Cox proportional hazards model of variables associated with reduced likelihood of survival

Variable	Coefficient	Standard error	Hazard ratio	95 % CI of the hazard ratio	*p* value
Packed cell volume on admission (%)	0.032	0.014	1.033	1.004–1.06	0.024
Heart rate on admission (beats/min) *"the linear effect"*	0.014	0.005	1.014	1.004–1.024	0.008
Duration of surgery (min)	0.0066	0.0025	1.007	1.002–1.01	0.008
Epiploic foramen entrapment	Ref				
No	−0.66	0.77	0.52	0.1–1.35	0.39
Yes					
Surgery duration × EFE	0.013	0.006	1.013	1.002–1.03	0.027

The data are from 318 horses that survived following laparotomy for treatment of small intestinal lesions; only 302 horses were included in the model due to missing data for some variables. The model is adjusted for the non-linear relationship between heart rate on admission and probability of survival. *CI* confidence interval, *Re* reference category

other prokinetic drugs such as metoclopramide and this was not taken into account in the analysis of the data. Therefore, the evidence for the use of perioperative lidocaine to improve intestinal motility in horses at high risk of developing POI remains of low quality [25] and supports the need for further investigation.

We acknowledge that one of the key limitations to this study is the fact that horses were not randomly assigned to lidocaine treatment. Lidocaine was instead assessed as an intervention, as this was the only major change in management of horses undergoing surgical treatment of small intestinal lesions causing colic in the study hospital between the two study periods. Other factors that may have differed between the two time periods and may have had a potential effect include the effect of surgeon and anaesthetist, but they were assessed in the model and were not significantly associated with outcome. It is also important to note that economic factors may influence the decision to perform surgery or to recover horses following general anaesthesia [50, 51] and consequently this may introduce bias into survival models. The costs of treatment, including lidocaine therapy, may have been a limiting factor for some owners, particularly when postoperative reflux persisted for a number of days with no evidence of clinical improvement. It is, therefore, possible that with longer duration of therapy that some of these horses may have survived. We did not specifically investigate whether insurance cover had an effect on the surgical outcome. However, we have previously found this to have no effect on survival of horses recovered following surgery (unpublished hospital data) and the estimated costs of treatment are the same regardless of whether the horse is insured or not. It is also important to note that the effect of lidocaine on postoperative pain could not be assessed due to lack of consistent scoring in pain. This was not one of the key aims of the present study, but the analgesic effects of lidocaine should also be taken into consideration in future prospective trials evaluating its use in horses following intestinal surgery for colic.

In the current study, horses that underwent surgery for treatment of ileal impaction had the greatest probability of survival which is consistent with previous studies [43]. IFEE lesions were also associated with high rates of postoperative survival, with a relatively stable probability of survival at around 0.8 throughout the follow-up period. In contrast, EFE had a poor prognosis for survival with a median survival time of 370 days, which is again consistent with previous studies [4, 33, 43, 52]. In the current study, PCV and heart rate measured on admission and prolonged surgery duration were significantly and positively associated with postoperative mortality. PCV and heart rate can be markers for the degree of dehydration and systemic inflammatory response syndrome (SIRS)/endotoxaemia on admission [35]. This emphasises the importance of early diagnosis and treatment of equine surgical colic patients before development of marked physiological derangements/SIRS in order to maximise the probability of survival following laparotomy.

Conclusions

In the current study, we found no effect of lidocaine therapy on frequency of POR, duration of reflux, nor was it a risk factor for, or associated with altered rates of postoperative survival. Despite the frequent use of lidocaine as a prokinetic agent in horses that develop or are at high risk of POI, the evidence for this still remains limited. Lidocaine therapy can add significantly to treatment costs making it important to fully evaluate the efficacy and cost-benefits of this drug. There is a need for a prospective, multicentre randomised clinical trial of lidocaine in horses with small intestinal lesions that has sufficient statistical power with well-defined inclusion criteria. There should also be a well-defined set of outcome measures including accurate measurement of POR duration and total reflux volume and use of objective and validated measures of postoperative pain, postoperative survival and complications.

Endnotes

[1]Centre for Disease Control (CDC), Atlanta, Georgia, USA

Additional files

Additional file 1: The form used for initial data collection on hospital admission of each of the horses.

Additional file 2: Continuous variables investigated for association with the risk of postoperative death. Data were collected from 318 horses that survived following general anaesthesia for treatment of small intestinal lesions and investigated for association with the risk of postoperative death using univariable Cox proportional hazards model. Descriptive data are presented as median (interquartile range).

Additional file 3: Categorical variables investigated for association with the risk of postoperative death. Data were collected from 318 horses that survived following general anaesthesia for treatment of small intestinal lesions and were investigated for association with the risk of postoperative death using univariable Cox proportional hazards model.

Additional file 4: Delta-betas plot of variables retained in the final Cox proportional hazards model. A single influential data point was evident for the variable packed cell volume (PCV) on admission.

Additional file 5: Complementary log-log Kaplan-Meier survival curve for epiploic foramen entrapment (EFE) and a deviance residual plot. The complementary log-log Kaplan-Meier survival curve of EFE on a logarithmic scale (a) suggests that the proportional hazards assumption is satisfied for this variable (Therneau-Grambsch non-proportionality test $p = 0.24$). A deviance residual plot from the final multivariable Cox proportional hazards model (b) demonstrates five outlying data points (deviance residuals >2.5).

Abbreviations

CRI, continuous rate infusion; EFE, epiploic foramen entrapment; EGS, equine grass sickness; HR, hazard ratio; IFEE, idiopathic focal eosinophilic enteritis; intra-op, intra-operatively; PCV, packed cell volume; PLO, pedunculated lipoma obstruction; POI, postoperative ileus; POR, postoperative reflux; post-op, postoperatively

Acknowledgements

The authors are grateful to Janet Smith for the assistance with the owner questionnaire, and to Philip Stratford for assistance with the project database design. We would like to thank all the staff at the Philip Leverhulme Equine hospital who assisted with the management of cases, the referring veterinary surgeons and the owners of the horses included in the study.

Funding

Salem SE's Ph.D. studies are funded by the Egyptian Ministry of Higher Education. The Liverpool colic survival study was funded by the Petplan Charitable Trust in 2004–2007.

Authors' contributions

SES contributed to the study design, collected the data, performed the statistical analysis and drafted the manuscript, CJP contributed to the study design, collected the 2004–2006 survival data and critically appraised the manuscript, DCA contributed to the study design, interpretation of the statistical results and writing of the manuscript. All authors gave their final approval of the manuscript.

Competing interests

None of the authors of this paper has a financial or personal relationship with other people or organisations that could inappropriately influence or bias the content of the paper.

Author details

[1]Institute of Infection and Global Health, Department of Epidemiology and Population Health, University of Liverpool, Wirral CH64 7TE, UK. [2]Department of Surgery, Faculty of Veterinary Medicine, Zagazig University, Zagazig, Egypt. [3]School of Veterinary Medicine, University of Surrey, Guildford GU2 7TE, UK. [4]Philip Leverhulme Equine Hospital, School of Veterinary Science, University of Liverpool, Wirral CH64 7TE, UK.

References

1. Morton AJ, Blikslager AT. Surgical and postoperative factors influencing short-term survival of horses following small intestinal resection: 92 cases (1994–2001). Equine Vet J. 2002;34(5):450–4.
2. Mair TS, Smith LJ. Survival and complication rates in 300 horses undergoing surgical treatment of colic. Part 2: Short-term complications. Equine Vet J. 2005;37(4):303–9.
3. Torfs S, Delesalle C, Dewulf J, Devisscher L, Deprez P. Risk factors for equine postoperative ileus and effectiveness of prophylactic lidocaine. J Vet Intern Med. 2009;23(3):606–11.
4. Archer DC, Pinchbeck GL, Proudman CJ. Factors associated with survival of epiploic foramen entrapment colic: a multicentre, international study. Equine Vet J. 2011;43:56–62.
5. Geest J, Vlaminck K, Muyelle E, Deprez P, Sustronck B, Picavet MT. A clinical study of cisapride in horses after colic surgery. Equine Vet Educ. 1991;3:138–42.
6. Gerring EL, King JN, Edwards GB, Pearson H, Walmsley JP, Greet TRC. A multicentre trial of cisapride in the prophylaxis of equine post operative ileus. Equine Vet Educ. 1991;3(3):143–5.
7. van der Velden MA, Klein WR. The effects of cisapride on the restoration of gut motility after surgery of the small intestine in horses; a clinical trial. Vet Q. 1993; 15(4):175–9.
8. Cohen ND, Faber NA, Brumbaugh GW. Use of bethanechol and metoclopramide in horses with duodenitis/proximal jejunitis: 13 cases (1987–1993). J Equine Vet Sci. 1995;15(11):492–4.
9. Dart AJ, Peauroi JR, Hodgson DR, Pascoe JR. Efficacy of metoclopramide for treatment of ileus in horses following small intestinal surgery: 70 cases (1989–1992). Aust Vet J. 1996;74(4):280–4.
10. Brianceau P, Chevalier H, Karas A, Court MH, Bassage L, Kirker-Head C, Provost P, Paradis MR. Intravenous lidocaine and small-intestinal size, abdominal fluid, and outcome after colic surgery in horses. J Vet Intern Med. 2002;16(6):736–41.
11. Malone E, Ensink J, Turner T, Wilson J, Andrews F, Keegan K, Lumsden J. Intravenous continuous infusion of lidocaine for treatment of equine ileus. Vet Surg. 2006;35(1):60–6.
12. Nieto JE, Rakestraw PC, Snyder JR, Vatistas NJ. In vitro effects of erythromycin, lidocaine, and metoclopramide on smooth muscle from the pyloric antrum, proximal portion of the duodenum, and middle portion of the jejunum of horses. Am J Vet Res. 2000;61(4):413–9.
13. Milligan M, Beard W, Kukanich B, Sobering T, Waxman S. The effect of lidocaine on postoperative jejunal motility in normal horses. Vet Surg. 2007;36(3):214–20.
14. Cook VL, Neuder LE, Blikslager AT, Jones SL. The effect of lidocaine on in vitro adhesion and migration of equine neutrophils. Vet Immunol Immunopathol. 2009;129(1–2):137–42.
15. Cook VL, Shults JJ, McDowell M, Campbell NB, Davis JL, Blikslager AT. Attenuation of ischaemic injury in the equine jejunum by administration of systemic lidocaine. Equine Vet J. 2008;40(4):353–7.
16. Okamura K, Sasaki N, Yamada M, Yamada H, Inokuma H. Effects of mosapride citrate, metoclopramide hydrochloride, lidocaine hydrochloride, and cisapride citrate on equine gastric emptying, small intestinal and caecal motility. Res Vet Sci. 2009;86(2):302–8.
17. Kranke P, Jokinen J, Pace NL, Schnabel A, Hollmann MW, Hahnenkamp K, Eberhart LH, Poepping DM, Weibel S. Continuous intravenous perioperative lidocaine infusion for postoperative pain and recovery. Cochrane Database Syst Rev. 2015 Jul 16;(7):CD009642. doi:10.1002/14651858.CD009642.pub2.
18. Harrison DC, Sprouse JH, Morrow AG. The antiarrythmic properties of lidocaine and procaine amide. Clinical and physiological studies for their cardiovascular effects in man. Circulation. 1963;28:486–91.
19. Traut U, Brügger L, Kunz R, Pauli-Magnus C, Haug K, Bucher HC, Koller MT. Systemic prokinetic pharmacologic treatment for postoperative adynamic ileus following abdominal surgery in adults. Cochrane Database Syst Rev. 2008 Jan 23;(1):CD004930. doi:10.1002/14651858.CD004930.pub3.
20. Cook VL, Blikslager AT. Use of systemically administered lidocaine in horses with gastrointestinal tract disease. J Am Vet Med Assoc. 2008;232(8):1144–8.
21. Rusiecki KE, Nieto JE, Puchalski SM, Snyder JR. Evaluation of continuous infusion of lidocaine on gastrointestinal tract function in normal horses. Vet Surg. 2008;37(6):564–70.

22. Tappenbeck K, Hoppe S, Reichert C, Feige K, Huber K. In vitro effects of lidocaine on contractility of circular and longitudinal equine intestinal smooth muscle. Vet J. 2013;198(1):170–5.
23. Tappenbeck K, Hoppe S, Hopster K, Kietzmann M, Feige K, Huber K. Lidocaine and structure-related mexiletine induce similar contractility-enhancing effects in ischaemia–reperfusion injured equine intestinal smooth muscle in vitro. Vet J. 2013;196(3):461–6.
24. Guschlbauer M, Feige K, Geburek F, Hoppe S, Hopster K, Propsting MJ, Huber K. Effects of in vivo lidocaine administration at the time of ischemia and reperfusion on in vitro contractility of equine jejunal smooth muscle. Am J Vet Res. 2011;72(11):1449–55.
25. Salem SE, Proudman CJ, Archer DC. Prevention of postoperative complications following surgical treatment of equine colic: current evidence. Equine Vet J. 2016;48:143–51.
26. Lefebvre D, Pirie RS, Handel IG, Tremaine WH, Hudson NPH. Clinical features and management of equine post operative ileus: Survey of diplomates of the European Colleges of Equine Internal Medicine (ECEIM) and Veterinary Surgeons (ECVS). Equine Vet J 2015. doi:10.1111/evj.12355
27. Proudman CJ, Edwards GB, Barnes J. Differential survival in horses requiring end-to-end jejunojejunal anastomosis compared to those requiring side-to-side jejunocaecal anastomosis. Equine Vet J. 2007;39(2):181–5.
28. Freeman DE. Post operative ileus (POI): another perspective. Equine Vet J. 2008;40(4):297–8.
29. Merritt AM, Blikslager AT. Post operative ileus: to be or not to be? Equine Vet J. 2008;40(4):295–6.
30. Stewart S, Southwood LL, Aceto HW. Comparison of short- and long-term complications and survival following jejunojejunostomy, jejunoileostomy and jejunocaecostomy in 112 horses: 2005–2010. Equine Vet J. 2014;46(3):333–8.
31. Gazzerro DM, Southwood LL, Lindborg S. Short-term complications after colic surgery in geriatric versus mature Non-geriatric horses. Vet Surg. 2015; 44(2):256–64.
32. French NP, Smith J, Edwards GB, Proudman CJ. Equine surgical colic: risk factors for postoperative complications. Equine Vet J. 2002;34(5):444–9.
33. Proudman CJ, Smith JE, Edwards GB, French NP. Long-term survival of equine surgical colic cases. Part 2: modelling postoperative survival. Equine Vet J. 2002;34(5):438–43.
34. Sauerbrei W, Royston P, Binder H. Selection of important variables and determination of functional form for continuous predictors in multivariable model building. Stat Med. 2007;26(30):5512–28.
35. Proudman CJ, Edwards GB, Barnes J, French NP. Modelling long-term survival of horses following surgery for large intestinal disease. Equine Vet J. 2005;37(4):366–70.
36. Therneau TM, Grambsch PM. Penalised models. In: Modelling sruvival data: extending the Cox model. New York: Springer; 2000. p. 120–6.
37. Therneau T: A Package for Survival Analysis in S_. version 2.38, URL:https://cran.r-project.org. 2015.
38. R Core Team: R. A language and environment for statistical computing. Vienna: R Foundation for Statistical Computing; 2014.
39. Grambsch PM, Therneau TM. Proportional hazards tests and diagnostics based on weighted residuals. Biometrika. 1994;81(3):515–26.
40. Fitrianto A, Jiin RLT. Several types of residuals in cox regression model: an empirical study. Int J Math Anal. 2013;7:2645–54.
41. Blikslager AT, Bowman K, Levine JF, Bristol DG, Roberts MC. Evaluation of factors associated with postoperative ileus in horses: 31 cases (1990–1992). J Am Vet Med Assoc. 1994;205(12):1748–52.
42. Cohen ND, Lester GD, Sanchez LC, Merritt AM, Roussel AJJ. Evaluation of risk factors associated with development of postoperative ileus in horses. J Am Vet Med Assoc. 2004;225(7):1070–8.
43. Proudman CJ, Smith JE, Edwards GB, French NP. Long-term survival of equine surgical colic cases. Part 1: patterns of mortality and morbidity. Equine Vet J. 2002;34(5):432–7.
44. Freeman DE, Hammock P, Baker GJ, Goetz T, Foreman JH, Schaeffer DJ, Richter RA, Inoue O, Magid JH. Short- and long-term survival and prevalence of postoperative ileus after small intestinal surgery in the horse. Equine Vet J Suppl. 2000;32:42–51.
45. Garcia-Seco E, Wilson DA, Kramer J, Keegan KG, Branson KR, Johnson PJ, Tyler JW. Prevalence and risk factors associated with outcome of surgical removal of pedunculated lipomas in horses: 102 cases (1987–2002). J Am Vet Med Assoc. 2005;226(9):1529–37.
46. van den Boom R, van der Velden MA. Short-and long-term evaluation of surgical treatment of strangulating obstructions of the small intestine in horses: a review of 224 cases. Vet Q. 2001;23(3):109–15.
47. Sun Y, Li T, Wang N, Yun Y, Gan TJ. Perioperative systemic lidocaine for postoperative analgesia and recovery after abdominal surgery: a meta-analysis of randomized controlled trials. Dis Colon Rectum. 2012;55(11): 1183–94.
48. Ventham NT, Kennedy ED, Brady RR, Paterson HM, Speake D, Foo I, Fearon KC. Efficacy of intravenous lidocaine for postoperative analgesia following laparoscopic surgery: a meta-analysis. World J Surg. 2015;39(9):2220–34.
49. Marret E, Rolin M, Beaussier M, Bonnet F. Meta-analysis of intravenous lidocaine and postoperative recovery after abdominal surgery. Br J Surg. 2008;95(11):1331–8.
50. Reeves MJ, Curtis CR, Salman MD, Hilbert BJ. Prognosis in equine colic patients using multivariable analysis. Can J Vet Res. 1989;53(1):87–94.
51. Christophersen MT, Dupont N, Berg-Sorensen KS, Konnerup C, Pihl TH, Andersen PH. Short-term survival and mortality rates in a retrospective study of colic in 1588 Danish horses. Acta Vet Scand. 2014;56:20.
52. Proudman CJ, Edwards GB, Barnes J, French NR. Factors affecting long-term survival of horses recovering from surgery of the small intestine. Equine Vet J. 2005;37(4):360–5.

15

A biomechanical comparison of conventional dynamic compression plates and string-of-pearls™ locking plates using cantilever bending in a canine Ilial fracture model

Allison R Kenzig[1], James R Butler[1*], Lauren B Priddy[2], Kristen R Lacy[2] and Steven H Elder[2]

Abstract

Background: Fracture of the ilium is common orthopedic injury that often requires surgical stabilization in canine patients. Of the various methods of surgical stabilization available, application of a lateral bone plate to the ilium is the most common method of fixation. Many plating options are available, each having its own advantages and disadvantages. The purpose of this study was to evaluate the biomechanical properties of a 3.5 mm String-of-Pearls™ plate and a 3.5 mm dynamic compression plate in a cadaveric canine ilial fracture model. Hemipelves were tested in cantilever bending to failure and construct stiffness, yield load, displacement at yield, ultimate load, and mode of failure were compared.

Results: The mean stiffness of dynamic compression plate (116 ± 47 N/mm) and String-of-Pearls™ plate (107 ± 18 N/mm) constructs, mean yield load of dynamic compression plate (793 ± 333 N) and String-of-Pearls™ plate (860 ± 207 N) constructs, mean displacement at yield of dynamic compression plate (8.6 ± 3.0 mm) and String-of-Pearls™ plate (10.2 ± 2.8 mm) constructs, and ultimate load at failure of dynamic compression plate (936 ± 320 N) and String-of-Pearls™ plate (939 ± 191 N) constructs were not significantly different. No differences were found between constructs with respect to mode of failure.

Conclusions: No significant biomechanical differences were found between String-of-Pearls™ plate and dynamic compression plate constructs in this simplified cadaveric canine ilial fracture model.

Keywords: SOP, String-of-pearls, DCP, Dynamic compression plate, Canine ilium, Ilial fracture, Plating, Biomechanics

Background

Fractures of the pelvis constitute approximately a quarter of all fractures in small animals [1–3]. The majority of these cases are due to high-energy trauma, such as vehicular trauma or falling from a height [1, 3–7]. Fractures of the ilial body account for 18–46% of pelvic fracture cases, with the majority being long oblique fractures, and they often occur concurrently with fractures of the ischium and pubis [1, 8]. Conservative management with cage rest may be utilized for minimally displaced fractures, but can result in sub-optimal long-term function if the fracture segments are displaced [3, 4]. Surgically treated ilial fractures are generally stabilized by open reduction and lateral application of appropriately contoured plates and screws [1, 4–8]. Various types of plates have been employed for the stabilization of ilial fractures, including dynamic compression plates, cuttable plates, T plates, miniplates, reconstruction plates, and double plates [4, 8].

The most common complication associated with ilial fracture repair is implant failure, which occurs in up to 62% of patients. The majority of these failures are due to screw pull-out, with one of the reasons for this high

* Correspondence: rbutler@cvm.msstate.edu
[1]Mississippi State University College of Veterinary Medicine, 240 Wise Center Drive, Mississippi State, MS 39762, USA
Full list of author information is available at the end of the article

incidence of screw loosening being poor bone quality in the cranial ilial wing [1, 8–12]. Conventional plating techniques rely on friction between the plate and bone to provide stability. The weakest point in this conventional plating system is the interface between the screw and the bone. Placing screws in poor quality bone, such as the cranial ilium, may result in an inability to generate adequate force to prevent implant and fracture motion [1]. Furthermore, the amount of compression needed to generate friction between a standard compression plate and bone has been shown to adversely affect the periosteal blood supply, which has been linked to delayed healing, non-union, and increased susceptibility to bacterial surgical site infections after fracture repair [13, 14]. Locking implant systems have been developed to provide more stable fracture repair, especially in poorer quality bone, and to minimize the negative impact on local vascularity during fracture healing [1]. These plating systems do not rely on plate-to-bone friction to provide stability, eliminating the need for high shear loads at the screw-to-bone interface [15]. Less plate-to-bone contact also decreases the need for precise plate contouring and helps preserve the blood supply to the bone [13–17].

The String-of-Pearls™ (SOP) implant is a stainless steel locking plate made up of repeating units of spherical pearls and cylindrical rods. Each pearl is designed to engage a standard cortical bone screw in a locking fashion by the screw threads engaging a ridge within the pearl, and the plate can be contoured by twisting along its longitudinal axis and bending in multiple planes without compromising its locking ability. The ability of the SOP locking plate to utilize standard cortical bone screws allows this construct to, in general, be considerably less expensive than more traditional locking plate constructs [13, 14]. In a 2014 study of Locking Compression Plates (LCP) versus Dynamic Compression Plates (DCP) in a canine ilial fracture model, there was no demonstrable difference between the constructs' performance in acute failure testing in vitro [1]. In a 2015 study comparing double SOP plating versus single DCP constructs in a synthetic bone model, the double SOP constructs had significantly greater bending stiffness, bending strength, bending structural stiffness, and torsional stiffness [13]. To the authors' knowledge, there have been no studies reported in the literature comparing the mechanical strength of SOP plating to DCP plating in a canine ilial fracture model.

The purpose of this study was to compare the stiffness, yield load, ultimate load at failure, displacement at yield, and mode of failure in cantilever bending of SOP and DCP constructs in an acute failure ilial fracture model. The hypothesis was that the SOP plates would have superior biomechanical properties compared to the DCP constructs of comparable size.

Methods

Pelves were harvested from 11 healthy, purpose-bred dogs,[1] weighing approximately 20–30 kg, that were humanely euthanized for reasons unrelated to orthopedic disease or this study. The dogs were part of an institutional approved teaching protocol unrelated to this study. The pelves were harvested by disarticulation at the sacroiliac joints within 12 h of euthanasia and stripped of all associated soft tissues. Visual inspection of the samples was performed to ensure they were free of pre-existing orthopedic disease. The samples were then stored at −20 °C after being wrapped in saline soaked towels and double bagged.

Prior to biomechanical testing, the samples were thawed at room temperature. The pelves were divided at the symphysis, and the paired ilia were randomly assigned to treatment with either a stainless steel six-hole 3.5 mm DCP[2] or a six-hole 3.5 mm SOP[3] construct such that the treatment groups were evenly distributed with respect to side. For both plating techniques, the plate was positioned with the cranial aspect of the plate centered within the wing of the ilium and the caudal aspect of the plate adequately cranial to the acetabulum so that no screws penetrated the joint. Three self-tapping cortical screws[4] were positioned cranial and three caudal to the osteotomy. For both plating systems, the plates were individually contoured to match the curvature of the respective ilium. Standardized long oblique osteotomies were performed using a sagittal saw. The osteotomy location was standardized at 40% of the distance from the cranial aspect of the acetabulum to the most cranial aspect of the ilial wing. Osteotomies were created such that the fracture line extended from the most caudal aspect of the ventral iliac spine to a point on the greater ischiatic notch which produced an osteotomy that was 1.5 times the length of the dorsoventral ilial shaft diameter. The osteotomies were then reduced, and the assigned constructs were applied using standard AO[5] technique (Fig. 1). All holes were drilled with a variable speed, hand-held, battery-powered drill[6] loaded with a 2.5 mm drill bit,[7] and using either a DCP drill guide[8] or an SOP drill guide[9] of the appropriate size, for the corresponding plates. Drill holes were not tapped due to the use of self-tapping cortical screws[4]. The screws were tightened by hand until they were "two-finger-tight" for the DCP construct, and until the screws locked into the SOP plates. The two screws adjacent to the osteotomy were placed eccentrically in the DCP constructs in order to provide fracture compression. The cranial aspect of each ilium was mounted in a custom-made steel rectangular pot using polymethylmethacrylate[10] such that pubic symphysis was perpendicular to the platform, and the long axis of the hemipelvis was 30 degrees from perpendicular to the platform (Fig. 2a and b). The plates and protruding ends of the screws were covered by a

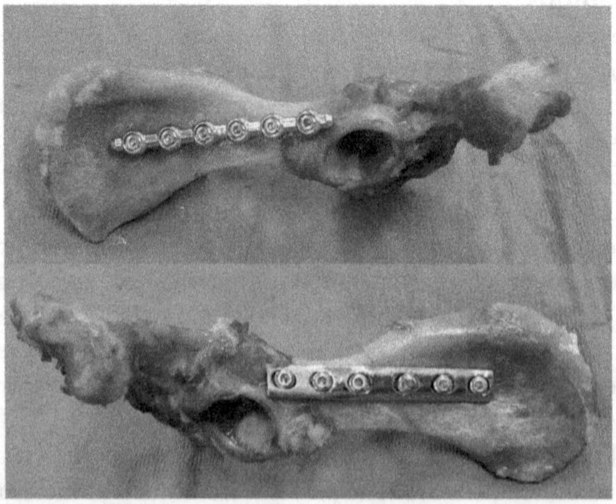

Fig. 1 Lateral String-of-Pearls™ plate and Dynamic Compression Plate application demonstrating osteotomy location, plate contouring, and fracture reduction

modelling compound[11] so that the acrylic would not adhere to or contact the implants during testing. The modelling compound was removed prior to biomechanical testing. The potted bone was fitted to a servohydraulic materials testing machine.[12] A 22 mm diameter stainless steel sphere[13] was placed in contact with the acetabulum prior to testing and used to transmit the load from the acetabulum to the load cell (Fig. 3). The angle of the potted ilia allowed for testing the constructs at 120°, which approximates hip angle during midstance [18]. Constructs were mounted for a bending stress state and tested to failure using a compression loading frame with a 50 kN load cell.[14] The constructs were preloaded to 5 N, and load was applied at 20 mm/min until failure was detected by an acute drop in load, concurrent with grossly detectable evidence of construct failure. Data were sampled at a rate of 100 Hz and stored electronically. Mode of failure, including screw pull-out, screw cut-out, and plate bending was recorded by observation during testing and inspection of the constructs after testing. Failure was classified as screw pull-out or screw cut-out when construct failure occurred with no observed bending of the plate. Screw cut-out occurred with damage to the surrounding bone, whereas screw pull-out occurred with no surrounding bony damage.

Data analyses

For each sample, a load-displacement curve was generated to determine ultimate load, stiffness, displacement at yield, and yield load. The maximum force applied during testing was the ultimate load (N). A linear trendline was obtained for the elastic portion of the load-displacement curve, and the slope of the line was defined as stiffness (N/mm). A 1 mm displacement offset method was used to determine displacement at yield (mm) and yield load (N).

Statistical analyses

Data were analyzed by paired t-tests and reported as mean ± standard error of the mean (SEM). Differences were considered significant when $p < 0.05$. All statistical testing was performed using a standard statistical software package.[15]

Results

Five left hemipelves and 6 right hemipelves were plated with a DCP construct. Six left hemipelves and 5 right hemipelves were plated with an SOP construct. In the DCP group, constructs failed through either screw pull-out in the cranial ilium (n = 9) or through plate bending at the osteotomy site (n = 2).

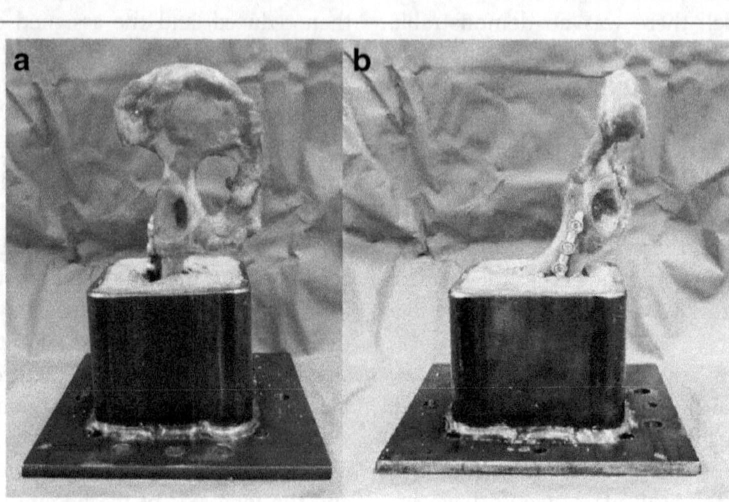

Fig. 2 a Mounting of hemipelvis with pubic symphysis perpendicular to platform. **b** Mounting of the hemipelvis with the long axis oriented 30 degrees from perpendicular to the platform

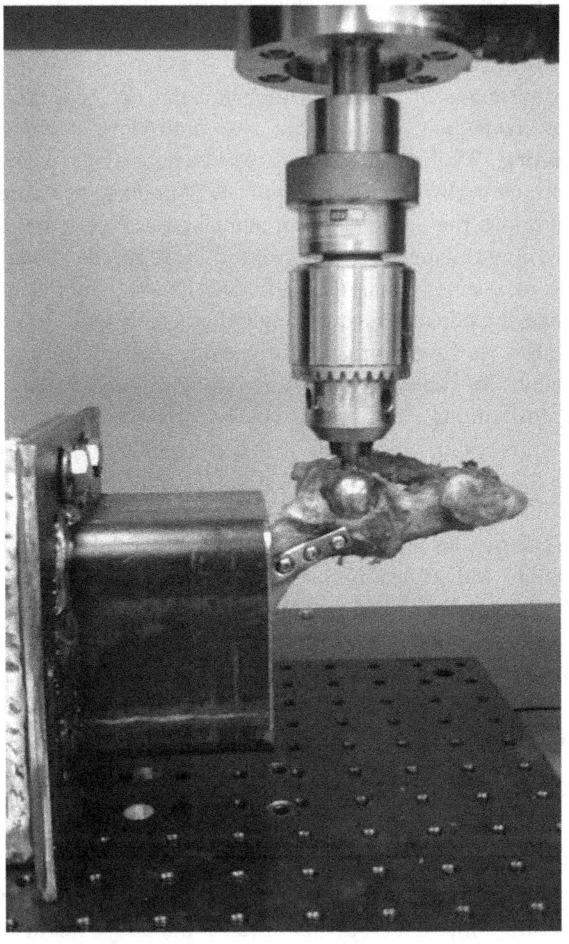

Fig. 3 Mounting of hemipelvis on testing platform

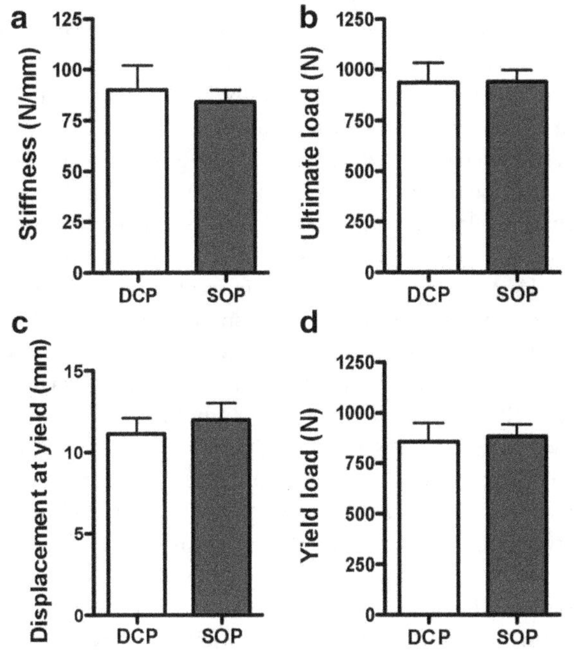

Fig. 4 Comparison of stiffness (**a**), ultimate load (**b**), displacement at yield (**c**), and yield load (**d**) for DCP and SOP constructs

In the SOP group, the constructs failed through either screw cut-out cranial to the ilium (n = 7) or through plate bending at the osteotomy site (n = 4). Screw cut-out for the SOP group occurred with apparent fracture of the ilium surrounding the screws, as opposed to the DCP group for which screw pull-out occurred without damage to the surrounding bone. In both groups, plate bending occurred at the osteotomy site without obvious screw loosening. No significant differences were found between groups for stiffness, ultimate load at failure, displacement at yield, or yield load (Table 1 and Fig. 4).

Table 1 Comparison of stiffness, ultimate load, displacement at yield, and yield load for DCP and SOP constructs

	Stiffness (N/mm)	Ultimate load (N)	Displacement at yield (mm)	Yield load (N)
DCP	116 ± 47	936 ± 320	8.6 ± 3.0	793 ± 333
SOP	107 ± 18	939 ± 191	10.2 ± 2.8	860 ± 207
p-value	0.69	0.98	0.53	0.79

DCP dynamic compression plate, *SOP* String-of-Pearls™ plate. Values are reported as mean ± SEM

Discussion

This study did not reveal any significant differences between SOP and DCP constructs in a cadaveric canine ilial fracture model in acute cantilever bending to failure. Previous studies comparing SOP plates, various forms of DCP constructs, and locking plate constructs have produced results that differ from the presented study. In 2008, DeTora and Kraus compared SOP, LCP, standard limited contact DCP (LC-DCP), and broad LC-DCP constructs. The results of that study showed that the broad LC-DCP was stronger in stiffness and bending compared to the SOP; however, the SOP was biomechanically superior to both the LCP and the LC-DCP [19]. In 2011, Blake et al. compared SOP to DCP, stainless steel and titanium LC-DCP, LCP, advanced locking plate system (ALPS), and Fixin plates in a validated bone model simulating bridging osteosynthesis. This study found that SOP constructs had significantly higher stiffness than all the other plates, and were significantly stronger than the titanium LC-DCP, ALPS, and Fixin constructs. The clinically relevant conclusion of this study stated that due to differing plate construct properties inherent to diverse implant systems, identical approaches to fracture management and plate application cannot be applied [20]. In 2012, Malenfant and Sod compared SOP to LCP constructs in a cadaveric tibial diaphyseal fracture gap model and found that the SOP construct was superior under bending static and cycling testing, but the LCP construct was superior in static and cycling torsion testing [21]. Hutcheson et al. compared bridging double plate SOP constructs to broad DCP constructs in a synthetic bone fracture gap model in 2015 and found that all biomechanical properties were significantly higher for the double SOP construct, but the actual differences were small [13].

The mechanical advantages of the SOP implant from the previous studies were often attributed to the circular profile of the implant and higher associated area moment of inertia compared to rectangular implants [13–15, 19–21]. The difference in fracture model configuration in the presented study compared to the multiple aforementioned studies likely allowed less demonstration of the previously observed biomechanical advantages of the SOP plating system. In our study the most common mode of failure was screw pullout from the cranial ilial wing. The diminished quality of bone in that portion of the ilium likely contributed to the lack of differences between the two constructs. Additionally, in previous studies, load application was purposefully oriented to examine the weakest plate direction. The current ilial fracture model tested the DCP oriented more with the width of the bone, rather than its thickness, resulting in an increase in the area moment of inertia, which places it at a mechanical advantage compared to the previous studies. The SOP plates are not affected by this change in force directionality as they are cylindrical implants.

A similar cadaveric ilial fracture model comparing 6-hole 3.5 mm DCP constructs to 3.5 mm LCP constructs also found no significant difference between the two constructs [1]. The anatomically reduced fracture permitted load sharing within the constructs and was one explanation of the minimal difference seen [1]. The interfragmentary compression achieved in DCP constructs likely benefited the DCP group in our study and may be an additional explanation for the lack of differences seen between constructs. Should interfragmentary compression not be clinically possible, the DCP construct *may* be weaker. However, additional mechanical studies would be required to validate that claim. The inherent characteristics of the SOP locking plate, including ease of contouring and decreased impact on vascularity due to decreased plate-to-bone contact, remain potential benefits despite the biomechanical similarity to the DCP constructs.

The oblique ilial osteotomy used in this fracture model is a similar method to the 2008 study by Fitzpatrick et al. which compared lateral ilial fracture plating to pelvic external skeletal fixators [4]. This fracture configuration was chosen due to its clinically relevant nature. Fractures of the ilium are most commonly long oblique fractures of the midbody with the obliquity oriented from cranioventral to caudodorsal [3, 5–8]. While it is known that the tension surface of the ilium is the ventral surface, and ventral plate fixation offers mechanical advantages compared to a lateral plate, we elected to evaluate lateral plating as the lateral surface of the ilium is more easily approached and is the most common method of internal fixation of pelvic fractures in dogs [1, 21–23].

Limitations of this study included the use of a cadaveric model and testing that was limited to cantilever bending. While cyclic testing would potentially provide more clinically applicable data, it is difficult to accurately reproduce the in vivo environment in a cadaveric model. To approximate the forces exerted on clinically repaired ilia, we elected to use a cantilever-bending model and tested the constructs at an angle that approximated midstance. However, the fracture model tested does not account for the various fracture configurations or patient conformations that may be encountered clinically. Fracture callus formation and bone remodeling following implant application may differ in SOP compared to DCP constructs due to the aforementioned effects on vascularity, which may in turn affect overall construct stability and/or healing rates. However, interfragmentary compression achieved with DCP constructs may also accelerate healing. This fracture model also does not account for potentially improved screw purchase with engaging the sacral wing, which has been studied previously with conflicting results [9, 10].

Conclusions

In this study, no significant differences were found in stiffness, yield load, ultimate load, displacement at yield, or mode of failure between 3.5 mm SOP and DCP ilial fracture constructs. Further studies, including further in vitro studies evaluating cyclical testing and the effect of sacral screw purpose, and prospective clinical trials, would be necessary to further evaluate any true mechanical or clinical benefit to SOP fixation compared to DCP fixation for oblique mid-body ilial fractures in the dog.

Endnotes

[1]Oak Hill Genetics, Ewing, Illinois, USA

[2]Dynamic Compression Plate (DCP): Orthomed, Halifax, West Yorkshire, UK

[3]String-of-Pearls™ (SOP): Orthomed, Halifax, West Yorkshire, UK

[4]3.5 mm cortical screws: Orthomed, Halifax, West Yorkshire, UK

[5]Arbeitgemeinschaft für Osteosynthesefragen / AO Foundation

[6]Makita drill: Makita, La Mirada, California, USA

[7]2.5 mm drill bit: Veterinary Orthopedic Implants, Saint Augustine, Florida, USA

[8]DCP drill guide: DePuy Synthes, West Chester, Pennsylvania, USA

[9]SOP drill guide: Orthomed, Halifax, West Yorkshire, UK

[10]Technovit: Jorgensen Labs, Loveland, CO, USA

[11]Play-Doh: Hasbro, Pawtucket, RI, USA

[12]MTI-2 K Universal Testing Machine: Measurements Technology, Inc., Marietta, GA

[13]316 Stainless Steel Precision Ball 7/8″ Diameter, product number 96415 K87: McMaster-Carr, Douglasville, GA, USA

[14]Universal Testing Instrument, Model 1011: Instron, Norwood, MA, USA

[15]GraphPad Prism 5: GraphPad Software, Inc., La Jolla, CA, USA

Abbreviations

ALPS: Advanced locking plate system; DCP: Dynamic compression plate; LC-DCP: Limited contact dynamic compression plate; LCP: Locking compression plate; SEM: Standard error of the mean; SOP: String-of-Pearls™

Acknowledgements

Not applicable.

Funding

This research project was partially funded by an internal research grant from Mississippi State University College of Veterinary Medicine. Implants for this study were generously donated by Orthomed, Halifax, West Yorkshire, UK.

Authors' contributions

ARK contributed to study design, construct assembly, construct testing, and manuscript writing. JRB contributed to study design, construct assembly, construct testing, and manuscript writing. LBP contributed to construct testing, data analysis, and manuscript writing. KRL contributed to construct testing and data analysis. SEE contributed to study design. All authors have read and approved the final version of this manuscript.

Consent for publication

Not applicable.

Competing interests

The authors declare that they have no competing interests.

Author details

[1]Mississippi State University College of Veterinary Medicine, 240 Wise Center Drive, Mississippi State, MS 39762, USA. [2]Mississippi State University College of Agricultural and Biological Engineering, Box 9632, 130 Creelman Street, Mississippi State, MS 39762, USA.

References

1. Bruce CW, Gibson T, Runciman RJ. A comparison of conventional compression plates and locking compression plates using cantilever bending in an ilial fracture model. Vet Comp Orthop Traumatol. 2014;27:430–5.
2. Zulauf D, Kaser-Hotz B, Hassig M, et al. Radiographic examination and outcome in consecutive feline trauma patients. Vet Comp Orthop Traumatol. 2008;21:36–40.
3. Denny HR. Pelvic fractures in the dog: a review of 123 cases. J Small Anim Pract. 1978;19:151–66.
4. Fitzpatrick N, Lewis D, Cross A. A biomechanical comparison of external skeletal fixation and plating for the stabilization of ilial osteotomies in dogs. Vet Comp Orthop Traumatol. 2008;21:349–57.
5. W.B. Saunders Company. Fractures of the pelvis. In: Piermattei D, Flo G, De-Camp C, editors. Brinker, Piermattei and Flo's handbook of small animal Orthopedics and fracture repair. 4th ed. Toronto: W.B. Saunders Company; 2006. p. 431 60.
6. DeCamp C. Fractures of the pelvis. In: Tobias K, Johnston S, editors. Veterinary surgery: small animal. 1st ed. Philadelphia: WB Saunders; 2011. p. 801–15.
7. DeCamp C. Fractures of the ilium. In: Johnson A, Houlton J, Vannini R, editors. AO principles of fracture Management in the dog and cat. 1st ed. Davos: AO Publishing; 2005. p. 170–7.
8. Breshears L, Fitch RB, Wallace LJ, et al. The radiographic evaluation of repaired canine ilial fractures (69 cases). Vet Comp Orthop Traumatol. 2004;17:64–72.
9. Bogoni P, Rovesti GL. Early detection and treatment of screw loosening in triple pelvic osteotomy. Vet Surg. 2005;34:190–5.
10. Doornink MTM, Nieves MAM, Evans RR. Evaluation of ilial screw loosening after triple pelvic osteotomy in dogs: 227 cases (1991–1999). J Am Vet Med Assoc. 2006;229:535–41.
11. Hamilton MHM, Evans DAD, Langley-Hobbs SJS. Feline ilial fractures: assessment of screw loosening and pelvic canal narrowing after lateral plating. Vet Surg. 2009;38:326–33.
12. Hosgood G, Lewis DD. Retrospective evaluation of fixation complications of 49 pelvic osteotomies in 36 dogs. J Small Anim Pract. 1993;34:123–30.
13. Hutcheson KD, Butler JR, Elder SE. Comparison of double locking plate constructs with single non-locking plate constructs in single cycle to failure in bending and torsion. Vet Comp Orthop Traumatol. 2015;28:234–9.
14. Kraus KH, Ness MG. Standard operating procedures for SOP fixation of fractures. West Yorkshire: Orthomed; 2007.
15. Egol KA, Kubiak EN, Fulkerson E, et al. Biomechanics of locked plates and screws. J Orthop Trauma. 2004;18:488–93.
16. Ahmad M, Nanda R, Bajwa AS, Candal-Couto J, Green S, Hui AC. Biomechanical testing of the locking compression plate: when dose the distance between bone and implant significnatly reduce construct stability? Injury. Int J Care Injured. 2007;38:358–64.
17. Case JB, Dean C, Wilson DM, Knudsen JM, James SP, Palmer RH. Comparison of the mechanical Behaviors of locked and nonlocked plate/screw fixation applied to experimentally induced rotational Osteotomies in the canine Ilia. Vet Surg. 2012;41:103–13.
18. Hottinger HA, DeCamp CE, Olivier NB, et al. Non- invasive kinematic analysis of the walk in healthy large-breed dogs. Am J Vet Res. 1996;57:381–8.
19. DeTora M, Kraus K. Mechanical testing of 3.5 mm locking and non-locking bone plates. Vet Comp Orthop Traumtol. 2008;21:318–22.
20. Blake CA, Boudrieau RJ, Torrance BS, et al. Single cycle to failure in bending of three standard and five locking plate and plate constructs. Vet Comp Orthop Traumatol. 2011;6:408–18.
21. Malenfant R-C, Sod GA. In vitro biomechanical comparison of 3.5 string of pearl plate fixation to 3.5 locking compression plate fixation in a canine fracture gap model. Vet Surg. 2014;43:465–70.
22. Vangundy T, Hulse D, Nelson J, et al. Mechanical evaluation of two canine iliac fracture fixation systems. Vet Surg. 1988;17:321–7.
23. Johnson AL, Houlton JE, Vannini R. AO principles of fracture Management in the dog and cat. Davos: AO Publishing; 2005.

16

Pilot, randomized, placebo-controlled clinical field study to evaluate the effectiveness of bupivacaine liposome injectable suspension for the provision of post-surgical analgesia in dogs undergoing stifle surgery

B. Duncan X. Lascelles[1,2,3,4*], Lesley C. Rausch-Derra[5], Jessica A. Wofford[5] and Margie Huebner[6]

Abstract

Background: Local anesthetics are an important component of perioperative pain management, but the duration of action of available products is limited. We hypothesized that a single local infiltration of a novel bupivacaine liposome injectable suspension (AT-003) would provide clinically effective analgesia over a 72-h period.
In a masked, randomized, placebo-controlled, multi-center pilot field study, dogs undergoing lateral retinacular suture placement for cranial cruciate insufficiency were randomly assigned to surgical site infiltration with AT-003 (5.3 mg/kg) or an equivalent volume of saline. Infiltration of the surgical site was done prior to closure. Primary outcome measure was the Glasgow Composite Measure Pain Scale (CMPS-SF) assessed prior to surgery and at 2, 4, 8, 12, 24, 30, 36, 48, 54, 60 and 72 h following surgery by trained individuals. Provision for rescue analgesia was employed. Repeated measures analysis of variance were utilized to test for possible differences between treatment groups and a success/failure analysis was also employed, based on the need for rescue analgesia.

Results: Forty-six dogs were enrolled and evaluated. For CMPS-SF scores there was a significant overall treatment effect ($p = 0.0027$) in favor of AT-003. There were significantly more successes in the AT-003 group compared to placebo over each time period ($p = 0.0001$ for 0–24 h, $p = 0.0349$ for 0–48 h, and $p = 0.0240$ for 0-72 h). No significant adverse events were seen.

Conclusions: AT-003 (bupivacaine liposome injectable suspension) provided measurable local analgesia over a 72-h period following post-stifle surgery surgical site tissue infiltration. Further work is indicated to develop this product for clinical use.

Keywords: Bupivacaine liposome injectable suspension, Dog, Pain, Cruciate surgery

Abbreviations: CCL, Cranial cruciate ligament; CMPS-SF, Glasgow composite measure pain scale (short form); EDC, Electronic data capture; IV, Intra-venous; SSMS, Surgical site manipulation scores

* Correspondence: duncan_lascelles@ncsu.edu
[1]Department of Clinical Sciences, Comparative Pain Research Laboratory, College of Veterinary Medicine, North Carolina State University, Raleigh, NC, USA
[2]Department of Clinical Sciences, Comparative Medicine Institute, College of Veterinary Medicine, North Carolina State University, Raleigh, NC 27606, USA
Full list of author information is available at the end of the article

Background

Perioperative analgesia has become recognized as an important ethical responsibility of veterinarians over the last three decades. Clinical evidence in dogs indicates that multimodal analgesia provides the most effective relief from postoperative pain [1]. One of the most effective means of preventing the transduction and transmission of nociceptive signals is through the use of local anesthetics. Indeed, it is the authors' opinion that the only currently available analgesics that can completely block perioperative pain are the local anesthetics. Despite their potential efficacy, the relief provided by currently available local anesthetics is of limited duration, and this may be one factor contributing to the currently relatively low use of local anesthetics in small animal practice [2]. Bupivacaine has the longest reported activity, potentially providing analgesia for as long as 6–7 h [3–5]. However, currently the only method in veterinary medicine to extend the action of bupivacaine beyond this involves using a wound catheter, and instilling bupivacaine approximately every 6 h into the wound [6, 7].

In 2011 the FDA approved an extended-release formulation of bupivacaine, DepoFoam® bupivacaine[1] for use as a single-dose infiltration into the surgical site to effect postsurgical analgesia in human surgical patients. The DepoFoam technology used in this product consists of multivesicular liposomes encapsulating aqueous bupivacaine. The liposomes are microscopic structures made of nonconcentric lipid bilayers designed such that bupivacaine is gradually released from vesicles over 96 h as the lipid bilayers break down. The lipids making up the bilayer structures consist of phospholipids, cholesterol and triglycerides, and importantly do not contain lecithin which has been associated with tissue necrosis and toxicity [8]. Bupivacaine liposome injectable suspension (Depofoam bupivacaine) has been extensively studied in dogs as part of the development for human use [9, 10]. Bupivacaine liposome injectable suspension, known as AT-003[2] is currently being investigated for use in veterinary patients. In a preliminary laboratory study to assess the analgesic properties of AT-003 following tissue infiltration around the site of stifle arthrotomy in beagle dogs, a dose of 5.3 mg/kg was determined to provide adequate analgesia for at least 24 h post-surgery (unpublished data). The current report describes a pilot field study evaluating the post-operative analgesia provided by AT-003 at a dose of up to 5.3 mg/kg administered by tissue infiltration just prior to closure following cranial cruciate ligament (CCL) surgery in client-owned dogs, using subjective, in-clinic assessments of pain.

We hypothesized that 5.3 mg/kg of bupivacaine liposome injectable suspension would provide clinically effective analgesia, as measured using subjective clinical assessment, over a 72-h period following stifle surgery in dogs, when compared to a saline placebo.

Results

Three (3) investigative sites screened and enrolled cases. There were forty-nine (49) dogs screened and forty-six (46) dogs enrolled in the study over the period April 2014 to September 2014 and the study concluded when the target number of dogs was enrolled. All forty-six (46) dogs enrolled in the study were included in both the efficacy and safety evaluation (see flow diagram, Fig. 1). Twenty-four (24) dogs were treated with AT-003 and twenty-two (22) dogs with saline. The mean (range) age was 7.47 years (2.1–13.3) for the AT-003 group and 6.71 years (1.0–10.4) for the saline placebo group. Group characteristics are summarized in Table 1.

CMPS-SF scores

The mean total CMPS-SF scores (+/− SEM) at the baseline (pre-surgery) evaluation were 1.58 (0.22) and 1.18 (0.20) for AT-003 and saline placebo, respectively. Following surgery, total CMPS-SF scores (Table 2) were consistently lower at all post-operative time points (except for 72 h) for the AT-003 treated dogs compared to saline placebo treated dogs, with a significant overall treatment effect ($p = 0.0027$) in favor of AT-003. At 72 h, the scores were similar, but only two dogs remained in the saline placebo group (note: at 60 h data were missing from one placebo dog). There was no treatment by time effect ($p = 0.8041$), however there were only a small number of subjects remaining in the saline placebo group after 12 h. When site effect and treatment by site interaction were entered into the model, the overall treatment effect was again statistically significant ($p = 0.0036$), with lower CMPS-SF scores in the AT-003 group.

Surgical site manipulation scores

The mean Surgical Site Manipulation Scores (SSMS) (+/−SEM) at the baseline (pre-surgery) evaluation were 0.42 (0.1) and 0.68 (0.21) for AT-003 and saline placebo, respectively. Following treatment, the mean scores for AT-003 were less than those for placebo at each evaluation time point except at 12, 54, 60 and 72 h (Table 3), however, there were only two placebo dogs left in the study at 54 h. The overall treatment effect showed no statistically significant difference between treatment groups ($p = 0.0941$), however when site effect and treatment by site interaction were entered into the model, the overall treatment effect was statistically significant ($p = 0.0312$), with lower surgical site manipulation scores in the AT-003 group.

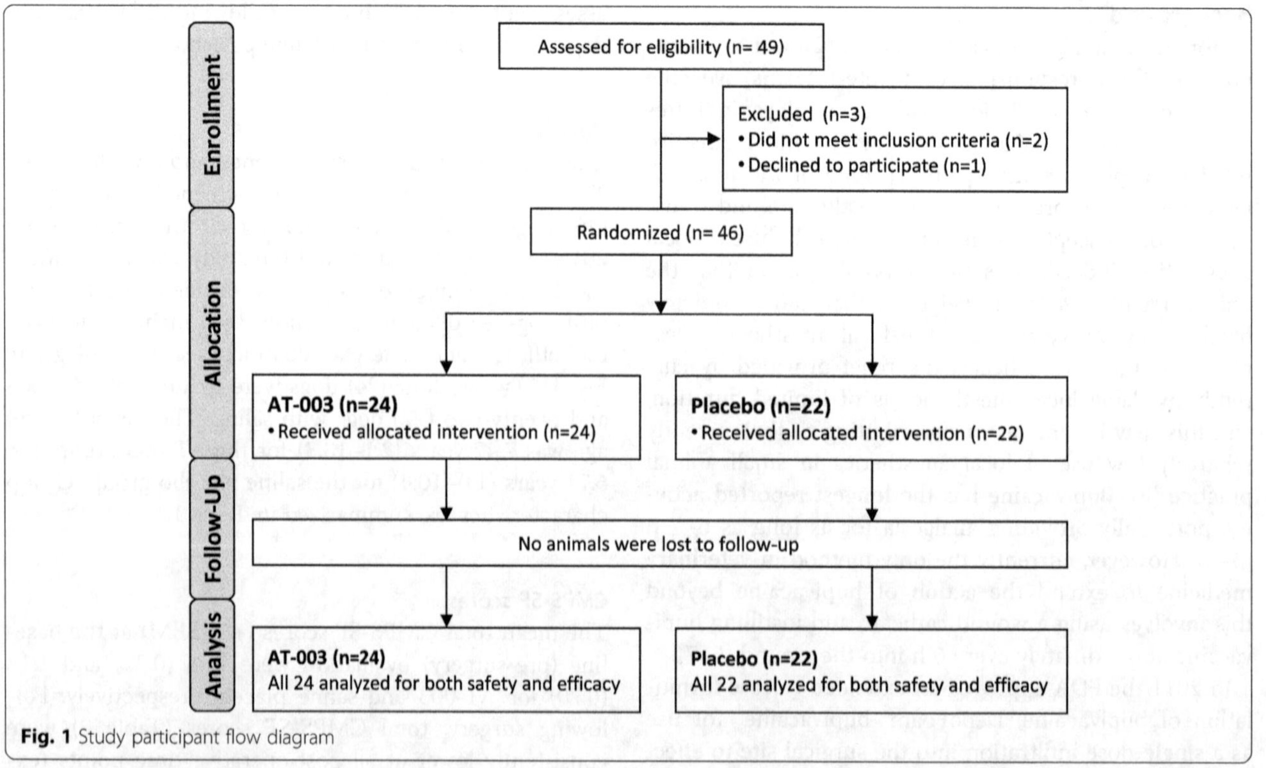

Fig. 1 Study participant flow diagram

Success/Failure analysis

Dogs receiving AT-003 were more likely to remain in the study (that is, not be rescued due to insufficient pain relief) following the surgical procedure than dogs receiving the saline placebo. At 72 h post-operatively, 9 of 24 AT-003 dogs and 2 of 22 placebo dogs remained in the study. Overall treatment success at each time period was statistically significantly different between the groups ($p = 0.0001$ for 0-24 h; $p = 0.0349$ for 0–48 h; and $p = 0.0240$ for 0–72 h) with more dogs being designated treatment successes in the AT-003 treatment group compared to the saline placebo group in each time period (Table 4). The odds of success were almost 13 times greater in the AT-003 group compared to the placebo group in the first 24 h; 4.5 times greater over the 0–48 h period, and 6 times greater over the 0–72 h period.

Table 1 Per protocol population demographics of enrolled dogs in the AT-003 and saline placebo groups

Characteristic		AT-003 ($n = 24$)	Saline placebo ($n = 22$)
Age (years)	Mean	7.47	6.71
	Min, Max	2.08, 13.33	1.00, 10.42
Weight (kg)	Mean	26.54	22.57
	Min, Max	3.2, 79.3	2.4, 44.8
Sex	Female	0	0
	Female spayed	13	11
	Male	1	0
	Male castrated	10	11

Adverse events

AT-003 appeared to be well tolerated. Adverse events were reported in 5 dogs during the study, three in the AT-003 group and two in the saline placebo group, all from a single site. All were classified with an "unlikely" or "unknown" relationship to study treatment. One dog in the AT-003 treatment group had mild bradycardia (heart rate was 56 beats per minute, as compared to 96 beats per minute at the pre-enrollment physical examination) detected 4 hours after surgery (at time of rescue). Another dog in the AT-003 treatment group vomited on a single occasion, and this resolved with no treatment. A third dog in the AT-003 group was found to have a small excoriated patch on its nose, considered unlikely to be treatment related, and rather resulting from trying to exit the cage. In the saline placebo group, a flea was found on one dog, and another had an episode of diarrhea with fresh blood, which resolved without treatment.

Discussion

The study hypothesis was supported, with the results indicating measurable analgesic effects of AT-003 (bupivacaine liposome injectable suspension) compared to placebo, over a 72-h period following surgical site tissue infiltration in 46 dogs undergoing cranial cruciate ligament (CCL) surgery. The odds of success (in terms

Table 2 Total mean (SEM) CMPS-SF scores by treatment group and time point

Time point (hours)	AT-003		Saline placebo	
	Number of dogs evaluated	Mean (+/SEM) CMPS-SF	Number of dogs evaluated	Mean (+/−SEM) CMPS-SF
0	24	1.58 (0.22)	22	1.18 (0.20)
2	24	4.38 (0.47)	22	6.82 (0.72)
4	22	3.36 (0.35)	16	6.56 (0.82)
8	21	4.24 (0.43)	9	7.00 (1.11)
12	19	4.21 (0.66)	5	6.20 (1.93)
24	14	3.50 (0.69)	4	4.50 (1.32)
30	11	2.64 (0.43)	3	5.67 (1.20)
36	10	2.20 (0.29)	3	3.33 (1.20)
48	10	2.30 (0.68)	3	4.67 (2.19)
54	9	2.44 (0.53)	2	3.00 (2.00)
60	9	2.00 (0.53)	1	5.00 (NA)
72	9	2.11 (0.48)	2	2.00 (0.00)

NA Not Applicable

of not needing rescue) were dramatically greater in the AT-003 group than the placebo group. It is possible that some dogs may have been inappropriately designated as comfortable when in fact pain was present, potentially due to the carry-over effects of the acepromazine sedation in the early postoperative period, or due to a lack of sensitivity of the pain assessment tool. However, in these respects, both groups should have been equally affected, making the comparison valid.

Pain is difficult to measure, and although the assessment tool used in the present study has been widely used, it has never undergone criterion validation. However, one measure of the success in measuring pain in placebo-controlled studies is the rescue rate in the placebo group. In the current study, it was 77 % within 24 h, and 91 % over the 72 h of the study, suggesting inadequate pain relief was being detected, and giving one further confidence that AT-003 provided clinically measurable pain relief. If one assumes surgery is associated with pain, then the lack of rescue of 2/22 dogs in the placebo group would be considered a failure of the assessment system. However, the approach to assessment and rescue in our study appears to have been comparatively successful when looked at other published studies. In a study of dogs undergoing cruciate surgery [11], only 11 % (1 of 9 dogs) was rescued in the 24 h following surgery. In a study of dogs undergoing soft tissue surgery [12], only 9 of 16 dogs were rescued over a 72-h period

Table 3 Total Mean (SEM) Surgical Site Manipulation Scores by Treatment Group & Time Point

Time point (hours)	AT-003		Saline Placebo	
	Number of dogs evaluated	Mean surgical site manipulation (SEM)	Number of dogs evaluated	Mean surgical site manipulation (SEM)
0	24	0.42 (0.10)	22	0.68 (0.21)
2	24	1.13 (0.31)	22	2.32 (0.30)
4	22	0.95 (0.27)	16	2.56 (0.32)
8	21	1.33 (0.30)	9	2.11 (0.45)
12	19	1.47 (0.30)	5	1.40 (0.51)
24	14	1.43 (0.39)	4	1.50 (0.50)
30	11	0.82 (0.33)	3	1.67 (0.67)
36	10	0.70 (0.30)	3	1.00 (1.00)
48	10	0.90 (0.35)	3	1.00 (1.00)
54	9	0.67 (0.37)	2	0.00 (0.00)
60	9	0.33 (0.24)	1	0.00 (NA)
72	9	0.67 (0.29)	2	0.00 (0.00)

SEM standard error of the mean, *NA* not applicable

Table 4 Summary results of the success/failure analysis. Dogs deemed failures in one time period were carried forward into the next time period, where they were also categorized as failures. The Odds of success (and 95 % Confidence Interval, CI) are tabulated

Time interval	AT-003		Saline placebo	Chi-square *p*-value	Odds ratio
0–24 h	Success	19 (79.2 %)	5 (22.7 %)	0.0001	12.92 (3.18, 52.48)
	Failure	5 (20.8 %)	17 (77.3 %)		
0–48 h	Success	10 (41.7 %)	3 (13.6 %)	0.0349	4.52 (1.05, 19.54)
	Failure	14 (58.3 %)	19 (86.4 %)		
0–72 h	Success	9 (37.5 %)	2 (9.1 %)	0.0240	6.0 (1.13, 31.94)
	Failure	15 (62.5 %)	20 (90.9 %)		

postoperatively. The lack of intra-operative analgesia provision (beyond preoperative hydromorphone, which all dogs received) was very deliberate due to how difficult pain is to measure. Given how insensitive our current assessment tools are, the more background treatments that are administered, the more difficult it becomes to assess whether a novel analgesic provides any benefit. Future work, hopefully with more sensitive, and ideally objective, outcome assessments, could evaluate the effect size of this product versus other treatments.

There are few data as to how long post-surgical pain persists in animals, and this time period will vary with the type of surgical procedure performed. The recommended time period for administration of analgesics post-operatively varies from days to weeks, depending on the surgery performed, but expert opinion emphasizes the first 72 h following surgery as a critical time period when analgesics should be administered [13]. Post-surgical pain can generally be well controlled while an animal is hospitalized using injectable opioids, ketamine, cyclooxygenase inhibiting NSAIDs and local anesthetics. However, with most veterinary patients being discharged from the veterinary hospital the same day, or within 24 h following surgery, there is a need to bridge between analgesics provided in the hospital and effective pain relief in the home environment. Currently in the United States, only oral cyclooxygenase inhibiting NSAIDs and transdermal fentanyl liquid[3] have been approved for post-surgical analgesia in dogs. Beyond these options, there are unapproved fentanyl patches manufactured for human use, which have been suggested to be efficacious [14] and tramadol is widely used, despite little evidence of efficacy [15–18].

Overall, there is a clear unmet need for effective analgesic products that can be administered in the clinic, and provide pain relief for the crucial first few days following surgery in the home environment. This pilot study suggests that bupivacaine liposome injectable suspension may directly address this unmet need, providing up to 72 h of analgesia. Though statistically greater than placebo, not all of the AT-003 dogs were successes out to 72 h. In this study, surgeons were not instructed to infiltrate around the anchor points of the suture material. In future studies, infiltration into all the tissue layers as well as around the anchor points for suture or around implants will be performed. Bupivacaine liposome injectable suspension will need to be administered as part of a multimodal approach as the anesthetic wears off, and indeed, this is consistent with the current recommendations for the treatment of postoperative pain [19, 20]. The prolonged duration of continuous action may also prevent episodes of breakthrough pain.

The current study was a pilot study, performed in dogs undergoing a single type of surgery, lateral retinacular suture placement for cruciate insufficiency. As such, the generalizability of these results to the larger population of dogs undergoing a variety of orthopedic surgeries and other surgical procedures is unknown. However, given the demonstrated efficacy in human clinical studies in both orthopedic [21] and soft tissue [22] surgery, it is highly likely that AT-003 will prove efficacious in dogs undergoing a wide variety of surgical procedures.

The current study employed direct injection of bupivacaine liposome injectable suspension into the surgical wound, and this may raise concerns about wound healing and wound infection. While there is some evidence that local anesthetics alter the cellular events of early tissue healing, there does not appear to be a clinically significant impact on wound healing or mechanical wound strength in preclinical animal studies [23] or humans. Infection rates following continuous local anesthetic installation into wounds found that reported wound infection rates were similar between active (0.7 %) and control groups (1.2 %) in humans undergoing surgery [24]. In the present study, no wound related adverse effects were seen, which mirrors the extensive pre-clinical work in dogs that has been performed with this product. In a dog model of inguinal hernia repair, bupivacaine liposome injectable suspension was infiltrated into the surgical site at doses ranging from 9 to 25 mg/kg and a mild granulomatous inflammatory response was seen histologically, that had not resolved by 2 weeks following infiltration, but was not considered indicative of any adverse effect on wound healing and the wound healing findings were similar to control (saline or bupivacaine HCL) treated animals [9]. In the present study, one dog was found to have bradycardia 4 h following administration of AT-003. In previous work, repeated doses of bupivacaine liposome injectable suspension were administered to dogs and the dogs evaluated for cardiotoxicity [25]. Doses of 9, 18 and 30 mg/kg bupivacaine liposome injectable suspension, 9 mg/kg bupivacaine HCl, or a volume-equivalent dose of saline, were administered into the subcutaneous tissue over the scapulae twice weekly for 4 weeks. No clinical signs consistent with central nervous system toxicity were seen and no electrocardiogram abnormalities were detected [25].

Dilution in this study was allowed based on the human experience and volumes used in previous canine knee surgery studies. Dilution does not impact efficacy in humans [26], and that appeared to be the case in this study as well. Most surgeons administered the drug in the undiluted state. The one surgeon who did dilute did so such that the total volume was divisible by four, facilitating a 25, 50 and 25 % tissue infiltration distribution.

Conclusions

Further work is indicated to develop this product for clinical use. This product has significant potential to address an important clinical need - the provision of extended duration local wound analgesia.

Methods

Design

The study was a masked, randomized, placebo-controlled, multi-center pilot field study, conducted under Good Clinical Practice Guidelines. The study was performed as part of the development program of AT-003 for FDA approval in dogs. The study was conducted according to the protocol and in compliance with Good Clinical Practice (VICH) Guideline GL9, International Cooperation on Harmonization of Technical Requirements for Registration of Veterinary Medicinal Products (VICH), June 2000, and the FDA Center for Veterinary Medicine (CVM) Guidance for Industry #85, May 2001. The study protocol was approved by Aratana's internal review board. Each owner gave written informed consent prior to dogs being enrolled into the study, and best practices for veterinary care and patient management were followed throughout the study.

Study population

Owned pet dogs of any breed or gender, greater than 5 months of age, deemed to require surgery for cruciate ligament insufficiency, were recruited to the study.

Inclusion criteria

Dogs were required to have been diagnosed with cranial cruciate ligament insufficiency within the previous 4 months, and not to have received systemic anti-inflammatories within 7 days of the surgical procedure. Dogs of a fractious demeanor, or who had an uncontrolled endocrine or systemic disorder, or who had had surgery within the previous 14 days were not eligible.

Study protocol overview

The study evaluated the post-operative analgesia provided by AT-003 at a dose of 5.3 mg/kg administered by tissue infiltration just prior to closure following unilateral cranial cruciate ligament (CCL) surgery in dogs. The study protocol is outlined in Fig. 2. Dogs were randomly assigned to one of the two treatment groups and AT-003 (5.3 mg/kg) or saline placebo (1.0 mL/kg) was administered into the wound bed at the end of surgery, prior to and during closure of the wound. Both AT-003 and saline were injected directly into tissues, using a moving needle technique.

All dogs underwent the lateral retinacular suture procedure, including stifle arthrotomy. The primary outcome measure was the Glasgow Composite Measure Pain Scale (CMPS-SF). Assessments were performed prior to premedication/surgery following a 2-h acclimation period, and at 2, 4, 8, 12, 24, 30, 36, 48, 54, 60 and 72 h following surgery by veterinarians and veterinary technicians trained on the use of the CMPS-SF. After the CMPS-SF assessment was completed, a Surgical Site Manipulation Score (secondary outcome measure) was assessed by standardized manipulation of the stifle joint that had undergone surgery (Table 5). Dogs were administered rescue analgesia (choice of rescue was at the discretion of the veterinarian) if the CMPS-SF score was greater than 8 or if the assessors felt additional analgesia was needed. Following either of these, dogs were removed from the study. Everyone involved in the assessments was trained in the use of the assessment tools through explanation and discussion of the tools during a single 'classroom' style training session run by the Contract Research Organization, and the document describing the definitions of expressions used in the CMPS-SF. All assessors had prior experience of using the CMPS-SF in clinical studies. No more than 3 assessors were permitted to do the assessments on any one dog. Different sites were not calibrated on the use of the CMPS-SF, and nor were any measures put in place to confirm consistency of scoring.

Safety assessments (secondary outcome measures) were made using clinical observations and behavioral observations at all assessment time points, and physical examination findings at 72 h or following rescue. No specific guidance on what to look for in the clinical observations was given; the physical examination was a standard physical examination covering evaluation of all body systems. Owners were also called within 4–7 days

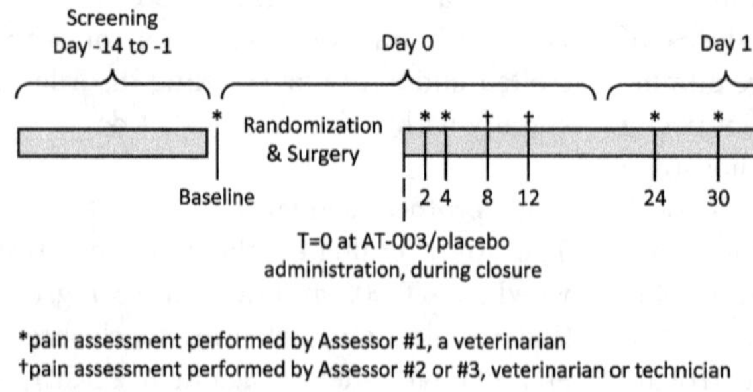

Fig. 2 Study Protocol Outline

following surgery to capture any adverse events that occurred following discharge.

Anesthetic protocol

Acepromazine (0.05 mg/kg) was administered intravenously (IV) or intramuscularly (IM) with a maximum total dose of 3.0 mg regardless of body weight. The doses of acepromazine used in the study were based on our experience with the drug. At least 15 min after acepromazine administration, hydromorphone (0.1 mg/kg) was administered IV. Anesthesia was induced with propofol, and maintained on isoflurane carried in oxygen, delivered via an endotracheal tube and a rebreathing circuit. Additional local/regional anesthesia (epidural, nerve block, intra-articular etc.) was not permitted, nor were any other analgesics. Fluids were administered intravenously during anesthesia.

Randomization to treatment groups

Dogs were randomly assigned to one of the two treatment groups and treated post-CCL surgery with AT-003 (5.3 mg/kg, equivalent to 0.4 mL/kg) or saline (1.0 mL/kg). Surgeons were allowed to dilute AT-003 up to 15 times, if needed, in order to cover the surgical area, with a recommended volume of 0.4–1.0 mL/kg based on previous studies. Randomization was performed using the Prelude Dynamics VISION™ electronic data capture (EDC) system. The VISION randomization framework generated each random treatment from a pre-computed table of treatments for each site. The randomization calculation maintained equal size groups per site and was calculated based on the current patient population. Subjects were randomized in blocks of two, stratified by site.

Table 5 Surgical Site Manipulation scoring system. At each relevant assessment time point, the joint was gently palpated around the surgical incision, and then the joint was put through a passive range of motion, flexing and extending the joint

Manipulate the joint through a normal range of motion, and score the patient as per below:

Score	Response
0	Does not notice manipulation.
1	Orients to site on manipulation, does not resist.
2	Orients to site, may lick, slight objection to manipulation
3	Withdraws from manipulation, may vocalize, excessive licking
4	Tries to escape from manipulation, or prevent manipulation, may bite or show aggression.

Masking procedures

One individual at each site was designated the Dispenser, and they documented the assignment of dogs to treatment group and kept the related documentation in a secure site, away from all other personnel. The Dispenser and the veterinarian performing the surgery had knowledge of which treatment group each dog was assigned. Blinded personnel were not given access to the treatment or randomization forms. The veterinarian or trained technician performing the assessments, sponsor, statistician and any other personnel involved in clinical evaluations and observations remained blinded to treatment during the study and until data base lock. The Owners were also blinded to treatment.

Tissue infiltration procedure

AT-003 or saline was injected slowly into the tissues using a 1–1.5 in. long needle, using a 'moving needle technique', in which the needle is inserted to near the hub and the material is injected as the needle is pulled out. The needle is inserted at varying angles depending on how the tissue is best approached in order to deposit the injectate within the tissues. In general, this means inserting the needle approximately parallel to the surface of the skin. The injections are repeated to create an area of infiltrated tissue around the whole wound, and at all levels of the wound. Approximately 25, 50 and 25 % of the AT-003 or saline was injected into the tissues around the joint capsule, the fascial tissue, and the sub-cuticular tissue, respectfully. The injections were performed such that the whole wound, at all levels, was infiltrated with AT-003 or saline. Dilution of AT-003 with normal saline was permitted and was utilized for 12 of the AT-003 treated dogs, all at one site, with a maximal dilution of 1:1 AT-003 to saline.

Outcome measures

The primary outcome measure was the Glasgow Composite Measure Pain Scale (Short Form) (CMPS-SF), and secondary outcome measures were a Surgical Site Manipulation Score and an evaluation of adverse events.

CMPS-SF

The Glasgow Composite Measure Pain Scale-Short Form (CMPS-SF), (http://www.newmetrica.com/acute-pain-measurement/download-short-form-painquestionnaire-for-dogs/) is a subjective clinical metrology instrument used by animal caretakers to evaluate perioperative pain in a practice setting that was developed at the University of Glasgow, UK [27, 28]. The expressions used in the CMPS-SF were defined in order to assist in training of sites, and are detailed in Additional file 1. Data were captured electronically, and thus the electronic version of the CMPS-SF differed from the published paper version. The layout of the electronic version is illustrated in Additional file 2: Figure S1.

Surgical site manipulation score (SSMS)

A simple descriptive scale, scored on a 0–4 scale (Table 5) was used for the assessment of surgical site pain associated with cruciate surgery. The scale was constructed by one of the authors, and is similar to wound palpation scoring systems used previously [7].

Adverse events

An adverse event was defined as any observation, undesirable experience, reaction or side effect in animals that was unfavorable and unintended and occurred after the use of AT-003 or placebo, whether or not considered to be treatment related. A serious adverse event was defined as any adverse event that resulted in death, was life-threatening, or resulted in persistent or significant disability/incapacity, although no serious adverse event occurred during this study.

Rescue analgesia

Dogs were removed from the study and administered rescue analgesia if the CMPS-SF score at a designated assessment time point was greater than 8 or at any time (assessment time point or at any time in between) if the assessing veterinarian felt additional analgesia was needed. The intervention score of 8 was based on one investigator's (BDXL) experience with the CMPS-SF, and a lack of data to substantiate the suggestion of an intervention score of 6 (http://www.newmetrica.com/acute-pain-measurement/download-short-form-painquestionnaire-for-dogs/). No dog in the study was removed for a reason other than rescue analgesia.

Data capture

Most data were captured electronically using an electronic data capture (EDC) system VISION developed and supported by Prelude Dynamics, LLC.

Power analysis and statistical analysis

The enrollment target was at least 40 evaluable cases (20 AT-003 and 20 placebo) per the study randomization schedule across all sites. An evaluable sample size of 20 AT-003 and 20 placebo cases was determined to be able to provide more than 90 % power (alpha = 0.05, 2-sided) to detect a difference between treatment groups of 0.37 (pooled standard deviation = 0.30) in the CMPS-SF assessment at 24 h post-administration. These calculations were based on results from a preliminary laboratory study to assess the analgesic properties of AT-003 following tissue infiltration around the site of stifle arthrotomy in beagle dogs.

To be eligible for the statistical analysis, each site must have enrolled and completed a minimum of 2 evaluable cases (at least 1 of each treatment). For total CMPS-SF and Surgical site manipulation scores, repeated measures analysis of variance were utilized to test for possible differences between treatment groups. SAS/STAT Proc MIXED were implemented with the model containing terms for treatment group, time point and the interaction of treatment by time point. The baseline value was included in the model as a covariate. If the treatment group by time point interaction was found to be statistically significant, then treatment effects were evaluated for each time point. The covariance structure that provided the smallest Akaike's Information Criterion value was used. Covariance structures that were tested include Compound Symmetry (CS), heterogeneous CS (CSH), first-order autoregressive [AR(1)] and heterogeneous autoregressive [ARH(1)]. Additionally, exploratory analysis used a repeated measures analysis of variance that included site effect and treatment by site interaction in the model.

A success/failure analysis was also employed, with success defined as no pain intervention over the intervals of 0–24 h, 0–48 h and 0–72 h. The number and percentage of dogs that were a success were presented for each time interval by treatment group. The chi-square test was utilized to test for possible differences between treatment groups, and odds ratios described.

Endnotes

[1]Exparel, Pacira Pharmaceuticals, Inc., Parsippany, NJ.
[2]Nocita, Aratana Therapeutics, Inc., Leawood, KS.
[3]Recuvyra™, Elanco.

Additional files

Additional file 1: Definitions of the expressions used in the CMPS-SF. In order to facilitate consistency in the way the CMPS-SF was used, the expressions used in the CMPS-SF were defined, and this file contains those definitions.

Additional file 2: Figure S1. Layout of the electronic version CMPS-SF. The electronic version CMPS-SF differed from the published paper version, and the layout of the electronic version is shown in this Additional file.

Acknowledgements
The authors wish to acknowledge AlcheraBio LLC, the Contract Research Organization that ran the study, and the individual site investigators: Dr. Sam Geller, Dr. Guy DeNardo, Dr. Matthew Barnhart, Dr. Shawn Kennedy, Dr. Roger Sifferman and Dr. Bert Shelley. Statistical analysis was performed by Margie Huebner, Biometrics, ClinData Services, Inc.

Funding
The study was funded by Aratana Therapeutics.

Authors' contributions
BDXL and LR-D designed the study; BDXL, LR-D and JAW drafted the manuscript. LR-D and JAW were responsible for overseeing the study. MH performed the statistical analysis. All authors reviewed and edited the manuscript. All authors read and approved the final manuscript.

Authors' information
The corresponding author (BDXL) is Professor of Surgery and Pain Management at North Carolina State University College of Veterinary Medicine, where he heads the Comparative Pain Research Laboratory, and is Associate Director of the Comparative Medicine Institute. He is actively involved in the Center for Pain Research and Innovation at the UNC Chapel Hill Medical School, and the Center for Translational Pain Medicine at Duke University Medical School.

Competing interests
Financial competing interests: The study was funded by Aratana Therapeutics, Inc., which own the rights to development of AT-003 for animals. BDXL is a paid consultant for Aratana; LR-D and JAW are both employees of Aratana. Non-financial competing interests: The authors declare that they have no other non-financial competing interests.

Consent for publication
Not applicable.

Ethics and consent to participate
The study was conducted according to the protocol and in compliance with Good Clinical Practice (VICH) Guideline GL9, International Cooperation on Harmonization of Technical Requirements for Registration of Veterinary Medicinal Products (VICH), June 2000, and the FDA Center for Veterinary Medicine (CVM) Guidance for Industry #85, May 2001. The study protocol was approved by Aratana's internal review board. Each owner gave written informed consent prior to dogs being enrolled into the study, and best practices for veterinary care and patient management were followed throughout the study.

Author details
[1]Department of Clinical Sciences, Comparative Pain Research Laboratory, College of Veterinary Medicine, North Carolina State University, Raleigh, NC, USA. [2]Department of Clinical Sciences, Comparative Medicine Institute, College of Veterinary Medicine, North Carolina State University, Raleigh, NC 27606, USA. [3]Center for Pain Research and Innovation, Dental School, UNC Chapel Hill, Chapel Hill, NC, USA. [4]Department of Anesthesiiology, Center for Translational Pain Medicine, Duke University, Durham, NC, USA. [5]Aratana Therapeutics, Inc., Leawood, KS 66211, USA. [6]ClinData Services, Inc., 6716 Holyoke Court, Fort Collins, CO 80525, USA.

References

1. Slingsby LS, Waterman-Pearson AE. Analgesic effects in dogs of carprofen and pethidine together compared with the effects of either drug alone. Vet Rec. 2001;148:441–4.
2. Hunt JR, Knowles TG, Lascelles BDX, Murrell JC. Prescription of perioperative analgesics by UK small animal veterinary surgeons in 2013. Vet Rec. 2015;176:493.
3. Sakonju I, Maeda K, Maekawa R, Maebashi R, Kakuta T, Takase K. Relative nerve blocking properties of bupivacaine and ropivacaine in dogs undergoing brachial plexus block using a nerve stimulator. J Vet Med Sci. 2009;71:1279–84.
4. Feldman HS, Arthur GR, Covino BG. Comparative systemic toxicity of convulsant and supraconvulsant doses of intravenous ropivacaine, bupivacaine, and lidocaine in the conscious dog. Anesth Analg. 1989;69:794–801.
5. Lemke KA, Dawson SD. Local and regional anesthesia. Vet Clin North Am Small Anim Pract. 2000;30:839–57.
6. Davis KM, Hardie EM, Lascelles BDX, Hansen B. Feline fibrosarcoma: perioperative management. Compend Contin Educ Vet. 2007;29:712–4. 716–20– 722–9 passim.
7. Hardie EM, Lascelles BDX, Meuten T, Davidson GS, Papich MG, Hansen BD. Evaluation of intermittent infusion of bupivacaine into surgical wounds of dogs postoperatively. Vet J. 2011;190:287–9.
8. Adams DH, Joyce G, Richardson VJ, Ryman BE, Wiśniewski HM. Liposome toxicity in the mouse central nervous system. J Neurol Sci. 1977;31:173–9.
9. Richard BM, Ott LR, Haan D, Brubaker AN, Cole PI, Nelson KG, Ross PE, Rebelatto MC, Newton PE. The safety and tolerability evaluation of DepoFoam bupivacaine (bupivacaine extended-release liposome injection) administered by incision wound infiltration in rabbits and dogs. Expert Opin Investig Drugs. 2011;20:1327–41.
10 Richard BM, Newton P, Ott LR, Haan D, Brubaker AN, Cole PI, Ross PE, Rebelatto MC, Nelson KG. The safety of EXPAREL ® (Bupivacaine Liposome Injectable Suspension) administered by peripheral nerve block in rabbits and dogs. J Drug Deliv. 2012;2012:962101–10.
11 Moak P, Hosgood G, Rowe E, Lemke KA. Evaluation of intra-articular and subcutaneous administration of meloxicam for postoperative analgesia following stifle surgery in dogs. Vet Comp Ortho Traumatol. 2011;24:32–8.
12 Bienhoff SE, Smith ES, Roycroft LM, Roberts ES. Efficacy and safety of deracoxib for control of postoperative pain and inflammation associated with soft tissue surgery in dogs. Vet Surg. 2012;41:336–44.
13 Mathews K, Kronen PW, Lascelles D, Nolan A, Robertson S, Steagall PV, Wright B, Yamashita K. Guidelines for Recognition, Assessment and Treatment of Pain. J Sm An Pract. 2014;55:E10–68.
14 Kyles AE, Hardie EM, Hansen BD, Papich MG. Comparison of transdermal fentanyl and intramuscular oxymorphone on post-operative behaviour after ovariohysterectomy in dogs. Res Vet Sci. 1998;65:245–51.
15 Rialland P, Authier S, Guillot M, del Castillo JRE, Veilleux-Lemieux D, Frank D, Gauvin D, Troncy E. Validation of orthopedic postoperative pain assessment methods for dogs: a prospective, blinded, randomized, placebo-controlled study. PLoS One. 2012;7:e49480.
16 Benitez ME, Roush JK, McMurphy R, KuKanich B, Legallet C. Clinical efficacy of hydrocodone-acetaminophen and tramadol for control of postoperative pain in dogs following tibial plateau leveling osteotomy. Am J Vet Res. 2015;76:755–62.
17 Davila D, Keeshen TP, Evans RB, Conzemius MG. Comparison of the analgesic efficacy of perioperative firocoxib and tramadol administration in dogs undergoing tibial plateau leveling osteotomy. J Am Vet Med Assoc. 2013;243:225–31.
18 Teixeira RC, Monteiro ER, Campagnol D, Coelho K, Bressan TF, Monteiro BS. Effects of tramadol alone, in combination with meloxicam or dipyrone, on postoperative pain and the analgesic requirement in dogs undergoing unilateral mastectomy with or without ovariohysterectomy. Vet Anaesth Analg. 2013;40:641–9.
19 Tomas A, Bledsoe D, Wall S, Davidson G, Lascelles BDX. Initial evaluation of a canine stifle arthrotomy post-operative pain model. The Vet J. 2015;204(3): 293–8.

20 Epstein ME, Rodanm I, Griffenhagen G, Kadrlik J, Petty MC, Robertson SA, Simpson W. AHAA, AAFP: 2015 AAHA/AAFP pain management guidelines for dogs and cats. J Fel Med Surg. 2015;2015:251–72.
21 Golf M, Daniels SE, Onel E. A phase 3, randomized, placebo-controlled trial of DepoFoam® bupivacaine (extended-release bupivacaine local analgesic) in bunionectomy. Adv Therapy. 2011. doi:10.1007/s12325-011-0052-y.
22 Gorfine SR, Onel E, Patou G, Krivokapic ZV. Bupivacaine extended-release liposome injection for prolonged postsurgical analgesia in patients undergoing hemorrhoidectomy: a multicenter, randomized, double-blind, placebo-controlled trial. Dis Colon Rectum. 2011;54:1552–9.
23 Abrão J, Fernandes CR, White PF, Shimano AC, Okubo R, Lima GB, Bachur JA, Garcia SB. Effect of local anaesthetic infiltration with bupivacaine and ropivacaine on wound healing: a placebo-controlled study. Int Wound J. 2014;11:379–85.
24 Liu SS, Richman JM, Thirlby RC, Wu CL. Efficacy of continuous wound catheters delivering local anesthetic for postoperative analgesia: a quantitative and qualitative systematic review of randomized controlled trials. J Am Coll Surg. 2006;203:914–32.
25 Richard BM, Rickert DE, Newton PE, Ott LR, Haan D, Brubaker AN, Cole PI, Ross PE, Rebelatto MC, Nelson KG. Safety evaluation of EXPAREL (DepoFoam Bupivacaine) administered by repeated subcutaneous injection in rabbits and dogs: species comparison. J Drug Deliv. 2011;2011:467429.
26 Hadzic A, Abikhaled JA, Harmon WJ. Impact of volume expansion on the efficacy and pharmacokinetics of liposome bupivacaine. Local Reg Anesth. 2015;8:105–11.
27 Reid J, Nolan AM, Hughes J, Lascelles D, Pawson P, Scott EM. Development of the short-form Glasgow Composite Measure Pain Scale (CMPS-SF) and derivation of an analgesic intervention score. Anim Welf. 2007;16(S):97–104.
28 Morton CM, Reid J, Scott EM, Holton LL, Nolan AM. Application of a scaling model to establish and validate an interval level pain scale for assessment of acute pain in dogs. Am J Vet Res. 2005;66:2154–66.

17

Femorotibial kinematics in dogs with cranial cruciate ligament insufficiency: a three-dimensional in-vivo fluoroscopic analysis during walking

Selena Tinga, Stanley E. Kim*, Scott A. Banks, Stephen C. Jones, Brian H. Park, Antonio Pozzi and Daniel D. Lewis

Abstract

Background: Cranial cruciate ligament (CrCL) insufficiency is a degenerative condition that is a common cause of pelvic limb lameness and osteoarthritis in dogs. Surgical therapies developed to treat dogs with naturally occurring CrCL insufficiency aim to address the resultant instability, but the in-vivo alterations in stifle kinematics associated with CrCL insufficiency have not been accurately defined. The objective of this study was to quantify the 3-dimensional femorotibial joint kinematics of dogs with naturally occurring cranial cruciate ligament (CrCL) insufficiency during ambulation. Eighteen client-owned dogs (20–40 kg) with natural unilateral complete CrCL rupture were included. Computed tomographic scans were used to create digital 3-dimensional models of the femur and tibia bilaterally for each dog. Lateral fluoroscopic images were obtained during treadmill walking and 3 complete gait cycles were analyzed. Stifle flexion/extension angle, craniocaudal translation, and internal/external rotation were calculated throughout the gait cycle using a previously described 3D-to-2D image registration process. Results were compared between the pre-operative CrCL-deficient and 6-month post-operative contralateral stifles (control).

Results: CrCL-deficient stifles were maintained in greater flexion throughout the gait cycle. Cranial tibial subluxation was evident in CrCL-deficient stifles at all time points throughout the gait cycle [9.7 mm at mid-stance ($P < 0.0001$); 2.1 mm at mid-swing ($P < 0.0017$)], and the magnitude of cranial tibial subluxation was greater at mid-stance phase than at mid-swing phase ($P < 0.0001$). Greater internal tibial rotation was present in CrCL-deficient stifles during stance phase ($P < 0.0022$) but no difference in axial rotation was evident during swing phase.

Conclusions: Naturally occurring CrCL rupture causes profound craniocaudal translational and axial rotational instability, which is most pronounced during the stance phase of gait. Surgical stabilization techniques should aim to resolve both craniocaudal subluxation and axial rotational instability.

Keywords: Femorotibial, Stifle, Kinematics, Cranial cruciate ligament

Background

Cranial cruciate ligament (CrCL) insufficiency is a degenerative condition [1, 2] that is a common cause of pelvic limb lameness [3] and osteoarthritis [4–8] in dogs. Pet owners were estimated to have spent over $1 billion treating dogs with CrCL insufficiency in 2003 [9]. Conservative medical management options are available and may result in improved function in some dogs, particularly dogs weighing less than 15 kg [10]. Surgical management, however, is typically recommended to address joint instability, mitigate the progression of osteoarthritis, and address concurrent meniscal pathology [10, 11].

Experimental transection of the CrCL invariably leads to stifle joint instability, [5, 12–14] and has been used to study the development of osteoarthritis [4–8]. The

* Correspondence: stankim@ufl.edu
Comparative Orthopaedics and Biomechanics Laboratory, College of Veterinary Medicine, and the Department of Mechanical & Aerospace Engineering, University of Florida, PO Box 100126, 2015 SW 16th Ave, Gainesville, FL 32610-0126, USA

presumed effects of CrCL insufficiency on joint motion during ambulation in-vivo are derived from 2 studies that were performed using invasive experimental techniques in normal dogs [5, 13]. Both studies measured joint kinematics before and after experimental unilateral CrCL transection by tracking metal implants (metal bone plates with removable spatial linkage [13] or implanted metal beads [5]) with biplanar radiophotogrammetry or fluoroscopy. However, acute experimental CrCL transection may not accurately replicate the pathology and biomechanics that are present in dogs with naturally occurring CrCL insufficiency. Additionally, there are logistical and ethical issues associated with the invasive nature of implanting metallic markers when studying the effects of CrCL insufficiency in client owned animals. A recent clinical study used lateral fluoroscopy to document stifle instability in a series of client owned dogs with natural CrCL insufficiency, but unfortunately the kinematic evaluation was limited to subjective qualitative assessments [15]. Recently, our group validated the use of single plane fluoroscopy (without the use of metal implants) for accurate quantification of bone motion in 3 dimensions [16] using methodology developed to study human knee kinematics [17–19]. While biplanar fluoroscopy is considered the most accurate modality for determining joint kinematics, this study demonstrated that the single plane modality was accurate to within 1.28 mm for translations and 1.58° for rotations [16].

Surgical therapies developed to treat dogs with naturally occurring CrCL insufficiency aim to address the resultant instability, [11] but the in-vivo alterations in stifle kinematics associated with CrCL insufficiency have not been accurately defined. Characterizing the kinematics of naturally diseased CrCL-deficient stifles would allow for more refined assessment of the efficacy of the currently advocated surgical stabilization techniques and guide the development of future treatment options. The objective of the current study was to quantify the 3-dimensional femorotibial joint kinematics of dogs with naturally occurring CrCL insufficiency during ambulation. We hypothesized that CrCL-deficient stifles would have increased femorotibial flexion, cranial tibial translation, and internal tibial rotation compared to each dog's unaffected contralateral stifle throughout the gait cycle.

Methods

Dogs presenting to the University of Florida Small Animal Hospital for CrCL insufficiency between July 2012 and March 2014 were evaluated for potential inclusion into the study. Adult non-chondrodystrophic dogs weighing between 20 to 40 kg with a history of unilateral lameness of less than 6-months duration were considered for enrollment. Inclusion was confirmed when (1) a unilateral complete CrCL rupture was diagnosed on orthopedic examination by a board certified surgeon based on cranial drawer and tibial compression tests (positive in the affected limb, negative in the contralateral limb), (2) stifle radiographs confirmed evidence of CrCL rupture in the affected stifle (stifle effusion ± osteoarthritis), and (3) complete CrCL rupture was confirmed at the time of surgery via arthroscopy or arthrotomy (surgeon preference). Dogs were excluded if concurrent clinical orthopedic disease was identified on physical examination, including palpable pain, effusion, or instability of the contralateral stifle. The study was approved by the University's Institutional Animal Care and Use Committee and owners signed informed consent at the time of enrollment.

Fluoroscopic image acquisition

Continuous lateral view fluoroscopic images centered on the stifle joints were acquired during treadmill walking using a ceiling-mounted fluoroscopic system with a flat panel detector.[1] Dogs were walked at a velocity of 2.0–2.5 mph (0.8–1.1 m/s), similar to previous studies [20]. The speed of the treadmill was set within this range at a speed that allowed a natural walking cadence. Images were acquired using a pulse rate of 30 frames/s, pulse width of 1 ms, and an image area of 410 × 300 mm, giving a 0.20 mm × 0.20 mm pixel resolution. The x-ray source was initially programmed to supply a 72 kV beam with a 50 mA beam current, with slight adjustments to parameters to optimize osseous definition for each subject. Fluoroscopic imaging was obtained for approximately 15 full gait cycles with the stifles centered in the field of view. Fluoroscopic sessions were also videotaped for later review to ensure a natural cadence was present and to aid in defining stance and swing phases of gait. Three representative gait cycles were chosen for processing. Radiation-associated risk was considered negligible.

3-dimensional model creation

Computed tomographic (CT) scans[2] were obtained extending from the hips through the tarsi. CT scans used a 512 × 512 image matrix, a 0.35 × 0.35 pixel dim, and 0.5 mm slice thickness with 0.3 mm overlap throughout the length of the femur and tibia. Radiation-associated risk was considered negligible. Bilateral femur/fabellae and tibia/fibula digital bone models were created using an open source 3D segmentation software program[3] followed by a reverse engineering program.[4] A 3-dimensional coordinate system based on anatomic landmarks was applied to each of the CT generated bone models similar to previous studies (Fig. 1) [16, 21–24]. Initially, femoral coordinates were applied such that the z-axis (mediolateral) passed through the center of the femoral condyles while remaining perpendicular to the

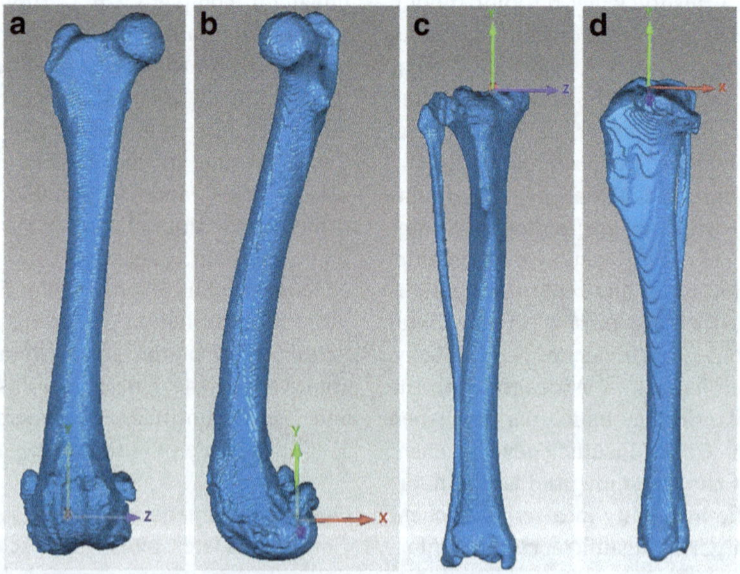

Fig. 1 Femoral and tibial coordinate systems. CT-generated 3-dimensional digital models of the femur (craniocaudal (1**a**) and lateral (1**b**) views) and tibia (craniocaudal (1**c**) and lateral (1**d**) views) with 3-dimensional coordinate system applied

longitudinal anatomic axis of the femur in the frontal plane. The y-axis (proximodistal) was perpendicular to the z-axis, along a plane that intersected the previously determined center of the femoral head and center of each medial and lateral femoral condyle, passing through the intercondylar notch in the frontal plane. Initially, tibial coordinates were applied such that the z-axis passed through the most prominent medial and lateral points of the tibial condyles, perpendicular to the longitudinal axis of the tibia in the frontal plane. The y-axis was perpendicular to the z-axis, along a plane that intersected the prominent medial and lateral points on the tibial condyles as well as a point mid-way between the medial and lateral malleoli. For both bones, the x-axes (craniocaudal) were determined by the right hand rule, which mandates that the 3rd axis be perpendicular to the first 2 axes. The origins of the femoral and tibial coordinate systems were then placed at the estimated center of the origin and insertion of the CrCL [21, 23].

3-dimensional to 2-dimensional image registration

A previously described [16–18, 23] 3D-to-2D image registration process was used to combine 3-dimensional bone model data with 2-dimensional fluoroscopic data to ascertain 3-dimensional kinematics of the femur and tibia throughout the gait cycle (Fig. 2). The digital femur and tibia models were projected onto each frame of the fluoroscopic gait cycle, and models were manually rotated and translated until the anatomic contours of the models precisely matched the underlying image.[5] The output of the software represents the individual model positions in space, and these results were converted to the relative positions of the bone models to each other using a custom computer program.[6]

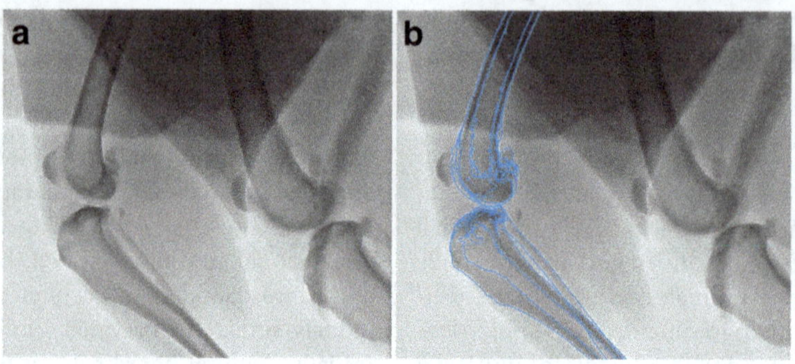

Fig. 2 Image registration process. Fluoroscopic image before (2**a**) and after (2**b**) 3-D to 2-D image registration process. In Fig. 2b, the bone models from Fig. 1 have been projected, edge-detected, and superimposed then precisely matched to the fluoroscopic image

Control kinematic data

Contralateral limb kinematics have been shown to be affected by the presence of lameness caused by CrCL insufficiency; [25] therefore, data for the contralateral limb was collected and evaluated 6-months following tibial plateau leveling osteotomy (TPLO) of the CrCL-deficient limb. A prior study has found no difference in force plate analysis between 6-month post-operative TPLO-treated naturally affected CrCL-deficient dogs and control dogs indicating that this time frame should allow return to soundness [26].

Kinematic data processing

The data were split into stance phase and swing phase and each phase was time normalized using a custom spline interpolation program[f] so that a data set of 101 data points was created (or 202 data points for the complete gait cycle). Every 10th data point was chosen for statistical comparison, so that in the final data set each stance cycle had 11 data points and each swing cycle had 11 data points. This allowed averaging within and between dogs, despite temporal differences. Kinematic data was compiled for flexion-extension angle, craniocaudal translation, and internal-external rotation for both the pre-operative CrCL-deficient and the 6-month post-operative contralateral stifle (internal control). Femorotibial kinematics after TPLO treatment will be reported in a separate study.

Statistical analysis

For each kinematic variable, 11 stance and 11 swing data points were averaged for 3 gait cycles for each dog and results were compared between affected and control stifles using a paired T-test followed by a Bonferroni correction with significance set at $P < 0.0025$. Repeated measures 2-way ANOVA was used to determine significance across the entire gait cycle for craniocaudal translation.

Results

Demographic information

Eighteen dogs were included in the study. Nine were mixed breed dogs, 5 were Labrador Retrievers, and the remaining dogs consisted of 1 Standard Poodle, 1 German Shepherd Dog, 1 English Springer Spaniel, and 1 Husky. Eleven dogs were spayed females and 7 were castrated males. Mean ± SD age was 6.7 ± 2.8 years. Mean ± SD body weight was 30.3 ± 5.8 kg with a median body condition score of 6/9 (range 4–8). The right stifle was affected in 10 dogs and the left in 8 dogs. Mean ± SD duration of lameness prior to presentation was 2.4 ± 2.3 months. Mean ± SD tibial plateau angle was 27.9 ± 3.0° for the CrCL-deficient stifle and 28.3 ± 2.9° for the contralateral control stifle ($P = 1$). On pre-operative radiographs, mild (9 dogs) to moderate (9 dogs) osteoarthritis of the affected stifle was noted. Ten dogs had no radiographic abnormalities noted in the contralateral stifle, while 8 dogs had mild osteoarthritis and effusion of the contralateral stifle detected on radiographs, despite the lack of abnormalities during clinical examination. At the time of surgery, median (range) Outerbridge scores [27] were 1 (0–3), 1 (0–2), 0.5 (0–3), and 1 (0–2) for the medial femoral condyle, medial tibial condyle, lateral femoral condyle, and lateral tibial condyle, respectively. Meniscal pathology was not identified in 8 dogs, while 10 dogs had injury to the caudal pole of the medial meniscus that required debridement. In addition to CrCL insufficiency, 5 dogs had unilateral mild to moderate osteoarthritis of the contralateral coxofemoral joint and 9 dogs had mild osteoarthritis detected in one or both tarsal joints; no pain or loss of range of motion of these joints was detected on clinical examination.

Flexion/extension angle (Fig. 3)

Over the 11 data points during stance phase, the control stifle had mean flexion/extension angles between 137 and 147° of extension, whereas the CrCL-deficient stifle

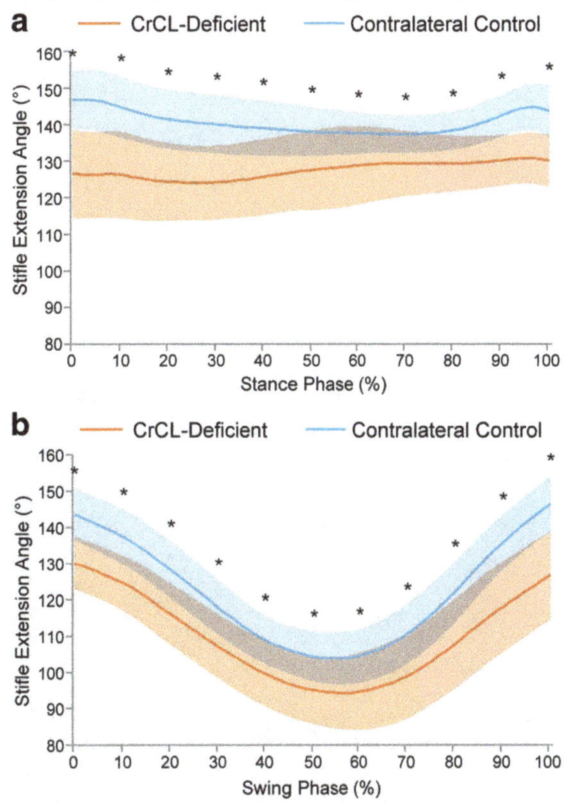

Fig. 3 Mean flexion/extension angle during **a**) stance and **b**) swing phase in CrCL-deficient and control stifles. Orange line = CrCL-deficient, Blue line = control. Error bars represent standard deviations and * represents a statistically significant difference (using paired T-test) at that time point. The CrCL-deficient stifle was more flexed throughout the gait cycle compared to the contralateral control stifle

was maintained in greater flexion ($P < 0.0007$) with means between 124 and 130° of extension. Over the 11 data points during swing phase, the control stifle had means between 104 and 146° of extension; the CrCL-deficient stifle was maintained in greater flexion ($P < 0.0001$), with a means between 95 and 130° of extension.

Craniocaudal translation (Fig. 4)

Craniocaudal translation was evaluated by measuring the distance between the femoral origin and tibial insertion of the CrCL along the craniocaudal axis at 10% increments throughout the phases of the gait cycle. *Range of craniocaudal motion,* defined as the maximum change in craniocaudal distance between the origin and insertion of the CrCL observed throughout the gait cycle, was a mean (±SD) of 1.6 ± 0.8 mm in the control stifle and 8.6 ± 2.9 mm CrCL-deficient stifle ($P < 0.0001$).

Cranial tibial subluxation was defined as a significant difference between the CrCL-deficient and control stifles, with respect to craniocaudal distance between the origin and insertion of the CrCL at an equivalent time point during the gait cycle. In CrCL-deficient stifles, there was significant cranial tibial subluxation at all time points throughout the gait cycle ($P < 0.0001$). At mid-stance, there was 9.7 ± 2.7 mm of cranial tibial subluxation ($P < 0.0001$) and at mid-swing there was 2.1 ± 1.7 mm of cranial tibial subluxation ($P < 0.0001$). The magnitude of cranial tibial subluxation was significantly greater at mid-stance phase than at mid-swing phase ($P < 0.0001$).

Internal/external rotation (Fig. 5)

Axial rotation was determined from the flexion-abduction-axial rotation ordered angle decomposition of the transformation matrix describing the tibial pose with respect to the femur [22]. This value can be thought of as the angular offset between the femoral and tibial x-axes. *Range of axial rotation* was defined as the difference between the maximum and minimum axial angular offsets throughout the gait cycle, within a joint. There was a mean (±SD) of 8.2 ± 4.4° of axial rotation range of motion in the control stifle and 8.0 ± 6.2° of axial

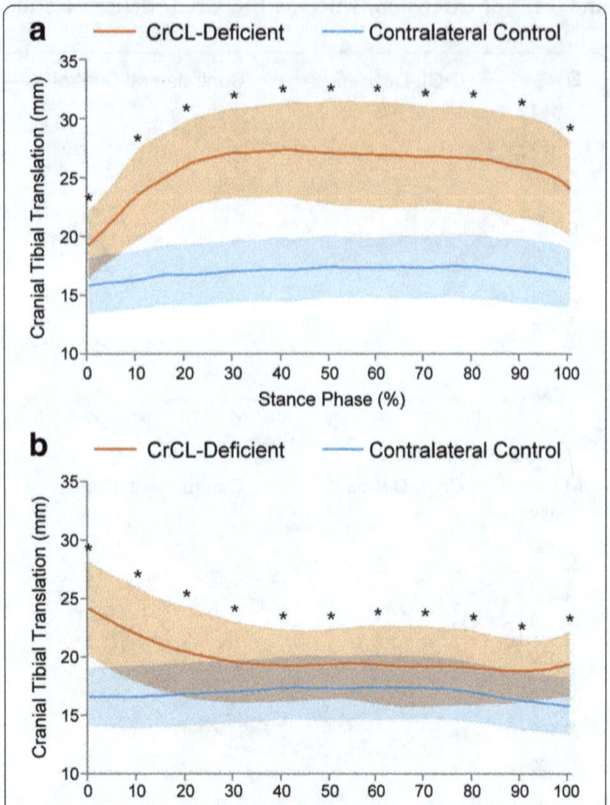

Fig. 4 Mean cranial tibial translation during **a**) stance and **b**) swing phase in CrCL-deficient and control stifles. Orange line = CrCL-deficient, Blue line = control. Error bars represent standard deviations and * represents a statistically significant difference (using paired T-test) at that time point. The CrCL-deficient stifle had more cranial tibial translation throughout the gait cycle compared to the contralateral control stifle

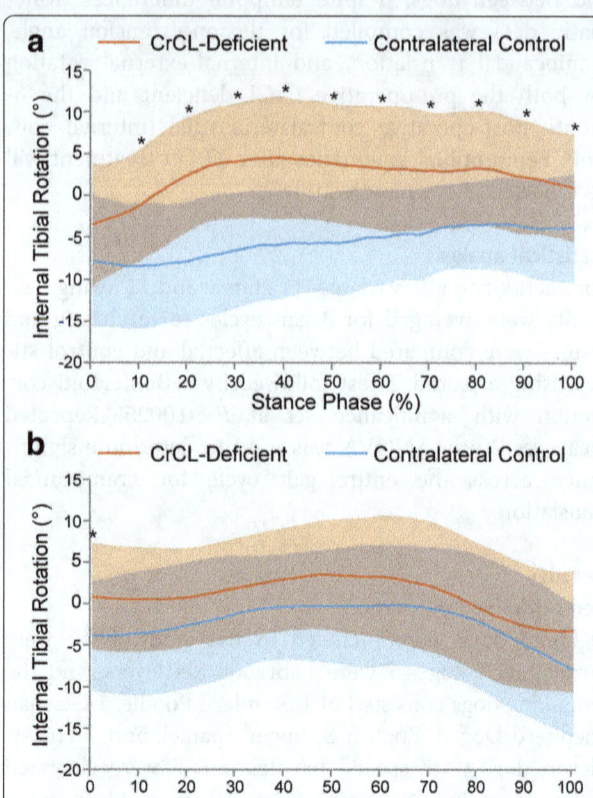

Fig. 5 Mean internal/external rotation during **a**) stance and **b**) swing phase in CrCL-deficient and control stifles. Orange line = CrCL-deficient, Blue line = control. Error bars represent standard deviations and * represents a statistically significant difference (using paired t-test) at that time point. The CrCL-deficient stifle had more internal tibial rotation throughout stance phase compared to the contralateral control stifle and there was no difference during swing phase

rotation range of motion in the CrCL-deficient stifle throughout the gait cycle ($P = 0.1085$). While the range of axial rotation was similar between control and CrCL-deficient stifles, the timing of rotation differed between limbs. Both the control and CrCL-deficient stifles were maximally externally rotated in early stance phase; however, the control stifles reached maximal internal rotation at mid-swing phase and the CrCL-deficient stifles reached maximal internal rotation at mid-stance phase.

Abnormal axial rotation was defined as a significant difference between the CrCL-deficient and control stifles, with respect to degree of axial rotation at a given equivalent time point during the gait cycle. In the CrCL-deficient stifles, the tibia was abnormally internally rotated for the majority of stance phase ($P < 0.0022$ between 10 and 100% stance phase). During the swing phase, there was no significant difference in axial rotational position between limbs.

Discussion

The objective of this study was to quantitatively define the 3-dimensional stifle motion in dogs with naturally occurring CrCL insufficiency. We found that flexion-extension angle and craniocaudal translation were abnormal throughout the walking gait cycle, and internal-external rotation was abnormal during the stance phase. We confirmed that naturally occurring CrCL insufficiency results in profound disturbance of stifle kinematics in dogs.

CrCL-deficient stifles were maintained in 8–20° greater flexion throughout the gait cycle when compared to control stifles. Prior in-vivo studies using optical motion capture [25, 28] and biplanar fluoroscopic 3D-2D image registration [5, 13] techniques have reported a similar magnitude of increased flexion in CrCL-deficient joints, ranging from 5 to 15° [5, 13, 25, 28]. Increased stifle flexion has been ascribed to joint effusion and pain, [29, 30] both of which are present in naturally occurring and experimentally induced disease states. Increased stifle flexion may also mitigate the magnitude of cranial tibial subluxation, as the angle formed between the patellar tendon and the femorotibial joint line decreases [31, 32]. Higher stifle flexion may be the result of a change in activity of the quadriceps, gastrocnemius, or hamstrings, or a combination of changes in activity of all 3 muscles. In humans with anterior cruciate ligament insufficiency, a proportion of the population ("copers") is able to stabilize the knee by altered muscular forces across the joint [33]. However, in contrast to human copers, dogs in our study were not able to completely overcome the cranial tibial subluxation despite increased stifle flexion.

The maximal magnitude of cranial tibial subluxation observed in our study was 9.7 mm, which occurred during the mid-stance phase. The mid-stance phase timing of maximal cranial tibial subluxation may be due to quadriceps and gastrocnemius muscle activity, which are required to support weight bearing during the stance phase [34, 35] in addition to maintaining joint extension, these muscles also exert a cranial force on the tibia (quadriceps) and caudal force on the femur (gastrocnemius), which may promote cranial tibial thrust [36]. Tashman, et al. reported a similar magnitude of subluxation (10 mm) in the in-vivo study of experimental CrCL transection, but Korvick, et al. reported a larger magnitude of subluxation (17 mm) in an earlier in-vivo study of experimental CrCL transection [5, 13]. We suspect that numerous factors could influence the maximal magnitude of cranial tibial subluxation, such as the degree of periarticular fibrosis, differences in study methodology (such as landmark identification), and dog size, breed, and activity level (e.g. type and speed of gait). Nevertheless, our results suggest that stifles with naturally occurring complete CrCL rupture have a comparable degree of cranial tibial subluxation to normal stifles subjected to experimental CrCL transection.

Despite the previous thought that the stability of the dog stifle is independent of the CrCL during stifle flexion, [12, 13, 31] mild cranial tibial subluxation was still present in CrCL-deficient stifles during the swing phase (when the stifle is in greater flexion). A similar phenomenon was found in the study by Tashman, et al., in which persistent cranial tibial subluxation was shown to develop over the 2 years following experimental CrCL transection [5]. The presence of persistent cranial tibial subluxation may be a reflection of a chronically thickened stifle that is unable to return to a completely reduced position. Furthermore, maximal hock flexion has been shown to occur during mid-swing phase, which may promote cranial tibial subluxation through increased tension on the gastrocnemius muscle [28]. Chronic CrCL insufficiency may also be associated with disruption of the balance of muscular forces (particularly quadriceps, hamstring, and gastrocnemius muscles), [37] meniscal degeneration, [38] and changes to the osseous anatomy of the joint [4, 13]. We suspect that some or all of these changes contribute to persistent cranial tibial subluxation during the swing phase, despite this being a "CrCL-independent phase" [12, 13, 31].

Stifles with CrCL insufficiency had significantly greater internal tibial rotation when compared to control stifles, occurring maximally at the mid-stance phase and therefore coinciding with maximal cranial tibial subluxation, consistent with both in-vivo [13] and ex-vivo [14, 39] studies. After CrCL loss, the collateral ligaments become the primary restraint against cranial tibial subluxation and because the lateral collateral ligament is not as taut as the medial collateral ligament in extension, [40] the lateral aspect of the tibial plateau has more latitude to translate cranially than the medial aspect of the plateau. The medial meniscus has been demonstrated to aid in resisting cranial tibial subluxation in CrCL-deficient stifles in canine cadavers, which could provide more craniocaudal stability to the medial compartment compared to the lateral compartment [41]. The differences in function between medial and lateral collateral ligaments and medial and lateral menisci likely contribute to the internal tibial rotation that occurs as the tibia translates cranially during stance phase in the absence of the CrCL [39, 40]. Surprisingly, the in-vivo study by Tashman, et al. did not report a difference in rotational alignment after CrCL transection [5]. The authors of this study postulated that bony geometry, muscular forces, or other soft tissue constraints were able to overcome the expected rotational laxity [5]. The cause of discrepant findings for axial rotational motion across in-vivo studies is unknown, but may be related to breed and conformational differences between study populations. Nevertheless, the prominence of rotational instability in dogs with CrCL insufficiency found in the current study supports clinical concerns that rotational instability may also need to be addressed during surgical treatment of CrCL insufficiency [42, 43].

There are several limitations associated with this investigation. We had narrow selection criteria based on body weight and obvious palpable stifle laxity; therefore, our results cannot be extrapolated to other populations such as small or giant breed dogs, chondrodystrophic dogs, dogs with excessive tibial plateau angles, dogs with partial CrCL tears, dogs with severe osteoarthritis, or dogs with purely traumatic CrCL ruptures. Additionally, data were collected at a single and likely variable time point from the onset of disease and thus we are unable to provide a definitive understanding of the temporal changes associated with the course of CrCL degeneration. Fluoroscopic imaging was obtained while dogs walked on a treadmill, which has been shown to result in slight variations in joint kinematics in dogs when compared to over-ground walking [44]. We did not assess activities other than walking, such as trotting or stair climbing, [23] which may have shown different results. We utilized a single-plane fluoroscopic technique, which is less precise than biplanar techniques and precludes the ability to accurately quantify translation in the mediolateral plane [17]. During modeling, there is subjectivity in coordinate assignation as well as determination of the stance and swing phases of the gait cycle; a single researcher (ST) performed these tasks to limit variability. We also recognize that stifle motion is a complex action and stifle stability is not controlled solely by the CrCL; additionally, in the face of CrCL deficiency there are likely multiple concurrent (primary or secondary) neuromuscular changes that could also affect our measured kinematic results.

Limitations also include the fact that our control data was collected from the contralateral limb 6-months following surgical treatment for CrCL insufficiency of the affected limb. The 6-month time point was chosen to mitigate the effects of lameness on contralateral limb kinematics; [26] however, the contralateral stifles may not have been normal themselves. The development of CrCL insufficiency is multifactorial [45] with one primary contributing factor being abnormal mechanical stresses secondary to variations from normal anatomy [46] and CrCL insufficiency is a bilateral disease in approximately 50% of dogs affected [47–51]. Despite some dogs having early (stable) contralateral CrCL disease, we considered the contralateral stifle to be a superior kinematic control than the alternative of using a separate population of dogs with normal stifles. Given that there was no lameness, pain, loss of range of motion, or instability associated with any joint other than the studied CrCL-deficient stifle at the time of initial and follow-up orthopedic examinations, we considered the influence of very early contralateral CrCL disease or concurrent hip or hock osteoarthritis would likely be minimal.

Conclusions

The femorotibial kinematic changes observed in dogs with naturally occurring CrCL insufficiency were largely consistent with previous experimental studies: we observed profound craniocaudal translational and axial rotational instability that was most pronounced during the stance phase of gait. Our investigation has provided an accurate, quantitative characterization of the instability that occurs with CrCL insufficiency. Based on our results, current surgical stabilization techniques should aim to address both craniocaudal translational and axial rotational instability with hopes to slow the progression of osteoarthritis and mitigate the likelihood of postoperative meniscal damage.

Endnotes

[1]Toshiba American Medical Systems, Inc., Tustin, CA.

[2]Toshiba Aquilon 8, Toshiba American Medical Systems, Inc., Tustin, CA.

[3]ITK-SNAP, https://sourceforge.net/projects/itk-snap/files/.

[4]Geomagic, Inc., Research Triangle Park, NC.

[5]JointTrack, University of Florida: http://sourceforge.net/projects/jointtrack/.

[6]MATLAB and Statistics Toolbox Release R2015a, The MathWorks, Inc., Natick, MA.

Abbreviations

CrCL: Cranial cruciate ligament; TPLO: Tibial plateau leveling osteotomy

Acknowledgements
The authors would like to acknowledge and thank Tim Vojt for assisting with production of graph figures and Debby Sundstrom, Cat Monger, Diane Downs, Matt Bolin, and Lisa McElveen for technical assistance.

Funding
This study was funded by a Hohn-Johnson Research Award from the Veterinary Orthopedic Society. Publication of this article was funded in part by the University of Florida Open Access Publishing Fund.

Authors' contributions
ST shape-matched the 3-D bone models of the femur and tibia onto the flat-panel images, analyzed the data, and drafted the manuscript. SK participated in the design of the study, assisted in data analysis, and helped draft the manuscript. SCJ trained ST in the methodology. BHP provided software assistance and custom software design for data analysis. SAB, DDL, and AP participated in study design and manuscript preparation. All authors read and approved the final manuscript.

Consent for publication
Not applicable.

Competing interests
The authors declare that they have no competing interests.

References

1. Vasseur P, Pool R, Arnoczky S, Lau R. Correlative biomechanical and histologic study of the cranial cruciate ligament in dogs. AJVR. 1985;46(9):1842–54.
2. Hayashi K, Frank JD, Dubinsky C, Hao Z, Markel MD, Manley PA, Muir P. Histologic changes in ruptured canine cranial cruciate ligament. Vet Surg. 2003;32:269–77.
3. Johnson JA, Austin C, Breur GJ. Incidence of canine appendicular musculoskeletal disorders in 16 veterinary teaching hospitals from 1980 through 1989. VCOT. 1994;7(2):56–69.
4. Pond MJ, Nuki G. Experimentally-induced osteoarthritis in the dog. Ann Rheum Dis. 1973;32:387–8.
5. Tashman S, Anderst W, Kolowich P, Havstad S, Arnoczky S. Kinematics of the ACL-deficient canine knee during gait: serial changes over two years. J Ortho Res. 2004;22:931–41.
6. Brandt KD, Myers SL, Burr D, Albrecht M. Osteoarthritic changes in canine articular cartilage, subchondral bone, and synovium fifty-four months after transection of the anterior cruciate ligament. Arthritis Rheum. 1991;34(12):1560–70.
7. Guilak F, Ratcliffe A, Lane N, Rosenwasser MP, Mow VC. Mechanical and biochemical changes in the superficial zone of articular cartilage in canine experimental osteoarthritis. J Orthop Res. 1994;12:474–84.
8. Marshall KW, Chan ADM. Bilateral canine model of osteoarthritis. J Rheumatol. 1996;23(2):344–50.
9. Wilke V, Robinson D, Evans R, Rothschild M, Conzemius M. Estimate of the annual economic impact of treatment of cranial cruciate ligament injury in dogs in the United States. JAVMA. 2005;227(10):1604–7.
10. Vasseur P. Clinical results following nonoperative management for rupture of the cranial cruciate ligament in dogs. Vet Surg. 1984;13(4):243–6.
11. Piermattei D, Flo G, DeCamp C: Brinker, Piermattei, and Flo's handbook of small animal orthopedics and fracture repair, 4 edn. St. Louis: Saunders Elsevier; 2006.
12. Arnoczky SP, Marshall JL. The cruciate ligaments of the canine stifle: an anatomical and functional analysis. AJVR. 1977;38(11):1807–14.
13. Korvick DL, Pijanowski GJ, Schaeffer DJ. Three-dimensional kinematics of the intact and cranial cruciate ligament-deficient stifle of dogs. J Biomech. 1994;27(1):77–87.
14. Warzee CC, Dejardin LM, Arnoczky SP, Perry RL. Effect of tibial plateau leveling on cranial and caudal tibial thrusts in canine cranial cruciate-deficient stifles: an in vitro experimental study. Vet Surg. 2001;30:278–86.
15. Rey J, Fischer MS, Bottcher P. Sagittal joint instability in the cranial cruciate ligament insufficient canine stifle: caudal slippage of the femur and not cranial tibial subluxation. Tierarztliche Praxis Kleintiere. 2014;42(K):151–6.
16. Jones SC, Kim SE, Banks SA, Conrad BP, Abbasi AZ, Tremolada G, Lewis DD, Pozzi A. Accuracy of noninvasive, single-plane fluoroscopic analysis for measurement of three-dimensional femorotibial joint poses in dogs. AJVR. 2014;75:477–85.
17. Banks SA, Hodge WA. Accurate measurement of three-dimensional knee replacement kinematics using single-plane fluoroscopy. IEEE Trans Biomed Eng. 1996;43(6):638–49.
18. Fregly BJ, Rahman HA, Banks SA. Theoretical accuracy of model-based shape matching for measuring natural knee kinematics with single-plane fluoroscopy. J Biomech Eng. 2005;127(4):692–9.
19. Komistek RD, Dennis DA, Mahfouz M. In vivo fluoroscopic analysis of the normal human knee. Clin Ortho and Related Res. 2003;410:69–81.
20. Piazza A, Binversie E, Baker L, Nemke B, Sample S, Muir P. Variance associated with walking velocity during force platform gait analysis of a heterogenous sample of clinically normal dogs. AJVR. 2017;78(4):500–7.
21. Tashman S, Anderst W. In-vivo measurement of dynamic joint motion using high speed biplane radiography and CT: application to canine ACL deficiency. J Biomech Eng. 2003;125(238–245)
22. Grood ES, Suntay WJ. A joint coordinate system for the clinical description of three-dimensional motions: application to the knee. J Biomech Eng. 1983;105:136–44.
23. Kim SE, Jones SC, Lewis DD, Banks SA, Conrad BP, Tremolada G, Abbasi AZ, Coggeshall JD, Pozzi A. In-vivo three-dimensional knee kinematics during daily activities in dogs. J Orthop Res. 2015;33(11):1603–10.
24. Jones SC, Kim SE, Banks SA, Conrad BP, Abbasi AZ, Tremolada G, Lewis DD, Pozzi A. Accuracy of noninvasive, single-plane fluoroscopic analysis for measurement of three-dimensional femorotibial joint poses in dogs treated by tibial plateau leveling osteotomy. AJVR. 2014;75(5):486–93.
25. Vilensky JA, O'Connor BL, Brandt KD, Dunn EA, Rogers PI. Serial kinematic analysis of the trunk and limb joints after anterior cruciate ligament transection: temporal, spatial, and angular changes in a canine model of osteoarthritis. J of Electromyography & Kinesiology. 1994;4:181–92.
26. Nelson SA, Krotscheck U, Rawlinson J, Todhunter RJ, Zhang Z, Mohammed H. Long-term functional outcome of tibial plateau leveling osteotomy versus extracapsular repair in a heterogenous population of dogs. Vet Surg. 2013;42:38–50.
27. Cameron ML, Briggs KK, Steadman JR. Reproducibility and reliability of the outerbridge classification for grading chondral lesions of the knee arthroscopically. Am J Sports Med. 2003;31(1):83–6.
28. DeCamp CE, Riggs CM, Olivier NB, Hauptman JG, Hottinger HA, Soutas-Little RW. Kinematic evaluation of gait in dogs with cranial cruciate ligament rupture. AJVR. 1996;57(1):120–6.
29. Kennedy JC, Alexander IJ, Hayes KC. Nerve supply of the human knee and its functional importance. Am J Sports Med. 1982;10(6):329–35.
30. Vilensky JA, O'Connor BL, Brandt KD. Serial kinematic analysis of the canine hindlimb joints after deafferentation and anterior cruciate ligament transection. Osteoarthr Cartil. 1997;5:173–82.
31. Kim SE, Pozzi A, Banks SA, Conrad BP, Lewis DD. Effect of cranial cruciate ligament deficiency, tibial plateau leveling osteotomy, and tibial tuberosity advancement on contact mechanics and alignment of the stifle in flexion. Vet Surg. 2010;39:363–70.
32. Nisell R. Mechanics of the knee. Acta Orthopaedica Scandanavica. 1985; 56(216):1–42.
33. Kaplan Y. Identifying individuals with an anterior cruciate ligament-deficient knee as copers and noncopers: a narrative literature review. J Orthop & Sports PT. 2011;41(10):758–66.
34. Goslow G, Seeherman H, Taylor C, McCutchin M, Heglund N. Electrical activity and relative length changes of dog limb muscles as a function of speed and gait. J Exp Biol. 1981;94(1):15–42.
35. Tokuriki M. Electromyographic and joint-mechanical studies in quadrupedal locomotion I. Walk. Japanese J Vet Sci. 1973;35:433–46.
36. Kanno N, Amimoto H, Hara Y, Harada Y, Nezu Y, Yogo T, Tagawa M. In vitro evaluation of the relationship between the semitendinosus muscle and cranial cruciate ligament in canine cadavers. AJVR. 2012;73:672–80.
37. Hayes GM, Granger N, Langley-Hobbs SJ, Jeffery ND. Abnormal reflex activation of hamstring muscles in dogs with cranial cruciate ligament rupture. The Vet J. 2013;196:345–50.

38. Bennett D, May C. Meniscal damage associated with cruciate disease in the dog. JSAP. 1991;32:111–7.
39. Kim SE, Pozzi A, Banks SA, Conrad BP, Lewis DD. Effect of tibial plateau leveling osteotomy on femorotibial contact mechanics and stifle mechanics. Vet Surg. 2009;38:23–32.
40. Vasseur P, Arnoczky S. Collateral ligaments of the canine stifle joint: anatomic and functional analysis. AJVR. 1981;42(7):1133–7.
41. Pozzi A, Kowaleski M, Apelt D, Meadows C, Andrews CM, Johnson K. Effect of medial meniscal release on tibial translation after tibial plateau leveling osteotomy. Vet Surg. 2006;35:486–94.
42. Boudrieau RJ. Tibial plateau leveling osteotomy or tibial tuberosity advancement? Vet Surg. 2009;38:1–22.
43. Fossum TW, Dewey CW, Horn CV, Johnson AL, MacPhail CM, Radlinsky MG, Schulz KS, Willard MD: Small animal surgery, 4 edn. St. Louis: Elsevier Mosby; 2013.
44. Torres B, Moens N, Al-Nadaf S, Reynolds L, Yu Y, Budsberg S. Comparison of overground and treadmill-based gaits of dogs. AJVR. 2013;74(4):535–41.
45. Hayashi K, Manley P, Muir P. Cranial cruciate ligament pathophysiology in dogs with cruciate disease: a review. JAAHA. 2004;40:385–90.
46. Ichinohe T, Kanno N, Harada Y, Yogo T, Tagawa M, Hara Y. Histological and immunohistological analysis of degenerative changes in the cranial cruciate ligament in a canine model of excessive tibial plateau angle. VCOT. 2015;28:240–9.
47. Buote N, Fusco J, Radasch R. Age, tibial plateau angle, sex, and weight as risk factors for contralateral rupture of the cranial cruciate ligament in Labradors. Vet Surg. 2009;38:481–9.
48. Fuller MC, Hayashi K, Bruecker K, Holsworth IG, Sutton JS, Kass PH, Kantrowitz BJ, Kapatkin AS. Evaluation of the radiographic infrapatellar fat pad sign of the contralateral stifle joint as a risk factor for subsequent contralateral cranial cruciate ligament rupture in dogs with unilateral rupture: 96 cases (2006-2007). JAVMA. 2014;244:328–38.
49. Bleedorn J, Greuel E, Manley P, Schaefer S, Markel M, Holzman G, Muir P. Synovitis in dogs with stable stifle joints and incipient cranial cruciate ligament rupture: a cross-sectional study. Vet Surg. 2011;40:531–43.
50. Grierson J, Asher L, Grainger K. An investigation into risk factors for bilateral canine cruciate ligament rupture. VCOT. 2011;24(3):192–6.
51. Cabrera S, Owen T, Mueller M, Kass P. Comparison of tibial plateau angles in dogs with unilateral versus bilateral cranial cruciate ligament rupture: 150 cases (2000-2006). JAVMA. 2008;232:889–92.

18

A laparoscopic approach for removal of ovarian remnant tissue in 32 dogs

Sebastiaan A. van Nimwegen[1*], Bart Van Goethem[2], Jeffrey de Gier[1] and Jolle Kirpensteijn[1,3]

Abstract

Background: Surgical treatment of ovarian remnant syndrome (ORS) in dogs usually necessitates large celiotomies and considerable manipulation of organs because of the relatively deep position of ovarian remnant tissue, large patient size, and often encountered adhesions. In women, laparoscopic treatment of ORS is successful and has significant advantages over laparotomy. Since laparoscopic ovariectomy has significant advantages over open ovariectomy in dogs, including reduced surgical stress and postoperative pain and shorter convalescence period, the rationale for a laparoscopic approach of canine ORS is evident. Feasibility and efficacy of a laparoscopic approach for treatment of ORS in dogs was prospectively evaluated using a standardized protocol for diagnosis, treatment, and follow-up. Treatment success was evaluated by histology of removed tissues, postoperative hormone testing, and long-term clinical follow-up.

Results: Thirty-two client-owned predominantly medium and large breed dogs diagnosed with ORS underwent abdominal ultrasound for ovarian remnant localization prior to laparoscopic surgery for removal of ovarian remnants. Tissue dissection and excision was performed using a vessel sealing forceps. Laparoscopy subjectively enabled detailed visibility and facilitated detection and removal of suspected ovarian tissue in all cases. Histology confirmed ovarian origin of removed tissue in all dogs. Additionally, a GnRH stimulation test was performed in fourteen dogs after a median follow-up of 10.5 months, which verified absence of residual functional ovarian remnant tissue in all dogs. Median surgery duration was 97.5 min and mean total convalescence duration, subjectively scored by owners, was 1.5 ± 0.7 days. No major complications occurred. Adhesions were observed in 79% of the dogs, complicated the surgical approach, and significantly affected surgery duration (85 versus 109 min; $p = 0.03$). Minor hemorrhage occurred in 12% and significantly increased surgery duration (95.5 versus 128 min; $p = 0.02$). Trendelenburg position and lateral tilting of the patient were essential for proper access to ovarian remnants. GnRH stimulation test results and/or absence of clinical signs indicative of ORS after a median follow-up period of 22.5 months confirmed treatment efficacy in all dogs.

Conclusion: Laparoscopic surgery for ORS in dogs is effective with minimal complications and short convalescence and can successfully replace the conventional, more invasive open surgical procedure.

Keywords: Ovarian, Remnant, Canine, Dog, Laparoscopy, Celiotomy, ORS, GnRH, Laparotomy, Ovariectomy

Background

Ovarian remnant syndrome (ORS) can occur as a complication after ovariectomy (OVE) or ovariohysterectomy (OVH). The syndrome is defined by clinical signs caused by hormone production by ovarian remnant tissue. Incidence rates of 0% (0/135), 0.1% (2/1880), and 0.5% (3/618) have been reported [1–3]. Despite anecdotal causes of ovarian remnant tissue, such as accessory or ectopic ovarian tissue or revascularization of ovarian tissue that dropped in the abdominal cavity during surgery, the only truly proven cause in dogs with ORS is iatrogenic, i.e. not removing the entire ovary during the OVE/OVH procedure [4, 5]. Possible risk factors for canine ORS are associated with accessibility of the ovaries during surgery and include large, deep-chested dogs, obesity, a too small and/or more caudal position of the celiotomy incision (OVH versus OVE) and seem to correspond with a

* Correspondence: S.A.vanNimwegen@uu.nl
[1]Department of Clinical Sciences of Companion Animals, Faculty of Veterinary Medicine, Utrecht University, Yalelaan 108, 3584CM, Utrecht, the Netherlands
Full list of author information is available at the end of the article

higher incidence of right-sided locations of ovarian remnant tissue [4–9]. Clinical signs from ovarian hormone production usually occur within several months after the initial procedure [7], although they can arise from as early as 1 week to as late as 11 years after the initial surgery [8]. Clinical signs of ORS can include symptoms associated with (pro) estrus, such as behavioral changes, attractiveness for male dogs, swelling of the vulva, serosanguineous vaginal discharge and receptivity to mating. Additionally, cystic endometrial hyperplasia, (stump) endometritis, pseudopregnancy, vaginitis, and ovarian neoplasia [4, 5, 7], and less commonly diabetes mellitus [10] and abdominal pain [11] are described. In contrast, ORS in humans is mainly associated with chronic inflammatory processes causing abdominal pain [12].

Diagnosis of ORS can be reliably made using a combination of history, clinical signs, vaginoscopic findings and vaginal cytology during (pro) estrus, measurement of the plasma progesterone (P_4) concentration during the expected luteal phase [7, 13]. When results of these tests are not diagnostic but suspicion of ORS remains, a GnRH stimulation test can be used to rule out or confirm the existence of an ovarian remnant [8].

Treatment of ORS consists of surgical excision of all the ovarian remnant tissue. The common approach is via midline celiotomy. After a thorough abdominal exploration, all suspicious tissue is excised, especially near the original OVE/OVH excision sites, as macroscopic distinction between ovarian remnant and fibrous (scar) tissue can be difficult. Because of the dorsal location of the ovarian pedicle and adhesions caused by the previous surgery, careful dissection is necessary to avoid damage to the ureters and other closely associated organs/structures. Performing surgery during estrus-like clinical signs aids the discovery of very small remnants or remnants covered by adhesions because of increased size and vascularization and the presence of developing follicles or *corpora lutea* [5, 8, 14]. Consequently, a large celiotomy incision and manipulation of organs are usually required for thorough exploration of the ovarian pedicle and uterine horn locations. All lesions including cystic abnormalities and foci of abnormal vascularity should be excised and histologically evaluated for ovarian remnant tissue. Recurrence of ORS after surgical intervention is common [15] and referral to a surgical specialist has been advised [16, 17].

Considering that surgery for ORS is accompanied by a larger celiotomy and considerably more manipulation of abdominal tissues than elective ovariectomy or ovariohysterectomy, the rationale for developing a minimally invasive approach was logical. Laparoscopic ovariectomy has become a routine procedure in dogs and cats with multiple studies showing reduced surgical stress response and post-operative pain and faster convalescence compared to an open celiotomy approach [18–25]. In women, laparoscopic treatment of ORS is generally successful [12, 26], has a low recurrence rate (up to 7%) [27–29], and is associated with decreased blood loss, a shorter hospital stay, and fewer postoperative complications compared to celiotomy [30]. Only a few case reports and three small retrospective case series exist of laparoscopic surgery for ORS in dogs and cats [15, 31–34]. Confirmation of full excision of ovarian remnant tissue was often made only by absence of clinical signs.

In the study reported here, a laparoscopic approach for removal of ovarian remnant tissue was prospectively investigated in dogs diagnosed with ORS, using a standardized protocol for diagnosis, treatment, and follow-up, including post-operative confirmation of the absence of any ovarian tissue using a GnRH stimulation test in a subset of 14 dogs. We hypothesized that a laparoscopic approach for removal of ovarian remnant tissue would be feasible in dogs without the need for conversion to a celiotomy, resulting in a high success rate and short convalescence period.

Materials and methods

Inclusion criteria

All dogs diagnosed with ORS, between July 2009 and February 2014, at the Department of Clinical Sciences of Companion Animals, Utrecht University and the Department of Small Animal Medicine, Ghent University, were offered a laparoscopic surgical approach for the same costs as a laparoscopic ovariectomy. A research grant by the Dutch Society for Veterinary Research in Companion Animals (Stichting D.O.G.) [35] enabled follow-up GnRH-testing in the first 13 dogs without additional costs for the owners. The study and associated protocol was approved by the local Ethical Committee of the Department of Clinical Sciences of Companion Animals, Utrecht University.

Diagnostic protocol

For inclusion in the study, ORS had to be proven by a combination of clinical history and clinical examination followed by functional endocrine tests if necessary. Signs of (pro) estrus, if present upon presentation to the clinic, were clinically investigated using vaginoscopy and vaginal cytology. In late follicular phase and suspected luteal phase, based on history and clinical examination, measurement of P_4 concentration was performed. Normal basal P_4 in ovariectomized bitches in our laboratory: median, 0.63 nmol/l (range: < 0.15–2.2 nmol/l). A P_4 concentration of higher than 3.36 nmol/l is diagnostic for ORS [36]. In cases in which these tests were negative, but suspicion of ORS remained, a GnRH stimulation test was performed.

Ultrasound imaging

Additionally, in all dogs an abdominal ultrasound was performed to search for abnormalities that could be related to ORS and to evaluate the ability to predict the location of ovarian remnant tissue by ultrasound. Ultrasound examination was performed using a C8–5 broadband curved array transducer at 8 MHz with a HD digital ultrasound system (HD11 XE, Philips, the Netherlands). If indicated, adjustment of ultrasound frequency in the individual patient was based on image quality and patient size.

Anesthetic protocol

Two different anesthetic protocols were used. Healthy ASA 1 and 2 patients received anesthesia according to a routine protocol consisting of dexmedetomidine (Dexdomitor, Orion Corporation, Finland) premedication (10–15 μg/kg IV), propofol (PropoFlo Plus, Abbott Logistics B.V., the Netherlands) induction (1–2 mg/kg IV to effect), and isoflurane (Isoflo, Abbott Laboratories, United Kingdom) in 50% O_2–50% air mixture as maintenance. Dogs were mechanically ventilated (IPPV) during surgery. Dexmedetomidine was routinely redosed at 5–7.5 μg/kg IV after 60 min of anesthesia. Additional analgesia consisted of carprofen (Rimadyl, Zoetis, België) (4 mg/kg IV) and buprenorphine (Buprecare, Animalcare ltd, United Kingdom) (10–15 μg/kg IV). After surgery, atipamezole (Antisedan, Orion Corporation, Finland) (50–75 μg/kg IM) was administered to reverse dexmedetomidine effects. Routine anesthetic monitoring consisted of esophageal temperature probe, capnography, pulse oximetry, end-tidal O_2, end-tidal CO_2, end-tidal isoflurane, ECG, heart rate, respiratory rate, tidal volume, airway pressure, non-invasive blood pressure. Dogs older than 7 years of age, or with increased risk of circulatory compromise received a different anesthetic protocol consisting of methadone (Comfortan, Eurovet Animal Health B.V., the Netherlands) (0.05 mg/kg IV) and midazolam (Dormicum, Roche B.V., the Netherlands) (0.4 mg/kg IV) premedication, followed by propofol induction (2–4 mg/kg IV to effect) and isoflurane in 50% O_2–50% air mixture maintenance. Additional analgesia consisted of constant rate infusion of fentanyl (Bipharma, the Netherlands) (10–20 μg/kg/hr) during maintenance of anesthesia, which is partially reversed during recovery by administering buprenorphine (10–15 μg/kg) while maintaining adequate postoperative analgesia. Postoperative analgesia consisted of 3 days of oral carprofen (2 mg/kg 2dd). Antibiotics were not part of the treatment protocol and were only sporadically administered as prophylaxis in cases of (partial) hysterectomy of suspected septic inflammation or contaminated contents of the uterus.

Surgery protocol

No attempt was made to plan the time of surgery to coincide with estrus for improved visualization of remnants. On the contrary, surgery was often postponed until anestrus for dogs that presented with overt estrus and a history of regularly occurring estrous cycles to decrease the chance of postoperative pseudopregnancy. For dogs that did not present with signs of regularly occurring estrous cycles, surgery was usually planned shortly after diagnosis. All surgeries were performed by three experienced laparoscopic surgeons with ECVS board certification (SvN, JK, BVG). The dogs were placed in 10-15° Trendelenburg position with alternate 20-30° lateral tilting. Surgery was performed through a standard 3-portal midline laparoscopic approach; using a modified Hasson approach with 6-mm outer diameter blunt tip threaded screw-in cannulas (Ternamian EndoTIP, Karl Storz Endoscopy, Germany). The first portal was midway between umbilicus and pubic rim. A 10 mm skin incision was made, followed by blunt dissection of subcutaneous tissue, revealing the linea alba. Two stay sutures were placed in the external abdominal fascia, bilaterally at 2 mm from the linea alba. The stay sutures were pulled up and a 4–5 mm stab incision was made in the linea alba. The cannula was placed under visual guidance of a 5 mm 0° or 30° telescope (Hopkins II, Karl Storz Endoscopy, Tuttlingen, Germany) inserted in the cannula [37]. After visual confirmation of proper abdominal entry, the abdomen was insufflated with CO_2 gas to an intra-abdominal pressure of 8 mmHg (Thermoflator, Karl Storz Endoscopy, Tuttlingen, Germany). Two additional 6-mm portals were placed 1–2 cm caudal and 1–2 cm cranial to the umbilicus, respectively. The telescope was then inserted through the middle portal and a routine inspection of the abdomen was performed. Surgery was commenced according to a preplanned routine: inspection of the left ovarian pedicle location and uterine remnant (if present) with the dog tilted to the right side; inspection of the right ovarian pedicle location and uterine remnant (if present) with the dog tilted to the left side; inspection of the cervical stump (if present). As a rule, adequate access to the ovarian pedicle area included at least proper visualization of both kidneys. Furthermore, any abnormalities and omental adhesions were inspected. In cases where remnants were not visually identified, existing omental adhesions were carefully inspected and followed towards any attachment site. Likewise, the round ligament of the uterus was identified at the inguinal ring and followed cranially. Any suspect looking tissues, adhesions, cystic structures or ligature scars were excised from the pedicle region and any cystic or inflammatory changes of the uterine remnant or locations of omental adhesions to the uterine remnant were also excised. A fourth portal for extra tissue manipulation was used if necessary. Manipulation of tissues was routinely performed using 5 mm diameter endoscopic instruments, including a Kelly dissection forceps and a self-retaining blunt grasping forceps. Additional instruments for tissue manipulation were optional, including fan retractors, Babcock forceps, endoscopic suction/irrigation device, and endoscopic scissors. All tissue dissection and excision was performed using a vessel sealing device (VSD; LigaSure, Covidien, Boulder, CO). Excised tissues were removed from the abdominal cavity either through a 10-mm cannula that was exchanged for the 6-mm cannula in the caudal portal, or through an enlarged caudal portal. Larger tissue specimens or fragments were removed using a 10-mm specimen retrieval bag. Uterine remnants with hormone-induced changes within the normal range were not excised. In cases of abnormal uterine changes, such as overt cystic endometrial hyperplasia or pyometra, the uterine remnants were excised intra-abdominally using the VSD, or laparoscopy-assisted hysterectomy was performed with removal of the uterus through an enlarged caudal portal and either ligated and transected with scissors or transected using VSD outside of the abdomen. Isolated uterine abnormalities, such as (para-) uterine cysts or adhesions were treated by local excision of the abnormal tissue. Closure of portals larger than 6 mm was done in 3 layers (external abdominal fascia, subcutis, and skin) using absorbable monofilament suture material. In portals < 6 mm where the external abdominal fascia was not easily accessible, only subcutis and skin were closed. Dogs were released from the hospital directly after recovery from anesthesia and owners were instructed the keep their dog on a leash with restricted exercise for 3–5 days.

Follow-up protocol

Owners were routinely contacted by telephone after 1 week to inform them of the histology results and a standardized questionnaire was used to obtain information on the immediate postoperative period, scoring the duration of convalescence (how long it took until the dog was acting as before the operation, seemingly not affected by the surgery or anesthesia, as subjectively scored by the owner), occurrence of pseudopregnancy, occurrence of wound complications, changes in appetite, behavior, and activity levels of the dog, and owner satisfaction with the treatment and outcome. For the first 13 dogs, a routine control visit was planned, preferably more than 3 months post-operatively, during which a GnRH stimulation test was performed in order to evaluate if all ovarian remnant tissue was removed during surgery. After the initial 13 cases, post-operative GnRH testing was only performed if clinical signs of possible recurrent ORS were suspected. Long-term follow-up consisted of several telephonic contact moments with the owners throughout the duration of the study, scoring any behavioral or clinical signs suggestive of ORS, and monitoring changes in appetite and activity level. Short- and long-term follow-up questionnaire forms were added as an additional file (see Additional file 1).

GnRH stimulation test

Blood samples were collected at − 40, 0, 10, 60, and 120 min by venipuncture. At $t = 0$, immediately after collecting the second blood sample, a GnRH analogue, 10 μg/kg body weight Gonadorelin (Fertagyl; Intervet/Schering-Plough Animal Health, Boxmeer, the Netherlands) was administered intravenously. Plasma hormone concentrations were measured as previously described [8], at the following time points: estradiol-17β (at − 40, 0, 60, and 120 min), LH and FSH (both at − 40, 0, 10, and 60 min). Before GnRH stimulation at $t = 0$, baseline hormone levels were measured twice with 40 min time interval and values were averaged for increased accuracy [8]. Previously established cut-off values were used to differentiate between dogs with and without residual ovarian tissue (Table 1) [8, 38]. LH measurements after GnRH stimulation, at 10 and 60 min, were routinely performed to confirm that GnRH stimulation was effective as indicated by a short-lived increase in plasma LH concentration at $t = 10$ min [39]. FSH measurements at $t = 10$ and 60 min were performed as an extra indication of the absence of functional ovarian tissue as indicated by no further increase in plasma FSH concentration [38].

Histologic evaluation

Histologic evaluation was performed through standard H&E stained sections of paraffin-embedded tissue labeled according to their location in the abdomen. In case of negative findings (i.e. fatty tissue without clear evidence of either suture material, inflammatory changes, or scar tissue, or with evidence of mesosalpinx-like structures or cystic structures without ovarian components), additional deeper sections were performed to rule out the possibility of skipping small ovarian remnants.

Initial diagnosis, ultrasound-predicted location, and treatment success were ultimately confirmed by histologic examination of all excised tissues.

Statistical analysis

Statistical analysis of the data was performed using IBM SPSS 23 data analysis software. Apart from general descriptive statistics, differences between sub-groups were evaluated using Student's t-test or Mann-Whitney U test if data were not normally distributed, as tested using Shapiro-Wilk test. Statistical relations or trends were evaluated using ANOVA and linear regression tests.

Table 1 Reference values for interpretation of GnRH stimulation test results after removal of ovarian remnants [8, 38]

plasma parameter	time point	cut-off value (ovariectomized)
LH	Basal (before GnRH)	> 3.4 μg/l
FSH	Basal (before GnRH)	> 11.0 μg/l
FSH: Estradiol-17β ratio	Basal (before GnRH)	> 0.66
Estradiol-17β	120 min after GnRH	< 21.3 pmol/L
Estradiol-17β	Basal (before GnRH)	< 7 pmol/l → no ORS 7–21.3 pmol/l → not diagnostic

Time point is relative to the administration of GnRH during a GnRH stimulation test. An animal was considered completely ovariectomized if the measured parameters were > or < the presented cut-off values as specified

Statistical significance was assumed when $p < 0.05$. Results are reported as means ± sd or median (Inter Quartile Range (IQR) and/or range).

Results

Patient population

Thirty-two dogs with ORS were included in the study. Mean age was 4.5 ± 2.7 years; mean body weight was 26.7 ± 12.4 kg (range 4.5–71.6 kg). Breeds included 12 (38%) crossbreed dogs, 8 (25%) Labrador Retrievers, 2 German Shepherds, 2 English Cocker Spaniels, a Labradoodle, Airedale Terrier, Boerboel, Dachshund, Flat-coated Retriever, Galgo Espangol, Rottweiler, and a Siberian Husky. Seventy-five percent of the patients had initially been spayed in the Netherlands and Belgium (countries in which the study was performed), 25% of the dogs were previously operated abroad, including Bulgaria, Greece, Turkey, Spain, and the USA. According to the clinical history, the initial surgery consisted of ovariectomy in 59%, and ovariohysterectomy in 31%, and was unknown for 10% of the dogs.

The exact date of initial surgery was known for 18 animals and the median interval between initial surgery and clinical signs of ORS was 8.5 months, (range 0.5–96 months; $n = 18$). Clinical signs that were most frequently reported by the owners were attractiveness to male dogs (96%), vulvar discharge (83%), and vulvar swelling (57%). Less frequently, swelling of mammary glands, occurrence of pseudopregnancy, decreased appetite, frequent urination, and weight loss were reported. Two dogs suffered from increased stress/anxiety that the owners attributed to the ORS. Abdominal pain was present in one dog, pain during defecating in one dog, occasional abdominal discomfort and vomiting in one dog, and a mammary tumor in another. In 6 dogs (19%), treatment of the ORS by exploratory celiotomy had already been attempted by the referring veterinary practitioner. The presence of residual ovarian tissue was confirmed by observation of overt clinical estrus, as confirmed by vaginoscopy and vaginal cytology or distinct endometritis in 56% of dogs. Clinical presentation and measurement of a plasma progesterone level of > 3.36 nmol/l confirmed ORS in 38% of the patients. The remaining 6% was solely diagnosed by means of a GnRH stimulation test.

Preoperative ultrasound findings

Ultrasound imaging was performed in 31/32 (97%) of the dogs. One dog did not undergo ultrasound imaging because the referring veterinarian knew that a right ovarian remnant was left behind during the ovariectomy procedure but had been unable to locate it and remove it at that time. Ultrasound evaluation indicated at least one suspect tissue in 30/31 dogs. Based on ultrasound evaluation a possible ovarian remnant was located only at the left ovarian pedicle area in 4/31 (13%), only at the right ovarian pedicle area in 16/31 (52%), and at both sides in 10/31 (32%) of dogs. No suspect tissue was found in one dog (3%). Uterine tissue was identified in 26/31 (84%) of the patients, which was abnormal in 14/26 (54%) of the cases (i.e. cystic, enlarged, fluid filled, or signs of endometritis). One coincidental finding was the absence of a left kidney in the presence of a left ovarian remnant in a Labradoodle that was spayed at the age of 8 weeks.

Surgical findings

All dogs successfully underwent laparoscopic surgery for ORS without the need for conversion to an open approach. Median duration of surgery, from skin incision to completion of wound closure, was 97.5 min (IQR 24.5; range 60–204 min). Adequate exposure of ovarian remnants sometimes necessitated tilting the dog > 30° laterally or up to 20° in Trendelenburg position. All suspect tissues were excised, including ligature scar tissue, especially if any adhesions, apparent vasculature, or cyst-like changes, even if only very small, were present. Ligature scars with only minimal fibrotic changes without apparent vasculature or other changes were not excised (Fig. 1).

Suspect or abnormal looking tissue was removed from the left pedicle area in 69%, from the right pedicle area in 91%, from the tip of the left uterine horn in 50%, and from the tip of the right uterine horn in 47% of dogs. Removal of the uterine body was performed in 9% of the dogs. The mean number of excised tissue specimens per

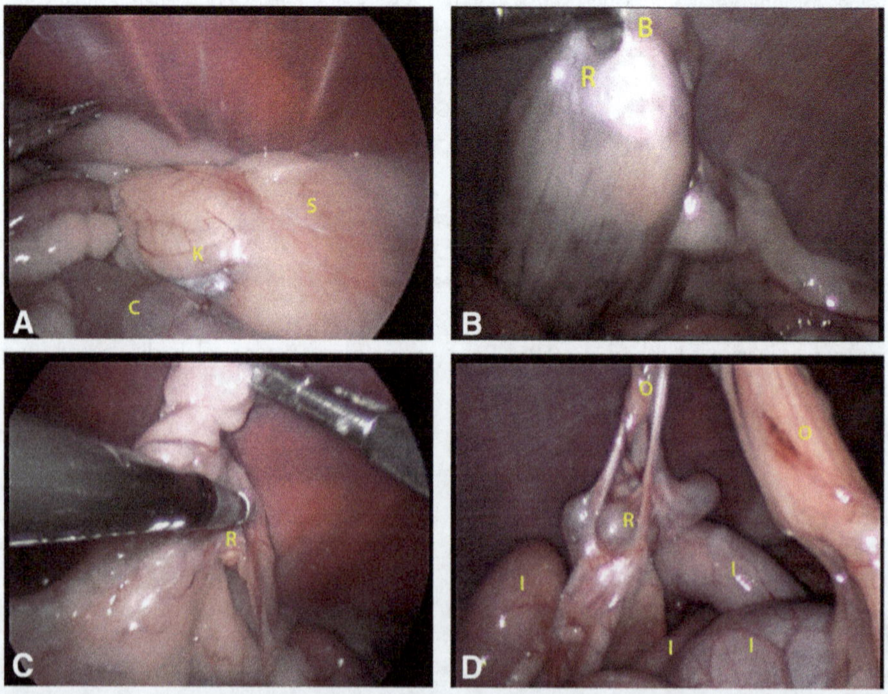

Fig. 1 Laparoscopic images of a normal ovarian pedicle scar and several examples of ovarian remnants. 1-**a**: Normal ligature scar in left ovarian pedicle area. 1-**b**: Large left-sided ovarian remnant with forceps in ovarian bursal opening. 1-**c**: Small right-sided ovarian remnant covered by fat and omental adhesions. 1-**d**: Right-sided ovarian remnant with omental adhesions and multiple cystic structures. S = scar; R = ovarian remnant; O = omentum adhesion; K = kidney; C = colon; I = intestine; B = bursal opening

dog was 2.5 ± 0.9. The size of excised tissues varied from < 1 cm to cystic structures of 5–6 cm in diameter.

Adhesions were found in 79% of the dogs (Fig. 2). Adhesions were located in the area of the left pedicle in 41%, in the area of the right pedicle in 67%, to the uterus in 48%, and to the mesoduodenum in 25% of the cases. Surgery duration was significantly faster in dogs without adhesions (median 85 (IQR 41.3) minutes, 18% of dogs) versus dogs with any form of adhesions (median 109 (IQR 36) minutes; 82% of dogs; $p = 0.03$). A fourth, paramedian, portal was placed in 2 dogs for improved access to the surgical area.

Complications

No major complications occurred. Minor complications consisting of intraoperative hemorrhage occurred in 4 dogs (12%). In one dog, hemorrhage occurred from a paramedian abdominal wall portal which was eventually controlled using a full-thickness abdominal wall suture. Minor bleedings occurred during tissue manipulation in 3 dogs: a splenic puncture by an instrument, several small bleedings occurring during dissection in the right pedicle area, and minor bleeding during dissection of extensive adhesions in the left pedicle area, respectively. All hemorrhages were successfully controlled laparoscopically, using either suction/irrigation or the application of a surgical gauze through a 10 mm portal to improve visibility and establishing hemostasis by plugging the splenic puncture site with a hemostatic gelatin sponge (Spongostan, Ethicon Inc., Somerville, NJ), or the application of the VSD. Total blood loss was considered minimal but the extra effort of evaluation and intervention caused a significant increase in surgery duration in cases of bleeding during ovarian remnant removal compared to non-bleeding cases (median 128 min (IQR 71.5) versus 95.5 (IQR 22) minutes respectively, $p = 0.02$).

Additional surgical procedures were performed in three dogs. One dog had a laparoscopic liver biopsy because of an increased level of circulating bile acids. Another dog had a partial mastectomy because of a concurrent mammary tumor. This turned out to be mammary carcinoma with lymph node metastasis and this dog died 3 months later because of generalized metastasis. A third dog (39 kg cross-breed) turned out to have a sub-clinical gastric volvulus of 270° with moderate dilation, which became apparent during routine laparoscopic inspection of the abdomen. This condition was corrected by deflating the stomach through gastric intubation and laparoscopic correction of the stomach position, followed by a laparoscopic-assisted gastropexy.

Histology results

Histologic evaluation identified removal of ovarian remnant tissue in all dogs. Ovarian remnant tissue was present only at the left ovarian pedicle area in 3 dogs (9%), only at the right ovarian pedicle area in 23 dogs

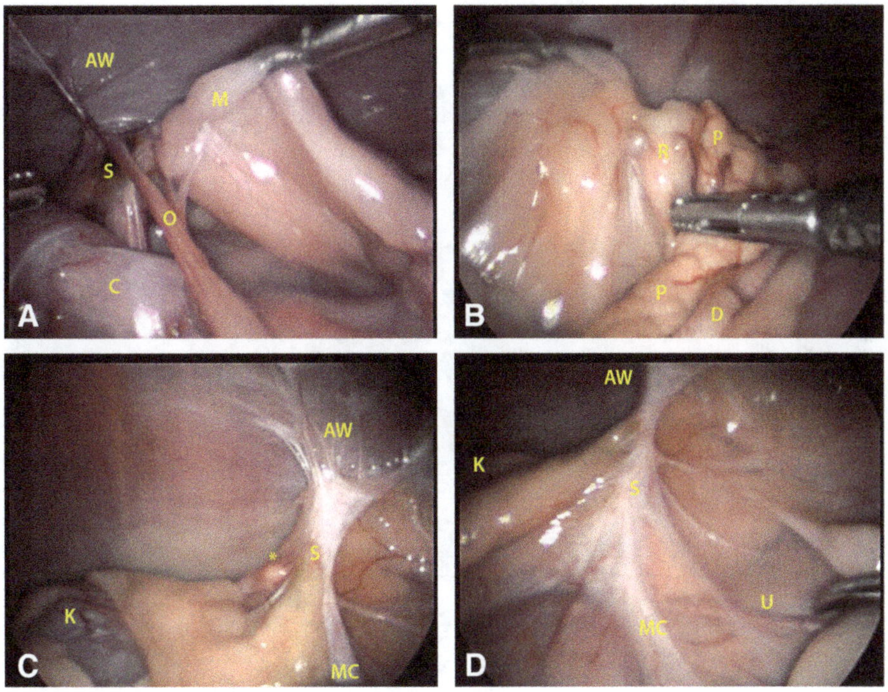

Fig. 2 Examples of adhesions in the ovarian pedicle area and visualization of the ureter. 2-**a**: Left-sided scar tissue with multiple adhesions, including abdominal wall. 2-**b**: Right-sided small cystic ovarian remnant adhered to mesoduodenum and pancreas. 2-**c**: . Left-sided ligature scar tissue with multiple adhesions, including abdominal wall and mesocolon. The suspicious looking nodular tissue* turned out to be reactive scar tissue on histologic evaluation. 2-**d**: The same ligature scar tissue as in Fig. 1C, visualizing the left ureter close to ovarian pedicle area. S = scar; R = ovarian remnant; O = omentum adhesion; K = kidney; C = colon; AW = abdominal wall adhesions; MC = mesocolon adhesions; M = mesometrium; P = pancreas; D = duodenum; U = ureter

(72%) and on both sides in 5 dogs (16%). Right-sided remnants were significantly overrepresented ($p = 0.01$). One dog (3%) had an ovarian remnant attached to the uterine horn without involvement of a pedicle area. In this dog, the tips of the uterine horns were adhered to each other and to omentum with a small ovarian remnant within the adhesions.

Several ovarian remnants contained small to large (up to 3 cm) cysts and/or areas representing corpora lutea. In two dogs (6%), the ovarian remnant contained a granulosa cell tumor. Uterine abnormalities consisted of cystic endometrial hyperplasia, endometritis, or localized large cysts (up to 6 cm).

When combining the results of preoperative ultrasound evaluation with the results of histology of excised tissues, the overall accuracy of abdominal ultrasound to predict the location of an ovarian remnant had a sensitivity of 94% and a specificity of 74%. Sensitivity and specificity were also determined for right-sided and left-sided remnant location apart (Table 2).

Postoperative parameters

Short-term follow-up

Median time interval from surgery to first follow-up contact with the owners was 7 days (range 3–17 days). Mean duration of recovery, as concluded from the telephone questionnaire with the owners, was 1.5 ± 0.7 days. Recovery duration significantly increased with increased surgery duration (linear regression, Fig. 3, $p < 0.01$). Pseudopregnancy was noted postoperatively by the owner in 4 dogs (12.5%) and resolved without medical intervention. Mild wound healing complications (minor swelling and serous discharge) were seen in 4% of the cases, without requiring medical attention. In the short term follow-up (during the first 2 months postoperative) 3 dogs (10%), one of which was also pseudopregnant, still showed increased attractiveness for male dogs. Another 3 dogs (10%) had an episode of minor vaginal discharge ranging from a white to bloody aspect. Owners reported to be very satisfied to have chosen the laparoscopic approach in 91% of the cases (range satisfied – very satisfied).

Table 2 Diagnostic accuracy of abdominal ultrasound to locate ovarian remnants in dogs

Ultrasound diagnosis	Sensitivity (95% CI)	Specificity (95% CI)
Left pedicle area	88% (48–99%)	70% (47–87%)
Right pedicle area	96% (81–99%)	100% (n.a.)
Overall	94% (81–99%)	74% (54–99%)

95% CI 95% confidence interval

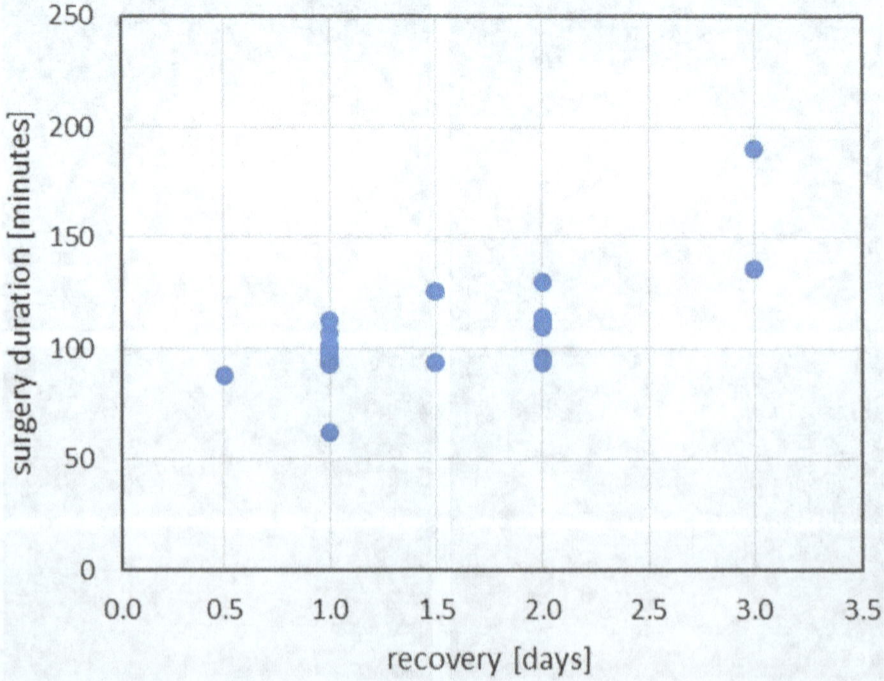

Fig. 3 Relation between recovery and surgery duration. Longer surgery duration was significantly related to an increased recovery duration, as subjectively scored by owners

GnRH stimulation test

GnRH stimulation testing was performed in 13 dogs without clinical signs of ORS. One additional dog was tested because of the occurrence of mild vaginal bleeding 11 months after surgery for ORS. No other clinical signs were apparent in this dog and the only abnormality found during clinical evaluation was a small vaginal septum remnant on vaginoscopy. Median time interval between ORS surgery and GnRH stimulation test was 10.5 months (range 1–25 months). Results of these tests

Table 3 Results of GnRH stimulation tests

Dog case nr.	interval OR - GnRH test [months]	basal E_2 [pmol/L]	E_2 t = 60	E_2 t = 120	basal LH [µg/L]	LH t = 10	LH t = 60	basal FSH [µg/L]	FSH t = 10	FSH t = 60	basal FSH/E_2
1	20	18.4	18.0	**16.5**	**25.3**	38.1	22.2	**24.2**	19.0	24.8	**1.31**
2	17.5	19.4	8.8	**8.6**	**19.8**	30.8	25.4	**31.0**	21.6	32.1	**1.60**
3	16.5	9.8	9.2	**11.2**	**11.3**	26.7	13.9	**15.1**	14.3	15.6	**1.54**
4	16	16.5	14.0	**17.6**	**10.1**	26.5	15.1	**11.3**	8.2	13.2	**0.68**
5	18	17.1	12.5	**14.3**	**16.6**	29.0	20.5	**20.6**	21.3	24.0	**1.20**
6	25	**3.2**		**4.5**							
7	12	**2.5**	**1.2**	**0.4**	**15.7**	22.2	12.2	**18.1**	18.3	17.5	**7.22**
8	6.3	**3.9**	**5.9**	**17.3**	**5.9**	10.7	6.6	**13.7**	12.7	15.1	**3.52**
9	9	**4.3**	**2.5**	**2.5**	**19.3**	36.0	15.4				
10	1.5	**3.7**	**1.5**	**0.6**	**14.7**	33.2	15.6	**14.4**	16.3	17.7	**3.88**
11	8.5	**1.8**	**6.4**	**2.0**	**20.8**	43.9	26.6	**20.0**	21.4	20.5	**11.08**
12	3	**3.7**	**3.7**	**5.9**	**10.4**	31.6	8.2	**13.2**	10.8	13.3	**3.56**
13	1	**2.4**	**1.9**	**0.3**	**11.6**	27.8	12.4	7.1[a]	7.9	8.1	**2.95**
14	7	**4.6**	**3.2**	**2.2**	**4.9**	13.1	7.2				

Basal plasma values of estradiol (E_2), LH and FSH are the average of two separate basal measurements at $t = -40$ and t = 0 min. All measured plasma values that indicate absence of functional ovarian tissue are displayed as bold text, based on previously published cut-off values (see Table 1). None of the values are consistent with the existence of functional ovarian tissue (see Table 1 for cut-off values). [a]The basal FSH of dog nr. 13 is below cut-off value which in this case was caused by a short time interval between surgery and GnRH stimulation test (see discussion section) confirmed that ovarian remnant tissue was not present after surgery in all tested dogs. Moreover, none of the measured blood plasma hormone levels could indicate the presence of ovarian tissue, while at least 2 measurements (median 4, range 2–5) per dog indicated the absence of functional ovarian tissue (Table 3). A peak in plasma LH concentration at $t = 10$ min confirmed effective GnRH stimulation in all cases.

Long-term follow-up

Median duration between surgery for ORS and last telephone follow-up was 22.5 months (range 6–53 months). After a follow-up period of 51 months, one dog remained to show increased attractiveness to male dogs according to the owners. This, despite not showing any other signs of ORS and having a negative GnRH stimulation test at 16 months postoperative. None of the other dogs, including the ones that were attractive to male dogs or had vaginal discharge in the short-term follow-up, had any signs of possible ORS in the long-term follow-up. Only one dog had no long-term follow-up because it died due to metastasis of mammary carcinoma 3 months after surgery. Two dogs with reported stress/anxiety, one with abdominal pain, and one with pain during defecation preoperatively had all markedly improved. In one dog, signs of occasional abdominal discomfort and vomiting preoperatively did not improve postoperatively, although the dog became more active and had a better appetite. Signs of ORS disappeared completely after surgery. Overall activity level was subjectively increased in 16% of the dogs, appetite had increased in 16% and was reduced in 1 dog compared to the preoperative situation.

Discussion

Ovarian remnant tissue was successfully removed by laparoscopic surgery in 32 dogs diagnosed with ORS. All had histologically confirmed ovarian tissue excised. All follow-up GnRH stimulation test results were consistent with the absence of ovarian tissue and all, but one dog, were completely free of clinical signs associated with ORS in the long-term follow-up.

The incidence of referral and type of dogs with ORS in the present study is comparable to previous studies [7, 8]. In a study by Okkens et al. [7], 76% of dogs weighed more than 20 kg which is similar to 75% weighing over 20 kg in the present study, supporting the theory that ORS is more often present in large dogs. Likewise, the significant overrepresentation of right-sided remnants in the present study population is also consistent with other reports of ORS in dogs and may be related to the deeper and more cranial position of the right ovary making it more difficult to access during a standard midline laparotomy approach, which theoretically may increase the risk for ORS [4, 5, 7, 9]. Furthermore, ovarian remnant tissue was found in the pedicle area in 97% of the dogs, which makes other causes for ORS besides surgical error unlikely. There might theoretically be an increased risk for ORS after OVE compared to OVH because OVE necessitates 2 incisions near the ovary (ovarian pedicle and proper ligament) versus only one incision for OVH (ovarian pedicle) [40]. The majority of dogs (59%) in the present study was ovariectomized, which is the most common surgical neutering procedure for female dogs in the Benelux area. Only one dog (3%) had an ovarian remnant attached to a uterine horn, making transection of the proper ligament as a risk factor for ORS less likely. An improper general surgical technique to remove ovaria due to either insufficient visibility or a minimalistic approach seems to be a more likely cause than the discussion surrounding removing the uterus or not as a reason for ORS [40].

A relatively high percentage of dogs (25%) was imported to the Netherlands from other countries and was originally spayed abroad. Although this has not been mentioned in other studies, it may indicate a much higher occurrence of ORS in imported dogs of certain regions. The fact that 20 % of the dogs already underwent surgery by a general practitioner in an unsuccessful attempt to treat the ORS before referral, stresses that surgery for ORS can be a challenge, especially in less experienced hands [16, 17]. The absence of a left kidney in the presence of an intact left-sided ovarian remnant in one dog in the present study that underwent initial spay surgery at the age of 8 weeks may indicate a grave surgical error: the accidental removal of a kidney during initial gonadectomy in this dog. The presence of a single solitary kidney or kidney agenesis cannot be fully ruled out in this dog, however. The absence of a kidney in a dog with ORS has been reported previously [4].

The laparoscopic approach was very effective for abdominal exploration and detection of ovarian remnants or suspect tissues. Being able to get a detailed close up image of selected tissues was subjectively considered advantageous over open surgery for ORS, in which detection and surgical access to an ovarian remnant can be very challenging. Access to the pedicle area was usually considered sufficient. Proper visualization, including visual access to the caudoventral aspect of the kidney, was in most cases achieved using the standard 20-30° lateral tilting and 10-15° Trendelenburg positioning of the patient. This also facilitated identification of the caudal part of the ipsilateral ureter in most dogs, which was helpful for dissection of remnants located near the level of the peritoneum in this area. Difficult access to the pedicle area was mainly caused by the existence of adhesions that would sometimes prevent the intestines, pancreas, or spleen to be dissected away from the area of interest. These cases were managed by increasing the Trendelenburg angle (up to 20°) and careful manipulation of adhesions. In two cases, an extra instrument portal was needed for additional retraction of organs to increase visibility of the area of interest. Most of the ovarian remnants could be revealed by locating, grabbing and lifting up the adhered ligaments and omentum. Many of the ovarian remnants were also retracted to some extent and could be recognized by their increased vasculature or bulky or cystic appearance. Gently lifting the ovarian remnant tissue allowed dissection from all surrounding attachments to ligaments, organs, omentum, and retroperitoneal fat. The greatest difficulty was experienced with small ovarian remnants extensively covered by adhesions. In a few cases, the remnant was located in a very dorsal, almost retroperitoneal position. In such 'retroperitoneal' cases, the remnant would be covered by fat and could not be manipulated by lifting adhered tissues but would be buried beneath them. Careful probe palpation and dissection was then applied to reveal and remove the ovarian remnant tissue without leaving parts behind or damaging the ureter, which often ran close to the plane of dissection. Adhesions to the mesoduodenum, which were observed in 25% of the cases, could also be challenging because of close proximity of pancreas and pancreaticoduodenal blood vessels.

The amount of adhesions observed in these ORS patients was subjectively considered to be relatively high. Most severe adhesions were usually associated with the ovarian remnant tissue, although the contralateral scar and uterine remnants were equally affected in several cases. ORS may cause or promote chronic inflammatory lesions of the female canine reproductive tract, such as stump pyometra, cystic endometrial hyperplasia, and cystic changes in the ovarian remnant itself [4, 5, 7], which all may contribute to formation of adhesions. In humans, ORS is usually associated with extensive adhesions. However, abdominal inflammatory lesions, mainly endometriosis, are pre-existing to the original oophorectomy in most human patients, and recurrence of these lesions are associated with the ovarian remnant [41], which is not the case in dogs.

The significant relation between surgery duration and postoperative convalescence duration has not been described before. In humans, postoperative convalescence is mainly affected by postoperative pain [42], which seems affected most by pneumoperitoneum pressure level through stretching of peritoneum and diaphragm and possibly chemical irritation of CO_2 gas [43]. One could argue that prolonged pneumoperitoneum might also increase postoperative pain and convalescence period in dogs. This was however not an objective of the present study and no attempt was made to quantify post-operative pain. Nonetheless, recovery duration was short and comparable to that of laparoscopic ovariectomy [44, 45].

Using a VSD for dissection of adhesions and excision of tissues was convenient and very effective. The VSD was often also used as a mechanical dissecting forceps for dissecting and sealing of tissues with only minimal hemorrhage. Because ovarian remnants may be just a few millimeters in size, we suggest to remove all abnormal tissue that has some noticeable vasculature, small cyst-like changes, clear discoloration, or adhesions.

The diagnostic value of preoperative ultrasound was higher in the present study than previously reported [4, 8]. However, ultrasound alone cannot be used to prove or rule out the existence of functional ovarian tissue. The variation in results in Table 2 between the left and right ovarian pedicle area is probably caused by the relatively low numbers of ovarian remnants on the left side. The relatively low value for overall specificity (74%) of ultrasound diagnosis of the position of an ovarian remnant is largely explained by the high numbers of false positive diagnoses for the left ovarian pedicle area. This may be due to a much lower incidence of ovarian remnant tissue on this side making the chance of false positive diagnosis higher for the left side than for the right side. On the other hand, false positive diagnosis is also affected by detection of scar tissue because ultrasound may not be able to reliably differentiate between scar tissue and an actual ovarian remnant in all cases. Since scar tissue can often not be reliably differentiated from small ovarian remnants by the naked eye and is therefore removed during surgery, the detection of a pedicle scar with ultrasound is considered helpful for ORS surgery. Knowing the location and approximate size of abnormalities seen with ultrasound may help deciding when to stop or go on with searching for abnormalities, especially in patients with extensive adhesions or obesity where only a small remnant was found during surgery. A thorough presurgical evaluation using ultrasonography will help in determining the location and number of abnormalities and thus the surgical strategy. We suggest to always have an ultrasound performed before surgery to lower the risk of an unsuccessful 'goose' hunt.

Histology proved that ovarian remnants were removed from all dogs in the present study. Sizes of remnants varied from several millimeters up to complete ovaries and cystic changes of several cm's. Occasionally, large uterine cysts (up to 6 cm) were encountered, possibly caused by retention of fluid in the uterine lumen cranial to the site of ligation of the uterine horn. Two ovarian remnants turned out to contain a granulosa cell tumor. Formation of granulosa cell tumors in ovarian remnants is relatively common [4, 36]. The true incidence and/or causes of tumor formation in ovarian remnants are unknown. It has been suggested that increased gonadotropin levels may increase the risk of ovarian tumor formation in humans. The same may be true in dogs [36].

All results of follow-up GnRH stimulation tests were consistent with absence of ovarian tissue. These findings were confirmed clinically by the absence of clinical signs of ORS in all, but one, dogs after a median follow-up period of 22.5 months. This one dog continued to show increased attractiveness to male dogs according to the owners. However, the dog was tested negative by GnRH stimulation test 16 months postoperative, was herself not interested in male dogs, and was free of any other sign of ORS after a follow-up period of 51 months. Therefore, attractiveness to male dogs in this animal is most probably caused by another reason. Follow-up clinical investigation other than a GnRH stimulation test was however not performed in this dog.

There was an apparent trend of higher mean basal estradiol values in the GnRH stimulation test results in the early cases (Table 3). These cases also had a longer interval between surgery and GnRH stimulation test. A certain low basal plasma estradiol concentration is normally seen in dogs after gonadectomy, which might be a consequence of endogenous estradiol from conversion of androstenediol from the adrenal cortex [46]. Although not reported before, this process may change in time after surgery, as is the case for LH and FSH plasma levels [38, 47]. Nonetheless, estradiol did not increase after GnRH administration and was below the cut-off value at all times as expected after OVE/OVH (Table 3). The basal FSH of dog nr. 13 could in theory fit with an intact dog (< 11.0 µg/l) [38]. However, more importantly, basal plasma estradiol was low and both FSH and estradiol levels did not increase after GnRH administration, which is consistent with absence of ovarian tissue. It has been described that gonadotrophic hormones are decreased between 4 to 10 weeks after OVE/OVH, after which they steadily increase until week 42 [47]. This is one of the reasons that we preferably performed GnRH stimulation tests after a longer time interval and may explain the low basal plasma FSH in this dog, since it was tested only 1 month after surgery.

Study limitations

This study prospectively evaluated the feasibility and efficacy of laparoscopic ovarian remnant removal in dogs. The laparoscopic approach provided a clear and detailed visibility of abdominal tissues combined with a short recovery period. However, several intraoperative observations were subjectively scored and because of the lack of a control group, statistical comparison with an open celiotomy approach was not possible.

Several follow-up data were subjectively scored by owners by means of telephone questionnaires, which may have been subject to bias and owner opinion.

Conclusion

Findings in the study reported here support the theory that ORS is caused by surgical error, with an overrepresentation of right-sided ovarian remnants in predominantly medium and large sized dogs.

A laparoscopic approach for the removal of ovarian remnants in dogs was feasible and effective. The ability to change the position of the patient during the procedure, tilting sideways and in steep Trendelenburg position, is a requirement for proper access to both pedicle areas. A VSD facilitated good tissue dissecting and excision ability. The high success rate of this approach makes laparoscopic treatment of ORS a valid and appealing alternative to open laparotomy.

Abbreviations

E_2: Estrogen; IQR: Inter quartile range; ORS: Ovarian remnant syndrome; OVE: Ovariectomy; OVH: Ovariohysterectomy; P_4: Progesterone; Sd: Standard deviation; VSD: Vessel sealing device

Acknowledgements

The authors would like to thank their colleagues of the department of Veterinary Diagnostic Imaging and the Veterinary Pathology Diagnostic Centre of the Faculty of Veterinary Medicine, Utrecht University, for their involvement in the present study; drs. C.H.Y. Oei from the Veterinary Diagnostic Laboratory for processing blood samples and determining plasma hormone levels for the GnRH stimulation tests; drs. L.N.F. van Hövell for his help with data accrual and GnRH stimulation testing for his master student thesis.

Funding

A research grant by the Dutch Society for Veterinary Research in Companion Animals (Stichting D.O.G.) [35] enabled follow-up GnRH-testing in the first 13 dogs without additional costs for the owners. Funding was granted based on the existing study proposal and was purely financial. Stichting D.O.G. was not involved in the design of the study and collection, analysis, and interpretation of data and in writing the manuscript.

Authors' contributions

SvN, JK, and BVG were all involved in the accrual of patients and surgical data and acted as primary surgeons of the cases in the present study. SvN wrote the main text and was primarily responsible for data accrual and analysis. JdG was involved in patient accrual, diagnostic work-up, and interpretation of GnRH stimulation test results. All authors made important specific contributions to and approved the final manuscript.

Consent for publication

Not applicable.

Competing interests

The authors declare that they have no competing interests.

Author details

[1]Department of Clinical Sciences of Companion Animals, Faculty of Veterinary Medicine, Utrecht University, Yalelaan 108, 3584CM, Utrecht, the Netherlands. [2]Department of Small Animal Medicine, Faculty of Veterinary Medicine, Ghent University, Salisburylaan 133, 9820 Merelbeke, Belgium. [3]Hill's Pet Nutrition, 400 SW 8th Ave, Topeka, KS 66603, USA.

References

1. Okkens AC, Kooistra HS, Nickel RF. Comparison of long-term effects of ovariectomy versus ovariohysterectomy in bitches. J Reprod Fertil Suppl. 1997;51:227–31.
2. Muraro L, White RS. Complications of ovariohysterectomy procedures performed in 1880 dogs. Tierarztl Prax Ausg K Kleintiere Heimtiere. 2014;42: 297–302.
3. Pope JFA, Knowles TG. Retrospective analysis of the learning curve associated with laparoscopic Ovariectomy in dogs and associated perioperative complication rates. Vet Surg. 2014;43:668–77.
4. Ball RL, Birchard SJ, May LR, Threlfall WR, Young GS. Ovarian remnant syndrome in dogs and cats: 21 cases (2000-2007). J Am Vet Med Assoc. 2010;236:548–53.
5. Wallace MS. The ovarian remnant syndrome in the bitch and queen. Vet Clin North Am Small Anim Pract. 1991;21:501–7.
6. Miller DM. Ovarian remnant syndrome in dogs and cats: 46 cases (1988-1992). J Vet Diagn Investig. 1995;7:572–4.
7. Okkens AC, Dieleman SJ, v d Gaag I. Gynaecological complications following ovariohysterectomy in dogs, due to: (1) partial removal of the ovaries. (2) inflammation of the uterocervical stump (author's transl). Tijdschr Diergeneeskd. 1981;106:1142–58.
8. Buijtels JJCWM, de Gier J, Kooistra HS, Naan EC, Oei CHY, Okkens a C. The pituitary-ovarian axis in dogs with remnant ovarian tissue. Theriogenology. Elsevier Inc. 2011;75:742–51.
9. Pearson H. The complications of ovariohysterectomy in the bitch. J Small Anim Pract. 1973;14:257–66.
10. Pöppl AG, Mottin TS, FHD G. Diabetes mellitus remission after resolution of inflammatory and progesterone-related conditions in bitches. Res Vet Sci. 2013;94:471–3.
11. Parker K, Snead E. Atypical presentation of ovarian remnant syndrome in a dog. J Am Anim Hosp Assoc. 2014;50:e1–5.
12. Kho RM, Abrao MS. Ovarian remnant syndrome: etiology, diagnosis, treatment and impact of endometriosis. Curr Opin Obstet Gynecol. 2012;24:210–4.
13. Post K. Canine vaginal cytology during the estrous cycle. Can Vet J. 1985;26: 101–4.
14. Howe LM. Surgical methods of contraception and sterilization. Theriogenology. 2006;66:500–9.
15. Naiman JH, Mayhew PD, Steffey MA, Culp WT, Runge JJ, Singh A. Laparoscopic treatment of ovarian remnant syndrome in dogs and cats: 7 cases (2010-2013). J Am Vet Med Assoc. 2014;245:1251–7.
16. Fransson BA. Ovaries and uterus. In: Tobias KM, Johnston SA, editors. Vet Surg Small Anim. 1st ed. Saunders; 2012. p. 1871–91.
17. Feldman EC, Nelson RW. Fertility, associated breeding disorders, and disorders of sexual development. In: Feldman EC, Nelson RW, editors. Canine feline Endocrinol Reprod. 3rd ed. St Louis: Saunders; 2004. p. 868.
18. Culp WTN, Mayhew PD, Brown DC. The effect of laparoscopic versus open ovariectomy on postsurgical activity in small dogs. Vet Surg. 2009;38:811–7.
19. Davidson EB, Moll HD, Payton ME. Comparison of laparoscopic ovariohysterectomy and ovariohysterectomy in dogs. Vet Surg. 2004;33:62–9.
20. Hancock RB, Lanz OI, Waldron DR, Duncan RB, Broadstone RV, Hendrix PK. Comparison of postoperative pain after ovariohysterectomy by harmonic scalpel-assisted laparoscopy compared with median celiotomy and ligation in dogs. Vet Surg VS off J am Coll. Vet Surg. 2005;34:273–82.
21. Devitt CM, Cox RE, Hailey JJ. Duration, complications, stress, and pain of open ovariohysterectomy versus a simple method of laparoscopic-assisted ovariohysterectomy in dogs. J Am Vet Med Assoc. 2005;227:921–7.
22. Case JB, Boscan PL, Monnet EL, Niyom SR, Imhoff DJ, Wallace ML, et al. Comparison of surgical variables and pain in cats undergoing ovariohysterectomy, laparoscopic-assisted ovariohysterectomy, and Laparoscopic Ovariectomy. J Am Anim Hosp Assoc. 2015;51:1–7.
23. Nickel R, Sturtzbecher N, Kilian H, Arndt G, Brunnberg L. Postoperative Rekonvaleszenz nach laparoskopischer und konventioneller ovariektomie: eine vergleichende studie. Kleintierpraxis. 2007;52:413–24.
24. Lee JY, Kim MC. Comparison of oxidative stress status in dogs undergoing laparoscopic and open ovariectomy. J Vet Med Sci. 2014;76:273–6.
25. Höglund OV, Olsson K, Hagman R, Öhlund M, Olsson U, Lagerstedt AS. Comparison of haemodynamic changes during two surgical methods for neutering female dogs. Res Vet Sci. 2011;91:159–63.
26. Nezhat F, Nezhat C. Operative laparoscopy for the treatment of ovarian remnant syndrome. Fertil Steril. 1992;57:1003–7.
27. Nezhat C, Kearney S, Malik S, Nezhat C, Nezhat F. Laparoscopic management of ovarian remnant. Fertil Steril. 2005;83:973–8.
28. Abu-Rafeh B, Vilos GA, Misra M. Frequency and laparoscopic management of ovarian remnant syndrome. J Am Assoc Gynecol Laparosc. 2003;10:33–7.
29. Kho RM, Magrina JF, Magtibay PM. Pathologic findings and outcomes of a minimally invasive approach to ovarian remnant syndrome. Fertil Steril. 2007;87: 1005–9.
30. Zapardiel I, Zanagnolo V, Kho RM, Magrina JF, Magtibay PM. Ovarian remnant syndrome: comparison of laparotomy, laparoscopy and robotic surgery. Acta Obstet Gynecol Scand. 2012;91:965–9.
31. Krauss Z, Krauss M. Magnetic resonance imaging and laparoscopic management of an ovarian remnant in a bitch. Tierarztl Prax Ausg K Kleintiere Heimtiere. 2015;43:111–4.
32. Finger BL, Brun MV, Colomé LM, Pimentel RO, Feranti JPS. Videolaparoscopia no diagnóstico e tratamento da síndrome do ovário remanescente em uma gata. Ciência Rural Universidade Federal de Santa Maria. 2009;39:2539–41.
33. Brückner M. Laparoscopy for the treatment of ovarian remnant syndrome in four dogs and two cats. Tierärztliche Praxis Ausgabe K, Kleintiere/Heimtiere. 2016;44:86–92.
34. Phipps WE, Goodman AR, Sullivan M. Ovarian remnant removal using minimally invasive laparoscopic techniques in four dogs. J Small Anim Pract. 2016;57:214–6.
35. Stichting Diergeneeskundig Onderzoek Gezelschapsdieren (D.O.G.). Available from: www.stichtingdog.nl
36. Buijtels JJCWM, de Gier J, Kooistra HS, Kroeze EJBV, Okkens AC. Alterations of the pituitary-ovarian axis in dogs with a functional granulosa cell tumor. Theriogenology. 2010;73:11–9.
37. Ternamian AM. A trocarless, reusable, visual-access cannula for safer laparoscopy; an update. J Am Assoc Gynecol Laparosc. 1998;5:197–201.
38. de Gier J, Buijtels JJCWM, Albers-Wolthers CHJ, Oei CHY, Kooistra HS, Okkens AC. Effects of gonadotropin-releasing hormone administration on the pituitary-gonadal axis in male and female dogs before and after gonadectomy. Theriogenology. 2012;77:967–78.
39. van Haaften B, Bevers MM, van den Brom WE, Okkens AC, van Sluijs FJ, Willemse AH, et al. Increasing sensitivity of the pituitary to GnRH from early to late anoestrus in the beagle bitch. J Reprod Fertil. 1994;101: 221–5.
40. Van Goethem B, Schaefers-Okkens A, Kirpensteijn J. Making a rational choice between ovariectomy and ovariohysterectomy in the dog: a discussion of the benefits of either technique. Vet Surg. 2006;35:136–43.
41. Kho RM, Abrao MS. Ovarian remnant syndrome: Etiology, diagnosis, treatment and impact of endometriosis. Curr Opin Obstet Gynecol. 2012;24:210–4.
42. Bisgaard T, Kehlet H, Rosenberg J. Pain and convalescence after laparoscopic cholecystectomy. Eur J Surg. 2001;167:84–96.
43. Donatsky AM, Bjerrum F, Gögenur I. Surgical techniques to minimize shoulder pain after laparoscopic cholecystectomy. A systematic review Surg Endosc. 2013;27:2275–82.
44. Van Nimwegen SA, Kirpensteijn J. Comparison of Nd:YAG surgical laser and remorgida bipolar electrosurgery forceps for canine laparoscopic ovariectomy. Vet Surg. 2007;36:533–40.
45. Van Nimwegen SA, Van Swol CFP, Kirpensteijn J. Neodymium:yttrium aluminum garnet surgical laser versus bipolar electrocoagulation for laparoscopic ovariectomy in dogs. Vet Surg. 34:353–7.
46. Nelson LR, Bulun SE. Estrogen production and action. J Am Acad Dermatol. 2001;45:S116–24.
47. Reichler IM, Pfeiffer E, Piché CA, Jöchle W, Roos M, Hubler M, et al. Changes in plasma gonadotropin concentrations and urethral closure pressure in the bitch during the 12 months following ovariectomy. Theriogenology. 2004; 62:1391–402.

19

Retrograde intubation in a dog with severe temporomandibular joint ankylosis

Verónica Vieitez[1*], Luis Javier Ezquerra[1], Víctor López Rámis[1], Massimo Santella[1] and Ignacio Álvarez Gómez de Segura[2]

Abstract

Background: Orotracheal intubation in dogs is a common and easily-performed procedure that provides a patent airway during anaesthesia. In dogs with temporomandibular joint ankylosis or pseudo-ankylosis, airway management can be a challenging procedure since these dogs have a limited ability to open their mouth. Methods to provide safe, uneventful intubation in such patients may include minimally invasive techniques such as retrograde intubation using a guide wire and fibre-optic-aided laryngoscopy.

Case presentation: We report a case of a 16-month-old, intact female Bull Terrier weighing 17 kg, admitted to the hospital for surgical treatment of bilateral ankylosis of the temporomandibular joint. Intubation was achieved, without direct observation of the larynx, by retrograde intubation using a vascular access catheter and a vascular wire guide through cricothyroid membrane. Bilateral condylectomy was performed and the dog recovered uneventfully.

Conclusions: In conclusion, retrograde intubation was relatively simple to perform with the guide wire technique and no specific training or equipment were necessary.

Keywords: Dog, Difficult airway, Retrograde intubation

Background

Orotracheal intubation in dogs is a routine procedure, providing a patent airway through which to deliver oxygen and inhalant anaesthetic while facilitating ventilation and preventing aspiration of regurgitated material. Orotracheal intubation in dogs is an easily performed technique when using an adequately sized endotracheal tube (ETT) and adequate lighting. However, the use of a laryngoscope is always advised [1].

The "difficult airway" has traditionally been used to describe endotracheal intubation in patients with anatomic characteristics than make visualization of the vocal cords and placement of the endotracheal tube challenging [2]. The difficult airway is a rare condition in dogs, but in other species such as rabbits [3], camelids [4], pig [5] or mice [6], endotracheal intubation is considered technically difficult due to specific anatomical characteristics including size, a long, narrow oropharynx, large tongue, and limited mobility of temporomandibular joint (TMJ), which limit visualisation of the larynx.

Intubation in dogs with restricted mouth opening does not allow the use of laryngoscope and visualisation of the glottis. In people, a variety of pathological conditions such as TMJ ankylosis, oral submucosal fibrosis, and infection of the head and neck region are associated with reduction in mouth opening, making the intubation process difficult [7]. A variety of endotracheal intubation techniques have been advocated to manage the difficult airway, which include blind nasal intubation, retrograde intubation (RI), fibre-optic laryngoscopy and tracheostomy [8]. The RI of the trachea is an established airway management technique that can be used to place an ETT when more conventional methods (e.g. direct laryngoscopy) have failed [9].

The RI was reported in the early 1960s [10] as an alternative tool for unplanned preoperative tracheostomies

* Correspondence: vvieitez@gmail.com
[1]Veterinary Teaching Hospital, University of Extremadura, Avda, Universidad s/n, 10003 Cáceres, Spain
Full list of author information is available at the end of the article

in humans. This technique has evolved and is considered an approved method by the American Society of Anesthesiologists for the management of the difficult airways [11]. The elective use of RI is well-documented in patients with angioedema [12] deep neck infection [13], burns [14], trismus [15], musculoskeletal disorders [16], and patients in the prehospital or emergency room [17] and trauma setting [18]. In veterinary medicine, RI has been proposed as an alternative to conventional orotracheal intubation in mice [6], llamas [4], and rabbits [19]. Contraindications to the procedure include coagulation abnormalities, infection at the intended site of puncture, pre-tracheal mass and poorly palpable landmarks in the neck [18].

The relevance of this report relies on the fact that management of the difficult airway in dogs is scarcely documented [1]. Although flexible fibre-optic guided endotracheal intubation is the technique of choice for managing the difficult airway, its cost and availability of the device has limited its use. Therefore, RI is a practical alternative to manage these patients, also when fibre-optic guided technique fails [20]. The objective of this report was to describe a case in which RI was used electively in a dog with difficult airway due to severe TMJ ankylosis and limited mouth opening.

Case presentation

A 16-month-old, intact female Bull Terrier weighing 17 kg was admitted to the hospital for the surgical treatment of bilateral ankylosis of the TMJ. The dog had been previously treated by the referring veterinarian with prednisolone (Dacortin 30 mg; Merck. Madrid, Spain) at a dose of 2 mg/kg orally once daily for 2 weeks. Clinical examination revealed a 4-mm mouth opening with minimal space between the maxillary and mandibular incisor teeth and atrophy of the temporal and masseter muscles. The results of physical examination, haematological and biochemical blood tests were unremarkable. A bilateral condylectomy was scheduled to treat the TMJ ankylosis.

Conventional orotracheal intubation was not considered, as direct visualization of the larynx would have been impossible due to the limited movement and opening of the TMJ. Therefore, RI was planned and the required equipment for RI and temporary tracheostomy were prepared.

Food, but not water, was withheld for 12 h prior to anaesthesia. A 20-gauge cephalic venous catheter (Insyte; Becton Dickinson. Singapore) was then aseptically placed. The dog was premedicated with intravenous acepromazine (Equipromacina; Labiana. Barcelona, Spain), 0.05 mg/kg and subcutaneous meperidine (Dolantina; Kern Pharma, Barcelona, Spain) 5 mg/kg, 30 min prior to induction. Following pre-oxygenation with 100% oxygen via a facemask (10 min), anaesthesia was induced with propofol (Vetofol; Esteve, Barcelona, Spain) titrated slowly to effect by administering initially as a bolus at 2 mg/kg over 30 s, followed by incremental doses at 0.5 mg/kg every 15 s with a total dose of 4 mg/kg. Then, a continuous rate infusion (CRI) of propofol (0.4 mg/kg/min) was started until the RI was performed (approximately 5 min later). Attempts at opening the mouth while the dog was anesthetized were unsuccessful and the maximum opening of the mouth only allowed the passage of a 6 mm (internal diameter, ID) endotracheal tube between the incisors.

For the RI technique, the dog was positioned in right lateral recumbency. The cricothyroid membrane was palpated and the skin over the trachea was clipped and aseptically prepared. A venous catheter 16-gauge (Insyte; Becton Dickinson. Singapore) and a Seldinger's wire guide 0.8 mm diameter (Cook medical Limerick, Ireland) were used for RI technique. The anaesthetist was positioned in front of the dog and the larynx palpated and stabilized with the left hand while the cricothyroid membrane was punctured with a 16-gauge over-the-needle vascular access catheter. The needle was partially withdrawn into the catheter while it was advanced with a 45° angle in rostral direction. Tracheal placement of the catheter was confirmed by a lack of resistance to air aspiration through the catheter with a 6 mL syringe. The needle was removed and the wire guide was inserted throughout the catheter and advanced to the mouth opening. Then, the cannula was removed and the cricothyroid end of the wire guide was grasped with forceps to secure it. A cuffed ETT (6 mm ID) was passed caudally over the guide and into the larynx. Simultaneously, the mouth was forced open slightly to facilitate the tube passage between the incisive teeth. Once the ETT reached the entrance of the wire guide (previously measured) at the cricothyroid membrane, the wire guide was removed while slightly pushing the ETT to maintain its tip in the larynx. Then, the ETT was advanced into the trachea as the hold of the guide was removed (Fig. 1). Correct position of the ETT was confirmed using sidestream capnography (S/5 Anesthesia monitor: General Electric. WI, USA). The cuff was inflated immediately and the tube fixed.

Once intubated, the ETT was attached to the anaesthetic rebreathing system and mechanical ventilation was started using a pressure-controlled mechanical ventilator (Stephan ABC: Gackenbach, Germany). Peak inspiratory pressure (PIP) was set between 10 and 12 cm H_2O, and f_R was adjusted to maintain normocapnia (partial pressure of expired carbon dioxide, $PE'CO_2$ = 35-45 mmHg). The propofol infusion was stopped and anaesthesia was maintained with isoflurane (Isoflo 100%: Abbott. UK) delivered in 100% oxygen. Midazolam (Dormicum; Roche, Madrid, Spain) 0. 5 mg/kg and fentanyl (Fentanest; Kern Pharma, Barcelona, Spain) 5 μg/kg were administered IV slowly over 60 s,

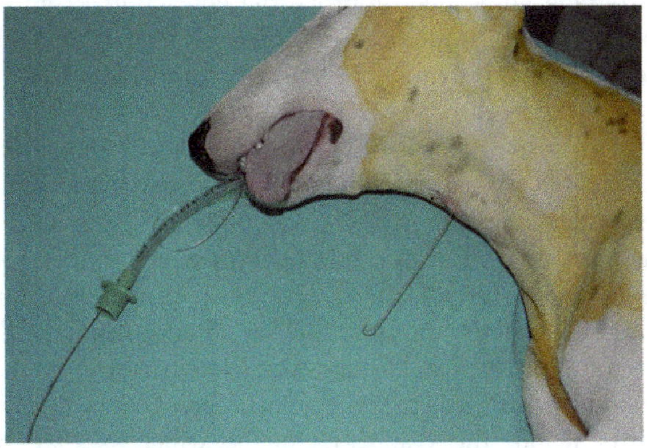

Fig. 1 Lateral view of the dog. A vascular guide wire, advanced through the cricothyroid membrane and the larynx, can be observed exiting the mouth. The tip of the endotracheal tube is advanced over the wire guide through the mouth opening and advanced beyond the vocal cords into the larynx

followed by a CRI of midazolam (0.15 mg/kg/h) and fentanyl (6 μg/kg/h) administered IV throughout surgery using infusion pumps (Perfusor; BBraun, Germany).

Continuous electrocardiography, HR, f_R, pulse oximetry (SpO_2), $PE'CO_2$, end-tidal isoflurane (F_E'Iso) and inspired fraction of oxygen (F_IO_2) were monitored throughout anaesthesia using a multiparametric monitor (S/5 Anesthesia monitor: General Electric. WI, USA). Arterial blood pressure was measured noninvasively using a Doppler monitor (811-B; Parks Medical, OR, USA) with the probe placed on the metacarpal artery and fixed with tape.

After monitoring instruments were applied, left and right mandibular and maxillary nerve blocks were performed with the dog in lateral recumbency. After aseptic scrubbing of both lateral aspects of the face and neck, an extra-oral approach was used for left and right mandibular nerve block; a 22-gauge needle was inserted at the lower angle of the jaw approximately 0.5 cm rostral to the angular process and was advanced 2 cm dorsally along the medial surface of the ramus of the mandible. Bupivacaine (Bupivacaina 0.5%; Fresenius, Barcelona, Spain) 1 mL was injected blindly, because intraoral palpation of the mandibular foramen was not possible due to the limited mouth opening. For the maxillary nerve block, the needle was placed percutaneously along the ventral border of the zygomatic process approximately 0. 5 cm caudal to the lateral canthus of the eye and advanced into close proximity of the pterygopalatine fossa. Bupivacaine 0.5% 1 mL was injected on each site. A total of 20 mg of bupivacaine (1.2 mg/kg) was administered.

Lactated Ringer's solution (Ringer Lactato: B.Braun. Barcelona, Spain) was infused IV during surgery at 10 mL/kg/h. Cefazolin (Cefazolina: Normon. Madrid, Spain) 22 mg/kg was administered IV 30 min prior to surgical incision and then every 90 min throughout surgery. During surgery, F_E'Iso ranged between 0.8 and 1. 2%, HR between 77 and 84 beats/min, and systolic blood pressure between 90 and 120 mmHg. The SpO_2 remained above 98% and $PE'CO_2$ was between 35 and 45 mmHg.

The bilateral condylectomy was performed successfully. After completion of surgery, isoflurane delivery, midazolam and fentanyl CRIs were stopped. Morphine (Morfina 1%: Fresenius. Barcelona, Spain) 0.5 mg/kg and dexamethasone (0.5 mg/kg) IV were administered. Mechanical ventilation was maintained until attempts to breathe spontaneously were observed. The ETT remained in place until laryngeal reflexes returned 30 min after the isoflurane was discontinued. The dog had a quiet, calm recovery, with no signs of anxiety or dysphoria, and was transferred to a quiet, warm room. Total anaesthesia time (from anaesthetic induction to cessation of isoflurane delivery) lasted 170 min. Postoperative assessment of pain (Short Form of the Glasgow Composite Pain Scale) and physiological parameters were conducted hourly until discharge with no detected complications related to RI.

Postoperative analgesia was provided with morphine 0. 5 mg/kg IV every 4-6 h as required for 24 h. Dexamethasone (Cortesona 2 mg mL^{-1}; Laboratorios Syva, León, Spain) 0.2 mg/kg was administered IV daily for 3 days. The dog was able to eat soft food, 4 h after extubation. Physical therapy 3-4 times daily included passive manually opening the jaw, holding it open for 5 s with moderate traction, and then closing the jaw. The diet was replaced with hard food immediately. One month after surgery the jaw opened correctly in an almost normal range.

Discussion

Alternative methods to orotracheal intubation are more commonly used in species other than dogs. Nasotracheal intubation has been described as an alternative method of intubation in rabbits [3], foals [21], calves [22], and llamas [23]. The RI has been evaluated in mice [6], llamas [4], and rabbits [19] and, briefly, as an alternative method of intubation in dogs [1].

In the present case, RI was preferred compared to other techniques or methods for several reasons. The laryngeal mask is an effective, non-invasive method of securing an airway in dogs, cats, pigs and rabbits [24–27]. It has been employed to provide a patent airway in a brachycephalic dog with suspected masticatory myositis and trismus (2 cm of mouth opened) [28]. However, in our case, a smaller mouth opening prevented its use.

Fibre-optic-assisted nasotracheal intubation is the technique of choice for difficult airway management in people [29]. However, the cost of the equipment and the required skills and expertise necessary for its use makes the RI technique preferable in veterinary medicine [7]. The main advantage of this latter technique over the more commonly employed anterograde techniques of tracheal intubation is that the laryngeal inlet does not have to be identified. It is a minimally invasive, feasible, and cost effective airway management technique in people with restricted mouth opening [7]. Unlike fibreoptic bronchoscope-guided endotracheal intubation, RI can be used when blood or secretions are present in the upper airway, where the former technique is difficult or impossible [30]. In this case, a flexible bronchoscopy device would have been an alternative for endotracheal intubation, but bronchoscope small enough to fit a 6 mm ETT is required and was not available.

A blind insertion airway device, the double lumen airway device (Combitube), has been evaluated in dogs [31] to provide ventilatory support. However, due to the inability to consistently seal the airway, the caudal aspect of the mouth is not fully protected for maxillofacial procedures including mandibular resection [31]. Additionally, the size of the device (11.1-12.1 mm in diameter) should have prevented its use.

In human another alternative method is fluoroscopic assisted airway intubation [32] using a nasal approach. Nasotracheal intubation has not been described in dogs, probably due to the small size of the nasal airways, which makes intubation traumatic or impossible. Also fluoroscopic guidance would unnecessarily expose personnel to radiation. Therefore, after considering all potential alternatives, RI was considered the most suitable way to establish and maintain a patent airway while avoiding tracheostomy.

The RI can be performed with minimal equipment. Although the RI set (Retrograde Intubation Set: Cook, Bloomington, IN, USA) is preferable, a standard venous catheter and epidural catheter or Seldinger's wire can be used for retrograde technique. This allows the technique to be employed by almost any clinical practice [7].

There are some differences in RI between humans and animals. In rabbits, the trachea is small, movable and more difficult to puncture and may require surgical exposure to insert the guide via direct puncture of the tracheal wall [19]. In llamas, incision of the skin over the trachea and between two tracheal rings has been performed [4]. However in humans like in dogs, the cricothyroid membrane is easy to localize and puncture, facilitating the introduction of the guide. Although the short distance between the cricothyroid membrane and the vocal cords allows the unattached wire to inadvertently be withdrawn above the cords, thereby losing tracheal access and increasing the risk of failed intubation [9]. In humans, the insertion of a catheter into the trachea before the removal of the guide wire may help to cope with this problem [20]. Anterograde over a retrograde guide may improve the efficacy of RI and is considered to be a more reliable and preferable technique for improving the success rate [33] without prolonging its duration [20].

In human medicine the RI encompasses several methods of translaryngeal guided non-surgical airway access to facilitate orotracheal or nasotracheal intubation. It has been used in awake, obtunded or apneic human patients when other methods have been unsuccessful, unavailable or contraindicated [34]. In an effort to make the technique more reliable and easier to perform, RI has undergone numerous modifications. Significant improvements include the Water's technique, which uses an epidural catheter to guide the ETT [35], the use of the Murphy's eye as a conduit for retrograde wire [36], and the pairing of the RI technique with other airway management techniques in an effort to increase the success of the procedure included the use of a fiberoptic bronchoscope [37], a light wand [38], a Combitube [39], a modified Eschmann stylet [40], a laryngeal mask airway [41], a Mini-Trach II kit [42], a Cook airway exchange catheter [43], a gastric tube [44], and even a Fogarty embolectomy catheter [38].

Although RI is reported as a simple and reliable method that can be performed easily and quickly in experienced hands, it has also been associated with a low success rate and a significant risk of complications [45]. In human medicine complications of RI are few; the most common is a sore throat, affecting 60% of the patients [45]. More severe complications are rare and the most common include hypoxemia, cough, laryngospasm/bronchospasm [46], development of hematoma, incorrect site of tube placement, procedure time greater than or equal to 3 min, unsuccessful tube placement, laryngeal fracture with permanent dystonia [33], pneumomediastinum [20], subcutaneous emphysema [47], infection, and bleeding [48].

In a recent retrospective report of 20 patients with restricted mouth opening receiving RI, three patients developed sore throat and cough after intubation, one bronchospasm, and another patient developed wound infection [7]. There are no reports of complications related to this technique in rabbits [19], mice [6], or llamas [4]. In the latter species, RI was evaluated as an alternative to traditional intubation with fewer attempts needed to place the tube and no relevant side effects were observed. Clinicians familiar with camelid and goat intubations considered the RI technique faster and easier, requiring fewer personnel compared with the traditional technique [4].

Conclusion

In conclusion, a dog with severe TMJ ankylosis and limited mouth opening was successfully intubated by RI without complications. The RI technique was considered safe, and minimally invasive, simple to perform and no specific training or equipment was required. Therefore, although new intubation techniques and devices have been developed, the RI remains useful in patients requiring blind orotracheal intubation due to inadequate mouth opening.

Abbreviations

CRI: Continuous rate infusion; ETT: Endotracheal tube; F_E'Iso: End-tidal isoflurane; F_iO_2: Inspired fraction of oxygen; f_R: Respiratory rate; HR: Heart rate; LM: Laryngeal mask; PE'CO_2: Expired carbon dioxide; PIP: Peak inspiratory pressure; RI: Retrograde intubation; SpO_2: Haemoglobin oxygen saturation; TMJ: Temporomandibular joint

Authors' contributions

All authors were implicated in the clinical management of the case. VV drafted the manuscript and provided the figures. All authors revised it critically, provided helpful discussions and final corrections on the manuscript. They read and approved the final version of this manuscript.

Consent for publication

The owner gave her written informed consent for publication by means of signing our official client acceptance form.

Competing interests

The authors declare that they have no competing interests.

Author details

[1]Veterinary Teaching Hospital, University of Extremadura, Avda, Universidad s/n, 10003 Cáceres, Spain. [2]Department of Animal Medicine and Surgery, Veterinary Faculty, University Complutense of Madrid, Avda. Puerta de Hierro, 28040 Madrid, Spain.

References

1. Hartsfield SM. Airway management and ventilation. In: Tranquilli WJ, Thurmon JC, Grimm KA, editors. Lumb & Jones' veterinary anesthesia and analgesia. 4th ed. Iowa: Blackwell. Ames; 2007. p. 495–531.
2. Mosier JM, Joshi R, Hypes C, Pacheco G, Valenzuela T, Sakles JC. The physiologically difficult airway. West J Emerg Med. 2015;16(7):1109–17.
3. Stephens Devalle JM. Successful management of rabbit anesthesia through the use of nasotracheal intubation. J Am Assoc Lab Anim Sci. 2009; 48(2):166–70.
4. Byers SR, Cary JA, Farnsworth KD. Comparison of endotracheal intubation techniques in llamas. Can Vet J. 2009;50(7):745–9.
5. Janiszewski A, Pasławski R, Skrzypczak P, Pasławska U, Szuba A, Nicpoń J. The use of a plastic guide improves the safety and reduces the duration of endotracheal intubation in the pig. J Vet Med Sci. 2014 Oct;76(10):1317–20.
6. Zhao X, Wu N, Zhou J, Yang Y, Fang Y, Cheng W, Ma R, Tian Y, Huang L. A technique for retrograde intubation in mice. Lab Anim. 2006;35(3):39–42.
7. Bhola N, Jadhav A, Borle R, Khemka G, Ajani AA. Awake endotracheal retrograde intubation in restricted mouth opening: a 'J'-tipped guide wire technique–a retrospective study. Oral Maxillofac Surg. 2014;18(4):393–6.
8. Vithal K. Retrograde intubation in temporomandibular joint ankylosis—a double guide wire technique. Indian J Anaesth. 2008;52(1):90–2.
9. Harris EA, Arheart KL, Fischler KE. Does the site of anterior tracheal puncture affect the success rate of retrograde intubation? A prospective, manikin-based study. Anesthesiol Res Pract. 2013;2013:354317.
10. Butler FS, Cirillo AA. Retrograde tracheal intubation. Anesth Analg. 1960; 39:333–8.
11. Collard V, Segura LG, Daaboul DG, Yuki K. Retrograde intubation during laryngeal cleft repair on cardiopulmonary bypass. J Anesth. 2012; 26(2):273–4.
12. Hill C, Martel M, Joing S. Retrograde intubation for ace inhibitor-induced angioedema. Acad Emerg Med. 2008;15(8):791.
13. Wolfe MM, Davis JW, Parks SN. Is surgical airway necessary for airway management in deep neck infections and Ludwig angina? J Crit Care. 2011; 26(1):11–4.
14. Hines MH, Meredith JW. Modified retrograde intubation technique for rapid airway access. Am J Surg. 1990;159(6):597–9.
15. Seavello J, Hammer GB. Tracheal intubation in a child with trismus pseudocamptodactyly (Hecht) syndrome. J Clin Anesth. 1999;11(3):254–6.
16. van Stralen D, Perkin RM. Retrograde intubation difficulty in an 18-year-old muscular dystrophy patient. Am J Emerg Med. 1995;13(1):100–1.
17. Burbulys D, Kiai K. Retrograde intubation. Emerg Med Clin North Am. 2008; 26(4):1029–41.
18. Ramsey CA, Dhaliwal SS. Retrograde and submental intubation. Atlas Oral Maxillofac Surg Clin North Am. 2010;18(1):61–8.
19. Corleta O, Habazettl H, Kreimeier U, Vollmar B. Modified retrograde orotracheal intubation technique for airway access in rabbits. Eur Surg Res. 1992;24(2):129–32.
20. Lenfant F, Benkhadra M, Trouilloud P, Marc F. Comparison of two techniques for retrograde endotracheal intubation in fresh human cadaver. Anesthesiology. 2006;104:48–51.
21. Webb AI. Nasal intubation in the foal. J Am Vet Med Assoc. 1984; 185(1):48–51.
22. Quandt JE, Robinson EP. Nasotracheal intubation in calves. J Am Vet Med Assoc. 1996;209(5):967–8.
23. Riebold TW, Engel HN, Grubb TL, Adams JG, Huber MJ, Schmotzer WB. Orotracheal and nasotracheal intubation in llamas. J Am Vet Med Assoc. 1994;204(5):779–83.
24. Reed F, Iff I. Use of a laryngeal mask airway in a brachycephalic dog with masticatory myositis and trismus. Can Vet J. 2012;53(3):287–90.
25. Kazakos GM, Anagnostou T, Savvas I, et al. Use of the laryngeal mask airway in rabbits: placement and efficacy. Lab Anim. 2007;36:29–34.
26. Braz JR, Martins RH, Mori AR, Luna SP. Investigation into the use of the laryngeal mask airway in pentobarbital anesthetized dogs. Vet Surg. 1999; 28:502–5.
27. Cassu RN, Luna SP, Teixeira Neto FJ, et al. Evaluation of laryngeal mask as an alternative to endotracheal intubation in cats anesthetized under spontaneous or controlled ventilation. Vet Anaesth Analg. 2004;31:213–21.
28. Patil VU, Fairbrother CF, Dunham BM. Use of the laryngeal mask airway for emergency or elective airway management situations in pigs. Contemp Top Lab Anim Sci. 1997;36:46–8.
29. Tüfek A, Uçan MC, Tokgöz O, Çelik F, Ağaçayak S. Evaluation of retrograde intubation in patients with limited mouth opening. J Anesth. 2013; 27(4):631–2.
30. Lama P, Shrestha BR. Retrograde intubation: an alternative way for the management of difficult airway. Kathmandu Univ Med J (KUMJ). 2008; 6(24):516–9.
31. James T, Lane M, Crowe D, Pullen W. A blind insertion airway device in dogs as an alternative to traditional endotracheal intubation. Vet J. 2015; 203(2):187–91.
32. Varughese I, Varughese PI, Soman T, Mathew J. Fluroscopic assisted airway intubation in temporomandibular joint ankylosis: a novel technique. Saudi J Anaesth. 2011;5(2):226–8.
33. Jain G, Singh DK, Yadav G, Gupta SK, Tharwani S. A modification in the tube guide to facilitate retrograde intubation: a prospective, randomised trial. Indian J Anaesth. 2011;55(5):499–503.
34. Rosenblatt WH, Wagner PJ, Ovassapian A. Practice patterns in managing the difficult airway by anesthesiologists in the United States. Anesth Analg. 1998;87:153–7.
35. Waters DJ. Guided blind endotracheal intubation. For patients with deformities of the upper airway. Anaesthesia. 1963;18:158–62.
36. Mahajan R, Sandhya X, Chari P. An alternative technique for retrograde intubation. Anaesthesia. 2001;56(12):1207–8.
37. Lechman MJ, Donahoo JS, Macvaughn H III. Endotracheal intubation using percutaneous retrograde guidewire insertion followed by antegrade fiberoptic bronchoscopy. Crit Care Med. 1986;14(6):589–90.
38. Sharma R. A technique to improve the success of light guided retrograde intubation. Paediatr Anaesth. 2008;18(12):1253–4.
39. Harrison WL, Bertrand ML, Andeweg SK, Clark JA. Retrograde intubation around an in situ combitube: a difficult airway management strategy. Anesthesiology. 2005;102(5):1061–2.
40. Freund PR, Rooke A, Schwid H. Retrograde intubation with a modified Eschmann stylet. Anesth Analg. 1988;67(6):605–6.
41. Arndt GA, Topp J, Hannah J, McDowell TS, Lesko A. Intubation via the LMA using a cook retrograde intubation kit. Can J Anaesth. 1998;45(3):257–60.

42. Slots P, Vegger PB, Bettger H, Reinstrup P. Retrograde intubation with a mini-trach II kit. Acta Anaesthesiol Scand. 2003;47(3):274–7.
43. Leissner KB. Retrograde intubation with epidural catheter and cook airway exchange catheter. Can J Anesth. 2007;54(5):400–1.
44. Gaszyński T. A modified technique of retrograde intubation using gastric tube—a manikin study. Anestezjol Intens Ter. 2009;41(4):230–3.
45. Gill M, Madden MJ, Green SM. Retrograde endotracheal intubation: an investigation of indications, complications, and patient outcomes. Am J Emerg Med. 2005;23(2):123–6.
46. American Society of Anesthesiologists Task Force on Management of the Difficult Airway. Practice guidelines for management of the difficult airway: an updated report by the American Society of Anesthesiologists Task Force on Management of the Difficult Airway. Anesthesiology. 2003;98(5):1269–77.
47. Bowes WA, Johnson JO. Pneumomediastinum after planned retrograde fiberoptic intubation. Anesth Analg. 1994;78:795–7.
48. Wijesinghe H, Gough J. Complications of a retrograde intubation in a trauma patient. Acad Emerg Med. 2000;7:1267–71.

20

Facilitation of arthroscopic visualization and treatment of meniscal tears using a stifle joint distractor in the dog

Gian Luca Rovesti[1], Veronica Devesa[2*], Laura Bertorelli[1] and Jesus Rodriguez-Quiros[3]

Abstract

Background: Stifle arthroscopy has been described to have high sensitivity and specificity in the evaluation of menisci in dogs, particularly for the medial meniscus. However, the visualization of menisci can be difficult. The use of femoral distractors in human medicine has been described to simplify demanding surgical procedures, such as meniscus transplantation. In veterinary medicine, stifle distraction has been reported to facilitate access to the joint and visualization of intra-articular structures, but there are no studies reporting the use of a stifle distraction technique while performing challenging surgical procedures, such as meniscal suture, in clinical patients.
The objective of this study was to evaluate the feasibility, effectiveness and safety of stifle distraction to achieve consistent visualization of menisci and to facilitate performing arthroscopic procedures in clinical patients with stifle disease. Initial arthroscopic evaluation of the stifle joint was performed without distraction in the study population consisting of 13 dogs with naturally occurring stifle disease. The criteria for inclusion was prospectively set as the observation of a frank disease or anomaly of the menisci that could not be further treated or clarified without the risk of damaging the joint cartilage due to the requested manoeuvres. After the first examination, distraction was applied in order to complete the assessment of menisci. After achieving an accurate diagnosis, partial meniscectomy or meniscal repair was performed as needed while maintaining the distraction.

Results: Complete visualization and assessment of menisci were achieved thanks to the use of distraction. This manoeuvre facilitated access to the required area of the involved meniscus, and meniscal treatment could be successfully performed without damaging the articular cartilage. During the follow-up period, no postoperative complication related to the distraction or to the arthroscopic procedure was observed.

Conclusions: Stifle joint distraction during arthroscopy in dogs improves visualization of both menisci, and particularly the caudal horn of the medial meniscus. Despite being a subjective assessment, it is the authors' opinion that this procedure also increases the ease of performing challenging procedures like meniscal suture, as it enlarges the space available to reach the correct working angulations.

Keywords: Arthroscopy, Stifle, Joint distraction, Meniscal surgery, Dog

Background

Stifle arthroscopy has been reported to be the most accurate diagnostic method for evaluating meniscal pathology and for carrying out its treatment, while arthrotomy has resulted in a higher incidence of missed diagnosis [1, 2]. Complete meniscal evaluation in the dog may be a challenging procedure, because adequate and complete visualization of the menisci can be difficult due to the narrow joint space. In addition, in chronic cases with severe synovitis, periarticular fibrosis and capsule thickening, external manipulation may be insufficient to facilitate access to the medial compartment, and visualization of the medial meniscus is difficult [3].

Furthermore, when conditions for treatment of meniscal lesions are present, it is mandatory to have enough room available to perform the requested procedure, particularly for partial meniscectomy and meniscal suture. The latter procedure, though quite demanding, has been described [4, 5],

* Correspondence: veronicadevesagarcia@gmail.com
[2]Madrid, Spain
Full list of author information is available at the end of the article

and the potential for developing the technique could be better if the risk of iatrogenic lesions is low.

Among the techniques used to improve the visualization of the joint compartments, the use of a motorized shaver for fat pad resection and electro cautery for bleeding control have been suggested for stifle arthroscopy [6]. Infrapatellar fat pad resection can cause intra-articular haemorrhage intraoperatively, which can complicate the procedure. Furthermore, the preservation of the infrapatellar fat pad has been associated with an improved outcome in a recent study [7].

Stifle joint distraction causes an increase in the joint space, making arthroscopy easier [8, 9] and reducing the need for fat pad debridement [10]. The use of a femoral distractor has been described to facilitate meniscal treatment in human medicine [11, 12]. It has been reported to be necessary during meniscal transplantation since it facilitates suture placement [12]. In veterinary medicine, a few studies have been published regarding the use of a joint distractor in the stifle joint during arthroscopy [3, 9, 10, 13]. Kim et al. [8] described the use of a stifle distractor in cadaveric joints of toy breed dogs for performing medial meniscal release; Böttcher et al. [3] described the use of a stifle distractor technique in a case series to improve visualization of the medial meniscus and to perform partial meniscectomy if needed; Gemmil and Farrell [10] evaluated a stifle distraction technique in cadaveric stifles and client-owned dogs and performed partial meniscectomy in five cases. Finally, Winkels et al. [9] have recently described the use of the Leipzig stifle distractor to evaluate the medial meniscus in large breed dogs. However, there are no studies reporting the use of a stifle joint distraction technique while performing challenging surgical procedures such as meniscal suture in clinical patients.

Joint distraction procedures have been described as causing potential complications in human medicine, such as soft tissue injuries, fractures or neurovascular damage [14, 15], so they need to be applied carefully. In veterinary medicine, intra-articular pin placement while using an invasive pin distractor in the stifle of two dogs has been described [3]. However, other studies report no complications, tissue damage or fractures when using an invasive joint distractor in different cadaveric joints [13, 16–18]. Complications were also not observed in a recent clinical study [9].

The aim of this study was to evaluate feasibility, effectiveness and safety of the use of a joint distractor in clinical patients, in order to perform arthroscopic meniscal visualization and treatment in a predictable way, reducing the risk of iatrogenic cartilage damage.

Methods

Study population

Dogs were presented to the Clinica Veterinaria M.E. Miller for evaluation for hind limb lameness of at least one month duration due to stifle disease. All patients that underwent stifle arthroscopy from March 26th, 2012 to June 28th, 2013 were examined without distraction as the standard examination. All owners signed the informed consent for stifle arthroscopic examination and potential meniscal treatment. When the menisci could not be seen properly or required treatment, the distractor was used to achieve sufficient intra-articular room either to perform the requested procedure or for further examination. Thirteen stifles in client-owned dogs undergoing stifle arthroscopy for spontaneously occurring stifle disease satisfied the criteria for inclusion.

Perioperative evaluation

Clinical and radiographic evaluations were performed, and stifle disease was diagnosed. All dogs were initially treated by the referring veterinarian with a non-steroidal anti-inflammatory drug, with no or limited improvement. The following clinical tests were performed to assess initial stifle stability: cranial drawer, tibial thrust, and varus/valgus stress. Some dogs showed no clinical stifle instability, though the clinical evaluation showed changes typical of chronic joint involvement. A procedure comprising radiographic study, arthroscopy evaluation and a potential surgical joint stabilization was scheduled in order to obtain either a final diagnosis or as part of a more complex treatment. Before the procedure, a preoperative physical examination and blood test were performed, and no concurrent abnormalities were found.

Distraction technique

Dogs were positioned in dorsal recumbency so that the pelvic limb to be examined could be maintained in its sagittal axis by an assistant. A dog's position was maintained with the use of a foam cushion. The unaffected hind limb was secured in the abducted position.

The distractor device was applied as described previously [13]. A 1.5-mm diameter K-wire was placed through the femoral condyles, halfway between the patella and the fibular head in a latero-medial direction and connected to a traction stirrup (Ad Maiora s.r.l., Cavriago, Italy). A second K-wire was inserted into the middle third of the tibial diaphisis, in a medio-lateral direction, to avoid any potential interference of the hole left by the K-wire when a stabilization procedure of the stifle involving the proximal metaphyseal area was necessary. This K-wire was connected with a second traction stirrup. Then, the distractor (Titan distractor, Ad Maiora s.r.l., Cavriago, Italy) was connected to the stirrups (Fig. 1) [13].

By rotating the distraction knob to lengthen the distractor, a light distraction was applied so as to allow easy entrance into the joint with the scope and instruments. During the procedure, the distraction was increased to achieve a visualization good enough to be able to examine

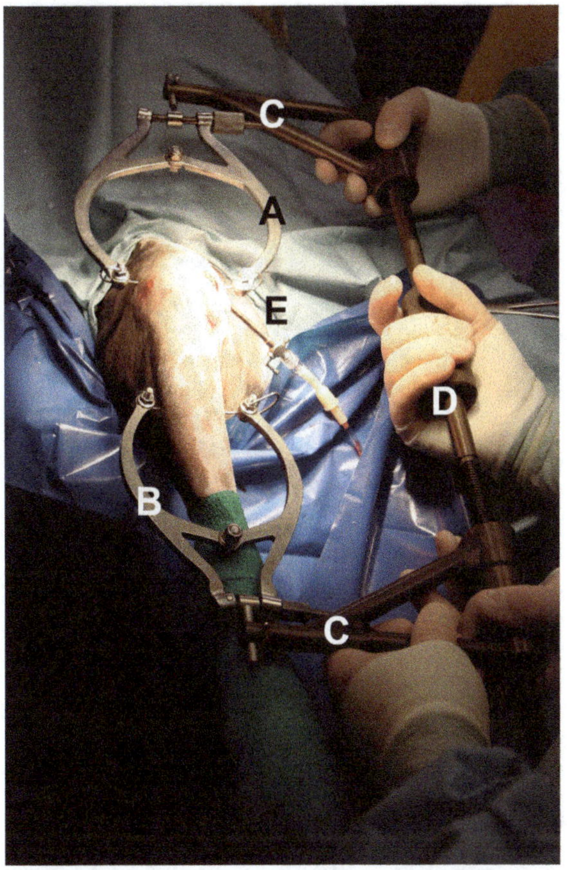

Fig. 1 Intraoperative picture of the applied stifle distractor. The proximal stirrup (**a**) was applied in the area of the femoral condyles, while the distal stirrup (**b**) was applied in the area of the proximal tibial metaphysis. They were both connected to the bone by means of a 1.5-mm K-wire. The stirrups were then connected to the distractor's arms (**c**), and the distraction load was increased as required by turning the knob (**d**) to achieve consistent visualization to perform a complete evaluation of the menisci and to perform the planned surgical procedure. An efflux cannula (**e**) was inserted in the proximo-medial area of the joint

the complete meniscus to achieve an accurate diagnosis and perform the manoeuvres needed in each patient.

Arthroscopic procedure

For the first examination without distraction, the aim was to visualize the proximal pouch, the patella, the femoral trochlea, femoral condyles, the cranial and caudal cruciate ligaments and both menisci, with a technique previously described [6]. After distraction was applied, the scope was introduced through a cranio-medial portal, and the palpation hook was introduced through a cranio-lateral portal (Fig. 1).

A 2.7 mm 30° fore-oblique scope was used to examine the stifle joint in medium and large breed dogs. In smaller dogs, a 2.4 mm 30° fore-oblique scope was used.

For each of the previous structures, a report of the findings was recorded.

Cartilage lesions were classified following a modified Outerbridge classification [19], while meniscal lesions were classified following the classification by Beale [6] (Table 1).

Meniscal treatment was performed accordingly with the diagnosed lesion and it included partial meniscectomy and/or meniscal suture. Partial meniscectomy was performed in cases where meniscal tissue was damaged and displaced and when the lesion was located in the two axial thirds of the meniscus [5, 20, 21]. Meniscal suture was performed in meniscal tears located in the abaxial third of the meniscus (red zone) when enough healthy tissue was present to have sufficient holding force for the suture. The suture of the caudal horn of the medial meniscus was performed following a modified out-in-out technique already described [4, 5]. A 22-G spinal needle was inserted through the cranio-lateral portal and was directed through the meniscal area axial to the lesion. It was then pushed so that it exited in the caudo-medial area of the stifle, where it could be palpated so that its tip was exposed through a stab wound by dissecting delicate soft tissues (Fig. 2). The mandrel of the needle was removed, and a 2-metric polypropylene suture was inserted through the tip of the needle and pushed until it exited the needle hub. The suture was then locked in the hub by a finger, and the needle was retracted until the suture was brought into the joint. Under arthroscopic guidance, the needle was redirected to the desired abaxial location and inserted again through the meniscus, bringing the suture out of the tip. Once the needle tip exited again in the previous caudo-medial area, the loop of the suture was retrieved from the needle tip, leaving the two extremities of the suture exiting from the wound, and the needle was removed from the joint. Once the two extremities of the suture were available through the caudo-medial area of the stifle, a stitch was carefully tightened to lie securely on the subcutaneous fascia. The procedure was repeated as many times as needed (Fig. 3).

Clinical information and time to complete the whole surgical procedure was recorded in each case, as well as the complications encountered in performing the meniscal treatment and in visualizing the intra-articular structures.

Postsurgical care

After surgery, pain management was performed by administration of buprenorphine (Buprenodale®, Dechra

Table 1 Beale's classification for meniscal lesions

a) Vertical longitudinal tears (bucket handle tears and variations)
b) Oblique or flap tears, single or double
c) Radial or transverse tears
d) Horizontal tears
e) Complex, degenerative or macerated tears

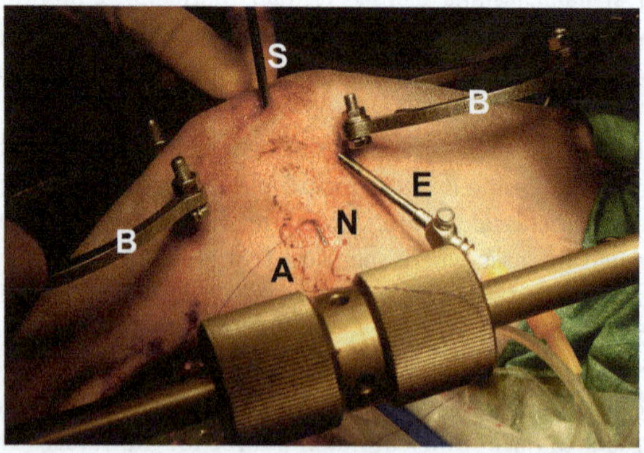

Fig. 2 Image showing the meniscal suture procedure while distracting the stifle joint. Note that the scope (**s**) was in the cranio-medial portal, the efflux cannula (**e**) was in the proximo-medial area and the 22-G spinal needle (**n**) was retrieved in the caudo-medial area of the stifle joint through a stab wound and with minimal soft tissue dissection. The polypropylene suture extremities (**a**) were retrieved through the needle in order to perform the meniscal suture. The distraction stirrups (**b**) did not interfere with the procedure

Limited, Stoke-on-Trent, United Kingdom; 0.01 mg/kg). The dogs were discharged as soon as they recovered from general anaesthesia and vital parameters were stable. They were given meloxicam (Meloxoral®, 0.1 mg/kg once daily, PO, A.T.I. s.r.l. Ozzano Emilia, Italy) for two weeks and tramadol (Altadol®, Formevet s.r.l., Milano, Italy; 3 mg/kg) for five days. Antibiotic therapy with cephalexin (ICF Vet®, I.C.F. Industria Chimica Fine s.r.l. Pignano, Italy; 20 mg/kg twice daily) was administered for one week.

Postsurgical evaluation

Radiographic evaluation was performed after the surgical procedure in all cases. The dogs were usually rechecked clinically and radiographically at 10 and 45 days, or up to bone healing in case an osteotomy technique was performed. In addition, all dogs were clinically evaluated for up to 6 months, and radiographic examination was repeated during this time at the surgeon's decision.

Results

The mean bodyweight of the dogs included in the study was 29 ± 10.4 kg (range, 9.5–53 kg) and the mean age was 5.8 ± 2.8 years old (range, 1–10 years). Six dogs were males and seven females. Four were left and nine were right stifle joints.

After joint distraction, the visualization and careful assessment of the involved structures or the arthroscopic treatment of the diagnosed tear were performed.

Cartilage and meniscal lesion classification

Cartilage and meniscal lesions were classified as described above.

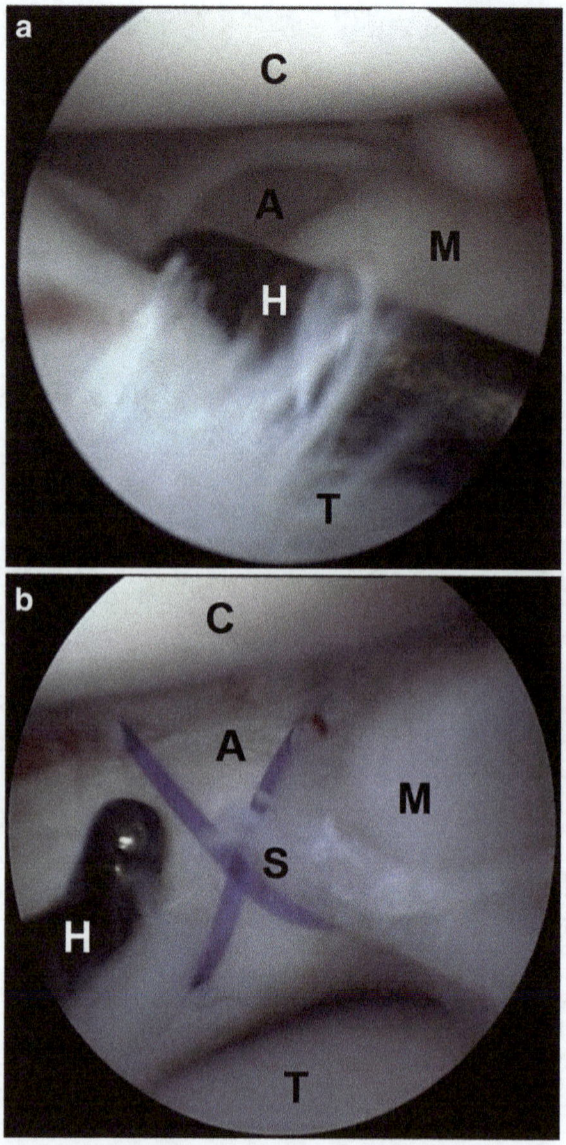

Fig. 3 Arthroscopic images showing a bucket handle lesion (**a**) of the caudal horn of the medial meniscus (**m**) before (**a**) and after (**b**) the out-in-out meniscal suture technique (**s**) in a cruciate pattern. The joint space was increased by means of the stifle distraction device. Note the change of ratio between the joint room and the palpation hook (**h**) and the distance from the femoral condyle (**c**) and the tibial plateau (**t**) before (**a**) and after (**b**) the application of the distraction

A focal cartilage lesion was observed in the medial femoral condyle in one case (case 9), which was classified as grade IV. The corresponding meniscus presented radial lesions that were curetted using a tissue ablator.

Meniscal lesions were also encountered in the remaining cases ($n = 12$). A bucket handle tear was present in seven dogs (lesion type a). The lesion was close to the caudal capsule in four dogs, thus a meniscal suture was performed. The remaining three dogs had a partial meniscectomy, since the location of the lesion was in the two axial thirds and not considered adequate for meniscal healing. Two dogs had meniscal flaps (lesion type b), which were treated by partial meniscectomy in one and meniscal suture in the other. Radial meniscal tears (lesion type c) were observed on both menisci in one dog, and this was treated by radiofrequency ablation of the affected area. Two dogs had complex lesions (lesion type e) of the caudal horn of the medial meniscus that were left untreated, since degenerative signs and macerated tissue were already present (Tables 1 and 2).

Treatment procedures

After the initial joint exploration, the distraction device was applied in order to complete the joint evaluation and perform the planned treatment. Its application took 11 min on average (range, 7–13 min, SD ± 1.9).

In three dogs, joint exploration revealed complex meniscal lesions or cartilage lesions that could not be repaired. In one of them, a focal radiofrequency ablation of the meniscal diseased tissue was performed (Table 2). In these dogs, the mean time to accomplish the entire procedure since the initial visualization without distraction was 58 min (range, 30–100 min; SD ± 30). The remaining dogs ($n = 10$) were diagnosed with a medial meniscal tear. Either partial meniscectomy or meniscal suture was performed according to the meniscal tissue condition. Partial meniscectomy of the medial meniscus was successfully performed in five stifles, while a meniscal suture was also successfully performed in five dogs. The mean time to complete the initial evaluation and the appropriate treatment technique was 117 ± 22 min (range, 85–145 min) (Table 2).

Surgical and postoperative complications

The only complication encountered during the procedures was the breakage of the suture while pushing it through the meniscus by means of a needle in one dog. The reason for this was attributed to calcification of the meniscal tissue, because it felt like a slight crepitus during needle insertion. The problem was managed by repeating the procedure until it was possible to achieve the suture passing through the meniscus. No complications related to the distraction manoeuvre were observed during the surgical procedures. The manipulation of the stifle joints after arthroscopy did not reveal soft tissue damage or instability caused by the distraction procedure in any case.

During the follow-up time, no postoperative complications related to the arthroscopic or distraction procedure were observed.

Discussion

Stifle arthroscopy has been described to have a high sensitivity and specificity in the evaluation of menisci in the dog, particularly for the medial meniscus [1]. However, the visualization of menisci can be difficult: stable joints or chronic cases may affect their evaluation. The use of a femoral distractor during arthroscopic procedures has been described in both human [11, 12] and veterinary medicine [3, 8–10, 13]. It has been reported that stifle joint distraction facilitates joint access, visualization of intra-articular structures, as well as the diagnosis and treatment required. Besides, it has been described to simplify demanding surgical procedures in human medicine, such as meniscus transplantation [12].

In this study, the preliminary arthroscopic examination of the stifle joint was performed without distraction, but detailed evaluation of intra-articular structures was not always possible in some patients until joint distraction was applied. With distraction, complete access to the menisci and their careful evaluation were possible. The distraction provided by such a device is very steady and progressive,

Table 2 Population data, clinical information, treatment and time to complete the whole surgical procedure

Case	Breed	Age (y)	Weight (kg)	Lesion found and meniscal procedure	Time (minutes)
1	Rottweiler	4	53	Complex lesion caudal horn of the medial meniscus. Not treated.	30
2	Labrador Retriever	3	39	Complex lesion and color change of the medial meniscus. Not treated.	100
3	Mixed	6	27	Radial lesions in both menisci. Focal radiofrequency ablation.	45
4	Labrador Retriever	3	30	Bucket handle caudal horn medial meniscus. Meniscal suture.	90
5	Mixed	8	22	Bucket handle caudal horn medial meniscus. Meniscal suture.	100
6	Golden Retriever	1	23	Bucket handle caudal horn medial meniscus. Meniscal suture.	120
7	Mixed	3	17	Bucket handle caudal horn medial meniscus. Meniscal suture.	140
8	Labrador Retriever	8	34	Flap lesion medial meniscus. Meniscal suture.	140
9	German Shepherd	8	32	Cartilage lesione grade IV medial femoral condyle and radial lesion medial meniscus. Partial meniscectomy.	85
10	Springer Spaniel	9	24	Axial bucket handle lesion medial meniscus. Partial meniscectomy.	95
11	Jack Russel Terrier	4	9,5	Axial bucket handle lesion medial meniscus. Partial meniscectomy.	120
12	German Shepherd	9	30	Axial bucket handle lesion medial meniscus. Partial meniscectomy.	140
13	German Shepherd	10	37	Flap lesion medial meniscus. Partial meniscectomy.	145

and it has been shown that the amount of distraction can be about 2 mm in the middle of the femoral condyles in a cadaveric study [13], following the mid-condyle method previously described. Though this distance was not consistently measured in this study, it can be assumed that it could be very similar, because the patients had muscle relaxation due to general anaesthesia. Stifle motion is possible during distraction: mild flexion and varus-valgus motion could be accomplished when the surgical procedure required it. The post-procedure radiographic tests performed for the cadaveric study [13] demonstrated that there are no changes in joint stability measured as varus-valgus stability. The clinical experience did not show any specific complication related to the use of the technique. All dogs were managed without bandages post-operatively – only an adhesive tape was applied to the surgical wound when present – and no local effusion, redness or pain were clinically evident. The presence of bone tunnels in the femur and tibia due to the K-wires used for application of the stirrup never showed fissures or cracks predisposing the bone to fracture.

Böttcher et al. [3] previously highlighted the usefulness of distraction in recognizing longitudinal meniscal tears, since a small joint space may make meniscal tear identification complicated. More recently, Winkels et al. [9] stated that some meniscal tears may be misdiagnosed when using external manipulation without instrumented distraction, since external manipulation limits access to the caudal pole of the medial meniscus.

In this study, after diagnosing the meniscal tear, the appropriate treatment was performed while maintaining the distraction. The selection of treatment was based on the diagnosed lesion, since the location of the lesion is important to achieve meniscal healing. With the abaxial third (red zone) being vascularized, the likelihood of meniscal healing is much higher than in the rest of the meniscal parenchyma [4, 20]. For this reason, meniscal suture was performed when the lesion was located in this vascular area.

Although partial meniscectomy could have been accomplished without the distraction manoeuvre, this procedure was performed in a more consistent and safe way due to the space provided by the distraction. The opening of the forceps used for this purpose or the introduction of a radiofrequency probe between joint surfaces is prone to contact with and damage of the joint cartilage. Moreover, radiofrequency ablation could be dangerous if it is performed too close to the joint cartilage [22]. Furthermore, joint evaluation and partial meniscectomy were completed without the need for a fat pad debridement, which may increase morbidity [10].

In the authors' opinion, meniscal suture could not have been performed without joint distraction. The narrow joint space makes it difficult to move the different instruments around, but using distraction provides safe and easy access to the caudal horn of the medial meniscus.

An important point for the meniscal suture technique is the correct angulation of the spinal needle. It is mandatory to position the scope in the cranio-medial portal and to insert the needle from the cranio-lateral portal, aiming to exit from the caudo-medial area of the stifle. If the needle is inserted in a sagittal direction, like it was if inserted from the cranio-medial portal, it would exit in the popliteal area, making its retrieval impossible.

The only intraoperative complication encountered was the breakage of suture during its passage through the meniscus in one case, but it was not related to the distraction or the amount of joint space. Though the distractor used here was much bulkier compared to other available distractors [3, 10], the force was applied in a more even way because of the bilateral K-wires held by stirrups, while the pin distractor works only on the medial side of the joint. In addition, wire placement in this technique does not interfere with intra-articular structures as is the case for intra-articular distractors. The small size of the wires does not create large bone tunnels, and they can be placed at a distance from the joint line. This is not the case for distractors that use pins, which should be placed quite close to the joint to be effective. A further advantage of this technique is that it can be used in joints other than the stifle [16–18].

The mean time to complete the evaluation and treatment in dogs that received a surgical meniscal treatment (partial meniscectomy and meniscal suture) was approximately double that of the group of dogs that were not treated. The time needed for completing the whole procedure was longer than that reported by Gemmill and colleagues [10], but a comparison cannot be made because the distraction device was different and they did not perform any treatment for the medial meniscus. Moreover, the surgery time is dependent on the skill of the surgeon, and it may be substantially reduced once the surgeon establishes proficiency in performing the procedure [23].

The distraction device used in this study did not cause fractures in a previous cadaveric study with loads of up to 200 N [13]. The clinical postoperative evaluation excluded complications to soft tissues that was not possible to evaluate in the previous cadaveric study.

Conclusions

Stifle joint distraction is a safe procedure to increase the intra-articular workspace during stifle arthroscopy in dogs. It facilitates joint access and makes possible and easier the consistent visualization of the joint structures and the diagnosis of meniscal pathology. The use of a stifle distractor device should be considered in order to perform partial meniscectomy and meniscal suture, since it facilitates access to the caudal horn of the medial meniscus and therefore suture placement. Although joint distraction is not exempt from complications, no problems related to the distraction procedure have been observed in this case cohort.

Abbreviations
K-wire: Kirschner wire

Acknowledgements
The authors would like to thank the staff of the Clinica Veterinaria M.E. Miller for their contribution.

Authors' contributions
GLR conceived and managed the study. He also performed all the interventions and participated in the writing. VD was responsible for evaluating the results and writing the paper. LB collected and analysed the data. JRQ participated in managing the study. All authors read and approved the final manuscript.

Competing interests
G.L. Rovesti owns shares of Ad Maiora company.

Author details
[1]Clinica Veterinaria M. E. Miller, Cavriago, Italy. [2]Madrid, Spain. [3]Department of Internal Medicine and Surgery, Veterinary Teaching Hospital, Veterinary School, Complutense University, Madrid, Spain.

References
1. Pozzi A, Hildreth BE, Rajala-Schultz PJ. Comparison of arthroscopy and arthrotomy for diagnosis of medial meniscal pathology: an ex vivo study. Vet Surg. 2008;37:749–55.
2. Plesman R, Gilbert P, Campbell J. Detection of meniscal tears by arthroscopy and arthrotomy in dogs with cranial cruciate ligament rupture. A retrospective, cohort study Vet Comp Orthop Traumatol. 2013;26:42–6.
3. Böttcher P, Winkels P, Oechtering G. A novel pin distraction device for arthroscopic assessment of the medial meniscus in dogs. Vet Surg. 2009;38: 595–600.
4. Cook JL, Fox DB. A novel bioabsorbable conduit augments healing of avascular meniscal tears in a dog model. Am J Sports Med. 2007;35:1877–87.
5. Thieman KM, Pozzi A, Ling HY, Lewis D. Comparison of contact mechanics of three meniscal repair techniques and partial meniscectomy in cadaveric dog stifles. Vet Surg. 2010;39:355–62.
6. Beale BS, Hulse DA, Schulz KS, Whitney WO. Arthroscopically assisted surgery of the stifle joint. In: Beale BS, Hulse DA, Schulz KS, Whitney WO, editors. Small animal arthroscopy. Philadelphia: Saunders; 2003. p. 114–57.
7. Moverley R, Williams D, Bardakos N, Field R. Removal of the infrapatella fat pad during total knee arthroplasty: does it affect patient outcomes? Int Orthop. 2014;38:2483–7.
8. Kim K, Leel H, Ragetly GR. Feasibility of stifle medial meniscal release in toy breed dogs with and without a joint distractor. Vet Surg. 2016;45:636–41.
9. Winkels P, Pozzi A, Cook R, Böttcher P. Prospective evaluation of the Leipzig stifle distractor. Vet Surg. 2016;45:631–5.
10. Gemmill TJ, Farrell M. Evaluation of a joint distractor to facilitate arthroscopy of the canine stifle. Vet Surg. 2009;38:588–94.
11. Jakob RP, Stäubli HU, Zuber K, Esser M. The arthroscopic meniscal repair. Techniques and clinical experience. Am J Sports Med. 1988;16:137–42.
12. Kurtz CA, Bonner KF, Sekiya JK. Meniscus transplantation using the femoral distractor. Arthroscopy. 2006;22:568.e1–3.
13. Rovesti GL, Devesa-Garcia V, Urrutia PG, SanRoman F, Rodríguez-Quirós J. Evaluation of a distractor to increase the joint space of the stifle joint in dogs: a cadaveric study. Vet Comp Orthop Traumatol. 2015;28:179–85.
14. Albert J, Reiman P, Njus G, Kay DB, Theken R. Ligament strain and ankle joint opening during ankle distraction. Arthroscopy. 1992;8:469–73.
15. Dienst M, Seil R, Gödde S, Brang M, Becker K, Georg T, Kohn D. Effects of traction, distension, and joint position on distraction of the hip joint: an experimental study in cadavers. Arthroscopy. 2002;18:865–71.
16. Rodríguez-Quirós J, Rovesti GL, Devesa V, Urrutia PG, SanRoman F. Evaluation of a joint distractor to facilitate arthroscopy of the tibio-tarsal joint in dogs. J Small Anim Pract. 2014;55:213–8.
17. Devesa V, Rovesti GL, Urrutia PG, SanRoman F, Rodriguez-Quirós J. Evaluation of a joint distractor to facilitate arthroscopy of the hip joints in dogs. J Small Anim Pract. 2014;55:603–8.
18. Devesa V, Rovesti GL, Urrutia PG, SanRoman F, Rodríguez- Quirós J. Evaluation of traction stirrup distraction technique to increase the joint space of the shoulder joint in the dog: a cadaveric study. Res Vet Sci. 2015; 100:283–90.
19. Outerbridge RE. The etiology of chondromalacia patellae. J Bone Joint Surg Br. 1961;43-B:752–7.
20. Barber FA, McGarry JE. Meniscal repair techniques. Sports Med Arthrosc Rev. 2001;15:199–207.
21. Thieman KM, Pozzi A, Ling HY, Lewis D. Contact mechanics of simulated meniscal tears in cadaveric canine stifles. Vet Surg. 2009;38:803–10.
22. Sasaki N, Tsuda E, Yamamoto Y, Maeda S, Ishibashi Y. Severe valgus knee deformity caused by chondronecrosis after using a radiofrequency device. J Orthop Sci. 2014;19:1046–50.
23. Beale BS, Hulse DA, Schulz KS, Whitney WO. History of arthroscopy. In: Beale BS, Hulse DA, Schulz KS, Whitney WO, editors. Small animal arthroscopy. Philadelphia: Saunders; 2003. p. 1–3.

Efficacy of buprenorphine for management of surgical castration pain in piglets

Abbie V. Viscardi* and Patricia V. Turner

Abstract

Background: Surgical castration is a painful procedure, performed routinely on commercial pig farms to prevent boar taint and reduce aggression. The objectives of this study were to assess the efficacy of 0.04 mg/kg buprenorphine (BUP) in reducing pain in castrated piglets, using behavioral indicators and vocalization analysis. This study also sought to further validate the Piglet Grimace Scale (PGS) as a pain assessment tool.
A pilot study first assessed the safety of BUP or 0.2 mg/kg butorphanol administration to piglets ($n = 4$ per treatment). When no side effects were noted with BUP, ten litters of 5-day old piglets ($n = 60$ total, 15 per treatment group) were used, and randomly assigned to one of four possible treatments: BUP (castrated or uncastrated), saline, or sham. Treatments were administered as an intramuscular injection 20 min prior to surgical castration. Piglets were video recorded 1 h pre-procedure, post-castration for 8 h and for another hour, 24 h post-procedure. Behaviors were scored continuously for the first 15 min of each hour and 511 still-images of piglet faces were scored using the PGS. Vocalizations were recorded from each piglet at three points in the study: at initial handling, injection, and castration.

Results: Butorphanol caused some piglets to become groggy and vomit and was not further evaluated. BUP-castrated piglets demonstrated significantly fewer pain behaviors and less facial grimacing compared to saline-treated pigs ($P < 0.0001$ and $P = 0.0073$, respectively). There was no difference between the pain behaviours displayed by BUP-castrated piglets compared to BUP-uncastrated and sham piglets ($P = 0.9986$ and $P = 0.7484$). There was also no difference in PGS score between BUP-castrated and BUP-uncastrated piglets ($P = 0.9376$). Piglets in the BUP-castrated group produced vocalizations of similar frequency, amplitude, power, and energy to saline-treated piglets.

Conclusions: Buprenorphine was highly effective in alleviating castration-associated pain behaviors and facial grimacing in piglets, without causing any obvious side effects. Its administration did not reduce piglet vocalizations at the time of castration. The PGS corresponded well to piglet pain behaviors and has utility as a pain assessment tool.

Keywords: Animal welfare, Analgesia, Buprenorphine, Pain assessment, Piglet, Castration, Behavior, Piglet grimace scale

Background

Surgical castration is a procedure performed routinely on piglets in North America to prevent boar taint and minimize agonistic behaviors [1]. It causes acute pain in piglets, as evidenced by behavioral and physiologic alterations after castration, including rump scratching, body spasms, high-frequency vocalizations, and increased blood cortisol levels [2–4]. However, piglets are generally not provided analgesia or anesthesia for pain relief. Canada and countries in the EU have recognized this as a significant piglet welfare concern and have guidelines that now require analgesia administration [5, 6]. Nonsteroidal anti-inflammatory drugs (NSAIDs), such as meloxicam and ketoprofen, are currently recommended for use in piglets to manage pain, yet previous research found the label dose (0.4 mg/kg) of meloxicam, a high dose (1.0 mg/kg) of meloxicam, or 6.0 mg/kg ketoprofen to be ineffective at alleviating surgical castration pain in piglets [4, 7]. The analgesic capacity of an NSAID is limited by the degree of tissue trauma caused by the surgical castration procedure, as a significant mechanism underlying NSAID-induced pain mitigation is suppression of pro-inflammatory prostaglandin synthesis [8]. Opioids, such as buprenorphine and butorphanol, are more potent analgesic drugs, binding to μ, δ, and κ opioid receptors in the brain, spinal cord, and peripherally to suppress central pain signal transmission [9]. Butorphanol has been used in combination with

* Correspondence: aviscard@uoguelph.ca
Department of Pathobiology, University of Guelph, 50 Stone Road E, Guelph, ON N1G 2W1, Canada

various drugs, such as xylazine-ketamine, medetomidine, azaperone-detomidine-ketamine, and midazolam-ketamine, in pigs to prolong sedation [10–13]. Butorphanol alone was found to be ineffective at reducing pain behaviors of piglets castrated at 8 weeks-old [14]. Buprenorphine has demonstrated efficacy in reducing pain and lameness in pigs [15, 16]. The ability of butorphanol and buprenorphine to alleviate pain in 5-day-old piglets following castration has not been assessed.

The Piglet Grimace Scale (PGS) is a novel pain assessment tool that examines specific facial feature alterations in piglets in response to an acutely painful event [17]. Similar species-specific scales have been developed for mice, rats, rabbits, horses, sheep, and lambs [18–23]. These scales are of interest for their non-invasive nature and ability to rapidly detect pain [24]. For appropriate validation of these scales, they must correspond well to known indicators of pain, such as behavior.

The objectives of this study were first to determine the safety of buprenorphine and butorphanol administration to piglets, and then to assess their efficacy in reducing pain in castrated piglets, using behavioral indicators and vocalization analysis. We hypothesized that piglets receiving an opioid pre-castration would show a significant reduction in vocalizations and pain behaviors. This study also sought to further validate the PGS by comparing it against castration-related pain behaviors. The findings of this work will be important for appropriate analgesic recommendations to alleviate piglet pain post-castration, leading to improved animal welfare, a topic of increasing societal concern [25].

Results

Part I- opioid pilot study

Behavioral observations

Approximately 30 min post-injection, piglets administered butorphanol became groggy, unable to stand or walk, and two of the four animals vomited. They remained in the farrowing pen, and the observers ensured there was enough distance between them and the sow to eliminate their risk of being crushed. Butorphanol-treated piglets did not experience any severe side effects to the drug (e.g., respiratory depression), and they fully recovered approximately 1.5 h post-injection. There were no side effects noted with buprenorphine administration.

Part II- buprenorphine definitive trial

Behavioral observations

Four individual behaviors (lying: $P < 0.0001$, standing: $P < 0.0001$, tail wagging: $P < 0.0001$, and walking: $P < 0.0001$) and both grouped behaviors (active: $P < 0.0001$, and pain: $P < 0.0001$), were affected by treatment across all time points. Piglets in the BUP-castrated and BUP-uncastrated treatment groups spent significantly less time lying and more time standing, walking, and engaged in more active behaviours than piglets in the saline and sham treatment groups ($P < 0.05$) (Fig. 1). Saline-treated piglets wagged their tails and demonstrated significantly more pain behaviors than piglets in all other treatment groups ($P < 0.05$) (Fig. 2).

Eight individual behaviors and both grouped behaviors (active and pain) were significantly affected by time across the observation period: awake inactive ($P < 0.0001$), lying ($P = 0.0016$), sleeping ($P < 0.0001$), standing ($P = 0.0004$), suckling ($P = 0.0288$), tail wagging ($P < 0.0001$), walking ($P < 0.0001$), chewing ($P = 0.0324$), active ($P = 0.0030$), and pain ($P < 0.0001$). Regardless of treatment, at 0 h post-castration, piglets were significantly more active, spending more time standing and walking, and less time lying and sleeping compared to piglets at 4 h, 5 h, and 7 h post-procedure ($P < 0.05$). No rump scratching or trembling behavior was observed from any piglet pre-procedure and there were no significant behavioral differences between any of the treatment groups pre-castration ($P > 0.05$) (Table 1). Suckling and chewing behaviors were not significant after the Tukey-Kramer adjustment.

A significant time x treatment effect was found for lying ($P = 0.0300$), standing ($P = 0.0228$), tail wagging ($P = 0.0488$), active ($P = 0.0259$), and pain ($P = 0.0002$). At 4 h post-castration, sham piglets were significantly less active, spending more time lying and less time standing than BUP-castrated piglets at 0 h, 2 h, and 3 h, and BUP-uncastrated piglets at 0 h and 1 h ($P < 0.05$) (Fig. 3). At 24 h post-castration, saline-treated piglets demonstrated significantly more tail wagging and pain behaviors than BUP-castrated piglets at 3 h, 5 h, 6 h, and 24 h, BUP-uncastrated piglets at 6 h and 24 h, and sham piglets at all post-castration time points ($P < 0.05$) (Fig. 4). Compared to themselves, saline-treated piglets displayed significantly more pain

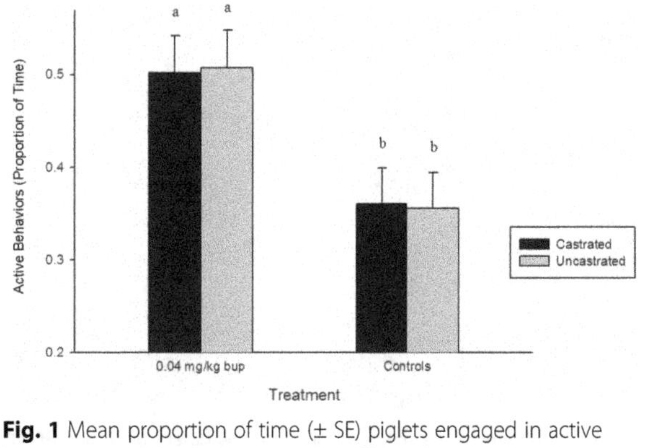

Fig. 1 Mean proportion of time (± SE) piglets engaged in active behaviors in each treatment group. Different letters indicated significance

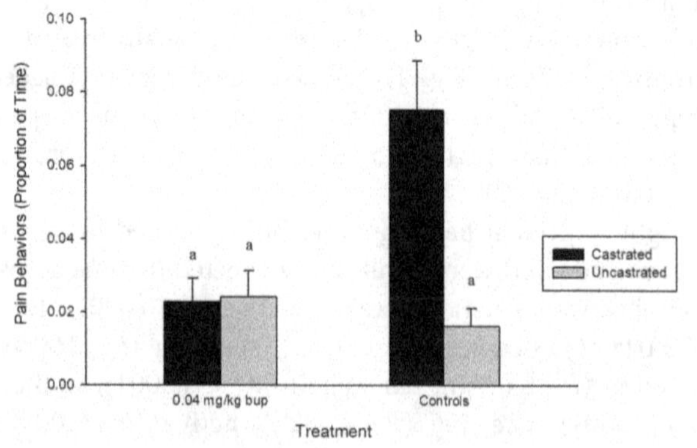

Fig. 2 Mean proportion of time (± SE) piglets displayed pain behaviors in each treatment group. Different letters indicated significance

behaviors at 24 h than at 0 h, 1 h, 3 h, and 5 h–7 h post-castration.

Piglet grimace scale

There was a significant treatment effect on PGS score (P = 0.0003) (Fig. 5). BUP-castrated and BUP-uncastrated piglets grimaced significantly less than both saline (BUP-castrated: P = 0.007, and BUP-uncastrated: P = 0.001) and sham (BUP-castrated: P = 0.049, and BUP-uncastrated: P = 0.013) treatment groups. Across all time points, there was no significant difference in PGS score between BUP-castrated and BUP-uncastrated piglets (P = 0.944), nor was there a difference found between piglets in the saline and sham treatment groups (P = 0.974).

Vocalization

For both castrated-treatment groups, the scrotal incision produced piglet vocalizations that were significantly lower in frequency, amplitude, and power compared to the IM injection (P = 0.0003, P = 0.007, and P = 0.0001, respectively). When compared to castration (i.e., pulling and tearing of the spermatic cord to remove testicles), the scrotal incision produced piglet vocalizations significantly lower in frequency and power (P < 0.0001 for both). Injecting piglets resulted in vocalizations that were significantly higher in frequency, amplitude and power compared to marking piglets (P = 0.02, P = 0.04, and P = 0.02, respectively) (Fig. 6).

Piglets in the BUP-castrated treatment group produced vocalizations significantly higher in frequency, power, and energy compared to piglets in the sham group (P = 0.04, P = 0.02, and P = 0.04, respectively) (Fig. 7). Buprenorphine administration did not reduce piglet vocalizations at the time of castration; piglets in the BUP-castrated group produced vocalizations of similar frequency, amplitude, power, and energy to saline-treated piglets (P = 1.00 for all).

Weight analysis

Sham piglets, with an average BW of 1.95 ± 0.14 kg, weighed significantly less than piglets in all other treatment groups (BUP-castrated: 2.48 ± 0.13 kg, P = 0.0044; BUP-uncastrated: 2.32 ± 0.12 kg, P = 0.045; saline: 2.44 ± 0.14 kg, P = 0.009).

Discussion

This study examined buprenorphine efficacy in mitigating post-castration pain in piglets. Buprenorphine significantly reduced piglet pain behaviors such that no differences were observed between BUP- castrated and BUP- uncastrated or sham piglets at any post-castration time point (up to 24 h). Castrated and uncastrated

Table 1 Behavioral analysis of piglets (n = 60) pre-treatment and post-treatment across all litters and timepoints. Values presented are the proportional means ± SE

	Behavior[c]	Pre-Castration		Post-Castration						
		Treatment P-value	Pre-Treatment	Treatment P-value	Time P-value	Time*Treatment P-value	0.04 mg/kg BUP cast	0.04 mg/kg BUP uncast	Saline	Sham
Proportion (duration)	Awake inactive	0.9704	0.64 ± 0.05	0.6749	*<.0001*	0.2277	0.53 ± 0.02	0.50 ± 0.02	0.54 ± 0.03	0.52 ± 0.03
	Lying	–	0.53 ± 0.08	*<.0001*	*0.0001*	*0.0300*	0.49 ± 0.04^{a}	0.44 ± 0.04^{a}	0.68 ± 0.04^{b}	0.67 ± 0.03^{b}
	Nosing udder	0.0551	0.23 ± 0.05	*0.0248*	*0.0047*	0.9439	0.15 ± 0.03	0.17 ± 0.03	0.23 ± 0.04	0.25 ± 0.04
	Sleeping	0.6062	0.28 ± 0.06	*0.0187*	*<.0001*	0.7070	0.35 ± 0.07	0.32 ± 0.07	0.45 ± 0.07	0.49 ± 0.07
	Standing	0.7142	0.44 ± 0.08	*<.0001*	*<.0001*	*0.0228*	0.48 ± 0.08^{a}	0.52 ± 0.07^{a}	0.28 ± 0.06^{b}	0.29 ± 0.06^{b}
	Tail wagging	0.4929	0.02 ± 0.00	*<.0001*	0.4166	*0.0488*	0.00 ± 0.00^{a}	0.00 ± 0.00^{a}	0.07 ± 0.01^{b}	0.01 ± 0.00^{a}
	Walking	0.2945	0.16 ± 0.04	*<.0001*	*0.0001*	0.3728	0.23 ± 0.03^{a}	0.25 ± 0.03^{a}	0.07 ± 0.01^{b}	0.09 ± 0.02^{b}
	Active[d]	0.6394	0.47 ± 0.07	*<.0001*	*<.0001*	*0.0259*	0.51 ± 0.06^{a}	0.56 ± 0.06^{a}	0.33 ± 0.06^{b}	0.33 ± 0.06^{b}
	Pain[e]	0.2859	0.02 ± 0.00	*<.0001*	*0.0329*	*0.0002*	0.02 ± 0.00^{a}	0.03 ± 0.00^{a}	0.08 ± 0.01^{b}	0.02 ± 0.00^{a}

[a,b]Means with different superscripts in the same row differ significantly (P < 0.05); entries in italic font are statistically significant
[c]Only behavior variables that were significant post-treatment are presented
[d]Active behaviors include: nosing, suckling, walking, chewing, playing, running
[e]Pain behaviors include: stiffness, trembling, spasms, tail wagging and scratching

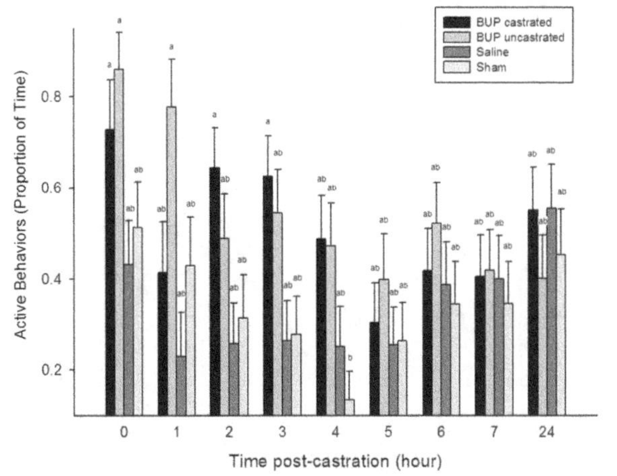

Fig. 3 Mean proportion of time (± SE) piglets engaged in active behaviors within each treatment group across the observation period. Different letters indicated significance

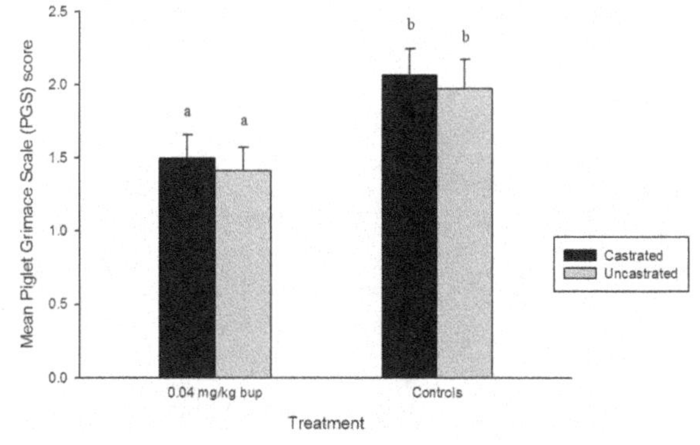

Fig. 5 Mean Piglet Grimace Scale (PGS) scores (± SE) in each treatment group. Different letters indicate significance

buprenorphine-treated piglets were significantly more active than saline-treated pigs, showing no sedative effect with the 0.04 mg/kg dose. Animals often become less active but more restless when in pain [26]. Restlessness was difficult to assess with the ethogram used, but increased pain behavior and decreased activity was noted in saline-treated piglets in this study. Results from the treatment control group (i.e., piglets given buprenorphine but uncastrated) also verified no negative behavioral side effects are associated with buprenorphine administration. Saline-treated piglets wagged their tails significantly more than all other treatment groups. An increase in tail wagging after a painful event, such as castration or dehorning, has been observed in piglets, lambs, and calves [2, 7, 27–30], suggesting that this may be a useful pain indicator. Note that piglets in this study had not been tail docked

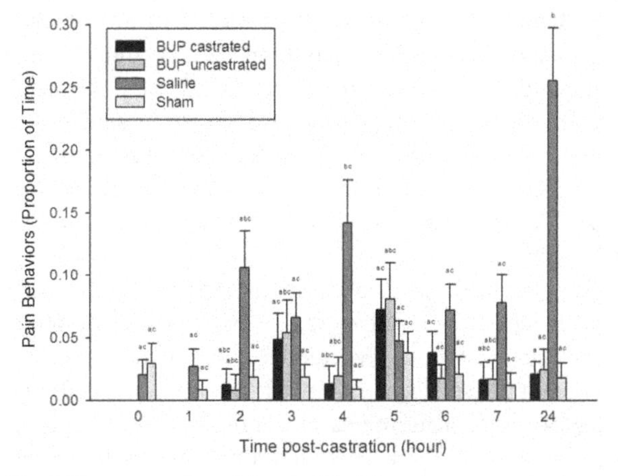

Fig. 4 Mean proportion of time (± SE) piglets demonstrated pain behaviors within each treatment group across the observation period. Different letters indicated significance

and thus increases in tail wagging could not be attributed to tail stump hyperalgesia [31].

Increased piglet activity was observed immediately post-castration (at 0 h). This may be attributed to the stress of repeated handling, the IM injection and separation from the sow for 20–30 min. Piglets are also generally more active in the early morning and early evening [32]. At 24 h post-castration, saline-treated piglets demonstrated significantly more tail wagging and pain behaviors than any other treatment group and at most other time points. This increase in pain may be due to progression of the inflammatory process [33]. Buprenorphine-castrated piglets might have been expected to display more pain behaviors at 24 h post-castration, since the maximum duration of action of buprenorphine in swine is 12 h [34], but this was not observed. Future work should assess piglet pain beyond 24 h post-castration, to determine whether a single dose of buprenorphine provides sufficient post-castration analgesia for piglets.

After observing the significant sedative and emetic effects associated with butorphanol administration to piglets in the pilot study, this drug was not tested further. The sedative effects put piglets at greater risk of hypothermia or being crushed if they are immediately placed back in their pen, making it an inappropriate opioid for use in piglets. Buprenorphine was determined to be safe and there were no evident side effects in the pilot or definitive studies.

NSAIDs, such as meloxicam and ketoprofen, are licensed for use in swine and are the most practical drugs available for producers to administer to piglets for pain relief [35]. In terms of efficacy, both NSAIDs have had variable success in significantly reducing post-castration pain [4, 36]. A review of the existing literature by a group of swine experts determined the quality of evidence to support NSAID use was low, and they gave a weak recommendation for the use of NSAIDs to mitigate surgical castration pain [37]. It is clear that a more

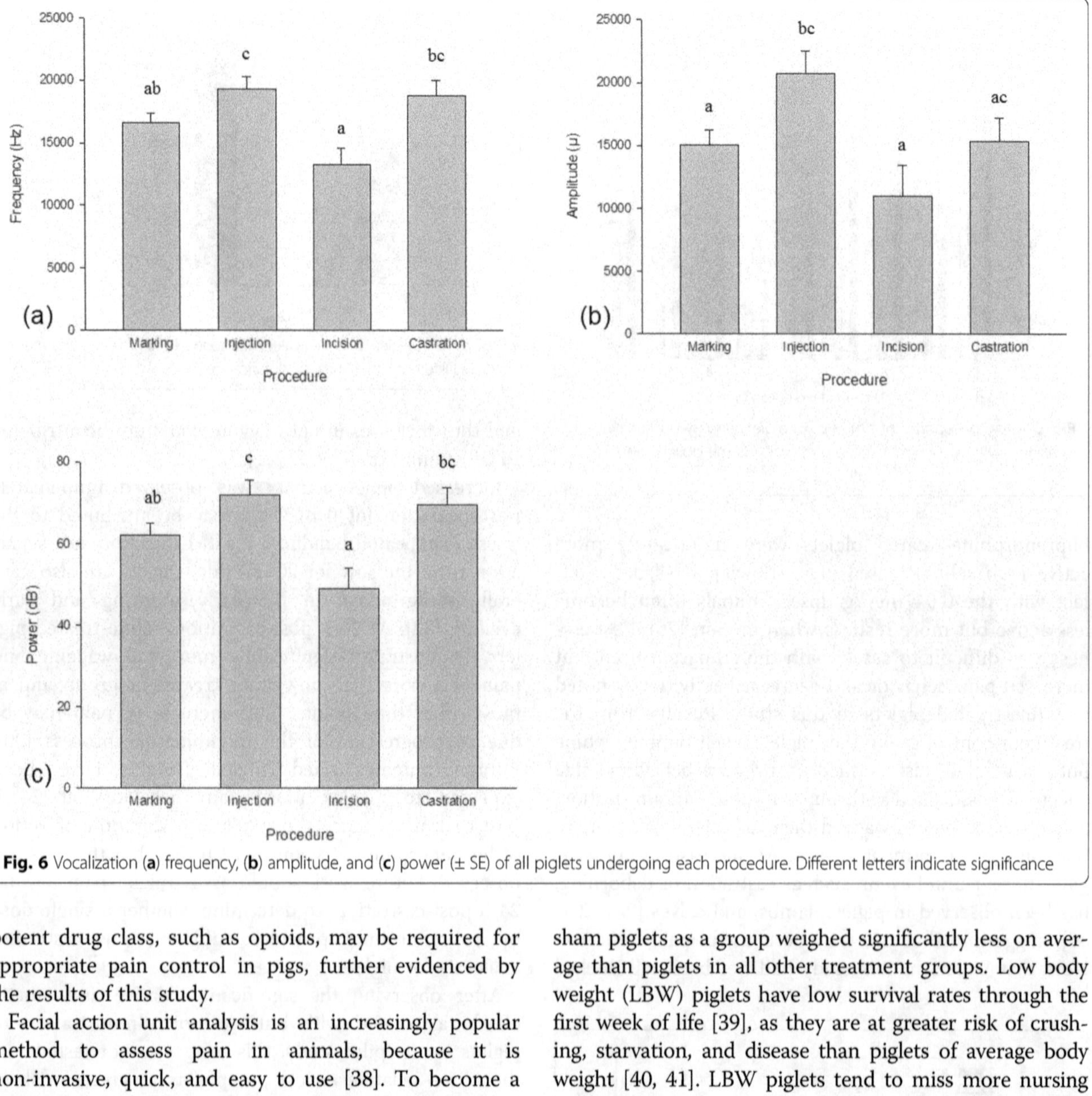

Fig. 6 Vocalization (**a**) frequency, (**b**) amplitude, and (**c**) power (± SE) of all piglets undergoing each procedure. Different letters indicate significance

potent drug class, such as opioids, may be required for appropriate pain control in pigs, further evidenced by the results of this study.

Facial action unit analysis is an increasingly popular method to assess pain in animals, because it is non-invasive, quick, and easy to use [38]. To become a validated pain assessment tool, the PGS must be comparable to known indicators of pain. In this study, we compared PGS scores to the pain behaviors displayed by piglets. The observed pain behaviors corresponded perfectly to PGS results for buprenorphine-castrated, buprenorphine-uncastrated, and saline-castrated piglets (e.g., an increase in pain behavior corresponded to higher facial grimacing), and buprenorphine significantly reduced facial grimacing in castrated piglets. However, this was not noted for the sham-uncastrated group. Sham piglets were expected to demonstrate low facial grimacing, high activity, and low pain behaviors, as this group did not receive an IM injection and were not castrated. Instead, they demonstrated high facial grimacing, low activity, and low pain behaviors. The post-study weight analysis revealed that sham piglets as a group weighed significantly less on average than piglets in all other treatment groups. Low body weight (LBW) piglets have low survival rates through the first week of life [39], as they are at greater risk of crushing, starvation, and disease than piglets of average body weight [40, 41]. LBW piglets tend to miss more nursing bouts and spend more time alone [42]. It may be that the increase in facial grimacing and decrease in activity level of these piglets was due to weakness and discomfort, not pain. This is a confounder in this study and future work should ensure piglet weights are balanced across treatment groups.

Piglets emit distinct vocalizations associated with castration that have been attributed to pain [3, 43]. Buprenorphine did not reduce the frequency, amplitude, power, or energy of these vocalizations at the time of castration. Therapeutic concentrations of buprenorphine (0.1 ng/mL) are reached rapidly in pigs after IM injection (between 5 and 30 min) [32] and piglets were castrated 20 min after its administration. This suggests that buprenorphine alone does not provide sufficient analgesia to fully mitigate pain

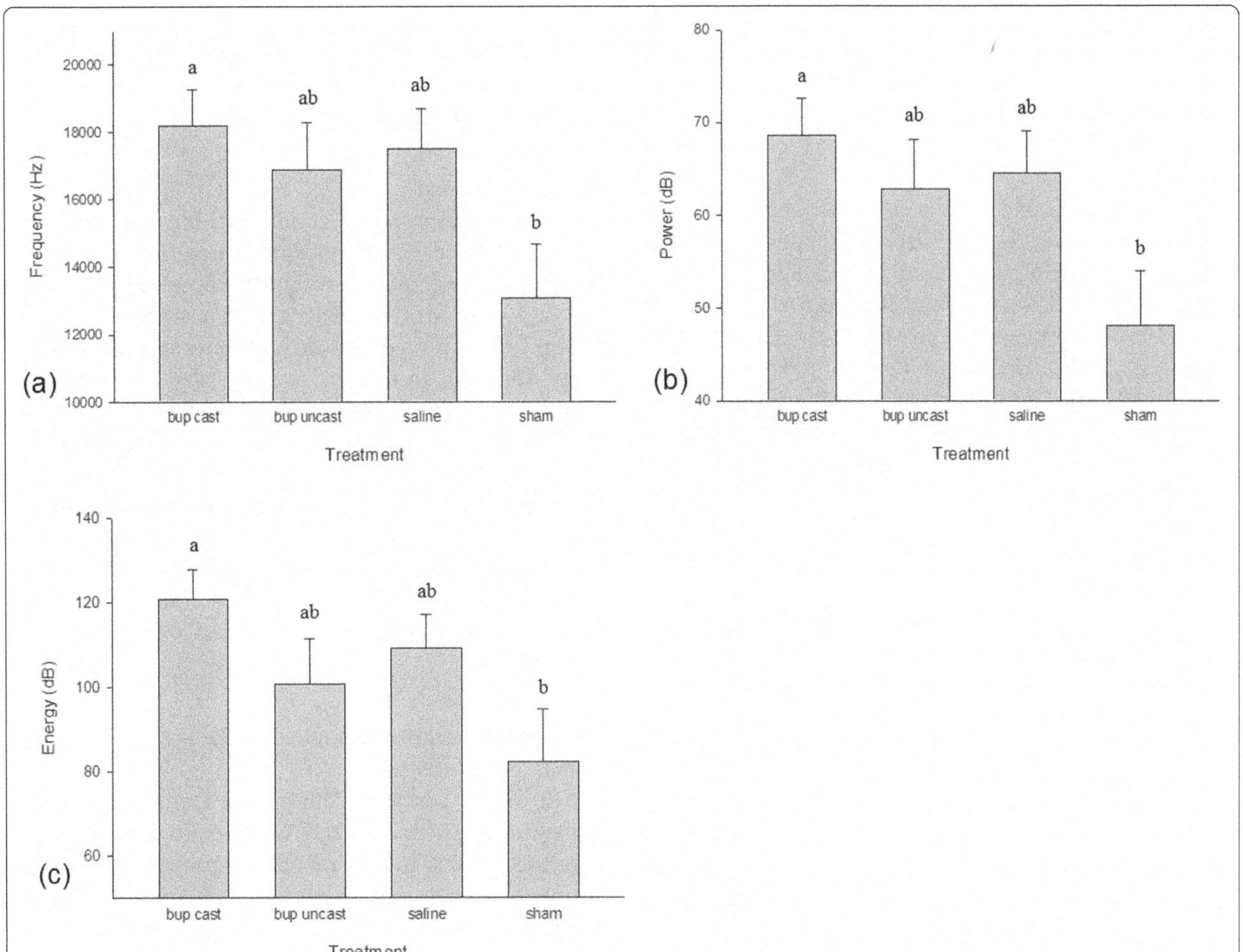

Fig. 7 Vocalization (**a**) frequency, (**b**) power, and (**c**) energy (± SE) of piglets in each treatment group. Different letters indicate significance

associated with surgical castration in conscious piglets. Previous studies have found that surgical castration-related stress vocalizations are reduced by CO_2 anesthesia, a combination of ketamine-climazolam-azaperone anesthesia or intratesticular lidocaine injection [44–46]. However, these agents or combinations provide minimal post-operative analgesia and present greater limitations for on-farm use (e.g., sedated piglets can not be returned to the sow until after drug recovery).

The practicality of buprenorphine use on-farm currently is low. While it was highly effective, easy to administer, and one injection provided pain relief for at least 24 h post-procedure, it is a controlled substance that must be administered by a veterinarian and its use is currently prohibited (illegal) in pigs or other food-producing animals [47, 48]. The opioid abuse epidemic is another issue to consider. With more than 42,000 deaths in the U.S. related to opioid drug overdose in 2016, veterinarians have had to make major adjustments to the type of drugs they send home with clients and carry in their practice to reduce the risk of human abuse [49, 50]. Farmers appear to be disproportionately at risk, with three-quarters of U.S. farmers and farm workers having reported being directly affected by opioid dependence [51]. While the idea of widespread opioid use on-farm is inconceivable, identification of buprenorphine as a drug that significantly reduced surgical castration pain may encourage other researchers to focus on how to make this highly effective option for piglet pain management practical for use in swine production (e.g., through novel formulation or administration that is safe and limits the risk of abuse).

Conclusions

Buprenorphine, when administered at 0.04 mg/kg IM, significantly reduced pain behaviors and facial grimacing in surgically castrated piglets for up to 24 h post-procedure, without evident adverse effects. It was not able to reduce vocalizations at the time of castration. The PGS corresponds well to the pain behaviors of piglets and has utility as a pain assessment tool. Future work should focus on potential solutions to the current limitations of using buprenorphine on-farm, as it is a highly effective analgesic agent that could improve the welfare of millions of piglets undergoing painful procedures each year.

Methods

This study was conducted at Arkell Swine Research Station, an active research facility supported by the University of Guelph and the Ontario Ministry of Agriculture, Food and Rural Affairs (OMAFRA). All animal use and procedures were approved by the University of Guelph Animal Care Committee (Animal Utilization Protocol #3350). The institution is registered under the Animals for Research Act of Ontario and holds a Good Animal Practice certificate issued by the Canadian Council on Animal Care.

Part I- opioid pilot study

Animals and treatments

A total of 8 Yorkshire-Landrace x Duroc male piglets (5-days-old, average BW = 2.19 ± 0.07 kg) from 2 different litters were used in this pilot study. Sows and piglets were housed in farrowing pens at the University of Guelph Arkell Swine Research Station (Arkell, ON, Canada). The floor space for each pen was 1.8 m × 2.4 m (6 ft. × 8 ft) and the farrowing crate was 0.8 m × 2.3 m (2.5 ft. × 7.5 ft). The farrowing rooms were maintained at ambient temperature (23 °C ± 0.5 °C) with lights on/off at 7:00 am/ 9:00 pm, and additional natural light was provided by windows in each room. Sows were fed ab lib 4 days after farrowing. The creep areas for piglets were heated to approximately 30–35 °C by means of a heat lamp.

Four piglets from each litter were used and randomly assigned one of two treatments: 0.04 mg/kg buprenorphine (Vetergesic 0.3 mg/mL; Champion Alstoe Animal Health Inc., Whitby, ON, Canada; extra-label use) or 0.2 mg/kg butorphanol (Torbugesic 10 mg/mL; Zoetis Inc., Kalamazoo, MI; extra-label use). Both drugs were administered intramuscularly (IM) and doses were derived from the literature [52]. Treatment groups were identified by a symbol ('C' or 'D') marked on the piglet's back with a permanent marker prior to injection, to ensure that those involved in post-castration observations were blinded to treatment. A number was also marked on the back leg of each piglet for individual identification purposes.

Processing procedure

Piglets were weighed approximately 24 h prior to the study start for drug dose calculations, and then marked with a symbol and number. On the day of castration, male piglets were removed from their pen, placed in a transport cart, and treatments were administered. Approximately 20 mins later, piglets were surgically castrated by making one vertical incision over each testicle using a scalpel and tearing the spermatic cords. The piglets were then returned to their home pen. Castrations occurred between 8:00 am and 8:30 am and were all done by the same individual (AVV).

Behavior recording

Live observations were conducted for the first 1 h post-injection; if piglets responded negatively to the administered drug, they were quickly removed from their pen and assisted. One experienced observer blinded to treatment was placed outside each litter of piglets in this study and was instructed to note any unusual piglet behavior (e.g. grogginess, vomiting, distress, or lying isolated from littermates for an extended period). Video cameras (JVC GZ-E200 full HD Everio Camcorder, Yokohama, Japan) were also placed on tripods outside of the farrowing pens and piglets were video recorded during and after the live observations for 7 h. An individual not involved in the live observations assessed the video footage for behavioral signs of distress related to opioid administration.

Part II- buprenorphine definitive study

Animals and treatments

A total of 60 Yorkshire-Landrace x Duroc male piglets (5-days-old, 1.07 to 3.34 kg BW) from 10 different litters were used in this study. Sows and piglets were housed in farrowing pens at the University of Guelph Arkell Swine Research Station.

Within each litter, piglets were randomly assigned to one of the following treatments: 0.04 mg/kg buprenorphine- castrated, 0.04 mg/kg buprenorphine- uncastrated, saline (castrated control), or sham (uncastrated control). Buprenorphine (BUP) was administered IM at 0.04 mg/kg (range: 0.2–0.5 mL/piglet). Saline was given IM at 0.2 mL/piglet. The sham treatment group was handled for approximately 30 s and did not receive an injection. Treatment groups were identified by a symbol ('V', 'X', circle or diamond) marked on each piglet's forehead and back with a black permanent marker prior to castration. This was to ensure that the individual involved in post-castration observations and behavior scoring was blinded to animal treatment. A number was also marked on the back leg of each piglet for individual identification purposes.

Processing procedure

Piglets were processed as described for the pilot study. Castrations occurred between 8:00 am and 10:00 am. The sham treatment group were the only non-castrated piglets that underwent a simulated castration. All handling and technical procedures were conducted by female researchers to eliminate the potential confound of increased stress and an altered pain response in piglets exposed to male researchers, as reported in mice [53].

Behavior recording and scoring

Video cameras were placed on tripods outside of the farrowing pens and piglets were video recorded pre-procedure for 1 h. Immediately post-castration, piglets were video recorded continuously for 8 h, and 24 h post-procedure, piglets were recorded for 1 h (10 h of video data were collected in total for each pen of pigs). Videos were randomized using a random number generator (random.org) and the behavior of each piglet was scored continuously by one experienced observer for the first 15 mins of every hour of video collected using the Observer XT program (Version 12.0: Noldus Information Technology, Wageningen, The Netherlands) according to a detailed ethogram adapted from Hay et al. [2] (Table 2). The observer was blinded as to time point, litter, and piglet treatment; however, castrated piglets could be clearly distinguished from those that had not been castrated. A total of 9000 min (150 h) of behavior recordings were scored and analyzed.

Piglet behaviors were analyzed individually and then grouped into active, inactive and pain categories, to assess the piglet's activity level throughout the observation period and the total amount of pain behaviors displayed [7]. Active behaviors included walking, running, playing, nosing, chewing, and suckling. Inactive behaviors included sleeping and awake inactive. Postures were used for this behavioral analysis; piglets that were standing or sitting were scored as active and lying piglets were scored as inactive. Sitting was scored in the active category because most piglets exhibited this posture when rump scratching or suckling and these were considered active behaviors. Pain behaviors included trembling, stiffness, spasms, tail wagging, and rump scratching [2].

Table 2 Ethogram used to score piglet behavior, grouped into feeding, locomotion, non-specific behaviors, pain-related behaviors, posture, and social cohesion (adapted from [2])

Behaviors	Description
Suckling	Teat in mouth and suckling movements
Nosing udder	Nose in contact with udder, up and down head movements
Playing	Springing, bouncy movements with littermates
Agonistic	Biting or fighting other littermates
Walking	Moving forward at a normal pace
Running	Trot or gallop
Awake inactive	No special activity, but awake
Sleeping	Lying down, eyes closed
Nosing	Snout in contact with a substrate
Chewing	Nibbling at littermates or substrates
Trembling	Shivering, as with cold
Spasms	Quick and involuntary contractions of the muscles
Scratching	Rubbing the rump against the floor, pen walls, or littermates
Tail wagging	Tail's movements from side to side (or up and down)
Stiffness	Lying with extended and tensed legs
Lying	Body weight supported by side or belly
Sitting	Body weight supported by hindquarters and front legs
Standing	Body weight supported by four legs
Kneeling	Body weight supported by front carpal joints and hind legs
Isolated	Alone or with one littermate at most, distance of 40 cm separates the animal(s) from the closest group of littermates
Desynchronized	Activity different from that of most littermates (at least 75%)

Table 3 Total number of piglet faces captured for Piglet Grimace Scale scoring

Time point (h)	Treatment				Total
	0.04 mg/kg BUP cast	0.04 mg/kg BUP uncast	Saline	Sham	
pre	17	14	17	9	57
0	18	17	15	11	61
1	12	21	3	10	46
2	18	19	11	6	54
3	23	12	7	8	50
4	12	15	7	5	39
5	19	19	10	7	55
6	14	15	10	8	47
7	12	13	9	2	36
24	18	21	15	12	66
Total	163	166	104	78	511

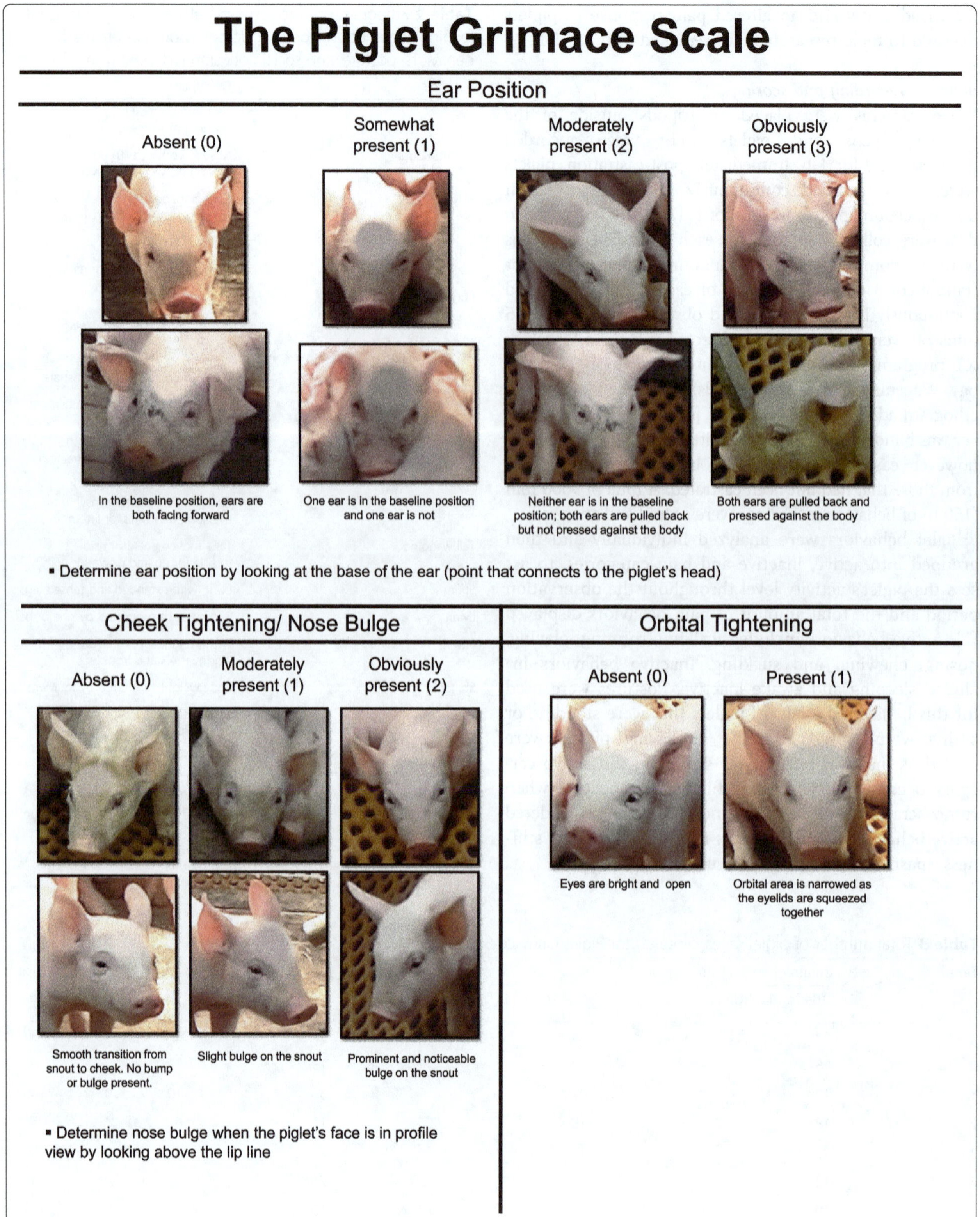

Fig. 8 The Piglet Grimace Scale (PGS) scores ear position, cheek tightening/nose bulge and orbital tightening. The maximum score is 6

Piglet grimace scale and scoring

Still images of piglet faces were taken from the first 30 min of every hour of video data by an individual blinded as to time point and animal treatment using the Everio MediaBrowser 4 program (Pixela Corporation, Osaka, Japan). Whenever a piglet face was in view, the video was paused, and the still image was captured (excluding times when piglets were lying with their head down or sleeping). Taking at least one facial image of each piglet per time point in this study was attempted. A total of 511 images were captured (Table 3). The images were uploaded to Photoshop (Adobe Systems Incorporated, San Jose, CA) prior to scoring to blur the symbol marked on each piglet's forehead. This was to ensure that those scoring the faces were blinded as to treatment. Faces were then randomized into files using a random number generator (random.org).

Four individuals with extensive animal experience were trained to use the Piglet Grimace Scale (Fig. 8) in a 30 min interactive training session prior to scoring study faces. If an image could not be scored reliably, those scoring were instructed to exclude it (3 images were removed in total because of poor image quality). The PGS score for each image was calculated by summing the scores given to each of the facial action units (ear position, cheek tightening/nose bulge and orbital tightening). If more than one image was pulled from the same piglet within one time point, the PGS scores were averaged across images prior to analysis, to prevent issues with pseudo-replication. The final PGS score of each piglet per time point was calculated as a mean of the scores from the four individuals.

Vocalizations

Vocalizations of each piglet were collected at three points during the study, at initial handling when they were marked with a symbol (marking), when they received their treatment injection (injection) and when they were surgically castrated (incision and castration). A video camera on a tripod was placed as close to the focal piglet's face as possible and recorded each procedure. Vocalizations from the recorded videos were analyzed using Raven Pro 1.5 (Cornell Lab of Ornithology, Ithaca, NY) by two individuals who were blinded as to procedure and piglet treatment. From the spectrograms, maximum frequency (Hz), maximum amplitude (μ), maximum power (dB) and energy (dB) of each call was determined [43, 54].

Data and statistical analysis

The total duration of behaviors was converted into a proportion of time that piglets spent demonstrating each behavior prior to analysis to account for periods of time when piglets were out of view and unable to be scored. Normality was evaluated using the univariate procedure in SAS (Statistical Analysis System 9.4, SAS Institute Inc., NC). Data was analyzed with a GLIMMIX procedure with a beta distribution, including time, treatment, litter, and the time x treatment interaction. Litter was included as a random effect and time was a repeated measure with piglet as the experimental unit. Post hoc tests were conducted on significant factors using the Tukey-Kramer adjustment. Statistical significance was set at $P < 0.05$.

The PGS scores were analyzed using a mixed model procedure, including litter, time, treatment, and time x treatment interaction. Litter was included as a random effect, time was a repeated measure, and piglet was the experimental unit. A post-hoc Tukey's test was conducted for significant outcomes.

Vocalization data was analyzed using a mixed procedure, including litter, treatment, and procedure in the model. Litter was included as a random effect and piglet was the experimental unit. Significant outcomes were further analyzed using a post-hoc Tukey's test. Behavior, PGS and vocalization data were used to assess the effectiveness of buprenorphine treatment in reducing surgical castration pain.

To determine if piglet weight was balanced across treatment groups, post-hoc analysis was performed using a GLM procedure, including litter and treatment in the model.

Abbreviations

BUP: Buprenorphine; BW: Body weight; IM: Intramuscular; NSAID: Nonsteroidal anti-inflammatory drug; PGS: Piglet Grimace Scale

Acknowledgements

The authors wish to thank Brianne Mercer, Stephanie Cervi, Anna Maystrenko, Tim Thalen, and personnel at the Arkell Swine Research Station for technical assistance.

Funding

Funding was provided by Ontario Pork (052367), National Pork (052457) and the Ontario Ministry of Agriculture Food and Rural Affairs (27295).

Authors' contributions

AW and PVT conceived of and designed the experiments. AW performed the experiments and analyzed the data. Both authors prepared and edited the final manuscript.

Consent for publication

Not applicable.

Competing interests

The authors declare that they have no competing interests.

References

1. Sutherland MA. Welfare implications of invasive piglet husbandry procedures, methods of alleviation and alternatives: a review. N Z Vet J. 2015;63:52–7.

2. Hay M, Vulin A, Genin S, Sales P, Prunier A. Assessment of pain induced by castration in piglets: behaviour and physiological responses over the subsequent 5 days. Appl Anim Behav Sci. 2003;82:201–18.
3. Leidig MS, Hertrampf B, Failing K, Schumann A, Reiner G. Pain and discomfort in male piglets during surgical castration with and without local anaesthesia as determined by vocalisation and defense behaviour. Appl Anim Behav Sci. 2009;116:174–8.
4. Kluivers-Poodt M, Houx BB, Robben SRM, Koop G, Lambooij E, Hellebrekers LJ. Effects of a local anaesthetic and NSAID in castration of piglets, on the acute pain responses, growth and mortality. Animal. 2012;6:1469–75.
5. European Commission. European declaration on alternatives to surgical castration of pigs. 2010. https://ec.europa.eu/food/animals/welfare/practice/farm/pigs/castration_alternatives_en. Accessed 15 Oct 2017.
6. National Farm Animal Care Council. Code of practice for the care and handling of pigs. 2014. http://www.nfacc.ca/pdfs/codes/pig_code_of_practice.pdf. Accessed 15 Oct 2017.
7. Viscardi AV, Mercer B, Whatley J, Hoffman H, Turner PV. NSAIDs do not mitigate piglet castration pain based on behavioural and activity monitoring. Proceedings of the 7th International Conference on the Assessment of Animal Welfare at Farm and Group level, Ede, The Netherlands, September 5–8. Wageningen, The Netherlands: De Jong, Koene, Wageningen Academic Publishers; 2017.
8. Papich MG. An update on nonsteroidal anti-inflammatory drugs (NSAIDs) in small animals. Vet Clin Small Anim. 2008;38:1243–61.
9. Chahl LA. Opioids- mechanism of action. Aust Prescr. 1996;19:63–5.
10. Nishimura R, Sakaguchi M, Mochizuki M, Sasaki N, Takahashi H, Tamura H, Takeuchi A. A balanced anesthesia with a combination of xylazine, ketamine and butorphanol and its antagonism by yohimbine in pigs. J Vet Med Sci. 1992;54:615–20.
11. Sakaguchi M, Nishimura R, Sasaki N, Ishiguro T, Tamura H, Takeuchi A. Enhancing effect of butorphanol on medetomidine-induced sedation in pigs. J Vet Med Sci. 1992;54:1183–5.
12. Heinonen ML, Raekallio MR, Oliviero C, Ahokas S, Peltoniemi OAT. Comparison of azaperone-detomidine-butorphanol-ketamine and azaperone-tiletamine-zolazepam for anaesthesia in piglets. Vet Anaesth Analg. 2009;36:151–7.
13. Schöffmann G, Winter P, Palme R, Pollak A, Trittenwein G, Golej J. Haemodynamic changes and stress responses of piglets to surgery during total intravenous anaesthesia with propofol and fentanyl. Lab Anim. 2009; 43:243–8.
14. McGlone JJ, Nicholson RI, Hellman JM, Herzog DN. The development of pain in young pigs associated with castration and attempts to prevent castration-induced behavioral changes. J Anim Sci. 1993;71:1441–6.
15. Hermansen K, Pedersen LE, Olesen HO. The analgesic effect of buprenorphine, etorphine and pethidine in the pig: a randomized double blind cross-over study. Acta pharmacol et toxicol. 1986;59:27–35.
16. Meijer E, van Nes A, Back W, van der Staay FJ. Clinical effects of buprenorphine on open field behaviour and gait symmetry in healthy and lame weaned piglets. Vet J. 2015;206:298–303.
17. Viscardi AV, Hunniford M, Lawlis P, Leach M, Turner PV. Development of a piglet grimace scale to evaluate piglet pain using facial expressions following castration and tail docking: a pilot study. Front Vet Sci. 2017;4:51.
18. Langford DJ, Bailey AL, Chanda ML, Clarke SE, Drummond TE, Echols S, Glick S, Ingrao J, Klassen-Ross T, LaCroix-Fralish ML, Matsumiya L, Sorge RE, Sotocinal SG, Tabaka JM, Wong D, van den Maagdenberg AMJM, Ferrari MD, Craig KD, Mogil JS. Coding of facial expressions of pain in the laboratory mouse. Nat Methods. 2010;7:447–9.
19. Sotocinal SG, Sorge RE, Zaloum A, Tuttle AH, Martin LJ, Wieskopf JS, Mapplebeck JCS, Wei P, Zhan S, Zhang S, McDougall JJ, King OD, Mogil JS. The rat grimace scale: a partially automated method for quantifying pain in the laboratory rat via facial expressions. Mol Pain. 2011;7:55.
20. Keating SCJ, Thomas AA, Flecknell PA, Leach MC. Evaluation of EMLA cream for preventing pain during tattooing of rabbits: changes in physiological, behavioural and facial expression responses. PLoS ONE. 2012. https://doi.org/10.1371/journal.pone.0044437.
21. Costa ED, Minero M, Lebelt D, Stucke D, Canali E, Leach MC. Development of the horse grimace scale (HGS) as a pain assessment tool in horses undergoing routine castration. PLoS One. 2014. https://doi.org/10.1371/journal.pone.0092281.
22. Guesgen MJ, Beausoleil NJ, Leach M, Minot EO, Stewart M, Stafford KJ. Coding and quantification of a facial expression for pain in lambs. Behav Process. 2016;132:49–56.
23. McLennan KM, Rebelo CJB, Corke MJ, Holmes MA, Leach MC, Constantino-Casas F. Development of a facial expression scale using footrot and mastitis as models of pain in sheep. Appl Anim Behav Sci. 2016;176:19–26.
24. Miller AL, Leach MC. The mouse grimace scale: a clinically useful tool? PLoS One. 2015. https://doi.org/10.1371/journal.pone.0136000.
25. Rollin BE. Annual meeting keynote address: animal agriculture and emerging social ethics for animals. J Anim Sci. 2004;82:955–64.
26. Berger N, Eeg PH. Pain management considerations for laser surgery procedures. In: Veterinary laser surgery: a practical guide. Ames, Iowa: Blackwell Publishing; 2006. p. 101–8.
27. Robertson IS, Kent JE, Molony V. Effect of different methods of castration on behavior and plasma cortisol in calves of three ages. Res Vet Sci. 1994;56:8–17.
28. Graf B, Senn M. Behavioural and physiological responses of calves to dehorning by heat cauterization with or without local anaesthesia. Appl Anim Behav Sci. 1999;62:153–71.
29. Rault JL, Lay DC. Nitrous oxide by itself is insufficient to relieve pain due to castration in piglets. J Anim Sci. 2014;89:3318–25.
30. Jongman EC, Borg S, Hemsworth PH. Assessment of pain responses associated with castration of 10-week-old lambs using the Callicrate 'WEE bander' compared with a standard elastrator. Appl Anim Behav Sci. 2016;179:46–52.
31. Di Giminiani P, Edwards SA, Malcolm EM, Leach MC, Herskin MS, Sandercock DA. Characterization of short- and long-term mechanical sensitisation following surgical tail amputation in pigs. Sci Rep. 2017;7:4827.
32. Park SY, van Oord R, van der Staay FJ, Nordquist RE. Social behaviour of pigs: Utrecht University Repository; 2010. https://dspace.library.uu.nl/handle/1874/204302.
33. Kumar V, Abbas A, Aster J. Robbins & Cotran Pathologic Basis of Disease, 9th ed. Amsterdam, NL: Elsevier; 2015.
34. Thiede AJ, Garcia KD, Stolarik DF, Ma J, Jenkins GJ, Nunamaker EA. Pharmacokinetics of sustained-release and transdermal buprenorphine in Göttingen minipigs (*Sus scrofa domestica*). J Am Assoc Lab Anim Sci. 2014;53:692–9.
35. Canadian Pork Council. Swine Health Ontario. Pain control information for swine. 2016. http://www.swinehealthontario.ca/About-Us/Latest-News-View/ArticleId/2563/Pain-Control-Information-for-Swine. Accessed 25 Jan 2018.
36. Keita A, Pagot E, Prunier A, Guidarini C. Pre-emptive meloxicam for postoperative analgesia in piglets undergoing surgical castration. Vet Anaesth Analg. 2010;37:367–74.
37. O'Connor A, Anthony R, Bergamasco L, Coetzee J, Gould S, Johnson AK, Karriker LA, Marchant-Forde JN, Martineau GS, McKean J, Millman ST, Niekamp S, Pajor EA, Rutherford K, Sprague M, Sutherland M, von Borell E, Dzikamunhenga RS. Pain management in the neonatal piglet during routine management procedures. Part 2: grading the quality of evidence and the strength of recommendations. Anim Health Res Rev. 2014;15:39–62.
38. Leach MC, Klaus K, Miller AL, Scotto di Perrotolo M, Sotocinal SG, Flecknell PA. The assessment of post-vasectomy pain in mice using behaviour and the mouse grimace scale. PLoS One. 2012;7:e35656.
39. Marchant JN, Rudd AR, Mendl MT, Broom DM, Meredity MJ, Corning S, Simmins PH. Timing and causes of piglet mortality in alternative and conventional farrowing systems. Vet Rec. 2000;147:209–14.
40. Herpin P, Damon M, Le Dividich J. Development of thermoregulation and neonatal survival in pigs. Livest Prod Sci. 2002;78:25–45.
41. Pedersen LJ, Berg P, Jørgensen G, Andersen IL. Neonatal piglet traits of importance for survival in crates and indoor pens. J Anim Sci. 2011;89:1207–18.
42. Bovey KE, Widowski TM, Dewey CE, Devillers N, Farmer C, Lessard M, Torrey S. The effect of birth weight and age at tail docking and ear notching on the behavioural and physiological responses of piglets. J Anim Sci. 2014;92:1718–27.
43. Marx G, Horn T, Thielebein J, Knubel B, von Borell E. Analysis of pain-related vocalizations in young pigs. J Sound Vib. 2003;266:687–98.
44. White RG, DeShazer JA, Tressler CJ, Borcher GM, Davey S, Waninge A, Parkhurst AM, Milanuk MJ, Clemens ET. Vocalization and physiological response of pigs during castration with or without a local anesthetic. J Anim Sci. 1995;73:381–6.
45. Axiak SM, Jäggin N, Wenger S, Doherr MG, Schatzmann U. Anaesthesia for castration of piglets: comparison between intranasal and intramuscular application of ketamine, climazolam and azaperone. Schweiz Arch Tierheilkd. 2007;149:395–402.

46. Sutherland MA, Davis BL, Brooks TA, Coetzee JF. The physiological and behavioural response of pigs castrated with and without anesthesia or analgesia. J Anim Sci. 2012;90:2211–21.
47. US Food & Drug Administration. BupreLab- for the control of post procedural pain in rats. 2014. https://www.fda.gov/downloads/AnimalVeterinary/DevelopmentApprovalProcess/MinorUseMinorSpecies/UCM373292.pdf. Accessed 24 Jan 2018.
48. US Food & Drug Administration. The index of legally marketed unapproved new animal drugs for minor species. 2017. https://www.fda.gov/AnimalVeterinary/DevelopmentApprovalProcess/MinorUseMinorSpecies/ucm125452.htm. Accessed 27 Jul 2018.
49. Centers for Disease Control and Prevention. Opioid overdose: understanding the epidemic. 2017. https://www.cdc.gov/drugoverdose/epidemic/index.html. Accessed 28 Jul 2018.
50. Shadle CC, Meyer JL. Pets, vets, and opioids. 2018. Am Vet. https://www.americanveterinarian.com/journals/amvet/2018/april2018/pets-vets-and-opioids?p=2. Accessed 27 Jul 2018.
51. U.S. Department of agriculture. Opioid misuse in rural America. 2018. https://www.usda.gov/topics/opioids. Accessed 28 Jul 2018.
52. Flecknell P. Analgesia and post-operative care. In: Laboratory animal anaesthesia. 4th ed. Amsterdam, NL: Elsevier; 2015. p. 174.
53. Sorge RE, Martin LJ, Isbester KA, Sotocinal SG, Rosen S, Tuttle AH, Wieskopf JS, Acland EL, Dokova A, Kadoura B, Leger P, Mapplebeck JCS, McPhail M, Delaney A, Wigerblad G, Schumann AP, Quinn T, Frasnelli J, Svensson CI, Sternberg WF, Mogil JS. Olfactory exposure to males, including men, causes stress and related analgesia in rodents. Nat Methods. 2014;11:629–32.
54. Taylor AA, Weary DM. Vocal responses of piglets to castration: identifying procedural sources of pain. Appl Anim Behav Sci. 2000;70:17–26.

22

Pelvic modelling and the comparison between plate position for double pelvic osteotomy using artificial cancellous bone and finite element analysis

William McCartney[1], Bryan MacDonald[2], Ciprian Andrei Ober[3*], Rubén Lostado-Lorza[4] and Fátima Somovilla Gómez[4]

Abstract

Background: Finite element analysis was used to compare fixation methods for double pelvic osteotomy (DPO). Using 3D scanning a stereolithography (stl) image was produced of a canine pelvis and this was subsequently refined in computer aided design (CAD). Using the CAD files, the images were imported in MSC Marc software to produce a working finite element (FE) model with 3 dimensional tetrahedral elements with linear shaped functions. The dimensions of a precontoured pelvic osteotomy plate with eight screws and a twisted seven screw straight plate were used to build the 2 fixations implants for the FE models. An equivalent load of 300 N was applied progressively on all FE models in order to facilitate its convergence. The load was applied in a distributed manner on the femur-hip joint contact area in order to simulate the actual behavior of the joint. The aim of the present study was to analyze the difference in stiffness and behavior under loading between a lateral vs ventral plate fixation, with unlocked screws and different gap scenarios, for stabilization of a pelvic osteotomy using finite element analysis.

Results: From both configurations the maximum displacement of the ventral plate with 7 screws without gap had a value of 1.988 mm, while in the DPO plate had a maximum displacement of 2.191 mm. The load applied for each of the different configurations studied when a gap of 1° was considered and also when a condition of no gap was considered. The ventral plate was stiffer than the lateral plate when a gap was not present. When the gap was closed in the ventral plate, the stiffness increased until a point that remained constant.

Conclusions: Ventral plate fixation can be as or more stiff as lateral plate fixation and provides flexible fixation. This behavior should reduce screw loosening. Using ventral plate fixation is recommended to reduce screw loosening or failure.

Keywords: Pelvic osteotomy, Hip dysplasia, Finite element analysis

Background

Triple pelvic osteotomy in dogs was first mentioned in the literature in 1969 [1]. Encouraging clinical and radiographic results were reported following triple pelvic osteotomy [2–6]. Thus, triple or double pelvic osteotomy has been used successfully to treat canine hip dysplasia [7, 8]. However, fixation complications are common in pelvic osteotomy repair and there has been little research into methods to reduce the rate of complications. Additional ventral fixation of the ilium decreased complications in a small group of dogs undergoing triple pelvic osteotomy and provided good stability for cadaveric oblique iliac osteotomy [9, 10]. In 2011, a study was undertaken to quantify the comparative benefit of using a ventral iliac plate in a double pelvic osteotomy model, and the effects of a gap in the fixation. Testing to compare the rigidity of the fixation methods were analyzed through the analysis of the degree of deformation under loading [11]. Anyway, complications rates for pelvic osteotomy can be very high with screw

* Correspondence: ciprian.ober@usamvcluj.ro
[3]Department of Surgery, Faculty of Veterinary Medicine, University of Agricultural Sciences and Veterinary Medicine, Calea Manastur 3-5, Cluj-Napoca, Romania
Full list of author information is available at the end of the article

loosening at up to 62% being the most common problem [12–14]. Recommendations on screw selection and use have been made to reduce the incidence of screw loosening [15–17]. Locking screw use in pelvic osteotomy reduces the incidence of loosening [18–20]. Using either a triple or double pelvic osteotomy achieves similar acetabular ventroversion and have in effect the same result [11]. The purpose of this study was to analyze the difference in stiffness and behavior under loading between a lateral and a ventral plate for stabilization of a pelvic osteotomy using finite element analysis.

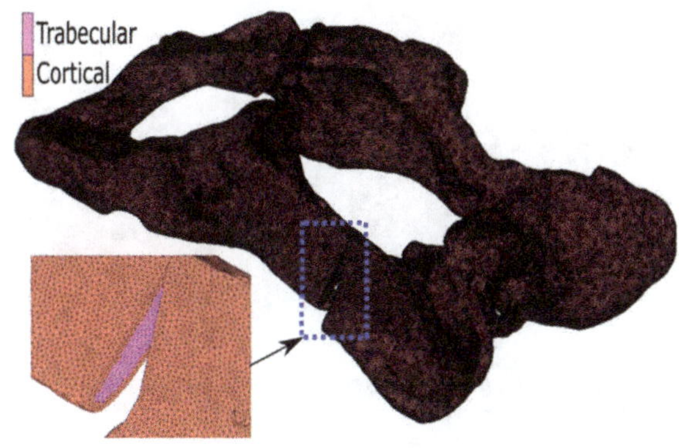

Fig. 1 FE model of pelvis proposed in which is appreciated in the osteotomy in the cortical and cancellous bone

Methods

Cadaver pelvis was used to scan and build pelvis model. Artificial bone was used in lab testing. Sourcing of materials was from a dog that died of natural causes and the artificial bones from Sawbones Company (Sweden). Using 3D scanning a stl image was produced of a canine pelvis (25 kg male Collie breed) and this was subsequently refined in CAD. Using the CAD files, the images were imported in MSC Marc software to produce a working finite element (FE) model with 3 dimensional tetrahedral elements with linear shaped functions. The dimensions of a precontoured pelvic osteotomy plate with eight 3 mm screws and a twisted seven 3 mm screw straight plate were used to build the 2 fixations implants for the FE models. The screws were fixed to behave as unlocked screws. Before the FE simulations were run validation bench tests were carried out using artificial cancellous bone blocks (Sawbones, Malmo). Osteotomy and plate fixation were set up in the 2 methods: 1. Ventral plate fixation 2. Lateral plate fixation. The load required to cause a deformation of set amount was recorded for 3 experiments for each plate position. This data was used to validate the FE simulation for all configurations.

Finite Element (FE) models for each of the plate configurations studied were built to determine and verify the joint stiffness according to the applied load. Each of the FE models proposed that formed each configuration considered the osteotomised pelvis, the different plates and the screws. The geometric models used in the FEM discretization process of each of the parts (pelvis, plates and screws) were generated by measurements from actual samples of plates and artificial osteotomised pelvis. Due to the fact that the surface of the artificial osteotomised pelvis is very irregular; a 3d scanner was used to obtain its geometrical model. The remaining parts (plates and screws) were modeled directly in the FE MSC Marc software used. For all plate configurations studied, three dimensional FE models with 4-node isoparametric tetrahedral elements were used to mode the pelvis, plates and screws. An average element size of 0.6 mm was used for the cortical and cancellous bone, while for the plates and screws element sizes were for 0.8 mm and 0.9 mm respectively. An outer thin cortical bone and an inner cancellous bone were used to model the pelvis according to the literature. The material properties used for the cortical bone were $E = 17,000$ MPa and $\nu = 0.25$, while for the cancellous values of $E = 150$ MPa and $\nu = 0.3$ were used. A titanium alloy with $E = 107,000$ MPa and $\nu = 0.34$ was used for modeling of the plates and screws. The cortical and cancellous bone topography in the osteotomised area of the FE pelvis model was the same for all plate configurations (Fig. 1). A segment-to-segment method with a coefficient of friction of 0.1 was used for detecting mechanical contact between the plates and pelvis for all studied configurations. The mechanical contact between the screws and the osteotomised pelvis was defined via a glue contact between the matching nodes in both contact bodies. The same boundary conditions were applied in all

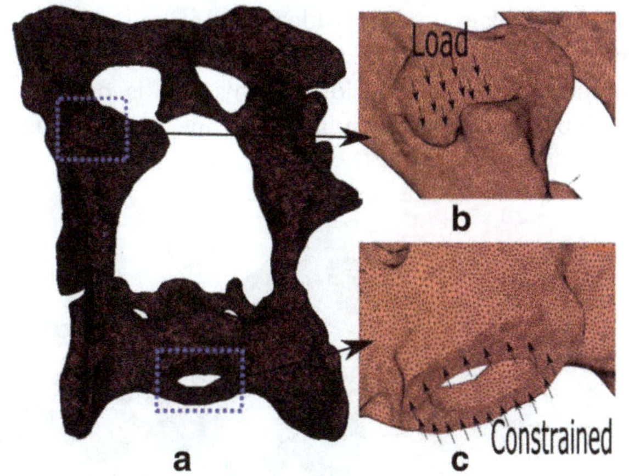

Fig. 2 a Boundary conditions applied to the FE model pelvis: load (**b**) and constraints (**c**)

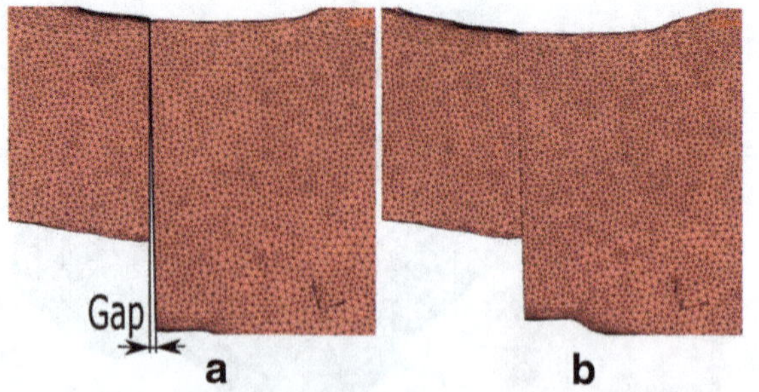

Fig. 3 Detail of the gap considered (**a**) and not considered (**b**)

finite element models in order to compare the different stiffness's obtained. An equivalent load of 300 N was applied progressively on all FE models in order to facilitate its convergence. The load was applied in a distributed manner on the femur-hip joint contact area in order to simulate the actual behavior of the joint. The movement of the nodes that connected the pelvis to the column were constrained in order to immobilize the pelvis. Figure 2 shows a model of the pelvis which details the area where the load was applied and the area of the spinal column in which the constraint was applied.

Also, for all configurations studied, the value of the joint stiffness depending on the applied load was calculated according to the following equation:

$$Stiffness = \frac{Applied\ Force}{Displacement\ Obtained}$$

In this study, two types of different plate configurations were studied. The first configuration studied was a DPO plate with eight screws on the lateral ilium. The final configuration studied was a ventral plate and was fixed to the pelvis with seven screws. In addition, a small gap in the osteotomised pelvis area was taken into consideration for all configurations studied in order to determine their influence on the stiffness of the joints. This gap is defined as the separation corresponding to a one angular degree (1°) between the different parts in which the osteotomised pelvis is divided. Figure 3 shows a configuration of plate in which the gap has been considered (Fig. 3a) and another in which it has not been considered (Fig. 3b).

Figure 4a shows the DPO plate mounted on the osteotomised pelvis. Four screws were used on one side of the osteotomy while another four screws were used on the opposite side (see Fig. 4b). The dimensions of the plate were 15 × 3 mm and the diameter of the screws was 3 mm. In this configuration, all screws pass through the entire pelvis, and mechanical contact between the plate & cortical bone and between the plate & screws is created in order to completely define the contact in the plate. Contact between the bone fragments is defined in the elements close to the osteotomy in order to detect when the osteotomy gap is closed or open.

Figure 5a shows the ventral plate mounted on the osteotomised pelvis. Four screws were used on one side of the fracture while three screws were used on the opposite side (see Fig. 6b). The dimensions of the plate were 6 × 2 mm and the diameters of the screws were 3 mm. Similar to the previous configuration, contact between the bone fragments is defined in the elements close to the fracture site in order to detect when the gap is closed or open.

Results

The maximum displacement obtained from the osteotomised pelvis by applying a maximum load of 300 N when a ventral plate of 7 screws without gap (Fig. 6a) and a DPO plate without gap (Fig. 6) are illustrated. From both configurations it is observed that the maximum displacement of the ventral plate with 7 screws without gap has a value of 1.988 mm. while in the DPO plate has a maximum displacement of 2.191 mm. Figure 7 shows the variation of the stiffness obtained Vs. the load applied for each of the different configurations studied when a gap of 1° is considered and when a condition of no gap is considered.

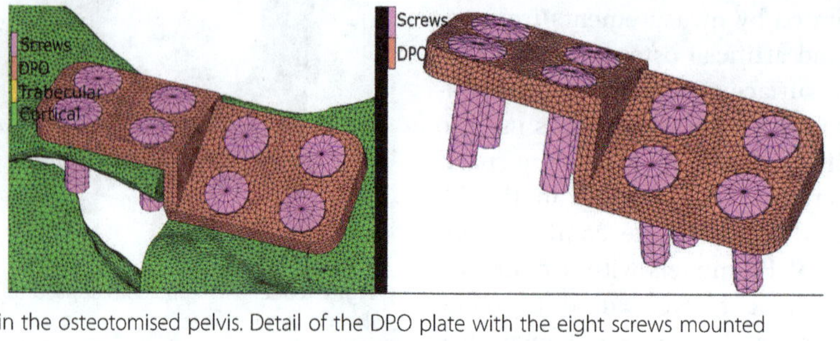

Fig. 4 DPO plate mounted in the osteotomised pelvis. Detail of the DPO plate with the eight screws mounted

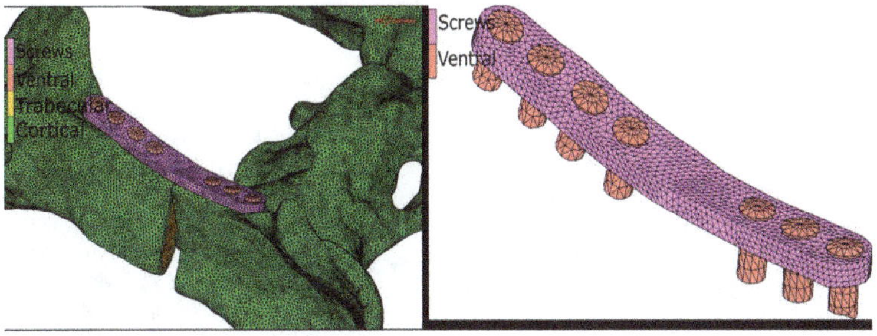

Fig. 5 Ventral plate mounted in the osteotomised pelvis. Detail of the ventral plate with the seven screws mounted

Discussion

The ventral ilium is the tension surface of the ilium and therefore is the natural choice for plating. During pelvic osteotomy the ventral ilium is exposed to allow retraction of the soft tissues medially, so there is no extensive extra tissue retraction to enable use of the ventral ilium for fixation. One of the authors (WMcC) routinely adds a ventral plate fixation to triple pelvic osteotomy fixation in giant breeds dogs, and this is a topic of further investigation.

Loss of fixation is the core issue in pelvic osteotomy complications. In non-locking plate fixation, the screws loosen in the cranial segment [15], whereas in locking plate fixation the loosening occurs in the caudal fragment. Although the number of reported cases repaired with locking plates is very low in the literature, the claim is that loosening is reduced overall by decreasing the stress on each individual screw. This is countered by the lower incidence of screw loosening in non-locking plates when the sacrum is included in the cranial screw fixation [15]. Another method to increase the overall stiffness of the fixation is to add a ventral plate [9]. Based on the results in this study, the addition of a ventral plate is theoretically justified and should lead to a reduced incidence of loss of fixation in any lateral plate fixation.

From this study it is observed that when a gap exists the fixation exhibits lower stiffness than the configuration that has no gap. Likewise, an increase in stiffness as the applied load increases is observed for ventral plate configurations. This variation in the stiffness is mainly due to the fact that the gap is closed at the ventral configuration as the load is applied, while in the DPO configurations type, this gap stays open as the load is applied. This means that DPO plates have a high stiffness in the area close to the fracture and prevent the gap from closing as the load increases. From these figures it can be deduced that the configuration of ventral plate of 7 screws without gap presents a higher stiffness than the configuration of DPO plate without gap. When the gap is closed in the ventral plate, the stiffness increases until a point that remains constant. The gap is important because depending on the dog size, the stiffness could take a low value or a high values and it is like a variable joint. The ventral plate has a dynamic aspect to its fixation. This effect does not occur on the pelvic osteotomy plate in which the stiffness keeps constant for

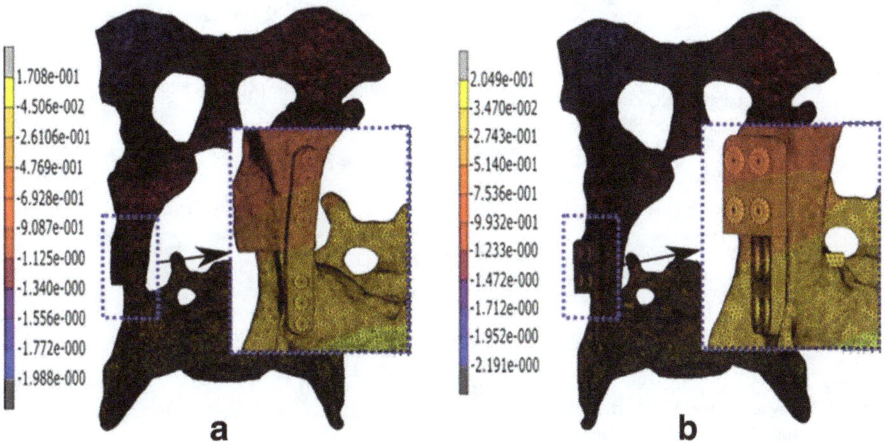

Fig. 6 Maximum displacement obtained for the ventral plate of 7 screws without gap configuration (**a**) and for the DPO plate without gap configuration (**b**)

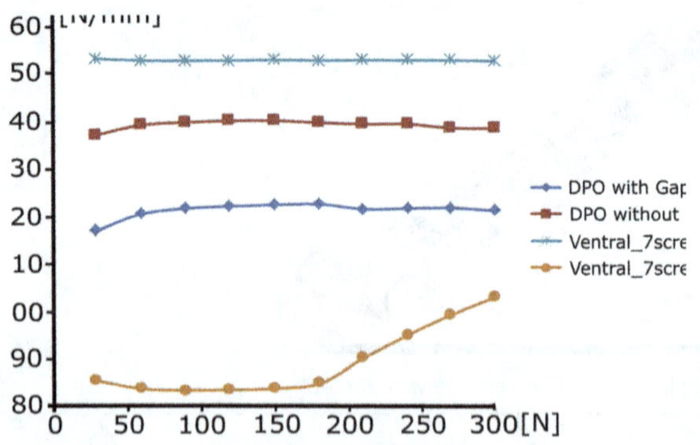

Fig. 7 Variation of the stiffness obtained Vs. the load applied for each of the different configurations studied

all loads studied. Therefore, there is increased risk of screw loosening in the lateral plate.

The limitations of this study are that finite element verification using artificial bones may not reflect actual behavior bone loading in vivo.

Conclusions

In conclusion, this study shows that ventral plate fixation can be as or more stiff as lateral plate fixation and provides flexible fixation. Using a ventral plate fixation is therefore recommended to reduce screw loosening or failure in double pelvic osteotomy to correct hip dysplasia in young dogs.

Abbreviations

3D: Three dimensional; CAD: Computer-aided design; DPO: Double pelvic osteotomy; FE: Finite element

Acknowledgements

N/A

Funding

N/A

Authors' contributions

WMcC and BMD were involved in preparation of specimens, analysis and interpretation of data and manuscript preparation. CO contributed to the preparation of specimens and writing the manuscript. RLL and FSG performed finite element analysis. All authors read and approved the final manuscript.

Consent for publication

Not applicable.

Competing interests

The authors declare that they have no competing interests.

Author details

[1]NOAH, 38 Warrenhouse Road, Baldoyle, Dublin 13, Ireland. [2]Dublin City University, Glasnevin, Dublin 9, Ireland. [3]Department of Surgery, Faculty of Veterinary Medicine, University of Agricultural Sciences and Veterinary Medicine, Calea Manastur 3-5, Cluj-Napoca, Romania. [4]Department of Mechanical Engineering, University of La Rioja, Avda. de la Paz, 93, 26006 Logroño, La Rioja, Spain.

References

1. Hohn RB, Janes JM. Pelvic osteotomy in the treatment of canine hip dysplasia. Clin Orthop. 1969;62:70–8.
2. Schrader SC. Triple osteotomy of the pelvis as a treatment for canine hip dysplasia. J Am Vet Med Assoc. 1981;178:39–44.
3. Schrader SC. Triple osteotomy of the pelvis and trochanteric osteotomy as a treatment for hip dysplasia in the immature dog: the surgical technique and results of 77 consecutive operations. J Am Vet Med Assoc. 1986;189:659–65.
4. Slocum B, Devine T. Pelvic osteotomy technique for axial rotation of the acetabular segment in dogs. J Am Anim Hosp Assoc. 1986;22:331–8.
5. McLaughlin RM, Miller CW, Taves CL, Hearn TC, Palmer NC, Anderson GI. Force plate analysis of triple pelvic osteotomy for the treatment of canine hip dysplasia. Vet Surg. 1991;20:291–7.
6. Slocum B, Devine T. Pelvic osteotomy for axial rotation of the acetabular segment in dogs with hip dysplasia. Vet Clin North Am. 1992;22:645–82.
7. Haudiquet PH, Guillon JF. Radiographic evaluation of double pelvic osteotomy versus triple pelvic osteotomy in the dog: an in vitro experimental study. In: Proceedings of the 13th European Society Of Veterinary Orthopaedics and Traumatology Congress. Munich; 2008.
8. Vezzoni A, Boiocchi S, Vezzoni L, Vanelli AB, Bronzo V. Double pelvic osteotomy for the treatment of hip dysplasia in young dogs. Vet Comp Orth Traumatol. 2010;23:444–52.
9. Fitch RB, Kerwin S, Hosgood G, Rooney M, Pluhar E, Pelsue D. Radiographic evaluation and comparison of triple pelvic osteotomy with and without additional ventral plate stabilization in forty dogs-part 1. Vet Comp Orthop Traumatol. 2002;15:164–7.
10. Vangundy T, Hulse D, Belson J, Boothe W. Mechanical evaluation of two canine iliac fracture fixation systems. Vet Surg. 1988;17(6):321–17.
11. Punke JP, Fox DB, Tomlinson JL, Davis JW, Mann FA. Acetabular ventroversion with double pelvic osteotomy versus triple pelvic osteotomy: a cadaveric study in dogs. Vet Surg. 2011;40:555–62.
12. Hosgood G, Lewis D. Retrospective evaluation of fixation complications of 49 pelvic osteotomies in 36 dogs. J Smll Anim Pract. 1993;34:123–30.
13. Koch D, Hazewinkel H, Nap R, Meij B, Wolvekamp W. Radiographic evaluation and comparison of plate fixation after triple pelvic osteotomy in 32 dogs with hip dysplasia. Vet Comp Orthop Traumatol. 1993;6:9–15.
14. Simmons S, Johnson AL, Schaeffer DJ. Risk factors for screw migration after triple pelvic osteotomy. J Am Anim Hosp Assoc. 2001;37:269–73.
15. Bogoni P, Rovesti GL. Early detection and treatment of screw loosening in triple pelvic osteotomy. Vet Surg. 2005;34:190–5.
16. Doornink MT, Nieves MA, Evans R. Evaluation of ilial screw loosening after triple pelvic osteotomy in dogs: 227 cases (1991–1999). J Am Vet Med Assoc. 2006;229:535–41.
17. Whelan MF, McCarthy RJ, Boudrieau RJ, Kraus KH. Increased sacral screw purchase minimizes screw loosening in canine triple pelvic osteotomy. Vet Surg. 2004;33:609–14.
18. Case JB, Dean C, Wilson DM, Knudsen JM, James SP, Palmer RH. Comparison of the mechanical behaviors of locked and nonlocked plate/screw fixation applied to experimentally induced rotational osteotomies in canine ilia. Vet Surg. 2012;41:103–13.
19. Rose SA, Peck JN, Tano CA, Uddin N, de Haan JJ. Effect of a locking triple pelvic osteotomy plate on screw loosening in 26 dogs. Vet Surg. 2012;41:156–62.
20. Rose SA, Bruecker KA, Petersen SW, Uddin N. Use of locking plate and screws for triple pelvic osteotomy. Vet Surg. 2012;41:114–20.

Retrospective evaluation of perioperative and short term clinical outcomes in appendicular long bone skeleton fractures repaired via the string of pearls (SOP) locking plate system

Matthew R. Field[1*], Ryan Butler[2], Robert W. Wills[2] and Wilburn M. Maxwell[3]

Abstract

Background: Internal plate fixation and, more recently, locking plate fixation are commonly used in the repair of fractures in small animal surgery. This retrospective study reviewed the use of the String of Pearls locking plate system in the fixation/repair of appendicular long bone skeleton fractures in 31 small animal veterinary patients (33 fractures).

Results: Major complications necessitating revision surgery occurred in 7/33 (21%), with implant failure as the inciting cause in all cases. Variables corresponding to an unsuccessful outcome were evaluated, and a correlation was found with plates placed in a bridging manner (placed without rigid anatomic reconstruction, $p = 0.02$) and length of follow-up ($p = 0.01$).

Conclusions: The SOP plating system can be used in the repair of appendicular longbone skeletal fractures, however, the authors propose that adjunct fixation, such as intramedullary pin, double plating, or external coaptation would likely improve results and should be considered imperative in cases in which anatomic reconstruction is either not desirable or achievable.

Keywords: Locking plate, SOP plate, String of pearls, Appendicular fracture

Background

Locking plates were first introduced in human surgery in the late nineteenth century. However, they did not gain widespread acceptance and use until Danis' work along with Arbeitsgemeinschaft fur Osteosynthesefragen (AO) in the 1960s [1]. Locking plate systems, while traditionally limiting screw insertion angles, offer several advantages that make them attractive alternatives to conventional plating systems. Locking plates act as "internal fixators," wherein the construct is created by screws locking to the plate and, thus, do not rely on plate-bone friction for stability. This is in contrast with conventional plating techniques in which plates are essentially compressed onto the bone by conventional screws in a lag fashion. Since locking plates do not rely on friction from compression for construct stability, they do not need to be contoured precisely to fit the bone. There are multiple advantages to this: shorter surgical time, reduced bone fragment handling, and, thus, easier maintenance of biologic osteosynthesis if desired [2–5]. Periosteal blood supply is preserved because of the lack of reliance on friction generated between bone and implant with conventional plating, and fractures can be stabilized more easily without interfering with biologic osteosynthesis [2–7]. Locking screws engaging with the plate are angle-stable and resist pullout when compared with non-locking screws [2, 8, 9]. When blood supply is preserved, faster healing times and lower risk of

* Correspondence: matthewfielddvm@gmail.com
[1]Arkansas Veterinary Emergency & Specialists, 11619 Pleasant Ridge Road, Little Rock, AR 72212, USA
Full list of author information is available at the end of the article

infection may result [2, 8]. Inserting screws in a monocortical fashion may further help to preserve blood supply at the fracture site and also allow the use of orthogonally placed plates [7, 10]. Monocortical screw placement, however, comes at the cost of increased construct compliance [11].

The SOP locking plate system (Orthomed, UK), a veterinary-specific locking plate, is composed of larger pearls (nodes) for screw insertion separated by internodes, such that the plate vaguely resembles the appearance of pearls on a string. (Figure 1) Plates are made of 316 L stainless steel and accept regular cortical bone screws, either self-tapping or non-self-tapping. Plate sizes are available in 2.0, 2.7, or 3.5 mm. Utilizing standard cortical bone screws is an advantage of the SOP system, as there is no extra inventory to keep on hand in the form of screws. The inside of the pearl portion of the plate is contoured in the shape of a ridge, which allows press-fit of the screw head into the plate. This helps to prevent screw loosening during cyclic loading of the plate [12].

Special plate bending irons are available that interface with the rounded nodes and allow the plates to be contoured in six degrees of freedom: medial to lateral bending, cranial to caudal bending, and torsion. When properly performed, contouring results in bending at the internode site, which helps to preserve the locking function of the pearl portion of the plate [12]. Temporary tee inserts are available for the 2.7 and 3.5 plates for use during contouring to further help preserve the locking function of the plate.

Previous research has shown the SOP plate to be stronger than the LC-DCP plate of comparable size when bending forces are applied [13–16]. SOP plates have also been found to have significantly higher perpendicular load at failure and were found to be stiffer than LC-DCP plates [17, 18]. In the nearly decade that it has been in use, we are only aware of ex vivo, in vitro, and case report studies on the use of SOP plates published in the scientific literature [11, 13–17, 19–31]. The purpose of the present study was to retrospectively evaluate the SOP system in a clinical setting when applied to appendicular skeletal fractures. We hypothesized that the SOP system would prove to be an adequate fixation method when addressing fractures involving the appendicular skeleton in small animal surgery.

Results

Complete data with follow-up ≥6 weeks were available for 31 patients (30 dogs, 1 cat, 35 SOP applications) consecutively treated for long bone fractures with SOP plate.

Signalment

Seventeen breeds of dogs (mean weight: 22.2 kg; range 4.5–50.2 kg) and one cat (domestic shorthair) were represented in the present study. Common dog breeds represented included mixed breed (12), Jack Russell Terrier

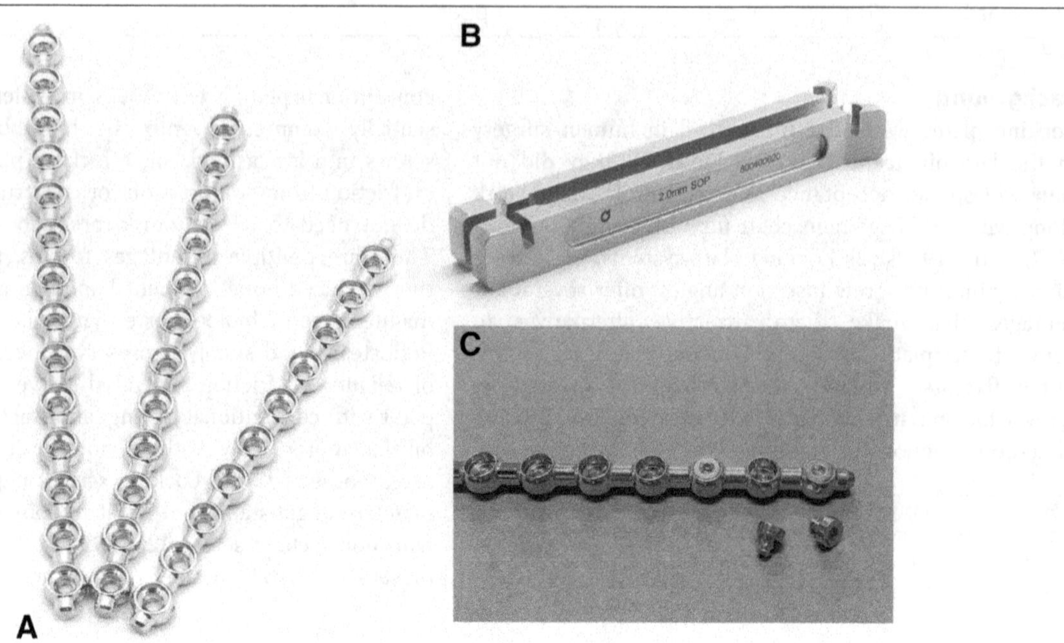

Fig. 1 a Photo of SOP plate, displaying node and internode areas (**b**) Specialized bending irons for SOP plate, allowing precision bending in multiple planes [**c**] SOP plate with associated bending tees (available for only 2.7 mm and 3.5 mm plates).

(2), Australian Shepherd (2), and one each of various other dog breeds.

Mean age of treated animals was 3.8 years (range 0.25–16 years). Nine intact males and six neutered males were represented, along with three intact females and thirteen spayed females. Mean follow-up time was 10.8 weeks (range 6.0–34).

Of 31 patients, all received non-steroidal anti-inflammatory drugs except for the feline patient.

Surgical results and complications

Thirty-one patients were treated for 33 appendicular longbone skeleton fractures. Fractures included femur (19), tibia (4), radius (4), ulna (2), and humerus (4). All patients' fractures were clinically healed at the end of the follow-up period. The two additional plate applications were orthogonally placed plates.

Fractures encountered included 13 "simple" fractures (classified as spiral, transverse, or oblique), eight "simple" comminuted fractures (defined as a comminuted fracture with four or fewer fragments), and 12 "complex" comminuted fractures (defined as a comminuted fracture with greater than four fragments).

Ten 2.0 mm plates were used in ten patients (median patient weight: 9.8 kg; mean: 16.1 kg; range 4.5 to 50.2 kg). In the largest patient, the 2.0 mm plate was placed as an adjunct fixation to a 3.5 mm SOP plate. Eleven 2.7 mm plates were used in nine patients (mean patient weight: 20.2 kg; range 8.3 to 30 kg). Fourteen 3.5 mm plates were used in 14 patients (mean patient weight: 30.8 kg; range 18.8 to 50.2 kg).

Adjunctive fixation was applied in 19/33 fractures. Sixteen of the 19 utilized cerclage wire, while two others incorporated an intramedullary pin as part of fixation, and one was and augmentation to a fissure fracture in a total hip revision. In one patient (a revision from a previous interlocking nail nonunion), the nail portion of the previous fixation was retained as an intramedullary pin following removal of the interlocking bolts. Two other cases with adjunctive fixation were large patients in which two orthogonally placed plates were used for fixation. All fractures of long bones occurred in the diaphyseal portion of the bone except one which occurred in the metaphysis of the femur. Twenty-three out of thirty-three fractures were repaired with anatomic reconstruction of all cortices and load sharing between the bone and implants ("neutralization"). The remaining ten were repaired without anatomic reconstruction ("bridging").

Seven of the 33 fractures (21%) sustained major complications, necessitating revision surgery with alternative fixation (one screw break with non-union, and six broken plates [two of which also had broken screws]). (Figure 2) Of the seven patients with implant failure, five were repaired in a "bridging" fashion. The remaining two were repaired with anatomic reconstruction and load-sharing.

One minor complication was noted in a patient who exhibited post-operative regurgitation which resolved with medical management. With the exception of one of the patients in which the plate broke, all patients were alive at final recheck, with minimal lameness noted. The deceased patient arrested during amputation of the fractured limb at another facility.

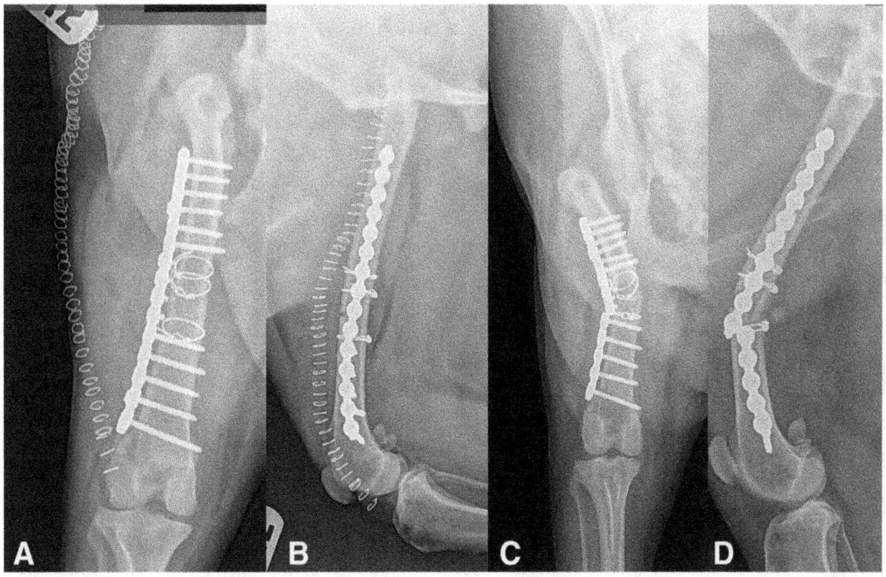

Fig. 2 Lateral and craniocaudal immediate postoperative views [**a**] & [**b**] of one of the major complication patients. **c** and **d** illustrate a plate fracture at one of the internode spaces. This patient was one of the "Bridging" patients and likely would have benefited from additional placement of an IM pin

Statistical analysis

After analyzing all variables with the aforementioned methods, the only variables which were statistically associated with higher rate of complication were bridging versus neutralization ($p = 0.02$) and length of followup time ($p = 0.01$). Fractures with longer followup time longer than 10 weeks were 1.5 times more likely to have an unsuccessful outcome. Fractures repaired in a "bridging" manner were 9.12 times more likely to have an unsuccessful outcome compared with those repaired in a "neutralization" manner.

Discussion

The purpose of our study was to report on the clinical application and outcome associated with SOP plate fixation of appendicular long bone fractures in small animals. The most common major complication reported in the present study was breakage of screws and/or plates. Broken screws were encountered near the plate/screw or the screw/bone interface. (Figure 3) We hypothesized that this was due to a stress riser effect at the SOP plate-screw shaft or screw shaft-bone interface, as has been hypothesized for screw breakage in previous studies [1, 32]. During plate application, stress risers are created at areas where there is a transition from an area with a relatively high area moment of inertia to an area with a lower area moment of inertia (AMI) [33]. AMI is a mechanical concept related to the bending strength of a construct. For solid objects, generally speaking, a larger AMI value means increased resistance to bending forces. In a standard LC-DCP plate, the transition of AMI points occurs at the screw-hole portion of the plate because this is the area with the lowest AMI, and screws are essentially inserted in lag fashion, and thus are not considered a part of the construct. With the SOP system, since the entire construct behaves as one unit, this happens at the transition point of the node (high AMI) and the screw shaft (lower AMI), thus leading to a stress riser effect at the proximal screw shaft. This, in turn, can predispose to breakage of the screw shaft. Additional stress risers exist at the screw-bone interface and at the internode portion of the plate, potentially accounting for breakage of plates at those locations.

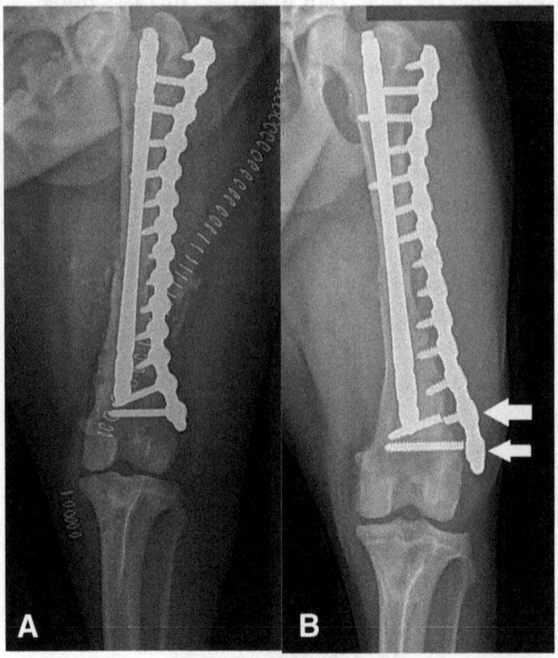

Fig. 3 Immediate postoperative radiograph [**a**] of a patient who had revision of a failed interlocking nail repair of a femur fracture. The repair was augmented with autogenous cancellous graft harvested from the proximal tibia and synthetic bone graft substitute. Screw breakage [**b**] (arrows) was noted in this patient six weeks postoperatively

It is worth mentioning that locking plates operate on the principle of angular stability, and all locking plates are technically inserted in "bridging" fashion unless other fixation is utilized to obtain significant load-sharing between the bone and the implants [33]. When significant load-sharing does not exist, even in a relatively simple fracture (such as a mid-diaphyseal oblique pattern), compliance of the construct can lead to excessive interfragmentary strain and cyclic loading, which would then result in delayed healing or non-union of fractures, placing more stress on the implant and thus making it more likely to fail. Load sharing between the implant and the bone can be difficult to assess intraoperatively in some cases and may be incorrectly judged. This also is acknowledged as a potential failure point in the patients examined in our study.

Other locking systems take advantage of the previously-mentioned AMI concept and use a screw with a larger screw core diameter [34], thus creating a higher resistance to bending forces on the screw and lessening the likelihood of screw failure. Although this improves the mechanical function of the construct, the additional screw inventory and need for varying drill bits and potentially taps increases the cost associated with the procedure and may increase surgical time. A major cost-saving advantage of the SOP system, as previously noted, is the ability to use standard cortical screws. However, the smaller core diameter of these screws may account for the higher incidence of construct failure (21%) seen in the present study when compared to studies evaluating other locking plate systems (0–9%) [34–37]. Additionally, if the SOP plating system has an unacceptably high failure rate, any cost savings gained in inventory may be negated by costs of additional surgery.

AO suggests differing guidelines in the treatment of non-reconstructable comminuted fractures in human trauma [38]. When a fracture is deemed "complicated," plate span width and plate screw density recommendations are different than a "simple" fracture. Recommendations in human medicine are that the plate length should be two to three times higher than the overall fracture length in comminuted fractures versus the eight to ten times higher recommended in simple fractures. Data from human studies suggests that plate-screw density should be below 0.5. It is unknown if these recommendations can be routinely applied to veterinary medicine, as our ability to control a patient's post-operative activity is understandably limited compared with human medicine. In the current study, neither plate-screw density nor plate span length comparisons reached statistical significance.

Other veterinary locking plate systems have had different results compared to our current findings with the SOP plating system. A recent study evaluating the use of a titanium locking plate did not find a major complication rate as high as the current study [34]. In that study, a 5.5% major complication rate was noted, contrasting with our complication rate of 21%. Other studies investigating the use of the locking compression plate on fractures have found major complication rates necessitating revision in 0–9% of fractures [35–37]. In these studies, the predominant modes of failure were screw pullout, bending of plates, and breakage of plates.

Failure of locking plates in human surgery has been noted from several standpoints. Physiological loads beyond plate-design parameters, screw disengagement due to cross-threading, insufficient screw torque, and excessive cyclical loading have all been noted as causes of failure [1]. The authors believe that the modes of failure for the current study were likely the result of cyclical loading or physiologic overloading due to patient excessive activity, although the other causes cannot be completely ruled out. In future studies, failed implants might be examined with scanning electron microscopy to evaluate for modes of failure, as has been done in human and veterinary medicine [39, 40].

Previous studies have indicated that the SOP plate is at least equivalent or stronger in bending, torsion, and when perpendicular loads are applied than a comparable conventional LC-DCP plate [13–16, 18]. However, it is prudent to keep in mind that kinetic variables measured ex-vivo (bending or torsional strength, etc.) only approximate forces that the implants will see during actual load bearing. Failure of surgical implants is more often a consequence of cyclic loading over time rather than a single large physiological force application [33]. In reality, our patients likely see a variety of force magnitudes on fracture repairs; none of the patients in this study reported any catastrophic events that could be associated with a large force application. Examples of such a force application might include slipping on the floor, being involved in motor vehicle trauma, or falling from a height.

Statistical analysis from our data indicated that follow-up times were longer in patients in which an unsuccessful outcome was noted. This is a somewhat expected outcome, and likely occurred because our follow-up times were necessarily increased in patients in which delayed healing and/or implant failure were noted and, subsequently, revision surgery was necessary.

Analysis of our data also indicated that fractures which were repaired in a "bridging" manner were greater than nine times as likely to fail as those repaired in a "neutralization" manner. The authors chose this terminology for ease of comparison and classification of fractures. As previously mentioned, all locking plates are technically placed in bridging fashion, though there can be varying levels of load sharing and interfragmentary strain depending on level of anatomic reconstruction and adjunct fixation utilized. Of the seven unsuccessful outcomes noted in the current study, five were in patients whose fractures were repaired in a "bridging" fashion. Three of the five had no adjunct fixation applied. Only four of the adjunct fixation cases utilized implants that would directly provide additional bending strength; the cerclage utilized most often instead relies on bone integrity to reduce strain on the SOP plate.

Both plate-screw density and plate:bone ratio were assessed for complication rates to look for the possibility of inappropriately repaired fractures (at least when compared to human recommendations for fractures repaired in bridging fashion). No correlation was found with regard to unsuccessful outcomes; this is potentially due to a type 2 statistical error.

The use of nonsteroidal anti-inflammatory drugs (NSAIDs) in human patients undergoing orthopedic surgery remains controversial. A recent literature review detected conflicting data on delayed bone healing in human and lab animal patients [37]. Due to the conflicting evidence in human medicine, the authors of this study wanted to include the administration of anti-inflammatory drugs as a potential confounding variable. Due to only one patient in the present study who did not receive NSAIDs, however, no meaningful conclusions could be drawn.

The mean follow-up time in this study classifies it as a perioperative to short-term study, as previously defined by Cook et al. [41] As an investigative study relating to the clinical applications of the SOP plating system for bone healing, it was beyond the scope of the current study to evaluate mid- and long-term outcomes. Further questions to be investigated in a longer-term study would include whether this plating system would have any effect on ambulation, scar tissue formation, or future occurrence of infection or neoplasia.

Potential solutions for the issue of implant failure noted in our study would be to augment fixation with implants that provide increased bending resistance, such as an intramedullary pin or a second, orthogonally placed, plate, particularly in patients with highly comminuted fractures that are unable to be neutralized or repaired anatomically. It has previously been shown that the addition of an intramedullary pin can decrease strain on a bone plate by as much as ten-fold [42]. As such, the addition of an intramedullary pin would greatly increase bending strength and may help prevent cyclical causes of failure. It is also difficult to predict the amount of activity a given patient will have and subsequent forces generated. Because of this, adjunct fixation could also be considered, whether in the form of adjunctive fixation (IM pin, orthogonal plating, etc.) or external coaptation such as splints, or temporary non-weight-bearing bandages (90–90, carpal flexion, etc.). However, the benefit of external coaptation must be weighed against potential complications.

It is possible that the method of fixation used in our study had an impact on fracture healing, and subsequently, implant failure. All SOP applications in this study utilized an open reduction with internal fixation method. The decision to repair the fractures in this manner was mainly dependent on surgeon experience with minimally invasive techniques and a lack of access to minimally invasive equipment. Minimally invasive plate osteosynthesis (MIPO) has gained favor in recent years, as it better preserves blood supply to the fracture site, and it has been shown to maintain viability of some smaller fractures segments [35]. The use of a radiopaque synthetic bone graft means it is possible that some plate applications involved less than ideal neutralization of load-bearing forces; these fractures (such as that shown in Fig. 2) may have been better suited to a "look but do not touch" open fracture stabilization technique and placement of the plate in a bridging fashion to better preserve the fracture blood-supply [33].

There were several limitations to the current study. Because of its retrospective nature and the lack of a comparison cohort, direct comparisons with other plating systems, especially locking systems, cannot be made. Indirect comparisons, therefore, were made with other systems when warranted. There were a limited number of cases in our study, especially considering the many variables that can affect the success of fracture fixation. It is possible with a higher number of patients, other variables associated with failure may reach statistical significance. With the exception of the two patients previously mentioned with two orthogonal plates, the patient in Fig. 3 with an interlocking nail revision, and one additional patient with an IM pin, none of the patients in the current study had adjunct fixation other than cerclage wire applied to the fracture. The manufacturer of the SOP system recommends the use of an intramedullary pin when used for long bone fractures and double plating for larger patients, but ultimately leaves the use of adjunct fixation up to the individual surgeon [12]. Given the ample biomechanical studies indicating the SOP plate stiffness [13–16, 18], we felt that such additional fixation might not be necessary. However, since the introduction of the SOP system, Rutherford et al. have found that adding an IM pin with 32% medullary canal diameter produced comparable construct compliance and angular deformation to a traditional plate-rod construct in a fracture gap model [19]. It is possible that the introduction of an intramedullary pin or other adjunct fixation would have improved construct durability in the current study.

Due to the use of radiopaque bone graft for all of the fractures in the current study, it is possible that the number of fractures repaired using plates in bridging fashion was underestimated. The opacity of the bone graft in some cases limited the assessment of reconstruction of the transcortex and might lead to an overestimation of load sharing between the bone and implant.

Another potential limitation is that we did not use a torque-limiter for screw insertion. The manufacturer of the SOP system recommends tightening screws so that the screw head seats firmly into the spherical component of the SOP plate [12]. This is practical advice, but it could potentially lead to under- or over-tightening of screws, which could fatigue the metal and also predispose to implant failure. We could not rule this out as a potential cause of implant failure.

Conclusions

Based on the results of the current study, we concluded that while the SOP plating system can be used to treat longbone fractures, precautions should be taken when using the plates in a bridging fashion, and adjunctive fixation that augments bending strength (in the form of intramedullary pin, orthogonal plating, external coaptation, etc.) is strongly recommended. Further in vivo study is recommended to further assess these adjunct fixations, as well as other potential confounding variables, such as plate span ratio or plate screw ratio.

Methods

Inclusion criteria

Medical records (May 2013–May 2016) from all consecutive dogs and cats with long bone fractures treated with SOP at Memphis Veterinary Specialists (MVS) were reviewed. Only clinical patients that had radiographic follow-up confirming bone healing after surgery were included in this study. For patients who had rechecks with the referring veterinarian, a copy of recheck radiographs was obtained and evaluated. Either a boarded surgeon or a surgical resident under the direct supervision of a boarded surgeon performed all surgeries. Radiographs were reviewed by a board-certified surgeon to assess post-operative and follow-up progress. For patients whose radiographs were obtained from the referring veterinarian, owners or referring veterinarians were questioned as to the patient's degree of function. Patients who were not considered clinically and radiographically healed at recheck were instructed to return every four weeks for an additional recheck until the fracture was considered healed.

Exclusion criteria

Patients with SOP applied for conditions other than fractures of long bones of the appendicular skeleton, those who did not return for follow up, and for whom no recheck data could be obtained (failed to return or deceased) were excluded from this study.

Data retrieved

Information retrieved from medical record and radiographs included: breed, body weight, age at time of surgery, gender, indication for surgery, plate size, plate length (measured as number of plate holes), manner repaired (defined as either "bridging" or "neutralization"), plate span ratio (ratio between the length of the fracture and the length of the plate [always > 1]), plate:bone ratio (ratio between the length of the bone and the length of the plate [always ≤1]), screw density (the ratio between number of holes in the plate and the number of screws used [always ≤1]), concurrent disease, follow-up time (in weeks), outcome, and complications.

Plates were considered placed in a "neutralization" fashion if, either through the use of adjunct fixation or a simple fracture configuration, anatomic reconstruction was possible such that absolute load sharing was achieved. All other plates applied to fractures in which strict anatomic reconstruction and load sharing could not be achieved, whether or not adjunct fixation was used, were considered placed in a "bridging" fashion.

Outcomes and complications were reported in a manner consistent with previous recommendations in outcome reporting in veterinary orthopedic surgery [41]. For the purpose of statistical analysis for this study, outcomes were assigned as either "Successful" or "Unsuccessful." Successful outcomes were defined as those fractures that healed without the need for revision (major complication) and no or mild lameness at recheck. All other outcomes were unsuccessful. A detailed case-by-case description is available as Additional file 1.

Surgical technique

All patients underwent open reduction with internal fixation of all fractures. Attempt at anatomic reconstruction was made for fractures oriented in a transverse, oblique, spiral, or mildly comminuted (≤4 large fracture fragments) pattern. Severely comminuted fractures were repaired by placing the SOP plate in a bridging fashion without attempt at anatomic reconstruction. Plates were contoured and fit as close to the bone surface as reasonably possible prior to application, and a minimum of three screws per fracture segment were inserted. Any remaining empty screw holes were filled with short screws (non-engaging) or bending tees to improve the strength of the overall construct. In some cases (at surgeon's discretion), adjunctive fixation was used in the form of cerclage wire, intramedullary pin, or double plating. Synthetic bone graft (Velosity Bioactive Synthetic Bone Graft, Securos, UK) was placed at all fracture sites prior to closure.

Statistical analysis

Variables evaluated for correlation with major complications or revisions included age at the time of surgery, gender, weight at the time of surgery, plate size, use of adjunct fixation, length of plate (measured by number of holes), bridging versus neutralization, bone segment in which the fracture occurred, fracture configuration (transverse, oblique, spiral, mildly comminuted [≤4 fragments], severely comminuted [> 4 fragments]), plate span width, plate:bone ratio, plate:screw density, and followup time in weeks. To determine the association between the occurrence of complications and each explanatory variable, separate univariable logistic regression models were fit with PROC LOGISTIC in SAS for Windows 9.4 (SAS Institute, Inc., Cary, NC). Penalized maximum likelihood estimation was used for the bone model due to quasi-complete separation of data points. Variables with a *p*-value of less than or equal to 0.26 were selected as candidates for a multivariable model. Collinearity was assessed by determining the correlation among quantitative variables using PROC CORR. A manual backward selection process was followed for variable selection, in which after fitting the model, the variable with the greatest *p*-values was removed and the model refit. This was continued until the final model contained only variables with a p-value of less than 0.05. Hosmer and Lemeshow Goodness-of-Fit Test was used to assess the model fit.

Abbreviations

AMI: Area Moment of Inertia; AO: Arbeitsgemeinschaft fur Osteosynthesefragen; IM: Intramedullary; LC-DCP: Limited Contact Dynamic Compression Plate; MIPO: Minimally Invasive Plate Osteosynthesis; MVS: Memphis Veterinary Specialists; SOP: String of Pearls; UK: United Kingdom

Acknowledgements

Not applicable.

Funding
The authors received no funding for this study in the form of money, grants, or equipment.

Authors' contributions
MF contributed the bulk of the research and manuscript preparation, while RB and WM provided guidance on manuscript format, research implementation, and much editing. RW provided full statistical analysis on all cases. All authors read and approved the final manuscript.

Consent for publication
Not applicable.

Competing interests
The authors declare that they have no competing interests.

Author details
[1]Arkansas Veterinary Emergency & Specialists, 11619 Pleasant Ridge Road, Little Rock, AR 72212, USA. [2]Mississippi State University, College of Veterinary Medicine, 240 Wise Center Drive, Starkville, MS 39762, USA. [3]Memphis Veterinary Specialists, 555 Trinity Creek Cove, Cordova, TN 38018, USA.

References

1. Kubiak E, et al. The evolution of locked plates. J Bone Joint Surg. 2006;88: 189–200.
2. Perren SM. Evolution of the internal fixation of long bone fractures. The scientific basis of biological internal fixation: choosing a new balance between stability and biology. J Bone Joint Surg Br. 2002;84:1093–110.
3. Voss K, Kull M, Hassig M, et al. Repair of long-bone fractures in cats and small dogs with the Unilock mandible locking plate system. Vet Comp Orthop Traumatol. 2009;22:398–405.
4. Miller DL, Goswami T. A review of locking compression plate biomechanics and their advantages as internal fixators in fracture healing. Clin Biomech (Bristol, Avon). 2007;22:1049–62.
5. Perren SM. Evolution and rationale of locked internal fixator technology. Introductory Remarks. Injury. 2001;32(Suppl2):B3–9.
6. Schwant CS, Montavon PM. Locking compression plate fixation of radial and tibial fractures in a young dog. Vet Comp Orthop Traumatol. 2005;18:194–8.
7. Boudrieau RJ. Advanced locking plate system (ALPS): rationale, biomechanics and early clinical use. Bologna: Proc World Vet Orthop Con; 2010. p. 77–82.
8. Sikes JW Jr, Smith BR, Mukherjee DP, et al. Comparison of fixation strengths of locking head and conventional screws, in fracture and reconstruction models. J Oral Maxillofac Surg. 1998;56:468–73.
9. Tepic S, Remiger AR, Morikawa K, et al. Strength recovery in fractured sheep tibia treated with a plate or an internal fixator: an experimental study with a two-year follow-up. J Orthop Trauma. 1997;11:14–23.
10. Keller MA, Voss K, Montavon PM. The ComPact UniLock 2.0/2.4 system and its clinical application in small animal orthopedics. Vet Comp Orthop Traumatol. 2005;18:83–93.
11. Demiariuk RM, Benamou J, et al. Effect of screw type and distribution on the torsional stability of 3.5 mm string of pearls locking plate constructs. Vet Surg. 2014;44:119–25.
12. Kraus KH, et al. Standard operating procedure for SOP plates. UK: Orthomed; 2008.
13. Ness MG. The effect of bending and twisting on the stiffness and strength of the 3.5 SOP implant. Vet Comp Orthop Traumatol. 2009;22:132–6.
14. Blake CA, et al. Single cycle to failure in bending of three standard and five locking plate and plate constructs. Vet Comp Orthop Traumatol. 2011;6: 408–18.
15. DeTora M, et al. Mechanical testing of 3.5 mm locking and non-locking bone plates. Vet Comp Orthop Traumatol. 2008;21:318–22.
16. Cabassu JB, et al. Single cycle to failure in torsion of three standard and five locking plate constructs. Vet Comp Orthop Traumatol. 2011;6:418–25.
17. Miller E, et al. Perpendicular pull-out force of locking versus non-locking plates in thin cortical bone using a canine mandibular ramus model. Vet Surg. 2011;40(7):870–4.
18. Benamou J, et al. Effect of bending direction on the mechanical behavior of 3.5 mm string-of-pearls and limited contact dynamic compression plate constructs. Vet Comp Orthop Traumatol. 2015;28:443–0.
19. Rutherford S, Demianiuk RM, et al. Effect of intramedullary rod diameter on a string of pearls plate-rod construct in mediolateral bending: an in vitro mechanical study. Vet Surg. 2015;44(6):737–43.
20. Segal U, Bar H, Shani J. Repair of lumbosacral fracture-luxation with bilateral twisted string-of-pearls locking plates. J Small Anim Pract. 2018. https://doi.org/10.1111/jsap.12857.
21. Kenzig AR, Butler JR, et al. A biomechanical comparison of conventional dynamic compression plates and string-of-pearls locking plates using cantilever bending in a canine ilial fracture model. BMC Vet Res. 2017;13(1): 222.
22. Hettlich BF, Fosgate GT, Litsky AS. Biomechanical comparison of 2 veterinary locking plates to monocortical screw/polymethylmethacrylate fixation in canine cadaveric vertebral column. Vet Surg. 2017;46(1):95–102.
23. Hurt RJ, Syrcle JA, et al. A biomechanical comparison of unilateral and bilateral string-of-pearls locking plates in a canine distal humeral metaphyseal gap model. Vet Comp Orthop Traumatol. 2014;27(3):186–91.
24. Malenfant RC, Sod GA. In vitro comparison of 3.5 string of pearl plate fixation to 3.5 locking compression plate fixation in a canine fracture gap model. Vet Surg. 2014;43(4):465–70.
25. Kim SE, Lewis DD. Corrective osteotomy for procurvatum deformity caused by distal femoral physeal fracture malunion stabilised with string-of-pearls locking plates: results in two dogs and a review of the literature. Aust Vet. 2014;92(3):75–80.
26. Acquaviva AE, Miller EI, et al. Biomechanical testing of locking and nonlocking plates in the canine scapula. J Am Anim Hosp Assoc. 2012;48(6): 372–8.
27. Fitzpatrick N, Yeadon R, et al. Shoulder arthrodesis in 14 dogs. Vet Surg. 2012;41(6):745–54.
28. Danielski A, Vanhaesebrouck A, Yeadon R. Ventral stabilization and facetectomy in a great Dane with wobbler syndrome due to cervical spinal canal stenosis. Vet Comp Orthop Traumatol. 2012;25(4):337–41.
29. Fitzpatrick N, Nikolaou C, et al. String-of-pearls locking plate and cerclage wire stabilization of periprosthetic femoral fractures after total hip replacement in six dogs. Vet Surg. 2012;41(1):180–8.
30. Fitzpatrick N, Bielecki M, et al. Total hip replacement with dorsal acetabular rim augmentation using the SOP implant and polymethylmethacrylate cement in seven dogs with dorsal acetabular rim deficiency. Vet Surg. 2012; 41(1):168–79.
31. Ness MG. Repair of Y-T humeral fractures in the dog using paired string of pearls locking plates. Vet Comp Orthop Traumatol. 2009;22(6):492–7.
32. Vallefuoco R, Le Pommellet H, et al. Complications of appendicular fracture repair in cats and small dogs using locking compression plates. Vet Comp Orthop Traumatol. 2016;29:46–52.
33. Johnson AL, et al. AO principles of fracture Management in the dog and cat. Davos: AO Publishing; 2005.
34. Guerrero TG, Kalchofner K, Scherrer N, Kircher P. The advanced locking plate system (ALPS): a retrospective evaluation in 71 small animal patients. Vet Surg. 2014;43:127–35.
35. Hudson CC, Pozzi A, Lewis DD. Minimally invasive plate osteosynthesis: applications and techniques in dogs and cats. Vet Comp Orthop Traumatol. 2009;22:175–82.
36. Gilbert, S, Ragetly, GR, Boudrieau. "Locking compression plate stabilization of 20 distal radial and ulnar fractures in toy and miniature breed dogs." Vet Comp Orthop Traumatol 2015; 28:441–447.
37. Pountos I, Georgouli T, et al. "Do nonsteroidal anti-inflammatory drugs affect bone healing? A critical analysis." Scientific World Journal 2012 (2012): 606404. *PMC* Web 21 June 2017.
38. Gautier E. Bridge plating. AO Dialogue. 2009:24–7.
39. Piatelli A, Piatelli M, et al. Light and scanning electron microscope report of four fractured implants. J Oral & Maxillofac Implants. 1998;13(4):561–4.
40. Charles EA, Ness MG, Yeadon R. Failure mode of transcondylar screws used for treatment of incomplete ossification of the humeral condyle in 5 dogs. Vet Surg. 2009;38(2):185–91.
41. Cook JL, et al. Proposed definitions and criteria for reporting time frame, outcome, and complications for clinical orthopedic studies in veterinary medicine. Vet Surg. 2010;39:905–8.

24

A novel tibial tuberosity advancement technique with cranial implant fixation (TTA CF)

Yauheni Zhalniarovich[1*], Marta Mieszkowska[1], Paulina Przyborowska-Zhalniarovich[1], Joanna Głodek[1], Andrzej Sobolewski[2], Grzegorz Waluś[2] and Zbigniew Adamiak[1]

Abstract

Background: Cranial cruciate ligament rupture is the most frequent orthopedic disorder in human and animals. An array of surgical techniques have been described to stabilize the stifle joint in dogs, including intraarticular stabilization, extraarticular stabilization, and tibial osteotomy techniques. Tibial plateau leveling osteotomy and tibial tuberosity advancement with a lot of modifications are the most common. In this study we report the possibility of fixing the novel titanium implant for tibial tuberosity advancement with two screws in a craniocaudal direction. The aim of our study was to improve the clinical benefit of the tibial tuberosity advancement surgical technique where an attempt was made to reduce the number of screws and obtain a strong implant fixation with minimal bone traumatization. This way of attachment allows to distribute the forces evenly on medial and lateral side of osteotomy gap.

Results: Tibial tuberosity advancement with cranial implant fixation was performed in four sheep. Complete radiographic and clinical follow up was recorded. All four sheep had a complete osteotomy line healing at a mean of 10 weeks postoperative (range 8–12 weeks). None of the animals had osteotomy gap healing grades of poor. Minor complication included the minimally cracked Maquet hole on the postoperative radiographs, without displacement of the tibial crest which occurred in 2 sheep. Major complication grade 1, major complication grade 2 and catastrophic were not found.

Conclusions: The novel surgical technique for tibial tuberosity advancement with cranial implant fixation is technically comparable to the recent trend in tuberosity advancement techniques, where partial osteotomy of the cranial tibial tuberosity crest is performed. A cranial implant fixation allows to distribute the forces evenly on medial and lateral side of osteotomy gap, which may result in less number of major complications in dogs. A novel titanium implant decreases the tibial traumatisation by reducing the number of screws.

Keywords: Cranial cruciate ligament, CCL, Stifle, Osteotomy, Maquet hole, Ovine model, Dynamic stabilization

Background

Cranial cruciate ligament (CCL) insufficiency is the most common orthopedic disorder in humans and dogs associated with pelvic limb lameness [1–4]. CCL rupture is one of the major contributors to the development of stifle joint osteoarthritis [2]. The CCL works as a primary stabilizer for both rotational and translational movements of the tibia, which is the main function to resist the cranial tibial thrust [5, 6]. Several surgical techniques have been described to stabilize the CCL ruptured stifle, including static intracapsular or static extracapsular [7–9] and dynamic techniques [10, 11]. Dynamic surgical methods provide stability during weight bearing by altering the geometry of the stifle joint [10–14]. Dynamic techniques are based on tibial osteotomies and the two most common of which are tibial plateau leveling osteotomy (TPLO) and tibial tuberosity advancement (TTA) [7].

* Correspondence: eugeniusz.zolnierowicz@uwm.edu.pl
[1]Department of Surgery and Radiologu with Clinic, Faculty of Veterinary Medicine, University of Warmia and Mazury in Olsztyn, Oczapowskiego 14, 10-718 Olsztyn, Poland
Full list of author information is available at the end of the article

Tibial tuberosity advancement was developed to reconstruct dynamic stability in CCL deficient stifles in dogs by reducing the patellar tendon angle (PTA). PTA is created by the tibial plateau and patella tendon [15, 16]. Stability is achieved by performing the mediolateral osteotomy and advancing the tibial tuberosity cranially [15, 16]. By changing the angle between patellar ligament and PTA to 90° during the stance phase of gait, shift forces are eliminated and the stifle is rendered dynamically stable [15]. Experimental in vitro studies attested the biomechanics of TTA [17–19], and clinical reports proved satisfactory limb function after surgery [20–23].

In the conventional TTA technique description, advancement of tibial tuberosity is achieved by using forks and cages of different sizes, which are introduced into the osteotomy line [20–24]. Cranial advancement of the tibial tuberosity varies from 3 to 12 mm depending on the cage size [15, 16]. As of 2010, > 80,000 conventional TTAs were performed by > 750 veterinary surgeons worldwide using one manufacturer's equipment [25]. In 2014 the TTA Rapid technique was reported, which was based on the Maquet technique. In this procedure the distal cortex of the tibial crest remains intact [26].

Animal models have been widely used in orthopedic biomedical research in human and veterinary medicine [27–31]. International standards established regarding the species corresponding for testing implantation of materials in bone, state that rabbits, pigs, dogs, goats, are suitable [27, 28]. The sheep is a species frequently used in orthopedic research, because of bones size, bone and joint structure, body weight, and bone healing processes [27, 28]. The ovine model is very useful to analyze the biomechanical characteristics of bones [27, 32].

Conventional TTA and TTA Rapid are based on fixing the cage from the medial side of the tibia [16, 21, 24, 26]. In both methods there are many implants (plate, fork, cage and screws) attached to the bone. This amount of material inside the bone can cause a lot traumatization to the bone and delay regeneration. It is also can cause bone weakness or affect the strength of the forming callus. In both surgical procedures mentioned above in case of postoperative complications, such as tibial tuberosity fracture, there are K-wires drilled cranially which are stabilizing the fracture [22, 25, 45, 46]. The aim of our study was to improve the clinical benefit of the TTA Rapid surgical technique by reducing the number of screws needed to obtain strong implant fixation with minimal tibial crest traumatization and, at the same time, to prevent tibial tuberosity fracture by screw placement in aa craniocaudal plane. Moreover, the aim was to check the possibility of fixing the novel titanium implant for TTA with screws in craniocaudal direction (TTA with cranial fixation [TTA CF]) on ovine model. Thanks to the dedicated implant guide the novel titanium implant is fixed with two screws in the proximal tibia.

Methods

Animals

This study was performed on four female Merino sheep, skeletally mature, between 2 and 4 years of age, with body weight (BW) of 40 kg (±5 kg). The sheep were obtained through the farm with registration nr PL 050649214001 (Barczewo, Poland). The animals were kept at 15 ± 2 °C under a 12 h/12 h dark/light cycle. The animals received water ad libitum and had free access to food. Patients were monitored at all times by a specialized veterinary surgeon. All animal procedures were conducted in accordance with the Local Ethical Committee for Experiments on Animals in OLSZTYN (NR 07/2015 Olsztyn, Poland). Animals were followed up for 6 months. After 6 month observation period the sheep were euthanized by intravenous injection of pentobarbital. Each animal was kept under the Good Laboratory Practice conditions and looked after by a specialist.

Anaesthesia

Animals were sedated with xylazine (0.1 mg/kg BW, Vetaxyl, Vet-Agro, Lublin, Poland) and general anaesthesia was induced with ketamine (3–5 mg/kg BW, Bioketan, Vetoquinol Biowet, Gorzów Wielkopolski, Poland), diazepam (0.1 mg/kg BW, Relanium, Polfa, Warsaw, Poland) and propofol (0.2–0.4 mg/kg BW, Scanofol, ScanVet, Gniezno, Poland) and maintained with intravenous administration of propofol constants rate infusion (1–5 mg/kg BW/h) with isolfurane inhalantion during the procedure (1.5–2% Aerane, Baxter, Warsaw, Poland). Carprofen (2 mg/kg BW, Carprodyl, Ceva Animal Health, Warsaw, Poland) as a painkiller and benzathine penicilline (4.5 mg/kg BW, Penicillin LA, ScanVet, Gniezno, Poland) was administered pre- and postoperatively.

Preoperative planning

Before surgery mediolateral and craniocaudal radiographs of the stifles were performed in each sheep to assure proper advancement of tibial tuberosity. Measurements were obtained using RadiAnt DICOM software. Common tangent TTA procedure was used to assess the degree of advancement [26, 33]. In all four animals 6 mm width titanium implants were used. The proximodistal height of the implant was 20 mm and the slope of the implant was 6° (Fig. 1). Using the TTA CF template the optimal Maquet hole position, the length of the osteotomy cut, and the thickness of the cranial cortex in the region of the Maquet hole were designated (Fig. 2). Detailed information about measurements are included in Table 1.

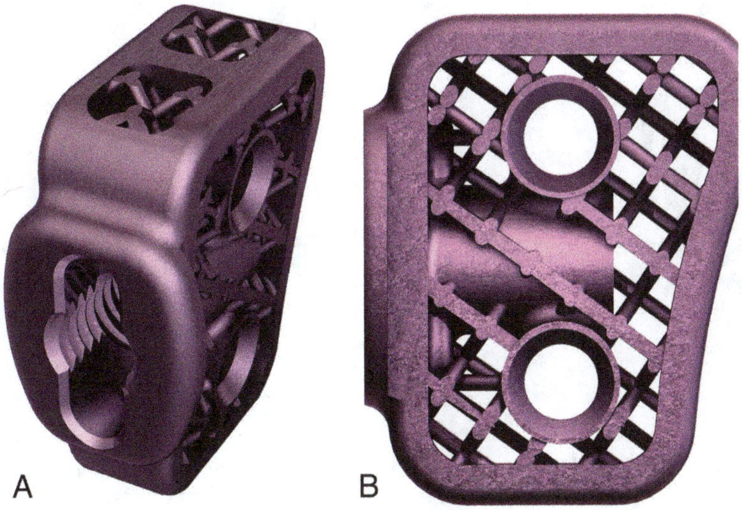

Fig. 1 Oblique (**a**) and lateral (**b**) view of 6 mm titanium implant for TTA CF

The titanium implants were designed with porous core and produced on a 3D printer with a Selective Laser Melting (SLM) technique. The printing process takes place in a closed, sealed machine chamber. The machine chamber was filled with an inert gas - argon, which protects the surface of the produced implant against reacting with moisture coming from the powder, oxygen and other elements that can change the composition and properties of the surface layers of the printout. Therefore, the powder was in a closed powder handling system, so that it does not change its properties during the printing process. The TTA-CF implants were made of biocompatible materials which chemical composition complies with the ISO 5832–3 standard.

Surgical procedures

The surgical technique was based on the Maquet procedure, which was firstly described in 1976 to allay pain related to osteoarthritis of the patellofemoral joint and in chondromalacia of the patella in people [34]. The sheep were located in lateral recumbency with the limb to be operated on the table with opposite limb removed from the surgery area. After the place of surgery had been shaved, the skin was disinfected completely, and a sterile surgical drape was applied.

A skin incision was made from the parapatellar region to the proximal tibia on the medial side using electrocautery to control bleeding. Fasciae were transected in line with the skin incision. A medial parapatellar mini-arthrotomy was performed and LCC was intersected using a #11 scalpel blade. For tibial osteotomy the designed drill and saw guide were positioned precisely in both craniocaudal and proximodistal planes of the tibia. In proximal part a 1.2 mm K-wire was inserted perpendicular to the straight patella ligament into the distal infra patellar bursa. This K-wire was inserted into the long leg of the designed drill and saw guide. The 0.9 mm needle was inserted into the short leg of the TTA CF drill and saw guide in the hole which is corresponding to the cranial cortical thickness of the tibial crest. The Maquet hole was drilled with a 3 mm drill bit (Fig. 3). The osteotomy was performed perpendicular to the craniocaudal plane of the tibia with a 0.7 mm saw blade with the use of a TTA CF drill and saw guide. After the osteotomy was performed the drill and saw guide were removed. A 3 mm bone spreader was inserted in the osteotomy line. The spreader has an adjustment screw, by which it is possible to precisely and at the same time slightly widening the osteotomy line. The spreader has been equipped with a scale that prevents the osteotomy line from opening excessively. Gentle rotation of the adjustment screw advanced the tibial tuberosity. When the desired tuberosity advancement was achieved, the 6 mm width TTA CF implant with screwed guide was inserted into the osteotomy gap (Fig. 4). The implant guide allows to drill 2 craniocaudal holes for implant attachment (Fig. 5). The TTA CF implants were fixed with two 2.7 mm titanium self-tapping cortical screws. The implant guide was unscrewed from the implant and removed. The wound was closed in layers, starting from deep fascia with interrupted absorbable suture. Subcutaneous tissue and skin was closed with continuous absorbable material. Immediately after surgery the operated leg was radiographed in mediolateral and craniocaudal projections to evaluate the implant position. A pressure bandage was applied for 24 h.

Radiography and clinical follow up

The operated leg was radiographed immediately postoperatively and then after every 2 weeks up to 6 months in

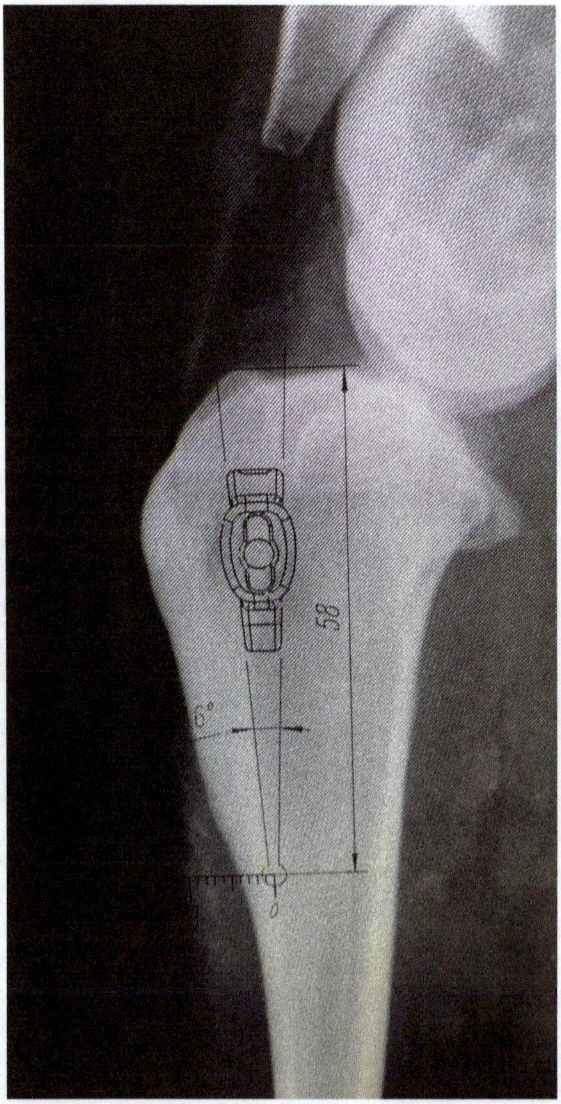

Fig. 2 Preoperative measurements. This image shows the measurement of cranial cortex of the tibial crest using 6 mm implant template for TTA CF. With the template the exact position of the Maquet hole along long axis of the tibia is determined. In this case 4 mm cranial cortical thickness was measured

both a craniocaudal and mediolateral projections. Positioning of the implant, position of the screws and callus formation were evaluated from the radiographs. Obtained images were evaluated by the specialized veterinary surgeon. Complete bone healing was defined when trabecular structures were visible in the osteotomy line [26]. A 5 level subjective numerical rating scale for lameness evaluation was used [31]. Lameness was graded as 0- sound lameness, 1- barely detectable, 2- mild, 3- moderate, and 4- severe lameness [31]. Postoperative complications were graded as minor, major grade 1, major grade 2 and catastrophic using a previously reported scale [35].

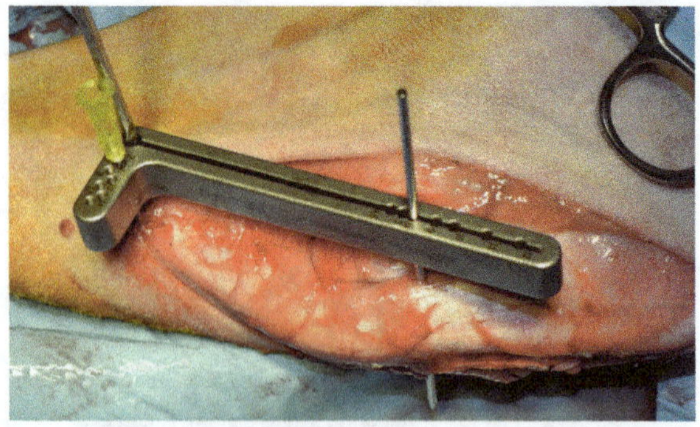

Fig. 3 Intraoperative use of drill and saw guide for TTA CF technique. The short leg of the guide corresponded to the cranial cortical thickness of the tibial crest measured with use of template (4 mm). The long leg of the drill and saw guide has numbers corresponded to the implant number (6 mm)

Results

TTA CF with the use of a 6 mm width titanium implant was performed in four sheep. All the sheep recovered from anesthesia and surgery without complications. Post-operative.

lameness was evaluated using the previously stated subjective 5-point grading scale (from 0 to 4). During the first 7 days after surgery, we observed in some animals an obvious mild lameness (degree 2) of the left hindlimb when walking, but it improved favorably to hardly detectable lameness (degree1) during the second week [31]. The normal gait was from third week since the end of the surgical procedure (Table 2).

The distance of the tibial tuberosity advancement and the appropriate titanium implant size were printed based on preoperative radiographic measurements. The TTA CF implant size used was 6 mm width. The dedicated implant guide allows the surgeon to drill and fix the implant with two 2.7 mm self-tapping titanium screws craniocaudally and a 2 mm drill bit was used to perform the screw holes. A 3 mm drill bit was used to perform the Maquet hole in all patients. Complete radiographic and clinical follow up was recorded. All four sheep had a complete bone healing at a mean of 10 weeks (range 8–12 weeks). None of the animals had osteotomy gap healing grades of poor.

After the surgery, osteotomy gaps were clearly visible. Radiographs taken during the experimental period of 6 months revealed gradual hyperplasia and progressive mineralization of bone callus at the following stages of healing (Fig. 6). Two weeks postoperatively the osteotomy line showed a clear contour. After 4 weeks small amounts of periosteal callus were observed. As a result of bone remodeling, the osteotomy gap began to disappear gradually after 6 weeks.

Minor complications included the minimally cracked Maquet hole on the 2 weeks postoperative radiographs,

Table 1 Preoperative measurements, surgery time and clinical observation

Animals	Cranial cortex thickness	Implant width	Body weight	Osteotomy length	Surgery time	Osteotomy healing time	Oservations
Sheep I	4 mm	6 mm	38 kg	58 mm	55 min	9 weeks	Minimally cracked Maquet hole on the 2 weeks postoperative radiographs
Sheep II	5 mm	6 mm	43 kg	58 mm	48 min	12 weeks	
Sheep III	5 mm	6 mm	42 kg	58 mm	40 min	11 weeks	Minimally cracked Maquet hole on the 2 weeks postoperative radiographs
Sheep IV	4 mm	6 mm	39 kg	58 mm	45 min	8 weeks	

without displacement of the tibial crest occur in 2 sheep (50%) (Fig. 7). Major complication grade 1, major complication grade 2 and catastrophic were not found. None of this sheep not required any additional treatment.

Discussion

Rupture of CCL is the most common orthopedic disorder [1–4]. The CCL stabilize both rotational and translational movements of the tibia [36, 37]. There are two common types of TTA procedure in dogs [15, 26]. TTA restore dynamic stability in CCL ruptured stifles by reducing the angle formed by the tibial plateau and the simple patellar ligament through the osteotomy of the tibial tuberosity in the dorsal plane and advancing the tibial crest. The dimension of advancement is based on the preoperative measurements of patellar ligament and plateau angle [15, 16, 22]. The TTA surgical technique is based on the Maquet procedure, which was presented to allay pain related to osteoarthritis of the patellofemoral joint and in chondromalacia of the patella in people [34]. Our modified TTA CF technique is a modification of conventional TTA and TTA Rapid technique, where an attempt is made to reduce the number of screws and obtain a strong implant fixation only with two screws in craniocaudal direction. In the current experiment, TTA with cranial implant fixation was investigated.

In the last two decades, conventional TTA and TTA Rapid have become a successful and respected surgical techniques for CCL insufficiency treatment [21, 22, 25, 26, 37, 38]. Both techniques have some limitations. In conventional TTA the surgeon has to ensure sufficient bone stock on the cranial part of tibial crest and sufficient space on the tibial shaft to allow attachment of the fork, plate and bone screws [22]. In TTA Rapid technique the cage is attached only on one side, all the screws are mounted from the medial side of the tibia. Therefore, mobility remains on the lateral surface of the osteotomy gap. This report describes the TTA CF technique, where the implant is attached with two 2.7 mm screws in a craniocaudal direction. The designed implant guide allows for the introduction of two screws through the center of cranial tibial crest.

We have reported the TTA CF technique on ovine model. Sheep are becoming popular as animal model in orthopedic research in both human and veterinary medicine [28, 32, 39, 40, 42]. In humans, the use dogs are reduced due to the emotional impact related to these kinds of animals [28]. Sheep were used to study repair of fractures and articular ligaments, limb lengthening, and treatment of osteoporosis and osteoarthrosis [28]. TTA CF titanium implants and special guides are dedicated for dogs affected by CCL insufficiency. The

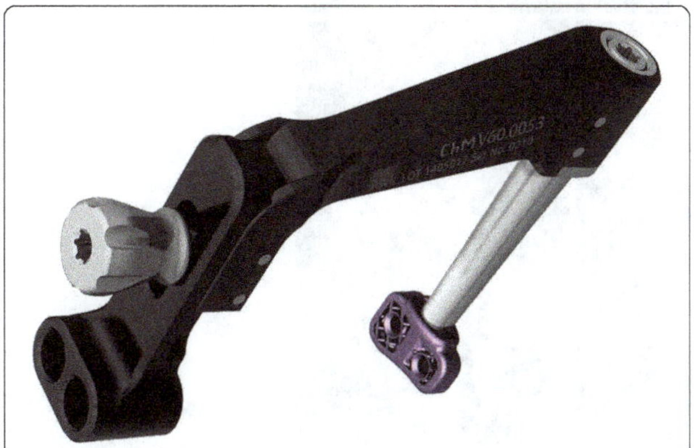

Fig. 4 Image of the 6mmTTA CF titanium implant with a screwed dedicated implant guide

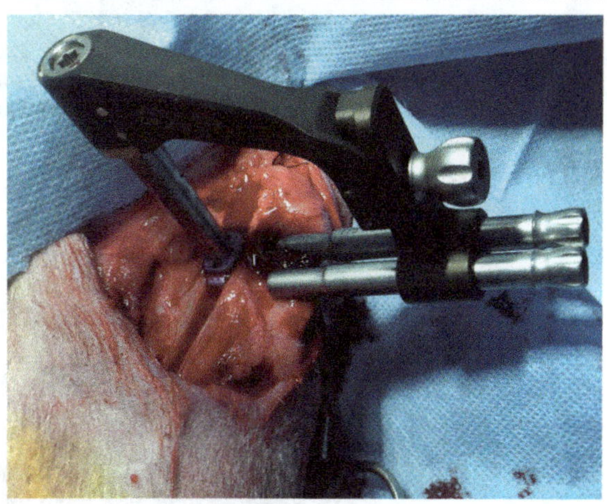

Fig. 5 Intraoperative use of dedicated implant guide for TTA CF technique. The implant guide allows to drill 2 craniocaudal holes throught the cranial tibial crest for implant attachment

Table 2 Summary of postoperative degree of lameness

Animals/days	1 day	2 day	3 day	4 day	5 day	6 day	7 day	8 day	9 day	10 day	11 day	12 day	13 day	14 day	15 day	16 day
Sheep I	3	3	3	3	3	3	3	2	2	2	2	2	2	1	1	0
Sheep II	3	3	3	3	3	3	2	2	2	2	2	2	1	1	1	0
Sheep III	3	3	3	3	2	2	2	2	2	2	1	1	1	1	0	0
Sheep IV	3	3	3	3	3	3	2	2	2	1	1	1	0	0	0	0

Lameness was graded as norm- normal gait, 0- sound lameness, 1- barely detectable, 2- mild, 3- moderate, 4- severe lameness. Lameness was evaluated starting from 1 day after surgery

sheep was chosen as a model animal because the anatomy and biomechanics of the stifle joint are similar to dogs [28, 32, 39, 40, 42].

Sheep reach sexual maturity between seven and 12 months of age. At sexual maturity, the animals are not mature from skeletal point of view yet. The proximal tibial ossification center closes between 20 and 26 months of age, and the distal tibia closes between 12 and 18 months. This report has been carried out on four female Merino sheep, skeletally mature between 2 and 4 years of age.

The TTA CF surgical technique is based on the Maquet procedure and has been derived from descriptions of the procedure in man [34]. With this surgical procedure in dogs, the osteotomy is performed in the frontal plane and left incomplete, so the tibial crest retains its distal attachment to the tibia [26, 41]. Once the osteotomy is made, the cranial tibial crest is advanced and held in position with implant [26, 41]. Our novel attachment method and the appropriate implant guide allow the firm fixation of the implant. Fixing the screws in a craniocaudal direction allows to distribute the forces evenly on medial and lateral side of osteotomy gap.

All Maquet holes were created with a 3 mm drill bit. In previous reports the diameter used for Maquet hole drilling varied from 2 to 3 mm [26, 43, 44]. A 3 mm hole allows for better force distribution throughout the osteotomy line [43], but on the other hand it creates a larger bone defect [26]. Because the size of implant is often related to the size of animal, a 2 mm and 2.5 mm drill bit can be used in animals under 20 kg of BW.

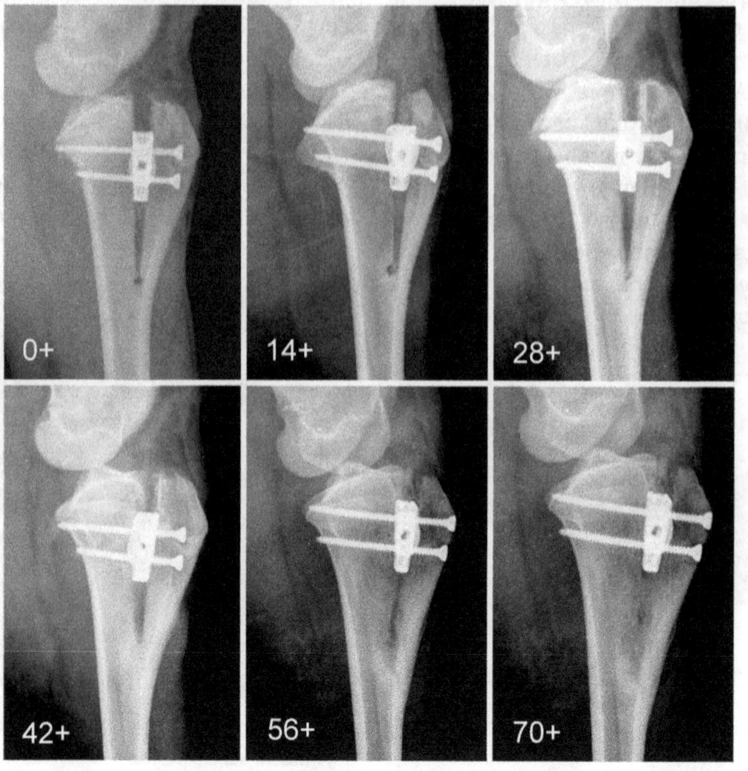

Fig. 6 Radiographic follow up. Mediolateral radiographs of the stifle immediate postoperative and on 14, 28, 42, 56, 70 day. As a result of bone remodeling, the osteotomy gap began to disappear gradually after 42 days

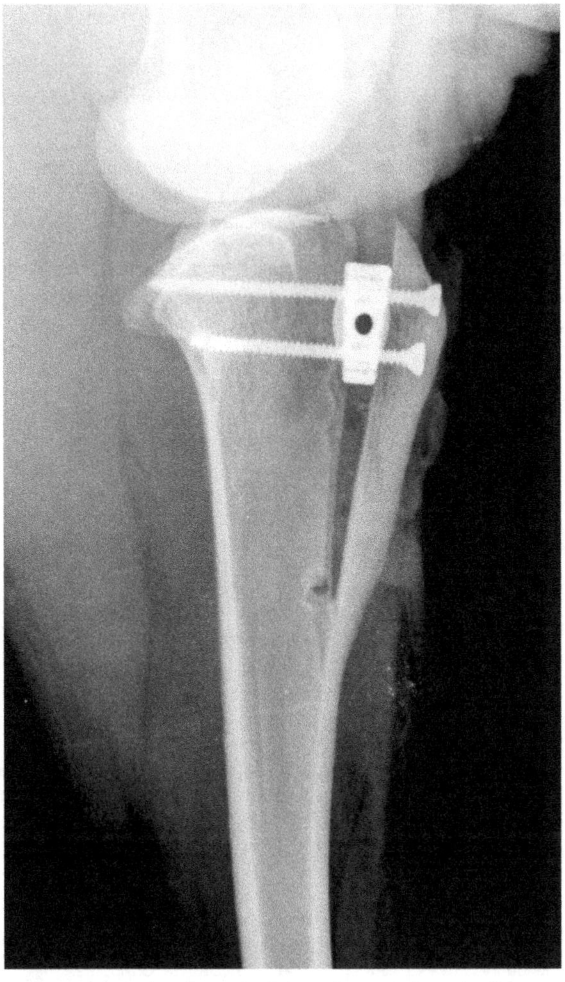

Fig. 7 Mediolateral radiograph of the stifle. A small crack of Maquet hole occurred 14 days postoperatively

We report the minor complication occurred in 2 sheep. The minor complication included the minimally cracked Maquet hole on the 2 weeks postoperative radiographs (Fig. 7). No major complication was noted. The TTA Rapid has an overall complication rate of 34%, based on limited case numbers [26]. Patellar ligament thickened and tibial fractures have been met most frequently at the level of distal cortical hinge [26]. Post-operative complications associated with conventional TTA technique include implant failure (0.8–2%), tibial fractures (1–5.1%), patellar luxation (0.8–1%) and infections (0.5–5.3%) [22, 25, 45, 46]. The presented TTA CF technique has the task to allow the firm fixation of the implant and prevent tibial tuberosity fractures.

Our report has some limitations. Experience of the surgeon was not taken into account. All TTA CF surgeries were performed by an experienced TTA surgeon. The number and type of complication might be higher or different with less experienced surgeon. Lameness evaluation was scored using a subjective scale of 0–4. Force plate analysis, would have been perfect, but was not available at the authors' institution. Further studies are needed to determine if the results remain the same in dogs and what kind of complications will occur. Another limitation is that post TTA patellar desmopathy has not been evaluated. Although the long time radiographic follow-up is needed to determine the progression of osteoarthritis of stifle joint, however this was not the objective in our study.

The novel surgical technique for tibial tuberosity advancement with cranial implant fixation is technically comparable to the recent trend in TTA, where partial osteotomy of the cranial tibial tuberosity crest is performed [26, 41, 47–49]. Accurate preoperative osteotomy planning is critical to achieve the perfect and good outcomes. TTA CF implant is fixing in tibia with two screws in craniocaudal direction, allowing to distribute the forces evenly on medial and lateral side of osteotomy gap. In addition, the novel titanium implant decreases the tibial traumatization by reducing the number of screws.

Conclusions

Our novel tibial tuberosity advancement technique with cranial fixation (TTA CF) is a modification of conventional TTA and TTA Rapid technique, where an attempt is made to reduce the number of screws and obtain a strong implant fixation only with two screws in craniocaudal direction. A cranial implant fixation allows to split the forces evenly on medial and lateral side of osteotomy gap, which may result in less number of major complications in dogs. A novel titanium implant decreases the tibial traumatisation by reducing the number of screws. Therefore this technique may be advantageous for surgeons and patients.

Abbreviations

BW: Body weight; CCL: Cranial cruciate ligament; h: Hour; kg: Kilogram; NR: Number, mg- milligram; PTA: Patellar tendon angle; TPLO: Tibial plateau leveling osteotomy; TTA CF: Tibial tuberosity advancement with cranial fixation; TTA: Tibial tuberosity advancement

Acknowledgements

We thank the "ChM sp. z o. o." company for their contribution to the design construction of implants and guides.

Funding

This work was supported and funded by The National Centre for Research and Development (Grant number: LIDER/10/0001/L-7/15/NCBR/2016). The role of the funding body was merely financial. The funders had no role in the study design, data analysis, and decision to publish, or preparation of the manuscript.

Authors' contributions

YZ, ZA, PPZ designed the study. Radiographic examinations, interpretation and surgeries was performed by YZ, MM, JG, PPZ and ZA. AS, GW designed and performed implants, instrumentation and graphics. All authors read and approved the final manuscript.

Competing interests

The authors declare that they have no competing interests.

Author details

[1]Department of Surgery and Radiologu with Clinic, Faculty of Veterinary Medicine, University of Warmia and Mazury in Olsztyn, Oczapowskiego 14, 10-718 Olsztyn, Poland. [2]ChM sp. z o. o, Lewickie 3b, 16-061 Juchnowiec Kościelny, Poland.

References

1. Ness MG, Abercromby RH, May C, Turner BM, Carmichael S. A survey of orthopedic conditions in small animal practice in Britain. Vet Comp Orthop Traumatol. 1996;9:43–52.
2. Elkins A, Pechman R, Kearney M. A retrospective study evaluating the degree of degenerative joint disease in stifle of dogs following surgical repair of the anterior cruciate ligament rupture. J Am Anim Hosp Assoc. 1991;27:533–40.
3. Lampman TJ, Lund EM, Lipowitz AJ. Cranial cruciate disease: current status of diagnosis, surgery, and risk for disease. Vet Comp Orthop Traumatol. 2003;16:122–6.
4. Gianotti SM, Marshall SW, Hume PA, Bunt L. Incidence of anterior cruciate ligament injury and other knee ligament injuries: a national population-based study. J Sci Med Sport. 2009;12:622–7.
5. Arnoczky S, Marshall J. The cruciate ligaments of the canine stifle: an anatomical and functional analysis. Am J Vet Res. 1977;38:1807–14.
6. Wilke VL, Robinson DA, Evans RB, Rothschild MF, Conzemius MG. Estimate of annual economic impact of treatment of cranial cruciate ligament injury in dogs in the United States. J Am Vet Med Assoc. 2005;227:1604–7.
7. De Angelis M, Lau RE. A lateral retinacular imbrication technique for the surgical correction of anterior cruciate ligament rupture in the dog. J Am Vet Med Assoc. 1970;157:79–84.
8. Arnoczky SP, Tarvin GB, Marshall JL, Saltzman B. Over-the-top procedure—technique for anterior cruciate ligament substitution in the dog. J Am Anim Hosp Assoc. 1979;15:283–90.
9. Shires PK, Hulse DA, Liu W. The under-and-over fascial replacement technique for anterior cruciate ligament rupture in dogs—a retrospective study. J Am Anim Hosp Assoc. 1984;20:69–77.
10. Slocum B, Slocum TD. Tibial plateau leveling osteotomy for repair of cranial cruciate ligament rupture in the canine. Vet Clin North Am Small Anim Pract. 1993;23:777–95.
11. Duerr FM, Martin KW, Rishniw M, Palmer RH, Selmic LE. Treatment of canine CCL disease. A survey of ACVS diplomates and primary care veterinarians. Vet Comp Orthop Traumatol. 2014;27:478–83.
12. Aragon CL, Budsberg SC. Applications of evidence based medicine: cranial cruciate ligament injury repair in the dog. Vet Surg. 2005;34:93–8.
13. Kowaleski MP, Apelt D, Mattoon JS, Litsky AS. The effect of tibial plateau leveling osteotomy position on cranial tibial subluxation: an in vitro study. Vet Surg. 2005;34:332–6.
14. Warzee CC, Dejardin LM, Arnoczky SP, Perry RL. Effect of tibial plateau leveling on cranial and caudal tibial thrusts in canine cranial cruciate deficient stifles: an in vitro experimental study. Vet Surg. 2001;30:278–86.
15. Tepic S, Damur DM, Montavon PM. Biomechanics of the stifle joint. Proceedings 1st world Orthopaedic veterinary congress. Munich: ESVOT-VOS; 2002. p. 189–90.
16. Montavon PM, Damur DM, Tepic S. Advancement of the tibial tuberosity for the treatment of cranial cruciate deficient canine stifle. In: Proceedings 1st World Orthopedic Veterinary Congress. Munich: ESVOT-VOS; 2002. p. 152.
17. Kim SE, Pozzi A, Banks SA, Conrad BP, Lewis DD. Effect of tibial tuberosity advancement on femorotibial contact mechanics and stifle kinematics. Vet Surg. 2009;38:33–9.
18. Kipfer NM, Tepic S, Damur DM, Guerrero T, Hässig M, Montavon PM. Effect of tibial tuberosity advancement on femorotibial shear in cranial cruciate-deficient stifles. An in vitro study. Vet Comp Orthop Traumatol. 2008;21:385 90.
19. Apelt D, Kowaleski MP, Boudrieau RJ. Effect of tibial tuberosity advancement on cranial tibial subluxation in canine cranial cruciate-deficient stifle joints: an in vitro experimental study. Vet Surg. 2007;36:170–7.
20. Stein S, Schmoekel H. Short-term and eight to 12 months results of a tibial tuberosity advancement as treatment of canine cranial cruciate ligament damage. J Small Anim Pract. 2008;49:398–404.
21. Hoffmann DE, Miller JM, Ober CP, Lanz OI, Martin RA, Shires PK. Tibial tuberosity advancement in 65 canine stifles. Vet Comp Orthop Traumatol. 2006;19:219–27.
22. Lafaver S, Miller NA, Stubbs WP, Taylor RA, Boudrieau RJ. Tibial tuberosity advancement for stabilization of the canine cranial cruciate ligament-deficient stifle joint: surgical technique, early results, and complications in 101 dogs. Vet Surg. 2007;36:573–86.
23. Voss K, Damur DM, Guerrero T, Haessig M, Montavon PM. Force plate gait analysis to assess limb function after tibial tuberosity advancement in dogs with cranial cruciate ligament disease. Vet Comp Orthop Traumatol. 2008; 21:243–9.
24. Montavon PM, Tepic S. Tibial tuberosity advancement: biomechanics and surgical procedure. San Diego CA: Proceedings American College of Veterinary Surgeons Symposium; 2005. p. 438–40.
25. Steinberg EJ, Prata RG, Palazzini K, Brown DC. Tibial tuberosity advancement for treatment of CCL injury: complications and owner satisfaction. J Am Anim Hosp Assoc. 2011;47:250–7.
26. Samoy Y, Verhoeven G, Bosmans T, Van der Vekens E, de Bakker E, Verleyen P, Van Ryssen B. TTA rapid: description of the technique and short term clinical trial results of the first 50 cases. Vet Surg. 2015;44:474–84.
27. Pearse AI, Richards RG, Milz S, Schneider E, Pearce SG. Animal models for implant biomaterial research in bone: a review. Eur Cell Mater. 2007;13:1–10.
28. Martini L, Fini M, Giavaresi G, Giardino R. Sheep model in orthopedic research: a literature review. Comp Med. 2001;51(4):292–9.
29. Liebschner MA. Biomechanical considerations of animal models used in tissue engineering of bone. Biomaterials. 2004;25:1697–714.
30. Leung KS, Siu WS, Cheung NM, Lui PY, Chow DH, James A, Qin L. Goats as an osteopenic animal model. J Bone Miner Res. 2001;16:2348–55.
31. Impellizeri JA, Tetrick MA, Muir P. Effect of weight reduction on clinical signs of lameness in dogs with hip osteoarthritis. J Am Vet Med Assoc. 2000;216: 1089–91.
32. Kitchen H. Sheep as animal models in biomedical research. J Am Vet Med Assoc. 1977;170:615–9.
33. Dennler R, Kipfer NM, Tepic S, Hassig M, Montavon PM. Inclination of the patellar ligament in relation to flexion angle in stifle joints of dogs without degenerative joint disease. Am J Vet Res. 2006;67:1849–54.
34. Maquet P. Advancement of the tibial tuberosity. Clin Orthop Relat Res. 1976; 115:225–30.
35. Cook JL, Evans R, Conzemius MG, Lascelles BD, McIlwraith CW, Pozzi A, Clegg P, Innes J, Schulz K, Houlton J, Fortier L, Cross AR, Hayashi K, Kapatkin A, Brown DC, Stewart A. Proposed definitions and criteria for reporting time frame, outcome, and complications for clinical orthopedic studies in veterinary medicine. Vet Surg. 2010;39:905–8.
36. Adamiak Z. Arthroscopy in dogs with cranial cruciate ligament injuries. Indian Vet J. 2002;79:177–8.
37. Adamiak Z, Brzeski W, Kalinowska K, Jaroszewicz A. Surgical repair of cranial cruciate ligament rupture in dogs by means of a surgical band - surgical loop. Med Weter. 2002;58:117–9.
38. Impellizeri JA, Tetrick MA, Muir P. Effect of weight reduction on clinical signs of lameness in dogs with hip osteoarthritis. J Am Vet Med Assoc. 2000; 216(7):1089–91.
39. Boudrieau RJ. Tibial plateau leveling osteotomy or tibial tuberosity advancement? Vet Surg. 2009;38:1–22.
40. Arican M, Parlak K, Sahin H. Evaluation and application of the TTA-rapid method in dogs with canal cruciate ligament rupture. Acta Vet Beograd. 2017;67:238–53.
41. Pape D, Madry H. The preclinical sheep model of high tibial osteotomy relaxing basic science to the clinics: standards, techniques and pitfalls. Knee Surg Sports Traumatol Arthrosc. 2013;21:228–36.
42. Tralman G, Andrianov V, Arend A, Mannik P, Kibur RT, Noupuu K, Uksov D, Aunapuu M. A novel combined method of osteosynthesis in treatment of tibial fractures: a comparative study on sheep with application of rod-through-plate fixator and bone plating. Anat Histol Embryol. 2013;42:80–9.
43. Etchepareborde S, Brunel L, Bollen G, Balligand M. Preliminary experience of a modified Maquet technique for repair of cranial cruciate ligament rupture in dogs. Vet Comp Orthop Traumatol. 2011;24:223–7.

44. Piorek A, Adamiak Z, Zhalniarovich Y, Jaskolska M. Treatment of tibial shaft fractures in sheep using interlocking nails, Schanz screws and type I external fixators. Pol J Vet Sci. 2012;15:651–9.
45. Black J. Practical aspects of material deformation. In: Orthopaedic biomaterials in research and practice. New York: Churchill Livingstone; 1988. p. 57–81.
46. Retallack LM, Daye RM. A modified Maquet-tibial tuberosity advancement technique for treatment of canine cranial cruciate ligament disease: short term outcome and complications. Vet Surg. 2018;47(1):44-51.
47. Nutt AE, Garcia-Fernandez P, San Roman F, San Roman F, Parkin T, Calvo I. Risk factors for tibial tuberosity fracture after tibial tuberosity advancement in dogs. Vet Comp Orthop Traumatol. 2015;28:116–23.
48. Hirshenson MS, Krotscheck U, Thompson MS, Knapp-Hoch HM, Jay-Silva AR, McConkey M, Bliss SP, Todhunter R, Mohammed HO. Evaluation of complications and short-term outcome after unilateral or single-session bilateral tibial tuberosity advancement for cranial cruciate rupture in dogs. Vet Comp Orthop Traumatol. 2012;25:402–9.
49. Kyon Pharma I: TTA-2. Zurich: KYON Pharma, Inc.; 2012. https://www.kyon.ch/current-products/tibial-tuberosity-advancement-tta.

25

The effect of bone allografts combined with bone marrow stromal cells on the healing of segmental bone defects in a sheep model

Marco Bernardo C Fernandes[1,2], João Antônio Matheus Guimarães[1], Priscila Ladeira Casado[1], Amanda dos Santos Cavalcanti[1], Natalia N Gonçalves[3,4], Carlos E Ambrósio[3*], Fernando Rodrigues[4], Ana Carolina F Pinto[4], Maria Angélica Miglino[4] and Maria Eugênia L Duarte[1,2]

Abstract

Background: The repair of large bone defects is a major orthopedic challenge because autologous bone grafts are not available in large amounts and because harvesting is often associated with donor-site morbidity. Considering that bone marrow stromal cells (BMSC) are responsible for the maintenance of bone turnover throughout life, we investigated bone repair at a site of a critically sized segmental defect in sheep tibia treated with BMSCs loaded onto allografts. The defect was created in the mid-portion of the tibial diaphysis of eight adult sheep, and the sheep were treated with *ex-vivo* expanded autologous BMSCs isolated from marrow aspirates and loaded onto cortical allografts (n = 4). The treated sheep were compared with control sheep that had been treated with cell-free allografts (n = 4) obtained from donors of the same breed as the receptor sheep.

Results: The healing response was monitored by radiographs monthly and by computed tomography and histology at six, ten, fourteen, and eighteen weeks after surgery. For the cell-loaded allografts, union was established more rapidly at the interface between the host bone and the allograft, and the healing process was more conspicuous. Remodeling of the allograft was complete at 18 weeks in the cell-treated animals. Histologically, the marrow cavity was reestablished, with intertrabecular spaces being filled with adipose marrow and with evidence of focal hematopoiesis.

Conclusions: Allografts cellularized with AOCs (allografts of osteoprogenitor cells) can generate great clinical outcomes to noncellularized allografts to consolidate, reshape, structurally and morphologically reconstruct bone and bone marrow in a relatively short period of time. These features make this strategy very attractive for clinical use in orthopedic bioengineering.

Keywords: Allografts, Segmental bone defect, Bone marrow stromal cell, Animal model

Background

Since the beginning of the last century, several reports have generated interest in orthopedics regarding the use of allografts for the treatment of lost or damaged bone. The incidence of fracture, non-union and resorption of allografts is still of great concern because each has an occurrence rate as high as 20%, 17% and 11%, respectively Though the use of allografts is well known and accepted for the treatment of large bone defects, it still has a great amount of complications [1].

It is estimated that more than 1.5 million bone graft operations, in human, will be performed in the United States to enhance the healing of spinal fusion, for the internal fixation of fractures, for maxillofacial reconstruction, and for bone restoration at sites of bone loss due to trauma, osteolysis or ablative surgery [2-4].

Autologous bone grafts have osteogenic, osteoconductive, and osteoinductive properties. They have an excellent success rate, low risk of disease transmission, and high

* Correspondence: ceambrosio@usp.br
[3]Department of Veterinary Medicine, FZEA, USP. Faculdade de Zootecnia e Engenharia de Alimentos, Departamento de Medicina Veterinária, Universidade de São Paulo, Av. Duque de Caxias Norte, 225, 13635-900 Pirassununga, São Paulo, Brazil
Full list of author information is available at the end of the article

histocompatibility [5]. However, for many patients, autologous bone grafts are insufficiently osteogenic, available in limited supply, and associated with additional surgical morbidity, such as blood loss, nerve and arterial injury, and pain at the donor site. The disadvantages of bone allografts include their reduced osteoinductive capacity and their limited capacity to incorporate with the host bone [1,5,6].

Studies must be performed on the use of allografts with ceramic biomaterial loading of bone marrow stromal cells to treat similar large bone defects. These studies must show that the correct microenvironment, i.e., oxygen and nutrient, is generated and supplied to support the quality of the reconstructed scaffold [7].

Due to the limited ability to replace lost or diseased bone, living functional tissue engineering technologies are being developed to try to incorporate autologous bone graft properties, such as osteogenesis, into bone allografts.

The aim of the present study was to verify whether cultured autologous bone marrow stromal cells (BMSCs) loaded onto irradiated bone allografts would result in effective bone repair at the site of a large segmental defect in sheep tibia.

Results

All animals experienced good postoperative recoveries: their surgical wounds healed well, and their microbiological tests showed no infection, because the implants were sterilized process by irradiated for sterilization. The cell samples from marrow aspirates (20–35 mL collected for each animal), for AOC 10 + and 14 + (animals with graft cellularized, ten and fourteen weeks before surgery), were obtained from the first pass, and for AOC 6 + and 18 + (animals with graft cellularized, six and eighteen weeks before surgery), were obtained from the second pass. In all cultures, regardless of the time of expansion, the cells had fusiform morphology characteristics of myofibroblastic cells. A similar process of culture isolation of bone marrow-derived mesenchymal stem cells was reviewed later and showed osteogenic and chondrogenic differentiation [8], which was different from the experimental cells.

The radiographic evolution of the grafts consolidation in the AOC 6+, 10 +, 14 +, and 18 + animals and the AOC 6 -, 10 -, 14 - and 18 - animals are illustrated in Figure 1. The parameters of the radiographic score of the two animals euthanized at 0, 4, 6, 10, 14 and 18 weeks are illustrated in Figure 2.

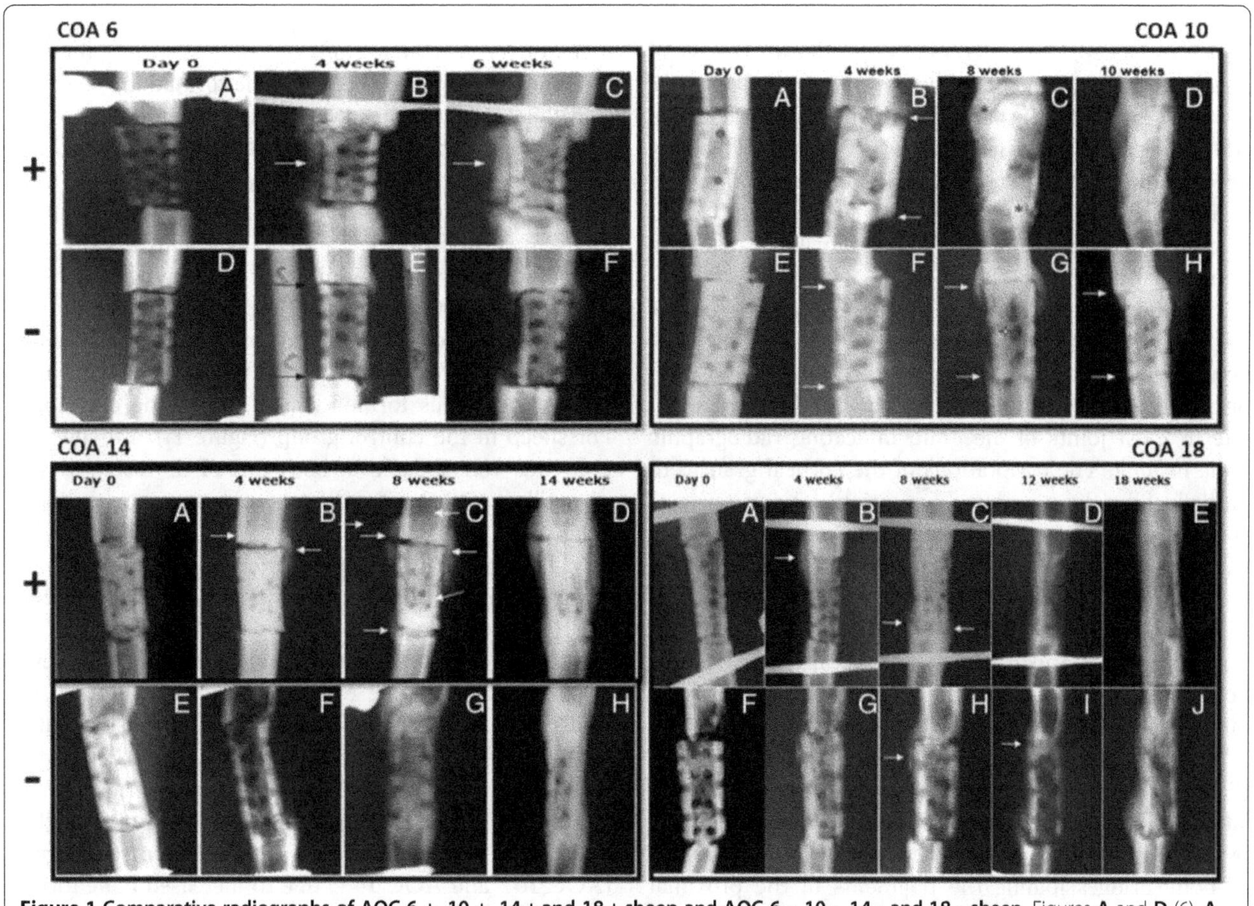

Figure 1 Comparative radiographs of AOC 6 +, 10 +, 14 + and 18 + sheep and AOC 6 -, 10 -, 14 - and 18 - sheep. Figures **A** and **D** (6), **A** and **E** (10), A and **E** (14) and **A** and **F** (18) illustrate the bone defect filled by a homologous bone graft over the weeks of the experiment.

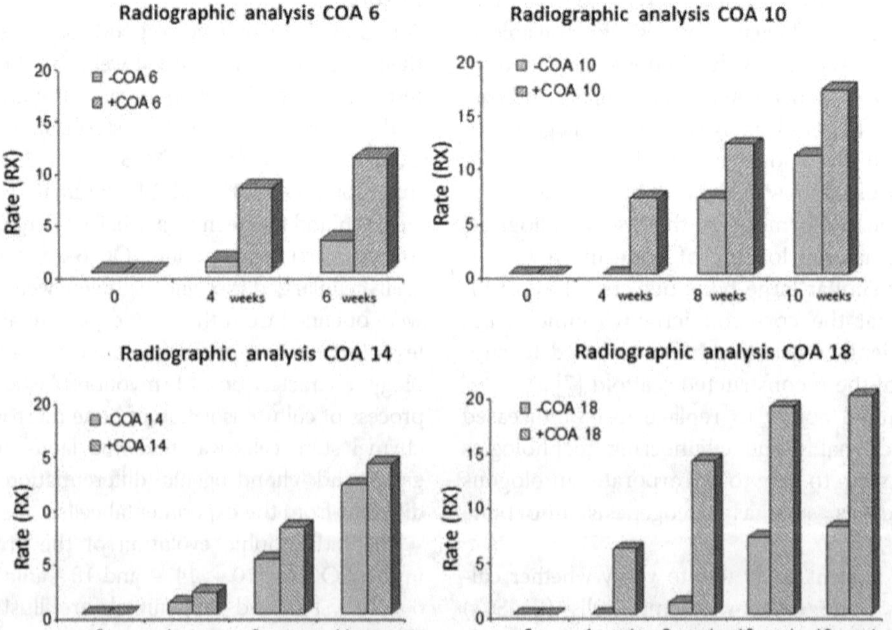

Figure 2 Graphic representation of the radiographic parameter scores for the AOC 6, 10, 14 and 18 animals in the evaluation points of 0, 4, 6, 10, 14, and 18 weeks.

In both sheep, the grafts were aligned with the distal and proximal fragments (Figure 1A and D). After 4 weeks, the radiotransparent lines were less clear in the AOC 6 + animals because they were partially filled by new bone formation (Figure 1B). Bone formation in this region of the graft was significantly higher in the AOC 6- animals (Figure 1C) than in the animals treated with noncellularized grafts (Figure 1F).

Two months after surgery, in the AOC 10 + animals (Figure 1C), the graft was completely covered by new bone formation on the entire lateral surface. The osteotomy line with the host bone was practically imperceptible in most joints of the graft, indicating radiographic bone healing. The perforations of the cortical graft were partially filled by new bone formation, leaving few unconcluded holes. In the same period, for the AOC 10 - sheep (Figure 1G), the holes in the cortical graft and bone formation around the graft remained patent, although osteotomy was not significant and no callus formed a bone bridge between the graft and the host bone. The radiotransparent line remained visible in both outbreaks of osteotomy.

Two months after surgery, the AOC 14 + sheep (Figure 1C) showed large bone formations involving the lateral and medial osteotomy of the graft. Although the osteotomy lines were still evident, there was a formation of bony bridges joining the fragments in the proximal and distal focus. In the AOC 14 - sheep (Figure 1G), the bone formation was small and limited to the lateral focus of the proximal graft, but the osteotomy line was difficult to see due to the new bone formation.

In the AOC 18 + sheep, after three months (Figure 1D) the graft was completely consolidated and remodeled: it was no longer possible to identify the focus of the osteotomy. In the AOC 18 - sheep (Figure 1I), the osteotomy focus was consolidated proximally and distally and remained fully visible, indicating delayed consolidation. At 18 weeks, the cellularized grafts (Figure 1E) showed an advanced process of remodeling, with the thickening of the cortical region and partial reduction of the thickness of the callus formed at the foci of the osteotomy. For sheep in the control group (Figure 1J), although the graft was consolidated at both foci of the osteotomy, it was still possible to visualize the radiotransparent line in distal focus.

At the first analysis point (6 weeks), perforations were clearly identified in the cortical grafts, and no difference was observed between the two animals with regards to the filling of the holes by new bone formation. However, as in the radiographic evaluation, the formation of the callus and the periosteal reaction were more evident in the animals with cellularized grafts (Figure 2A and B, AOC 6 + and 6 -). At 10 and 14 weeks, the animals treated with cellularized grafts (AOC 10 + and 14 +) had holes that were less patent than the control animals (AOC 10 - and AOC 14 -) due to increased bone formation and, consequently, greater obliteration of the perforations (Figure 2A, B, C and D).

After 18 weeks, the perforations of the cortical bone of the recipient cellularized grafts (AOC 18+) were completely filled by new bone formation and were no longer displaying tomographic sections (Figure 3A to 3G following complete healing of the bone and comparative disappearance of holes dependent of therapy and 3H as gross cross section of new formed bone structure, AOC 18 + and 18 -).

Histopathological evaluation was performed on the entire length of the graft, including the interface with the host bone. To standardize the results and thus facilitate the comparative analysis of the bone repair process in the presence and absence of AOC, the histological findings were correlated between the animals euthanized at each of the four observation points.

After 6 weeks, in the AOC 6 + animal, the holes of the compact bone graft were filled and consisted largely of bone formation and structured thick beams interconnected with marked osteoblastic activity. In the peripheral portion of the hole, the neoformation of immature bone tissue predominated and was related with high osteogenic cell activity. In the compact bone graft, there were frequent outbreaks of osteoclastic resorption of both the Haversian and cortico-endosteal surface. Haversian resorption occurred in an organized manner, and the presence of cutting-cones was characteristic of bone remodeling. The main components of the medullary filling at this vantage point were tissues and beams of neoformed bone in similar proportions. The peri-trabecular tissue in the general aspect was loose and highly vascularized, morphologically similar to the bone marrow stroma (Figure $4A^+$ to D^+).

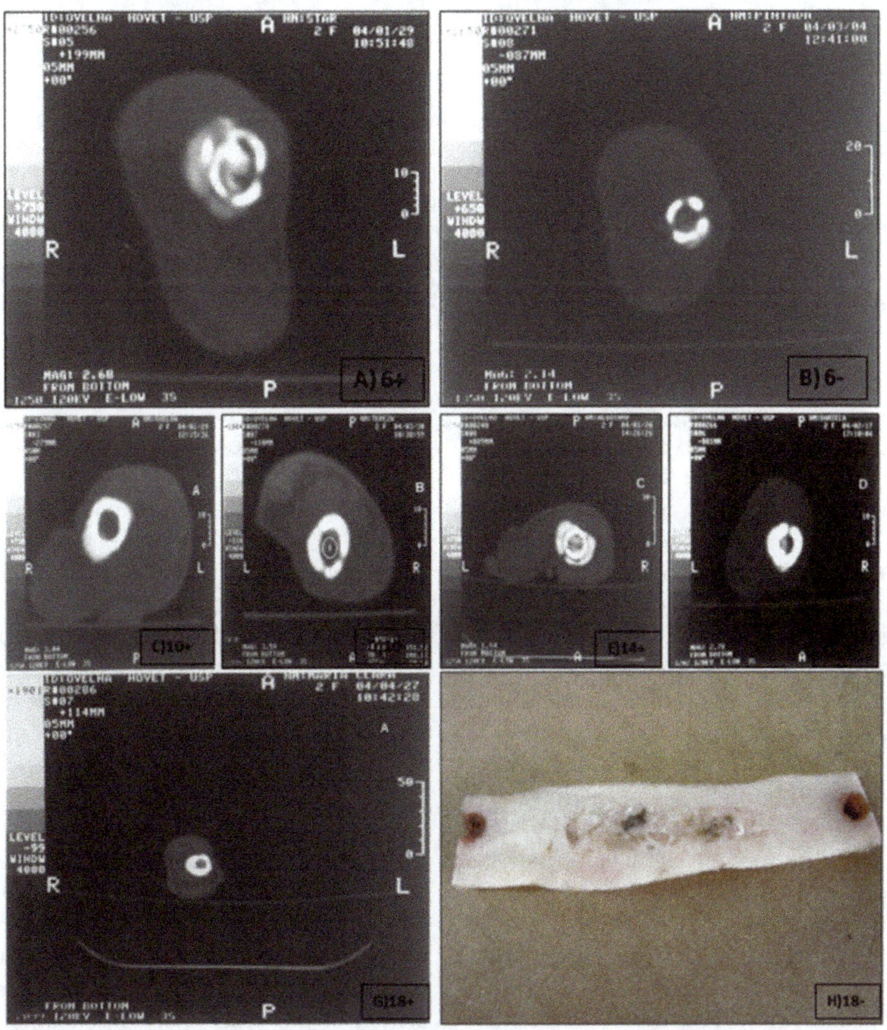

Figure 3 Tomography analyses during bone healing, after stem cell therapy, performed in the medial plane of the grafts of animals euthanized at 0, 6, 10, 14 and 18 weeks after the correction of diaphyseal segmental defects with cellularized homologous (A) and noncellularized homologous (B) grafts. The holes corresponding to the holes in the compact cortical bone are apparent in both animals. (Figure 3**A** to 3**G**). Gross piece of bone corresponding to the macroscopic analyses of the AOC 18 + animal (3**H**).

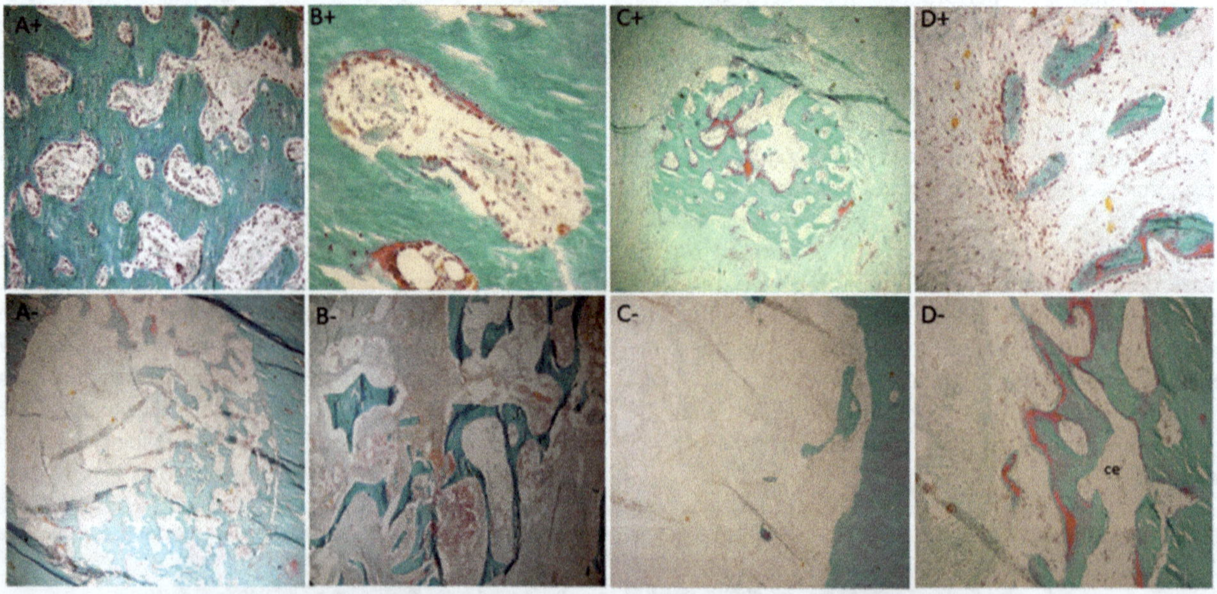

Figure 4 Histological appearance of the graft in AOC 6 - sheep. (A) Orifice corresponding to the perforation of the cortical graft only partially filled with new bone formation. **(B)** Intact allogeneic bone graft represents most of the filling of the inner portion of the graft. **(C)** Portions of the filling of the graft are represented mostly by connective tissue with no evidence of active osteogenesis. **(D)** Osteogenesis, when identified in the inner portion of the implant, is represented by partially mineralized bone trabeculae (osteoid seams stained in red). Masson-Goldner trichrome stain; 5-mm-thick undecalcified sections. Magnification **(A-D)** - 4×. Histological appearance of the graft in AOC 6 + sheep. **(A)** The site of the perforation in the cortical graft is filled by well-connected thick bone trabeculae displaying high osteoblastic activity through practically the entire length of the trabecular surfaces. **(B)** Cortical graft undergoing remodeling (*cutting cone*). **(C)** Focal area of active osteogenesis localized in the connective tissue that fills the central portion of the graft. **(D)** Bone formation in close association with loose connective tissue featuring characteristics of bone marrow supporting stroma. Masson-Goldner trichrome stain; 5-µm-thick undecalcified sections. Magnification 10× **(A and B)**, 4× **(C and D)**.

For the AOC 6 - animal, interfaces with the host bone graft were filled by dense connective tissue and bone formation inside the hole penetrated into the medullary cavity. However, the main difference observed by the comparison of the AOC 6 - animal with the AOC 6 + animal was the composition of the tissue filling the medullary space (Figure 4A$^-$ to D$^-$).

After 10 weeks of observation, the animals treated with cellularized grafts (AOC 10 +) had bone continuity in the region of the distal osteotomy. The compact bone graft was in the process of remodeling, and morphological structures of osteons were often identified. Although much of the graft that filled the medullary cavity consisted of bone formation, this was not uniform, and the beams filling the cavity were not structured because the interconnected distal edge of the graft and the host bone were joined by trabecular bone (Figure 5A$^+$ to D$^+$).

In the AOC 10 + animal, most of the tissue present in the marrow cavity of the graft was replaced by new bone. In the animal treated with a noncellularized graft (AOC 10 -), extensive areas of connective tissue and fbro-vascular tissue was observed and just a little or no osteogenic activity, differently from results found for AOC 10+ (Figure 5A$^-$ to D$^-$).

In the AOC 14 + animal, both interfaces of the graft were filled by newly formed bone, which established the union between the grafted bone and native bone. In the AOC 14 - animal, the medullary filling was not consistent and differed depending on the proximity to the edges of the host bone. In the regions immediately adjacent to the interfaces of the graft, the marrow space was filled mostly by dense connective tissue containing empty cavities and newly formed vessels (Figure 6A$^+$ to D$^+$ and A$^-$ to D$^-$).

After 18 weeks, in the animals treated with cellularized grafts (AOC 18 +), the regions of the graft interfaces were no longer histologically identifiable. The compact bone graft in this region comprised morphological structures with deposits of osteons, concentric lamellar bone osteocytes and round vascular structures. With the completion of the process of consolidation and remodeling of the callus, the endosteal and periosteal surfaces showed no more cellular activity, lying covered with thin ledge osteoid unrelated osteoblasts that featured inactive or latent state bone surfaces (Figure 7A$^+$ to D$^+$).

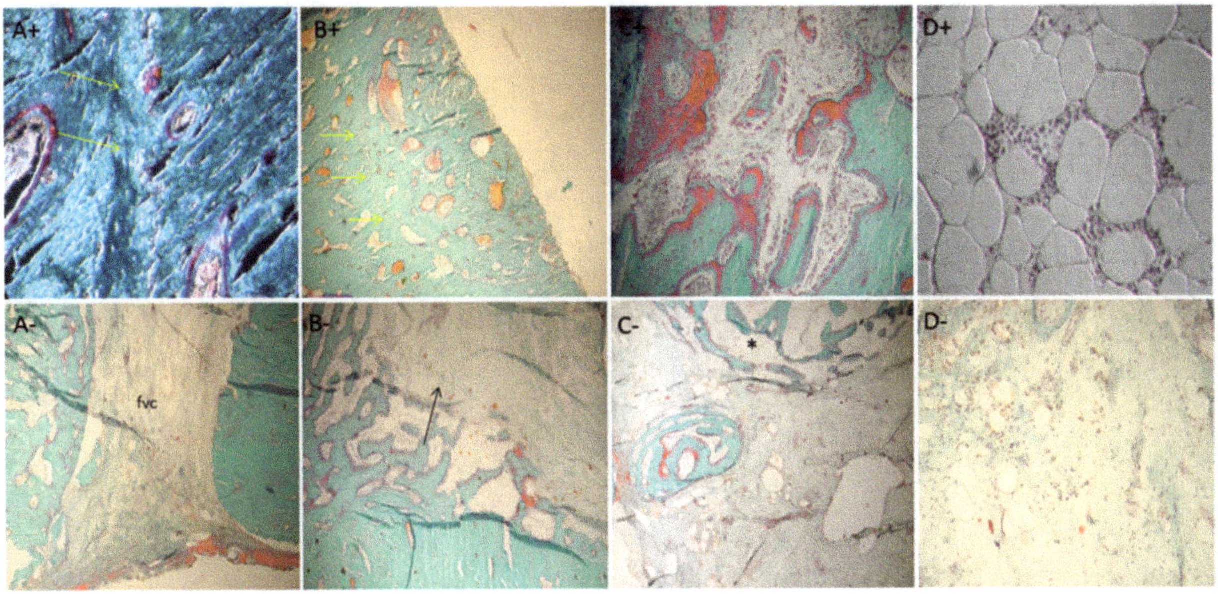

Figure 5 Histological appearance of the grafts in AOC 10 + sheep. (A) Line of fusion (arrows) in the interface between the distal portion of the cortical graft (right) and the host bone (left). **(B)** Corresponding site of a perforation of the cortical graft completely filled by well-organized bone formation. Arrows indicate the boundary of the former orifice. **(C)** Osteogenesis occurring in the inner portion of the graft. Bone trabeculae are covered by osteoid seams in close relationship with numerous active plump osteoblasts. **(D)** Adult adipocytes and classical hematopoietic cells are observed within the graft in the restored bone marrow. Masson-Goldner trichrome stain; 5- μm -thick undecalcified sections. Magnification 10× (**A**, under polarized light and **C**), **(B)** 4×, **(D)** 20×. Histological appearance of the graft in AOC 10 - sheep. **(A)** Gap between host bone and allograft containing fibrous connective tissue with no evidence of osteogenesis. **(B)** Interface between host bone and allograft displaying bone formation towards the inner portion of the medullary cavity (arrow). **(C)** The connective tissue that partially fills the central portion of the graft displaying a focal area of active osteogenesis intimately related with loose connective tissue, with the morphology of bone marrow supporting stroma (*). **(D)** Remainder of cancellous graft being actively resorbed by osteoclasts, without evidence of active bone formation. Masson-Goldner trichrome stain; 5- μm -thick undecalcified sections. Magnification **(A-D)** - 4×.

The comparison between the two animals euthanized after 18 weeks showed significant differences in the pattern and temporal evolution of the bone healing process at the graft site. Unlike what was observed in AOC 18 + animals, where the remodeling of the bone callus had been completed, the AOC 18 – animal (Figure $7A^-$ to D^-) exhibited a periosteal reaction covering a large part of the graft, including the region of the osteotomies. This finding confirmed that the process of graft consolidation was still in progress.

Inside the graft tissue, there was no uniformity in the filling composition. In the central portion, the tissue was represented by beams of bone formed from the cortico-endosteal surface and the intramedullary tissue and by fibrovascular tissue unattached to osteogenesis. The filling in the less central tissue alternated between beams with thick bone cell activity foci, a good standard of connectivity and related connective tissue stroma with features of bone marrow fat and areas represented exclusively by intensely vascularized tissue, unrelated to training of bone.

Discussion

The results of this study demonstrate that large diaphyseal defects can be effectively treated with irradiated homologous grafts in combination with external fixation and autologous osteoprogenitor cells, which, when added to these grafts, accelerate bone formation and the incorporation and remodeling of the graft in segmental diaphyseal defects and do not trigger local or systemic adverse reactions. The results also showed that the addition of the precipitating cells of the bone graft substituted for cancellous bone, cortical bone and bone marrow. In this study, in an experimental mammalian model, the treatment of allografts augmented with bone marrow stromal cells proved to be an effective option for ameliorating bone loss extending into the tibial shaft.

The results of pre-clinical studies [9-13] and clinical trials [14,15] using autologous mesenchymal cells and osteoprogenitors isolated from bone marrow and expanded in vitro to treat hydroxyapatite associated with diaphyseal defects were highly favorable. The recovery of the injuries occurred through the complete repair of the bone defects, with no history of local or systemic complications directly related to the implant or cellular components.

The alternative use of adipose tissue to isolate the osteoprogenitor cells may lead to insufficient bone formation, as observed in a previous study [16]. It is fairly

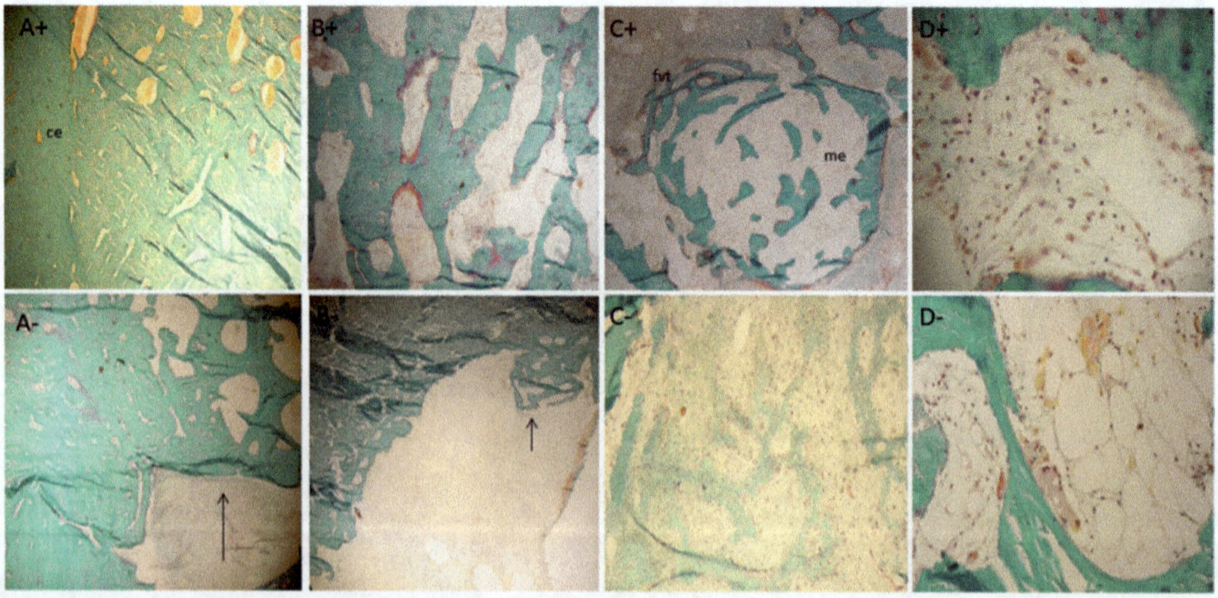

Figure 6 Histological appearance of the graft in AOC 14 + sheep. (A) Solid union between the allograft and the host bone depicted by well-organized and well-connected thick bone trabeculae. **(B)** Inner portion of the allograft filled mostly by mature bone trabeculae with sites of active new bone deposition represented by the presence of osteoid seams stained in red and covering portions of the trabecular surface. **(C)** Osteogenesis in the connective tissue that fills the allograft. Note the similarity of the loose connective tissue associated with the newly formed bone trabeculae and the supporting stroma of normal bone marrow. This aspect is histologically distinct from the clearly non-osteogenic fibro-vascular connective tissue that surrounds the site of osteogenesis. **(D)** Restoration of the bone marrow microenvironment with the colonization of the supporting marrow stroma by hematopoietic cells. Masson-Goldner trichrome stain; 5- μm -thick undecalcified sections. Magnification **(A-C)** 4× and **(D)** 20×. Histological appearance of the graft in AOC 14 - sheep. **(A)** Despite the osseous union achieved between the host bone and the allograft, the inner portion of the graft is devoid of osseous filling. **(B)** Inner portion of the cortical graft occupied by connective tissue with little or no osteogenic potential. **(C)** Most of the osteoforming response in this graft was represented by woven bone in an initial state of formation. **(D)** Remnants of cancellous graft are being actively resorbed by multinucleated osteoclasts without signs of restoration of the bone marrow microenvironment. Masson-Goldner trichrome stain; 5- μm -thick undecalcified sections. Magnification **(A-C)** 4× and **(D)** 10×.

well established that the growth of pluripotent cells isolated from adipose tissue generate a large number of progenitors committed to the adipogenic lineage with little or no ability to trans-differentiate into osteogenic cells [16].

Much of the observations of the pioneer study [17] are in agreement with our results. The authors of the pioneer study filled bone defects with a cylinder of hydroxyapatite and tri-calcium phosphate cellularized with mesenchymal cells that were expanded in vitro. Some disadvantages and complications of using this type of synthetic material, such as slow absorption and the occurrence of fractures, were infrequent in animals treated with cellularized grafts. As in our study, the most significant result from the histological point of view was the ability of cells added to the graft to induce bone formation.

As suggested in a previous study [18], mesenchymal cells that are in the process of osteogenic differentiation secrete factors that induce the recruitment of new cells and mesenchymal differentiation in the osteogenic lineage. The exuberance of the periosteal reaction in the host animals treated with cellularized bone grafts could be explained, at least in part, by the paracrine effects of these factors synthesized by the implanted cells. Pluripotent mesenchymal cells, in both the periosteum and the bone, respond to these factors, differentiating into osteoblasts and mature bone matrix producing cells. This hypothesis also applies to the slower bone formation and reduction of defects in the animals treated with noncellularized grafts. Recent studies complement this hypothesis [19] by demonstrating that TGF, BMP, FGF, IGF and PDGF are the main growth factors able to influence the proliferation and differentiation of mesenchymal cells into osteoprogenitors and osteoblasts [20].

There are other case studies on bone grafts in sheep that deserve special attention [20-23]. Furthermore, a clinical study on the use of mesenchymal cells expanded in vitro and associated with a synthetic implant was performed in four patients with segmental defects [24]. Monitoring these patients for 6–7 years after surgery showed that there were no early or late complications. There were no reports of pain, swelling, infection or fracture. The integration of the implant observed after 5–7 months was maintained 6–

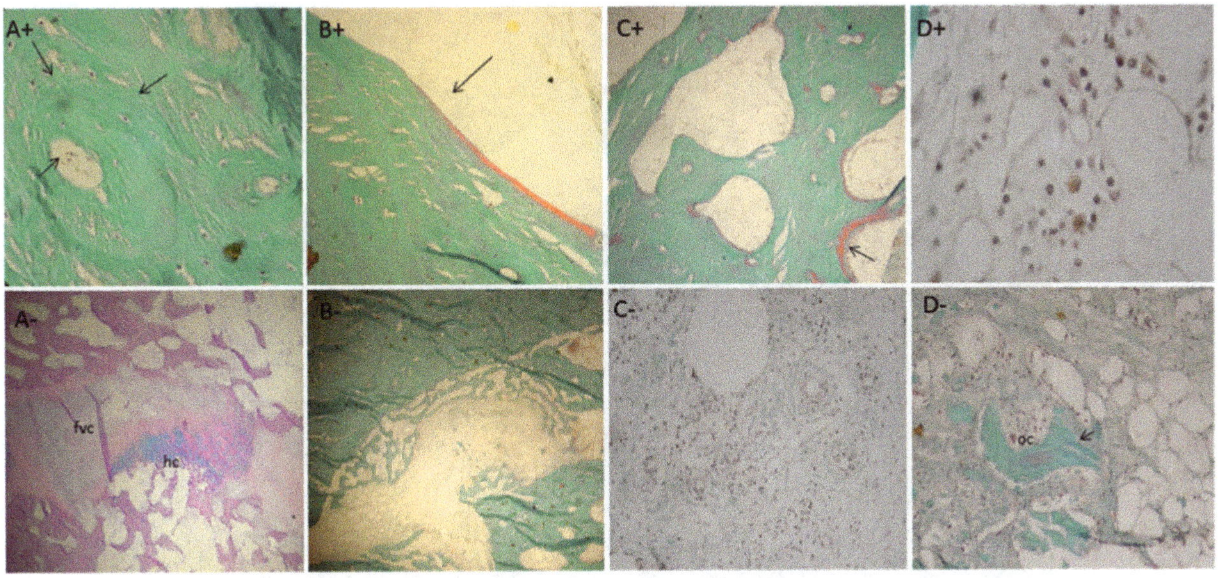

Figure 7 Histological appearance of the graft in AOC 18 + sheep. **(A)** Complete remodeling of cortical graft resulted in well-organized cortical bone with osteons displaying the classical concentric arrangement of the bone lamellae in close association with osteocytes. **(B)** Cortico-endosteal surface in a resting state, covered by a thin inactive osteoid seam (arrow) indicating that the remodeling process at this site was accomplished. **(C)** Structural restoration of the marrow cavity is evidenced by the presence of well-organized mature bone trabeculae undergoing remodeling (arrow). **(D)** The restoration of the bone marrow microenvironment can be confirmed by the presence of hematopoietic cells. Masson-Goldner trichrome stain; 5- µm -thick undecalcified sections. Magnification **(A-C)** 4× and **(D)** 20×. Histological appearance of the graft in AOC 18 - sheep. **(A)** Although an osseous union was accomplished at both interfaces with the host bone in CMA 18 + sheep, in CMA 18 - sheep, cartilage (ha) remnants and connective tissue (fvc) were still present at this location. This finding characterizes the incomplete incorporation of the graft. **(B)** Orifice corresponding to the perforation of the cortical graft incompletely filled with bone, suggesting that bone formation is not yet complete. **(C)** Despite the formation of highly vascular connective tissue in the inner portion the graft, there is no evidence of osteogenesis. **(D)** Compared with CMA 18 + sheep, the delay in the process of consolidation and remodeling of the allograft can be exemplified by the presence of residual cancellous graft (arrow) undergoing osteoclastic resorption (oc). Masson-Goldner trichrome stain; 5- µm -thick undecalcified sections. Magnification **(A and B)** 4×, **(C and D)** 10×.

7 years after surgery. Though the results were favorable, despite the low degree of resorption and mechanical stability of the hydroxyapatite compounds, we suggest that superior clinical outcomes can be achieved through the association of allografts of osteoprogenitor cells as autologous cells.

Conclusions

Allografts cellularized with AOCs (allografts of osteoprogenitor cells) can generate great clinical outcomes to non-cellularized allografts to consolidate, reshape, structurally and morphologically reconstruct bone and bone marrow in a relatively short period of time. These features make this strategy very attractive for clinical use in orthopedic bioengineering and open new venue for veterinary medicine bone surgery.

Methods

Experimental design

Ten (eight formed the experimental and control group and 2 animals is donors) adult female sheep (26–28 months) weighing 36 ± 2.7 kg were used in the present study after approval of the Ethical Committee for Animal Research at The University of São Paulo (authorization 317/2003). In all the animals, a central 30 mm bone segment was resected from the mid-portion of the right tibial diaphysis. The defect was replaced with a cylindrical graft of homologous cortical bone containing internal fragments of spongy bone. In four animals, osteoprogenitor cells were added to the autologous bone grafts (AOC 4+, n = 4); control animals were treated with cell-free allografts (AOC 4-, n = 4). Before the beginning of the experiment, two animals of the same age, sex and breed from the group of experimental animals were euthanized with an overdose of thiopentone and were used as bone (long bones mainly) allograft donors.

All animals were monitored with radiographs in the immediate postoperative period and monthly thereafter. Six, ten, fourteen, and eighteen weeks (AOC 6+/−, 10+/−, 14+/ 18+/−) after surgery, the animals were euthanized, and after removal of the external fixator, their right hind limb was evaluated by computed tomography. After the completion of CT and plain radiographs, the right tibia, which contained the bone graft, was resected and subsequently processed for histological analysis.

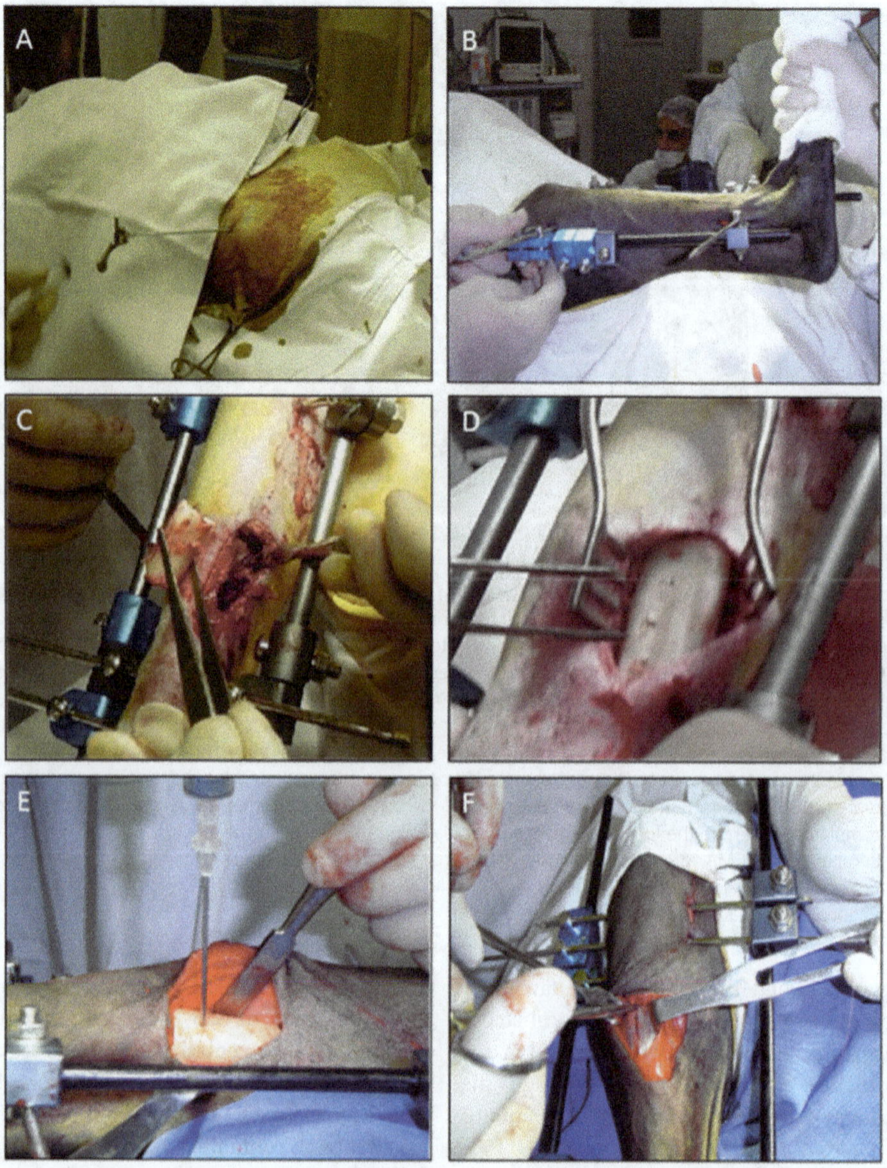

Figure 8 Procedures for bone marrow collection and surgical techniques for segmental defects establishment and stem cell transplantation. **A)** Puncture procedure of the left iliac crest for obtaining bone marrow aspirate. **B)** Monoplanar assembly positioned bilateral to external fixator. **C)** Creation of a 3.5 cm segmental defect in the middle third of the right tibial shaft. **D)** Cells were injected through the holes in the cortical graft to fill the bone defect. **E)** Cell suspension injection through the holes in the cortical graft. **F)** Suture of the incision of the periosteum at the end of the surgical procedure to prevent overflow of cell suspension.

Preparation of the allograft

After skeletonization, 30 mm cortical cylinders were obtained from the long bones of two donor sheep of the same breed, sex and age as the receptor sheep. Under sterile conditions, a central canal was bored through the length of the entire cylinder with the use of an 8 mm electrical drill. Cortical allografts were further perforated with a 3.2 mm high-speed drill to form equidistant holes along the entire surface, with approximately 4 mm between each hole. All bone grafts used, consisting of approximately 10×5 mm bone fragments were obtained from iliac crests and metaphyses of the long bones of the donor sheep. Both types of allografts were washed throughout this process with saline and were then placed for 10 minutes in a saline solution containing 0.02 g/ml of cephalotin and stored individually in plastic bags. Both types of allografts were kept frozen at −70°C, including during the sterilization process by γ-radiations (25,000 gray). Immediately before use, the samples were thawed in sterile saline.

Surgical procedure

Under general anesthesia and using endotracheal intubation, the right hind limb was shaved, and the area over the tibia was aseptically prepared. Mechanical stability was achieved with static external fixation (Baumer, São Paulo, Brazil) using a bilateral monoplanar frame with six parallel pins inserted from the lateral to the medial side of the tibia. With the animal placed on its left side, a 30 mm diaphyseal segment between the proximal and distal groups of pins was dissected subperiosteally, osteotomized and explanted, creating a segmental bone defect. The defect was replaced with a cortical sterile allograft and filled with scaffolds previously harvested from the donor sheep. In the experimental animals, autologous expanded BMSCs were subsequently loaded onto the scaffolds by injecting 2 mL of the cell solution with a 5 mL syringe through the 3.2 mm screw holes. Unrestricted weight bearing was allowed for all animals immediately after the operation (Figure 8A-F). Non-steroidal anti-inflammatory drugs were given for two days postoperatively, and after a week in isolated cages, the sheep returned to regular housing facilities, where they were monitored daily. The animals were euthanized by an intravenous injection of potassium chloride under sodium pentobarbital anesthesia 6, 10, 14 and 18 weeks after surgery.

Anesthesia and post-surgical procedures

After 24 hours of no intake food and 12 of not drinking water, animals were pre-medicated with midazolam maleate (0.6 mg/kg) and meperidine hydrochloride (2 mg/kg) intravenously (IV). Anesthesia was induced by propophol (3 mg/kg) associated to fentanyl hydrochloride (2.5 μg/kg) and maintained with isoflurorane. Post-surgical analgesia was provided with 1 mg/kg of flunixin meglumine and 25 mg/kg of sodium dipyrone IV and maintained with 2 mg/kg of tramadol twice a day until 10 days. Antibacterial prophylaxis was obtained with penicillin 40000 UI/kg for 10 days [25].

Isolation and culture of sheep BMSCs

20–30 mL of bone marrow aspirates was harvested from the iliac crest of the experimental sheep. The animals were anesthetized, and under sterile conditions, a 15-gauge trephine was used to aspirate the bone marrow into a 10 mL syringe rinsed with 1000 UI/mL heparin. Marrow samples were diluted into Dulbecco's modified Eagle's medium (DMEM) and filtered through a 150 μm cell strainer. Nucleated cells were plated at a density of 6×107 in DMEM supplemented with 10% fetal bovine serum (FBS) and 1% antibiotics in 150-cm^2 flasks at 37°C in a humidified atmosphere of 5% CO_2. After 24 hours, non-adherent cells were washed out, and adherent cells were then fed with fresh medium twice a week. When the cells were nearly confluent, they were harvested with 0.05% trypsin/0.01% EDTA, counted and seeded at a density of 6×107 in 150 cm^2 tissue-culture flasks.

Autologous BMSCs were expanded until passage 2 and suspended in 2.0 mL of implantation media (DMEM containing 10% FBS). From the time of preparation until the implantation procedure (4–5 hours), the cell suspension was kept at 4°C. In the operating room and immediately before use, the cell suspension was submitted to gentle mechanical homogenization, aspirated in 5 mL syringes and introduced into the positioned allograft through the cortical perforations.

Radiographic and tomographic analysis

All animals were regularly monitored radiographically after surgery and every month during the experimental period. The healing process was evaluated by antero-posterior and lateral radiographs and by computed tomography after *post-mortem* removal of the external fixator. Two observers (M. B. C. F and M. E. L. D) independently and blindly evaluated the presence of the periosteal reaction, host-graft union and the general graft appearance, which included

Table 1 Radiographic criteria for evaluating the consolidation of adapted bone grafts [19]

	Points	
A. Periosteal reaction	Forelimb	Hindlimb
Absent	0	0
Minimum	1	1
Medium (<50%)	2	2
Moderate (50-75%)	3	3
Complete (>75%)	4	4
B. Graft host bone union	Proximal limb	Distal limb
Radiotransparent line (total)	0	0
Radiotransparent line (partial)	2	2
Absent radiotransparent line	4	4
C. Graft changes		
Reaction absent	0	
Partial absorption	1	
Moderate remodeling	2	
Complete remodeling	3	
Total organization	4	
D. Complications (fracture or graft resorption)		
Total points	0	

partial absorption and graft remodeling according to a previously established scoring system (Table 1).

Histological analysis of retrieved allografts

The tibia was explanted at the time of euthanasia, and the middle part of the diaphysis, including the allograft and both host bone-implant interfaces, was excised. After removal of the surrounding soft tissues, tibial diaphysis specimens were obtained from the entire length of the allograft and from the osteotomy sites including the host bone with an oscillating saw. Macroscopic slices were fixed in 70% ethanol and dehydrated at 4°C by sequential changes in ascending concentrations of ethanol, cleared in xylene and embedded in methyl-methacrylate. Five-micron undecalcified bone sections were obtained using a Leica RM 2155 microtome (Leica, Nussloch, Germany) equipped with a disposable carbide-tungsten knife. Approximately 15–20 undecalcified histological sections taken from each animal were stained with Goldner´s Trichrome and PAS/Alcian Blue stain and examined with the use of a light microscope (Nikon Eclipse E800, Nikon Corporation, Japan). The reparative process in retrieved allografts was qualitatively assessed in both gaps at the osteotomy site, at the external and internal cortical surfaces of the grafted bone and internally in the medullary canal.

Competing interests

The authors declare that they have no competing interests.

Authors' contributions

MBCF, MELD designs the experiment. With first MBCF and MELD, JAMG, PLC, ASC, NJG, CEA, FR, ACFP, MAM prepared the animals, performed the surgery and material analysis consisting radiographic, sectioned and stained the bones, reviewed the literature and prepared the manuscript. All authors read and approved the final manuscript.

Acknowledgements

The authors acknowledge the National Institute of Traumatology and Orthopedics at Rio de Janeiro, FAPESP (2007-51222-2)and CNPq.

Author details

[1]Basic and Clinical Research Division, National Institute of Traumatology and Orthopedics, Rio de Janeiro, Brazil. [2]Institute of Biomedical Sciences, Federal University of Rio de Janeiro, Rio de Janeiro, Brazil. [3]Department of Veterinary Medicine, FZEA, USP. Faculdade de Zootecnia e Engenharia de Alimentos, Departamento de Medicina Veterinária, Universidade de São Paulo, Av. Duque de Caxias Norte, 225, 13635-900 Pirassununga, São Paulo, Brazil. [4]Department of Surgery, College of Veterinary Medicine and Animal Science, University of São Paulo, São Paulo, Brazil.

References

1. Trafton PG: **Tibial Shaft Fractures.** *Elsevier Science* 2003, **57:**2131–2255.
2. Solomon LB, Callary SA, Boopalan PR, Chakrabarty A, Costi JJ, Howie DW: **Impaction bone grafting of segmental bone defects in femoral non-unions.** *Acta Orthop Belg* 2013, **79:**64–70.
3. Katsenis D, Triantafillis V, Chatzicristos M, Dendrinos G: **The reconstruction of tibial metaphyseal comminution using hybrid frames in severe tibial plafond fractures.** *J Orthop Trauma* 2013, **27:**153–157.
4. Lin CC, Chen CM, Chiu FY, Su YP, Liu CL, Chen TH: **Staged protocol for the treatment of chronic tibial shaft osteomyelitis with Ilizarov's technique followed by the application of intramedullary locked nail.** *Orthopedics* 2012, **35:**1769–1774.
5. Nandi SK, Roy S, Mukherjee P, Kundu B, De DK, Basu D: **Orthopaedic applications of bone graft & graft substitutes: a review.** *Indian J Med Res* 2010, **132:**15–30.
6. Laurencin C, Khan Y, El-Amin SF: **Bone graft substitutes.** *Expert Rev Med Devices* 2006, **3:**49–57.
7. Giannoni P, Mastrogiacomo M, Alini M, Pearce SG, Corsi A, Santolini F, Muraglia A, Bianco P, Cancedda R: **Regeneration of large bone defects in sheep using bone marrow stromal cells.** *J Tissue Eng Regen Med* 2008, **5:**253–262.
8. Grässel S, Stöckl S, Jenei-Lanzl Z: **Isolation, culture, and osteogenic/chondrogenic differentiation of bone marrow-derived mesenchymal stem cells.** *Methods Mol Biol* 2012, **879:**203–267.
9. Bruder SP, Kraus KH, Goldberg VM, Kadiyala S: **The effect of implants loaded with autologous mesenchymal stem cells on the healing of canine segmental bone defects.** *J Bone Joint Surg Am* 1998, **80:**985–996.
10. Kon E, Muraglia A, Corsi A, Bianco P, Marcacci M, Martin I, Boyde A, Ruspantini I, Chistolini P, Rocca M, Giardino R, Cancedda R, Quarto R: **Autologous bone marrow stromal cells loaded onto porous hydroxyapatite ceramic accelerate bone repair in critical-size defects of sheep long bones.** *J Biomed Mater Res* 2000, **49:**328–337.
11. Arinzeh T, Peter S, Archambault M, Van Den Bos C, Gordon S, Kraus K, Smith A, Kadiyala S: **Allogeneic mesenchymal stem cells regenerate bone in a critical-sized canine segmental defect.** *J Bone Joint Surg Am* 2003, **85:**1927–1935.
12. Marcacci M, Kon E, Moukhachev V, Lavroukov A, Kutepov S, Quarto R, Mastrogiacomo M, Cancedda R: **Stem cells associated with macroporous bioceramics for long bone repair: 6- to 7-year outcome of a pilot clinical study.** *Tissue Eng* 2007, **13:**947–955.
13. Michael RJ, Ellis SJ, Roberts MM: **Tibial plateau fracture following proximal tibia autograft harvest: case report.** *Foot Ankle Int* 2012, **33:**1001–1005.
14. Follmar KE, Prichard HL, De Croos FC, Wang HT, Levin LS, Klitzman B, Olbrich K, Erdmann D: **Combined bone allograft and adipose-derived stem cell autograft in a rabbit model.** *Ann Plast Surg* 2007, **58:**561–565.
15. Reichert JC, Cipitria A, Epari DR, Saifzadeh S, Krishnakanth P, Berner A, Woodruff MA, Schell H, Mehta M, Schuetz MA, Duda GN, Hutmacher DW: **A tissue engineering solution for segmental defect regeneration in load-bearing long bones.** *Sci Transl Med* 2012, **141:**141–193.
16. Viateau V, Guillemin G, Bousson V, Oudina K, Hannouche D, Sedel L, Logeart Avramoglou D, Petite H: **Long-bone critical-size defects treated with tissue-engineered grafts: a study on sheep.** *J Orthop Res* 2007, **25:**741–749.
17. Kern S, Eichler H, Stoeve J, Kluter H, Bieback K: **Comparative analysis of mesenchymal stem cells from bone marrow, umbilical cord blood, or adipose tissue.** *Stem Cells* 2006, **24:**1294–1301.
18. Bruder SP, Jaiswal N, Ricalton NS, Mosca JD, Kraus KH, Kadiyala S: **Mesenchymal stem cells in osteobiology and applied bone regeneration.** *Clin Orthop Relat Res* 1998, **355:**56–S247.
19. Lieberman JR, Daluiski A, Einhorn TA: **The role of growth factors in the repair of bone.** *J Bone Joint Surg Am* 2002, **84:**1032–1044.
20. Sánchez Hidalgo R, Forriol F: **Bone-tendon integration of autologous grafts using different diameter tunnels. An experimental study on sheep.** *Rev Esp Cir Ortop Traumatol* 2012, **56:**216–223.
21. Duygulu F, Demirel M, Atalan G, Kaymaz FF, Kocabey Y, Dülgeroğlu TC, Candemir H: **Effects of intra-articular administration of autologous bone marrow aspirate on healing of full-thickness meniscal tear: an experimental study on sheep.** *Acta Orthop Traumatol Turc* 2012, **46:**61–67.
22. Reichert JC, Woodruff MA, Friis T, Quent VM, Gronthos S, Duda GN, Schütz MA, Hutmacher DW: **Ovine bone- and marrow-derived progenitor cells and their potential for scaffold-based bone tissue engineering applications in vitro and in vivo.** *J Tissue Eng Regen Med* 2010, **4:**565–576.
23. Taira H, Moreno J, Ripalda P, Forriol F: **Radiological and histological analysis of cortical allografts: an experimental study in sheep femora.** *Arch Orthop Trauma Surg* 2004, **124:**320–325.

26

Long-term functional outcome after surgical repair of cranial cruciate ligament disease in dogs

Sari H Mölsä*, Heli K Hyytiäinen, Anna K Hielm-Björkman and Outi M Laitinen-Vapaavuori

Abstract

Background: Cranial cruciate ligament (CCL) rupture is a very common cause of pelvic limb lameness in dogs. Few studies, using objective and validated outcome evaluation methods, have been published to evaluate long-term (>1 year) outcome after CCL repair. A group of 47 dogs with CCL rupture treated with intracapsular, extracapsular, and osteotomy techniques, and 21 healthy control dogs were enrolled in this study. To evaluate long-term surgical outcome, at a minimum of 1.5 years after unilateral CCL surgery, force plate, orthopedic, radiographic, and physiotherapeutic examinations, including evaluation of active range of motion (AROM), symmetry of thrust from the ground, symmetry of muscle mass, and static weight bearing (SWB) of pelvic limbs, and goniometry of the stifle and tarsal joints, were done.

Results: At a mean of 2.8 ± 0.9 years after surgery, no significant differences were found in average ground reaction forces or SWB between the surgically treated and control dog limbs, when dogs with no other orthopedic findings were included (n = 21). However, in surgically treated limbs, approximately 30% of the dogs had decreased static or dynamic weight bearing when symmetry of weight bearing was evaluated, 40-50% of dogs showed limitations of AROM in sitting position, and two-thirds of dogs had weakness in thrust from the ground. The stifle joint extension angles were lower ($P < 0.001$) and flexion angles higher ($P < 0.001$) in surgically treated than in contralateral joints, when dogs with no contralateral stifle problems were included (n = 33). In dogs treated using the intracapsular technique, the distribution percentage per limb of peak vertical force (DPVF) in surgically treated limbs was significantly lower than in dogs treated with osteotomy techniques ($P = 0.044$).

Conclusions: The average long-term dynamic and static weight bearing of the surgically treated limbs returned to the level of healthy limbs. However, extension and flexion angles of the surgically treated stifles remained inferior to healthy joints, and impairment of AROM and weakness in thrust from the ground in the surgically treated limbs were frequently present. Ground reaction forces may be inadequate as a sole method for assessing functional outcome after cranial cruciate ligament repair.

Keywords: Cranial cruciate ligament, Surgical outcome, Force plate analysis, Goniometry, Long-term, Dog

Background

Cranial cruciate ligament (CCL) rupture is a common cause of canine pelvic limb lameness and stifle joint osteoarthritis. Surgical treatment is advocated to stabilize the stifle joint, alleviate pain, treat any concurrent meniscal pathology, and decelerate the development of osteoarthritis [1]. Numerous surgical techniques have been developed and can be broadly classified as intracapsular ligament replacements, extracapsular suture techniques and neutralizing dynamic osteotomy techniques [2]. The search for the most beneficial surgical technique is ongoing.

The surgical outcome after CCL surgery has often been evaluated through clinical examination, radiography, and owner assessment. Force plate analysis has been the gold standard for objective evaluation of dynamic weight bearing, and it has also been used to evaluate outcome of CCL repair [3-12]. All studies report significant improvement of dynamic weight bearing after surgery, but the results are more variable when return to the level of healthy limbs is considered. In clinical patients, some studies have reported return of dynamic weight bearing to the level of healthy limbs after extracapsular repair [5] and tibial

* Correspondence: sari.molsa@helsinki.fi
Department of Equine and Small Animal Medicine, Faculty of Veterinary Medicine, University of Helsinki, Helsinki, Finland

plateau leveling osteotomy (TPLO) [6,10], whereas in others the ground reaction forces in surgically treated limbs or pelvic limb symmetry indices have remained inferior to full function after repair with extracapsular [6,7,10], intracapsular [7], TPLO [7], and tibial tuberosity advancement (TTA) [11] techniques. Few studies directly comparing different surgical techniques by using force plate analysis exist. Conzemius et al. [7] reported that the results of limb function in Labrador Retrievers treated with extracapsular and TPLO techniques were similar but superior to the intracapsular technique 6 months after surgery. Also in another study, no significant differences were found in limb function between TPLO and extracapsular repair 2 years after surgery [3]. On the other hand, two recent studies indicate that TPLO leads to limb function that is superior to that produced by extracapsular surgery [8,10].

In most dogs, despite the surgical technique chosen, osteoarthritic changes progress after CCL surgery [3,13-15] and this may cause deterioration of the dog's clinical condition later in life. However, only a few true long-term (>1 year) CCL repair outcome studies, using objective and validated outcome evaluation methods, have been published [3,16,17]. Au. et al. [3] evaluated ground reaction forces, stifle joint range of motion and thigh circumference of the surgically treated limbs 2 years after surgery. Peak vertical forces increased significantly after surgery, but the focus of the paper was to compare surgical techniques, not to evaluate the return of limb function to the preinjury level. However, after initial improvement, stifle joint range of motion started to decrease. Also in another study, stifle joint range of motion and thigh circumference in the surgically treated limbs remained significantly decreased relative to contralateral limbs 1-5 years after surgery [16]. In the third study 30% of the surgically treated dogs were found to have signs of chronic pain when long-term outcome was evaluated at a mean of 2.7 years after surgery using a validated pain index [17].

In veterinary orthopedic patients, the use of rehabilitation by physiotherapists that are specialized in animal physiotherapy has increased substantially during the last decade. Animal physiotherapists often use goniometric measurements, subjective or objective evaluation of muscle atrophy, and evaluation of weight bearing, posture, and thrust from the ground to evaluate the patient's functional condition and response to given treatment. In cruciate disease research, stifle joint goniometric measurements and thigh circumference measurements have been used to evaluate surgical outcome in several studies [3,8,16,18-23]. However, according to our knowledge, a thorough evaluation of the stifle joints done by a professional animal physiotherapist to assess surgical outcome after CCL surgery has not been reported.

The primary purpose of our study was to evaluate surgical outcome at a minimum of 1.5 years after CCL surgery. This was done by combining force plate analysis, clinical orthopedic and physiotherapeutic evaluations, and radiography. The secondary purpose was to compare surgical techniques used to repair CCL rupture. Our hypothesis was that in the long term, the function of the surgically treated limb would remain inferior to the healthy limb.

Methods

Study group

Based on a questionnaire study [17] and an another unpublished questionnaire data, owners were invited to bring their dogs to a clinical evaluation, including general, orthopedic, physiotherapeutic, and radiographic examination and force plate analysis. The inclusion criteria for dogs were surgically treated unilateral CCL rupture, a minimum time interval of 1.5 years between surgery and evaluation, and body mass over 17 kg. Patients with bilaterally treated CCL rupture, other known concomitant stifle problems (i.e. patellar luxation, septic or immune-mediated arthritis), or owner-reported significant orthopedic or neurologic problems, were excluded. In addition, possible nonsteroidal anti-inflammatory drug (NSAID), opioid or corticosteroid pain medication, and nutraceutical and fatty acid supplements were withdrawn at a minimum of 7 days, long-term corticosteroids 30 days, and pentosan polysulphate 90 days before the evaluation. The study protocol was approved by the Ethics Committee of Viikki campus, University of Helsinki, and written consent was obtained from all owners. During the evaluation the members of the research team were unaware of which pelvic limb had been operated on and the surgical technique used.

Building subgroups

Two additional subgroups were formed. Subgroup 1 dogs were used when force plate, static weight bearing, active range of motion and muscle atrophy results were evaluated. For these evaluations, only study group dogs with no signs of other orthopedic disease were included to minimize the effect of other conditions on the test results. On the other hand, when goniometric results in surgically treated limbs were compared to contralateral limbs, the study group dogs that did not have any findings in the contralateral stifle/tarsal joints, i.e. subgroup 2, were included. Subgroup 2 dogs were allowed to have hip dysplasia, elbow OA etc. because these findings were regarded to have no effect on the results of stifle or tarsal goniometry.

Control group

For the force plate and physiotherapeutic evaluation, a group of 21 clinically healthy Labrador Retrievers and

Rottweilers, voluntarily presented by their owners, was used [24]. Inclusion criteria were: age 1-8 years, no known orthopedic problems, and radiographic screening results free of elbow and hip dysplasia according to the Fédération Cynologique Internationale screening protocol.

Review of medical records

With permission from the owners, the surgical records were reviewed to ascertain the surgical date, technique used, and the surgically treated limb and to obtain information about the meniscal tear and possible complications or revision surgery needed.

Orthopedic examination

A full orthopedic examination was done to all dogs and included lameness evaluation on a scale from 0 to 4 (no/mild/moderate/severe weight bearing/non-weight bearing) [25] and palpation of the thoracic and pelvic limbs and spine as well as evaluation of conscious proprioception and withdrawal reflex. The stifle joints were palpated for pain (no/mild/moderate/severe), crepitation (no/mild/moderate/severe), periarticular swelling (no/mild/moderate/severe), decrease in range of motion (ROM) (no/mild/moderate/severe), and patellar luxation (grade 0/1/2/3/4) and also evaluated for a positive tibial compression test (negative/positive) and, under sedation with medetomidine 10-20 µg/kg (Dorbene, Syva, Leon, Spain) and butorphanol 0.1 mg/kg (Butordol, Intervet International, Unterschleissheim, Germany) for the cranial drawer test (no/mild/moderate/severe drawer sign). The spine was evaluated for pain and all other joints for pain, crepitation, swelling, decreased ROM and instability (no/yes). While sedated, an Ortolani test was used to evaluate hip joint laxity (negative/positive).

Radiography

The stifle, hip, and elbow joints bilaterally as well as the lumbar spine of the study group dogs were radiographed under sedation. The amount of osteoarthritis in stifle joints was evaluated from mediolateral and craniocaudal views (no/mild/moderate/severe) [26] in hip joints from an extended ventrodorsal view (no/mild/moderate/severe), and in elbow joints from 45° flexed mediolateral and craniocaudal views on a scale from 0 to III [27]. In addition, the lumbar spine was evaluated from laterolateral and ventrodorsal views for the amount of spondylosis deformans on a scale from 0 to IV [28], and the amount of osteoarthritis (no/mild or moderate/severe).

Force plate analysis

Gait was evaluated using a piezoelectric force plate (Kistler force plate, type 9286, Kistler Instrumente AG, Winterthur, Switzerland) embedded in a 14 m runway and computer-based software program (Acquire 7.3, Sharon Software Inc., DeWitt, MI). Three pairs of photoelectric cells, positioned 1 m apart from each other, were used to measure the velocity and acceleration of the dogs. Dogs were guided over the force plate by the owner or a member of the research team at a trotting velocity of 2.10-2.50 m/s and a maximum acceleration of ±0.5 m/s^2.

Data from five valid trials for each side were normalized for the dog's body mass and averaged. Peak vertical forces (PVFs) and vertical impulses (VIs) in thoracic and pelvic limbs were evaluated. In addition, distribution percentages per limb of peak vertical forces (DPVFs) was calculated using the equation

$$DPVF_{STPL} = 100\ PVF_{STPL} / (PVF_{STPL} + PVF_{CPL} + PVF_{ITL} + PVF_{CTL})$$

where PVF_{STPL} is the PVFs recorded in the surgically treated limbs, PVF_{CPL} in the contralateral pelvic limbs, PVF_{ITL} in the ipsilateral thoracic limbs and PVF_{CTL} in the contralateral thoracic limbs. The DPVFs were calculated similarly for contralateral pelvic and thoracic limbs of surgically treated dogs as well as thoracic and pelvic limbs of control dogs.

A symmetry index (SI) [29] was calculated for the pelvic limb PVF and VI in surgically treated and control dogs using the equation

$$SI = 200\left(X_{CPL/L} - X_{STPL/R}\right) / \left(X_{CPL/L} + X_{STPL/R}\right)$$

where $X_{CPL/L}$ is the value recorded in the contralateral (study group) or left (control group) pelvic limb and $X_{STPL/R}$ is the value recorded in the surgically treated (study group) or right (control group) pelvic limb. In surgically treated dogs, a symmetry index value of 0 indicates perfect symmetry; a positive value indicates decreased dynamic weight bearing on the surgically treated limb and a negative value decreased dynamic weight bearing on the contralateral pelvic limb. The symmetry indices were calculated similarly for control group dogs, but absolute values of the symmetry indices were used. Thus, only the magnitude of the symmetry index value was evaluated, while side (right or left pelvic limb) of deviation from perfect symmetry was disregarded. The control group values were used to determine the cut-off value for differentiation between normal and lame dogs by using the equation: Mean + Standard deviation. Based on the cut-off value, the surgically treated dogs were assigned to have normal gait symmetry if SI was between the negative and positive cut-off values, lame on the surgically treated limb if SI was greater than cut-off value, or lame on the contralateral pelvic limb if SI was lower than negative cut-off value.

Physiotherapeutic examination

A physiotherapeutic examination was done by a physiotherapist specialized in veterinary physiotherapy, as previously described [30]. The full assessment consisted of a visual evaluation of lameness and possible diagonal movement during it, movement on stairs, functional active range of motion (AROM) and thrust from the ground, manual evaluation of muscle atrophy of pelvic limbs, manual evaluation and quantitative measurement of static weight bearing (SWB), and a measurement of passive range of motion (PROM) in stifle and tarsal joints [30]. Of all the physiotherapeutic examination tasks used, the results of AROM, symmetry of thrust between pelvic limbs, muscle atrophy, quantitative SWB of pelvic limbs, and PROM in stifle and tarsal joints are presented here.

When evaluating functional AROM and symmetry of thrust, the dog was led over a 20-m distance and asked to sit and sit-to-move 3 times, and similarly lie-down and lie-to-move 3 times within equal distances. The position of pelvic limbs during sitting and lying was observed, and possible functional limitations or compensations of the pelvic limbs in sitting or lying position (external rotation or abduction of the limb, and limited flexion of stifle and/or tarsal joints) or weakness of pelvic limbs in thrust from sitting or lying positions were recorded [30]. Subjective manual evaluation of muscle atrophy was done by palpating the symmetry of the muscle bulk of pelvic limbs and recorded as either symmetrical muscle mass in pelvic limbs or decreased muscle mass in either the left or right pelvic limb [30].

Quantitative measurement of SWB in pelvic limbs was done using digital bathroom scales, as previously described [31]. Two identical commercially available bathroom scales were used under each limb and the thoracic limbs were placed on a custom-made platform of the same height as the scales. The owner held the dog from the front, keeping it in a straight, square-standing position and the examiner placed the pelvic limbs symmetrically onto the scales, and recorded the measurements for both limbs. The results of four measurements for each limb were averaged and converted from kilograms to percentages proportional to the dog's body mass (SWB%). In addition, difference in static weight bearing between the pelvic limbs (DiffSWB%) was calculated using the following equation:

$$100\,(SWB_{CPL}(kg) - SWB_{STPL}(kg))/\text{ body mass (kg)}$$

where SWB_{CPL} is the value recorded in the contralateral pelvic limb and SWB_{STPL} the value recorded in the surgically treated limb [31]. Based on the published DiffSWB% cut-off value of 6% in healthy control dogs [31], the surgically treated dogs were divided into groups with symmetrical SWB, decreased SWB on the surgically treated limb, or decreased SWB on the contralateral pelvic limb.

PROM was measured in un-sedated dogs from both stifle and tarsal joints in extension and flexion using a universal goniometer with a five-degree scale. The measurements were taken in lateral recumbency three times and averaged [30]. In addition, the extension and flexion results of the surgically treated limbs were reported as percentages of the contralateral limbs. Because flexion angles had a tendency to be smaller (higher in number) in the surgically treated limbs, for calculation of percentages the flexion angles were subtracted from 180°.

Statistical analysis

Statistical analysis was done using the SPSS software program (version 21 for Windows; SPSS Inc., Chicago, IL). Kolmogorov-Smirnov and Shapiro-Wilk tests were applied to determine whether the data were normally distributed. Results from nominal and ordinal data (surgical technique, condition of the meniscus, stifle joint palpation and radiographic findings, AROM, muscle atrophy), symmetry index and DiffSWB% are reported as frequencies and percentages. For continuous data (age at time of surgery, body mass at time of evaluation, follow-up, force plate data, SWB%, PROM), the results are summarized as mean ± SD, and for age, body mass, and follow-up also as range.

The Kruskall-Wallis test with pairwise comparisons was used to evaluate differences in age, follow-up, stifle joint palpation findings, and amount of radiographic osteoarthritis between surgical techniques, and Independent samples t-test or one-way ANOVA was used to evaluate differences in body mass between study group and control dogs or surgical techniques. The Mann-Whitney rank sum test for non-normally distributed and Independent samples t-test for normally distributed force plate, SWB%, and PROM data were used to evaluate differences between surgically treated limbs and contralateral limbs (force plate, SWB%, PROM) or control dog limbs (force plate, SWB%). Similarly, the Kruskall-Wallis test with pairwise comparisons for non-normally distributed and one-way ANOVA with Bonferroni and Tukey post hoc analyses for normally distributed force plate, SWB%, and PROM data were used to evaluate differences between surgical techniques. $P < 0.05$ was considered significant.

Results

Study group

From the 278 questionnaire results, 47 dogs (25 females, 22 males) with owners willing to bring their dog to the evaluation fulfilled the inclusion criteria. The breeds of these dogs were Labrador Retriever (15), Rottweiler (6), mixed breed (4), Golden Retriever (3), Bernese Mountain Dog (2), Doberman Pincher (2), Newfoundland Dog

(2), Nova Scotia Duck Tolling Retriever (2), and one each of Beauceron, Black Russian Terrier, Bordeaux Dog, Bullmastiff, Collie, Dalmatian, Giant Schnauzer, Karelian Bear Dog, Short-Haired German Pointer, South African Boerboel and Wheaten Terrier. The mean ± SD (range) age of the dogs and their body mass at the time of evaluation were 6.9 ± 2.7 (1.8-13.0) years and 38.2 ± 9.5 (17.5-60) kg, respectively.

Of the pelvic limbs (31 left, 16 right), 19 limbs (40.4%) had been surgically treated using a modification of the original intracapsular technique [32], with an autograft that was passed over the top of the lateral femoral condyle, 7 limbs (14.9%) using variations of the original modification of the extracapsular technique [33], with a nylon leader line or polyester sutures, and 21 limbs (44.7%) using the TPLO (9) [34], the TTA (7) [35], or triple tibial osteotomy (TTO, 5) [18] techniques. Diagnosis of the CCL rupture and inspection of the joint had been done via arthrotomy in all dogs. The condition of the meniscus was reported in 23 dogs (48.9%), with damage in 10 and an intact meniscus in 13 dogs. Postoperative complications were reported in two dogs. One dog had loosening of the screws after TPLO surgery and was treated successfully with revision surgery, and the other dog had excessive scar tissue formation in the surgical wound after intracapsular repair. Mean ± SD (range) time interval between surgery and evaluation visit (follow-up) was 2.8 ± 0.9 (1.5-4.4) years. No significant difference was present between the surgical technique groups in the age of the dogs or body mass of the dogs at the time of evaluation. The mean follow-up was significantly shorter in the osteotomy technique group (2.2 ± 0.6 years) than in the intracapsular (3.3 ± 0.8 years, P =0.001) or extracapsular (3.6 ± 0.4 years, P =0.002) technique groups.

Control group

The mean ± SD age and body mass of the healthy control dogs (14 females, 7 males) were 3.2 ± 1.6 years and 35.5 ± 8.2 kg, respectively. The healthy control dogs were significantly younger than the dogs in the study group (P <0.001). No significant difference was found in body mass between the healthy control group and study group dogs.

Orthopedic and radiographic examination

At follow-up, grade 1/4 lameness of the surgically treated limb was seen in 8 dogs (3 intracapsular, 1 extracapsular, 4 osteotomy). One dog treated with the intracapsular technique had grade 2/4 lameness. In addition, 7 dogs had signs of lameness in the contralateral pelvic limb (grade 1/4 in 6 dogs, grade 2/4 in one dog) and 2 dogs in both front limbs (grade 1/4). The gait could not be evaluated in one surgically treated dog due to lack of cooperation. The 21 healthy control dogs did not show any signs of orthopedic disease or lameness.

Orthopedic and radiographic findings in the surgically treated stifle joints are presented in Table 1. The radiographs were unavailable for one dog. The severity of stifle joint crepitation was significantly lower in the osteotomy group than in the extracapsular (P =0.030) or intracapsular (P =0.028) group, and amount of periarticular swelling was significantly lower in the osteotomy than in the extracapsular group (P =0.047). No significant differences were found between surgical techniques in pain response to stifle flexion/extension. Of 12 dogs with positive drawer sign, 5 had been treated with intracapsular and 7 with osteotomy techniques. Tibial compression test was negative in all stifle joints. The amount of radiographic osteoarthritis was lower in the osteotomy group than in the intracapsular group (P =0.007).

In the contralateral stifle joints clinical findings were recorded in 9 dogs, including crepitation in all dogs, periarticular swelling in 8, pain in 3, and decreased ROM in 2 dogs. Radiographic signs of osteoarthritis were seen in 11 dogs, and drawer sign was positive in 3 dogs. Concurrent clinical findings were also seen uni- or bilaterally in hip joints of 17 dogs, elbow joints of 8 dogs, and shoulder joints of 6 dogs. Pain on palpation of the spine was found in 19 dogs. Radiographic findings of osteoarthritis were seen uni- or bilaterally in the hip joints of 21 dogs, elbow joints of 4 dogs, and the lumbosacral spine of 13 dogs.

Based on orthopedic and radiographic examinations, 21 dogs were included in subgroup 1 and 33 dogs in subgroup 2.

Force plate analysis

In 6 dogs the force plate analysis could not be performed due to lack of cooperation or inability to maintain adequate trotting speed. Mean ± SD trotting velocity and acceleration of the study group (n = 41), subgroup 1 (n = 21) and control group dogs (n = 21) were 2.25 ± 0.07, 2.27 ± 0.07 and 2.26 ± 0.06 m/s, and - 0.05 ± 0.12, - 0.09 ± 0.13 and - 0.05 ± 0.14 m/s^2, respectively. Body mass, trotting velocity or acceleration did not differ significantly between the study group or subgroup 1 and the control group dogs, between the surgically treated and the contralateral limbs or between the surgical technique groups.

When force plate results for the study group were evaluated, no significant differences emerged when comparing the surgically treated limb with the contralateral pelvic limb or with the pelvic limbs of control dogs.

In subgroup 1, surgically treated limbs had significantly lower PVF (P =0.040) and DPVF (P =0.005) than contralateral pelvic limbs, but no significant differences were found when surgically treated limbs were compared with control dog limbs (Table 2). The symmetry index cut-off values, 7.1% for PVF and 8.1% for VI were rounded up to 8% and 9%, respectively, to improve the specificity of the cut-off value. Based on the cut-off

Table 1 Stifle joint findings of the surgically treated limb; orthopedic and radiographic examination

	Severity of stifle joint findings			
	No findings	Mild	Moderate	Severe
Pain response to stifle flexion/extension (n = 47)	68.1% (32)	25.5% (12)	6.4% (3)	-
Periarticular swelling (n = 47)	-	36.2% (17)	53.2% (25)	10.6% (5)
Crepitation (n = 47)	6.4% (3)	34.0% (16)	51.1% (24)	8.5% (4)
Cranial drawer sign (n = 39)	69.2% (27)	15.4% (6)	12.8% (5)	2.6% (1)
Radiographic OA (n = 46)	2.2% (1)	19.6% (9)	45.6% (21)	32.6% (15)

Results are expressed as percentages (number) of dogs. n, number of dogs evaluated; OA, osteoarthritis.

values, the symmetry index for PVF was <8% in 13 dogs (61.9%), indicating normal gait symmetry, and ≥8% in 7 dogs (33.3%), indicating lameness. In one dog, the symmetry index indicated lameness of the contralateral pelvic limb (≤ -8%). Similarly, the symmetry index for VI was <9% in 15 dogs (71.4%), indicating normal gait symmetry, and ≥9% in 6 dogs (28.6%), indicating lameness. Of the 7 dogs in which one or both symmetry indices indicated lameness, 3 had been treated with intracapsular, 2 with extracapsular and 2 with osteotomy techniques.

When force plate results of different surgical technique groups were evaluated, no significant differences were found in study group between intracapsular, extracapsular and osteotomy techniques, or either in study group or subgroup 1 when surgically treated limbs in each technique group separately were compared with pelvic limbs in control dogs. Subgroup 1 dogs that had been treated with the intracapsular technique had significantly lower DPVF in the surgically treated limb than the dogs treated with osteotomy techniques (P =0.044). The dogs that had been treated with the intracapsular technique (n = 7) had significantly lower VI (P =0.035) and DPVF (P =0.018) in the surgically treated limb than in their contralateral pelvic limb. No significant differences were seen when limbs treated with the osteotomy technique (n = 11) were compared with their contralateral pelvic limbs. The number of dogs treated with the extracapsular technique (n = 3) was too low to be analyzed.

Physiotherapeutic examination

In visual evaluations of functional AROM, the most frequent findings were in the sitting position. In subgroup 1, decreased flexion of the tarsal joint was seen in 12 dogs (57.1%) (2 intracapsular, 10 osteotomy), decreased flexion of the stifle joint in 10 dogs (47.6%) (2 intracapsular, 1 extracapsular, 7 osteotomy), and abduction of the limb in 9 dogs (42.9%) (1 intracapsular, 1 extracapsular, 7 osteotomy). Except for one dog, the positive findings were always localized in the surgically treated limbs. Thrust from the sitting position was weaker in the surgically treated limb in 14 dogs (66.7%) (3 intracapsular, 1 extracapsular, 10 osteotomy). When evaluating muscle atrophy in subgroup 1, altogether 16 dogs (76.2%) had decreased muscle mass of the surgically treated pelvic limb on palpation (5 intracapsular, 2 extracapsular, 9 osteotomy), while only 4 dogs (19.0%) had symmetrical muscle mass (2 intracapsular, 1 extracapsular, 1 osteotomy), and one dog (4.8%) had decreased muscle mass in the contralateral pelvic limb.

In 2 dogs the SWB could not be performed due to lack of cooperation. When results of SWB were evaluated, all dogs in both the study group and subgroup 1 had a significantly lower SWB% in the surgically treated limb than in the contralateral pelvic limb (P =0.010 and P =0.006, respectively), but no significant differences were found when surgically treated limbs were compared with control dog limbs (Table 2). Based on the

Table 2 Dynamic and static weight bearing in subgroup 1, surgical technique groups and control dogs

	Subgroup 1 (n = 21)				Intra (n = 7)		Extra (n = 3)		Osteo (n = 11)		Control group (n = 21)	
	CTL	ITL	STPL	CPL	STPL	CPL	STPL	CPL	STPL	CPL	TL	PL
Force plate analysis												
PVF (%N/N)	117.8 (7.2)	117.1 (6.7)	70.6 (7.0)#	75.3 (7.3)	67.2 (7.6)	75.1 (6.7)	NA	NA	73.2 (6.8)	75.2 (8.9)	121.4 (10.2)	72.2 (4.0)
VI (%Ns/N)	16.2 (1.5)	16.1 (1.5)	8.7 (1.2)	9.4 (1.0)	8.3 (0.9)#	9.5 (1.0)	NA	NA	9.2 (1.3)	9.5 (1.1)	16.2 (1.1)	8.7 (0.8)
DPVF (%)	31.0 (1.1)	30.8 (1.1)	18.5 (1.3)#	19.8 (1.4)	17.8 (1.5)#*	19.9 (1.3)	NA	NA	19.2 (0.9)	19.7 (1.7)	31.3 (1.1)	18.7 (1.1)
Static weight bearing												
SWB%	NE	NE	15.5 (5.6)#	19.7 (3.6)	13.8 (7.3)#	21.2 (3.3)	NA	NA	16.8 (5.0)	19.4 (3.9)	NE	17.7 (2.8)

Results are expressed as mean (SD). #Significant (P <0.05) difference present between the surgically treated and contralateral pelvic limbs. *Significant (P <0.05) difference present in the measured value between the limbs treated with intracapsular and osteotomy techniques.

CTL, contralateral thoracic limb; ITL, ipsilateral thoracic limb; STPL, surgically treated pelvic limb; CPL, contralateral pelvic limb; TL, thoracic limb; PL, pelvic limb, PVF, peak vertical force; VI, vertical impulse; DPVF, percentage distribution of peak vertical forces on each limb; SWB%, static weight bearing reported as percentages proportional to body mass; NA, not analyzed due to the low number of dogs in extracapsular group; NE, SWB% is not evaluated for thoracic limbs.

previously reported 6% cut-off value in DiffSWB%, of 21 dogs, 13 (61.9%) had symmetrical weight bearing, 6 (28.6%) had decreased weight bearing in the surgically treated limb, and 2 dogs (9.5%) bore less weight on the contralateral pelvic limb. Of the dogs with decreased weight bearing in the surgically treated limb, 3 had been treated with intracapsular and 3 with osteotomy techniques.

In the study group, no significant differences emerged when SWB in surgically treated limbs was compared between surgical techniques or separately in each surgical technique group with either contralateral or control dog limbs. Similarly, in subgroup 1 dogs, no significant differences were found between surgical techniques. When each surgical technique group in subgroup 1 was evaluated separately and surgically treated limbs were compared with the contralateral and control dog limbs, no significant differences were observed in the osteotomy group (n = 11), but in the intracapsular group (n = 7) the SWB% in the surgically treated limb was significantly lower than that in the contralateral limb (P =0.030) (Table 2). The number of dogs in the extracapsular group (n = 3) was too low to be analyzed.

The PROM was not evaluated in 3 dogs due to lack of cooperation and in one dog due to concurrent orthopedic findings in the tarsal joint. When PROMs of surgically treated limbs in subgroup 2 were compared with contralateral limbs, stifle extension angles (P <0.001) were significantly lower and stifle flexion (P <0.001) and tarsal flexion (P =0.002) angles were significantly higher (loss of flexion) in the surgically treated limb (Table 3). Similar differences were present also in the intracapsular and osteotomy groups when each surgical technique was evaluated separately and the surgically treated limb was compared with the contralateral limb. In the extracapsular group, stifle flexion angles (P =0.045) were significantly higher (loss of flexion) than in contralateral limbs. No significant differences were found between the surgical techniques.

Discussion

We evaluated overall long-term surgical outcome at a mean of 2.8 years after CCL repair using a combination of force plate analysis, orthopedic and radiographic examinations and as a new aspect, a physiotherapeutic evaluation performed by a veterinary physiotherapist.

Force plate analysis

Force plate analysis showed no significant differences in ground reaction forces (PVF and VI) between the surgically treated limbs and the pelvic limbs of control dogs as well as in VI between the surgically treated and the contralateral limbs. However, the PVF of surgically treated limbs was significantly lower than the corresponding value for the contralateral pelvic limbs. The mean (SD) difference in PVF between the surgically treated and contralateral limbs was 4.7% (7.9), but it must be taken into account that load distribution from the injured to the contralateral pelvic or other limbs often occurs and artificially increases the difference between limbs [36]. Furthermore, the PVF of the surgically treated limbs was only 1.6% (8.5) lower than the corresponding value for the control dog limbs and mean VIs were exactly the same (SD 1.5) in surgically treated and control dog limbs.

When the differences are interpreted, the clinical importance of changes must be considered. Our results indicate that the mean differences between the surgically treated and healthy limbs were minor and dynamic weight bearing of the surgically treated limbs had returned to the level of healthy limbs. Similar long-term studies have not been reported before, but these results are in accordance with those of previous short- and mid-term force plate studies where the function of the surgically treated limb was at the level of the contralateral or control dog limbs 7 months after an extracapsular repair [5], or 4 and 12 months after TPLO surgery [6,10].

Although the average differences in ground reaction forces between surgically treated and healthy limbs were minor, the SIs for PVF and VI were greater than cut-off

Table 3 Stifle and tarsal joint flexion and extension in subgroup 2 and in surgical technique groups

	Subgroup 2 (n = 33)			Intra (n = 11)			Extra (n = 6)			Osteo (n = 16)		
	STPL(°)	CPL(°)	%	STPL(°)	CPL(°)	%	STPL(°)	CPL(°)	%	STPL(°)	CPL(°)	%
Stifle joint												
Ext	149.2 (8.6)*	160.3 (6.6)	93.1	148.2 (7.5)*	163.0 (2.5)	90.9	144.7 (10.9)	155.3 (11.1)	93.2	151.7 (8.0)*	160.3 (5.6)	94.6
Flex	47.9 (7.2)*	41.1 (6.5)	95.1	48.0 (5.4)*	40.3 (8.5)	94.5	49.7 (5.2)*	44.2 (2.0)	95.9	47.1 (8.9)*	40.4 (6.0)	95.2
Tarsal joint												
Ext	173.0 (7.5)	172.9 (6.3)	+0.1	176.5 (5.4)	174.1 (5.8)	+1.4	174.4 (6.3)	173.3 (6.8)	+0.6	170.0 (8.2)	172.0 (6.8)	98.8
Flex	46.7 (11.9)*	37.6 (9.1)	93.6	42.4 (10.8)*	32.6 (6.0)	93.5	52.0 (12.7)	43.6 (10.7)	93.8	47.7 (12.1)*	38.9 (8.9)	93.8

Results are expressed as mean (SD).*Significant (P <0.05) difference in the measured angle between the surgically treated limb and contralateral pelvic limb. STPL, surgically treated pelvic limb; CPL, contralateral pelvic limb. In percentage results, positive (+) value indicates higher extension angles in surgically treated limbs than in contralateral limbs.

values in almost one-third of dogs, indicating clinically relevant problem of weight bearing in these dogs and revealing considerable variation between the evaluated dogs. By using the SIs, more differences were revealed than what was discovered when the mean ground reaction forces between the surgically treated and healthy limbs were compared.

Physiotherapeutic examination

A physiotherapeutic examination concentrating on the stifle joints and performed by a veterinary physiotherapist was included in our study. To our knowledge, evaluation of AROM, thrust of pelvic limbs, or SWB has not been used to evaluate surgical outcome after CCL repair. Interestingly, compensations of AROM were seen in 40-50% of the dogs. In addition, the compensations of AROM were almost always localized to the surgically treated limb, not to the contralateral healthy limb.

Static weight bearing of the pelvic limbs was measured using commercial bathroom scales, and validity study of their results has been reported elsewhere [31]. The mean (SD) SWB% of the surgically treated limbs was 4.2% (8.5) lower than that of the contralateral limbs, reaching statistical significance. It can be assumed that, similar to dynamic weight bearing, load distribution to other limbs occurs also when measuring SWB. The difference between surgically treated and control dog limbs was only 2.2% (6.2) and not statistically significant. Similar to the variation seen in dynamic weight bearing, in almost one-third of dogs also the DiffSWB% indicated decreased static weight bearing in the surgically treated limb.

Goniometry of the stifle joints has been evaluated after CCL repair in several studies [3,8,16,18-23]. CCL rupture causes pain and disuse of the affected limb, resulting in decreased stifle ROM and muscle atrophy [23]. The stifle ROM improves after surgical repair [3,8,18,20,22], and the improvement can be enhanced by intense postoperative physiotherapy [23]. However, in some studies the stifle joint ROM has been shown to decrease with time after surgery [3,8,18,22]. Au et al. [3] reported that stifle joint ROM angles in surgically treated limbs were below the preoperative values 2 years after TPLO or extracapsular repair. Our results are also in accordance with another study, in which significant loss of extension and flexion of the surgically treated stifle joint, compared with the contralateral joint, was reported 1-5 years after TPLO surgery [16]. The most probable cause for the decrease of ROM over time is the progression of osteoarthritis, causing functional impairment due to pain and mechanical restriction of joint mobility due to fibrous tissue and new bone formation in the joint and its periarticular tissues. The clinical relevance of a loss of 5% in flexion and 7% in extension of the stifle joint ROM in our study is unknown. Jandi and Schulman [21] reported that loss of flexion or extension ≥10° was associated with higher lameness scores, but we did not find any correlation between goniometric results and dynamic or static weight bearing.

In addition to loss of extension and flexion of the stifle joint, also flexion of the tarsal joint was significantly decreased in the surgically treated limbs. Loss of flexion in the tarsal joint might be explained by the anatomical fact that in order to measure full flexion of the tarsus a full flexion of the stifle joint is required and thus the limitations in the stifle joint flexion also may affect ipsilateral tarsal joint flexion angles.

Pain

An interesting aspect in the long-term assessment of CCL repair is the occurrence of pain. In our study, in almost one-third of dogs the symmetry indices for PVF and VI indicated lameness and the DiffSWB% indicated decreased weight bearing in the surgically treated limb, likely not only reflecting the functional outcome, but also pain in the surgically treated limb. Moreover, in the orthopedic examination, lameness was seen in almost 20% and pain response on flexion and/or extension of the surgically treated stifle joints in one-third of dogs. These findings resonate well with our previous report of chronic pain after CCL surgery, which is based on a validated questionnaire filled out by 253 dog owners and includes the 42 dogs serving as subjects here. In that report, almost one-third of the dogs had signs of chronic pain at a mean of 2.7 years after CCL surgery [17]. Recognition of chronic pain can be challenging for owners [37], and these dogs may often go undiagnosed and untreated. It's therefore important for clinicians to be aware that CCL-deficient dogs may experience chronic pain, and owners should be educated about recognizing signs of pain so that pain management can be initiated promptly.

Limitations

There are limitations in our study. Our patient material was very heterogeneous, with many confounding factors. Due to the retrospective study design we were unable to control such variables as conformation and age of the dog, duration of clinical signs before surgery, completeness of the cruciate ligament tear, meniscal pathology, and treatment or postoperative rehabilitation and medications. However, our patient material can be used to assess general surgical outcome and it better reflects a real-life situation with heterogeneity in patient material, surgical procedures, and postoperative treatments. The confounding factors may nevertheless have caused bias in the comparison of surgical techniques. Therefore the results must be interpreted with some caution.

The number of patients was unfortunately low. Due to the limitations set by the force platform, only dogs with a body mass exceeding 17 kg were included. For force plate and physiotherapeutic evaluation, we only included dogs with no other concurrent orthopedic problems (subgroups 1 and 2) in order to minimize the effect of concomitant problems on dynamic or static weight bearing, AROM, and PROM. Although only the dogs with unilaterally treated CCL rupture and no other owner-reported significant orthopedic or neurologic problems were originally included in the study group, during the evaluation surprisingly many of them were diagnosed with bilateral stifle joint pathology or other concurrent orthopedic problems, resulting in a low number of dogs for final evaluation. To detect a statistical significance in PVF between the surgically treated and control dogs using the data generated from this study, 400 dogs would have been needed (using α =0.05 and 80% power). On the other hand, it may be speculated that even if a statistical significance had been shown, a difference of 1.6% in PVF between the surgically treated and control dog limbs might anyway not be clinically significant.

In force plate analysis, we decided to compare the ground reaction forces to both contralateral and control dog limbs, both of which have some disadvantages. Due to weight redistribution to the contralateral pelvic limb or thoracic limbs, the use of the contralateral pelvic limb as a reference has been questioned [36]. On the other hand, when force plate results are compared with data obtained from other individuals, in addition to controlling the velocity, acceleration, and body mass of the dog, the conformation and size of the dogs have an effect on ground reaction forces [24,38,39]. In our study, there were no significant differences in body mass of the dogs between the groups, but although there were many Rottweilers and Labrador Retrievers in the study group, it also included several other breeds with different body conformations, while the control group of healthy dogs included only Rottweilers and Labradors. As a compromise, we compared the results with both contralateral and control dog limbs, and after taking into account the weight distribution, the results were in accordance with each other. Similar comparisons were made for static weight bearing.

In the physiotherapeutic examination, only a subjective assessment of muscle mass symmetry was used when evaluating muscle atrophy. We could have improved the test by measuring atrophy with a tape measure, thus quantifying the measurement and increasing the objectivity of the method. On the other hand, in a recent study [30], the subjective evaluation of muscle atrophy was shown to be sensitive for detecting functional pelvic limb problems. Interestingly, 16 of the 21 dogs evaluated in our study (76%) had decreased muscle mass in the surgically treated limb.

The postoperative treatment did not include any special rehabilitation program and only one of the dogs had had postoperative rehabilitation by a physiotherapist. Previous studies have shown that postoperative rehabilitation significantly improves the surgical outcome [23], and nowadays, rehabilitation is recommended to all CCL-deficient dogs. However, at the time the dogs in our study were treated, postoperative rehabilitation was not yet widely used.

Comparison of surgical techniques

The dogs treated with osteotomy techniques had less crepitation in the surgically treated limb than dogs treated with intra- or extracapsular techniques. In addition, the amount of radiographic osteoarthritis was lower in the osteotomy group than in the intracapsular group. These results must be interpreted with caution because of potential initial preoperative differences in the orthopedic or radiographic examination between the surgical technique groups. On the other hand, it could be speculated that the preoperative differences in radiographic osteoarthritis between groups might level off in the long run. Also, in two recent studies the preoperative amount of osteoarthritis was reported to correlate negatively with the progression of osteoarthritis postoperatively, meaning that dogs with severe pre-existing osteoarthritis would have less potential for osteoarthritis to worsen, compared with dogs with only minor pre-existing osteoarthritis [40,41].

The low number of dogs treated with extracapsular technique did not allow comparison of ground reaction forces or SWB of this group to other technique groups. The ground reaction forces and SWB% in the osteotomy group had a tendency to be higher than in the intracapsular technique and to reach control dog values. The dogs that had been treated with the intracapsular technique had significantly lower DPVF in the surgically treated limb than the dogs treated with the osteotomy technique. No other significant differences emerged between surgical technique groups when dynamic and static weight bearing or goniometric results were evaluated. No significant differences between surgically treated and contralateral or control dog limbs were found in the osteotomy group, whereas in the intracapsular group statistically significant differences in VI, DPVF and SWB between the surgically treated and contralateral limbs were achieved. Parallel results have been reported also in two previous force plate studies. Conzemius et al. [7] stated that the limb function after intracapsular repair was inferior to limb function after TPLO surgery 6 months postoperatively. Also in another experimental study the limb function after intracapsular repair remained significantly lower than the preoperative function at a 20-week follow-up [9]. In goniometry, stifle joint extension and flexion as well as tarsal joint flexion angles were decreased relative to the contralateral limb both in intracapsular and osteotomy technique groups.

Conclusions

The average long-term dynamic and static weight bearing of the surgically treated limbs returned to the level of healthy limbs. However, when symmetry of weight bearing was evaluated using cut-off values, approximately 30% of dogs had decreased static or dynamic weight bearing in the surgically treated limb, and almost one-third of dogs showed pain in stifle joint palpation. In addition, the extension and flexion angles of the surgically treated stifles remained inferior to healthy joints, and many dogs showed impairment of AROM and weakness in thrust from the ground in the surgically treated limbs. In sum, measurement of ground reaction forces may be inadequate as a sole method for assessing functional outcome and thus more objective outcome assessment methods should be included in evaluation of CCL repair.

Abbreviations

AROM: Active range of motion; CCL: Cranial cruciate ligament; CPL: Contralateral pelvic limb; CTL: Contralateral thoracic limb; DiffSWB%: Difference in static weight bearing between the pelvic limbs; DPVF: Percentage distribution of peak vertical force; ITL: Ipsilateral thoracic limb; L: Left; OA: Osteoarthritis; PL: Pelvic limb; PROM: Passive range of motion; PVF: Peak vertical force; R: Right; ROM: Range of motion; SI: Symmetry index; STPL: Surgically treated pelvic limb; SWB: Static weight bearing; SWB%: Static weight bearing as percentages proportional to dogs body mass; TL: Thoracic limb; TPLO: Tibial plateau leveling osteotomy; TTA: Tibial tuberosity advancement; TTO: Triple tibial osteotomy; VI: Vertical impulse.

Competing interests

All authors declare that they have no competing interests. No funding was received for the study.

Authors' contributions

Orthopedic and radiographic examinations and force plate analysis were done by SHM and physiotherapeutic examination by HKH. AKHB and OMLV evaluated and interpreted the radiographs. SHM performed the statistical analyses and drafted the manuscript with the aid of HKH, AKHB and OMLV. All authors read and approved the final manuscript.

Acknowledgements

The authors thank orthopedic surgeons Per Axelson, Esa Eskelinen, Pauli Keränen, Heikki Putro, Jan Räihä and Kai Skutnabb for providing the patient material.

References

1. Piermattei DL, Flo GL, DeCamp CE: **The stifle joint.** In *Brinker, Piermattei, and Flo's Handbook of Small Animal Orthopedics and Fracture Repair.* 3rd edition. Edited by Piermattei DL, Flo GL, DeCamp CE. Philadelphia: Saunders; 2006:562–632.
2. Kowaleski MP, Boudrieau RJ, Pozzi A: **Stifle Joint.** In *Veterinary Surgery Small Animal. Volume 1.* Edited by Tobias KM, Johnston SA. St. Louis: Saunders; 2012:906–998.
3. Au KK, Gordon-Evans WJ, Dunning D, O'Dell-Anderson KJ, Knap KE, Griffon D, Johnson AL: **Comparison of short- and long-term function and radiographic osteoarthrosis in dogs after postoperative physical rehabilitation and tibial plateau leveling osteotomy or lateral fabellar suture stabilization.** *Vet Surg* 2010, **39:**173–180.
4. Ballagas AJ, Montgomery RD, Henderson RA, Gillette R: **Pre- and postoperative force plate analysis of dogs with experimentally transected cranial cruciate ligaments treated using tibial plateau leveling osteotomy.** *Vet Surg* 2004, **33:**187–190.
5. Budsberg SC, Verstraete MC, Soutas-Little RW, Flo GL, Probst CW: **Force plate analyses before and after stabilization of canine stifles for cruciate injury.** *Am J Vet Res* 1988, **49:**1522–1524.
6. Böddeker J, Drüen S, Meyer-Lindenberg A, Fehr M, Nolte I, Wefstaedt P: **Computer-assisted gait analysis of the dog: Comparison of two surgical techniques for the ruptured cranial cruciate ligament.** *Vet Comp Orthop Traumatol* 2012, **25:**11–21.
7. Conzemius MG, Evans RB, Besancon MF, Gordon WJ, Horstman CL, Hoefle WD, Nieves MA, Wagner SD: **Effect of surgical technique on limb function after surgery for rupture of the cranial cruciate ligament in dogs.** *J Am Vet Med Assoc* 2005, **226:**232–236.
8. Gordon-Evans WJ, Griffon DJ, Bubb C, Knap KM, Sullivan M, Evans RB: **Comparison of lateral fabellar suture and tibial plateau leveling osteotomy techniques for treatment of dogs with cranial cruciate ligament disease.** *J Am Vet Med Assoc* 2013, **243:**675–680.
9. Jevens DJ, DeCamp CE, Hauptman J, Braden TD, Richter M, Robinson R: **Use of force plate analysis of gait to compare two surgical techniques for treatment of cranial cruciate ligament rupture in dogs.** *Am J Vet Res* 1996, **57:**389–393.
10. Nelson SA, Krotscheck U, Rawlinson J, Todhunter RJ, Zhang Z, Mohammed H: **Long-term functional outcome of tibial plateau leveling osteotomy versus extracapsular repair in a heterogeneous population of dogs.** *Vet Surg* 2013, **42:**38–50.
11. Voss K, Damur DM, Guerrero T, Haessig M, Montavon PM: **Force plate gait analysis to assess limb function after tibial tuberosity advancement in dogs with cranial cruciate ligament disease.** *Vet Comp Orthop Traumatol* 2008, **21:**243–249.
12. Wucherer KL, Conzemius MG, Evans R, Wilke WL: **Short-term and long-term outcomes for overweight dogs with cranial cruciate ligament rupture treated surgically and nonsurgically.** *J Am Vet Med Assoc* 2013, **242:**1364–1372.
13. Hoffmann DE, Miller JM, Ober CP, Lanz OI, Martin RA, Shires PK: **Tibial tuberosity advancement in 65 canine stifles.** *Vet Comp Orthop Traumatol* 2006, **19:**219–227.
14. Lazar TP, Berry CR, Dehaan JJ, Peck JN, Correa M: **Long-term radiographic comparison of tibial plateau leveling osteotomy versus extracapsular stabilization for cranial cruciate ligament rupture in the dog.** *Vet Surg* 2005, **34:**133–141.
15. Vasseur PB, Berry CR: **Progression of stifle osteoarthrosis following reconstruction of the cranial cruciate ligament in 21 dogs.** *J Am Anim Hosp Assoc* 1992, **28:**129–136.
16. Moeller EM, Allen DA, Wilson ER, Linerberger JA, Lehenbauer T: **Long-term outcomes of thigh circumference, stifle range-of-motion, and lameness after unilateral tibial plateau levelling osteotomy.** *Vet Comp Orthop Traumatol* 2010, **23:**37–42.
17. Mölsä SM, Hielm-Björkman AK, Laitinen-Vapaavuori OM: **Use of an owner questionnaire to evaluate long-term surgical outcome and chronic pain after cranial cruciate ligament repair in dogs: 253 cases (2004-2006).** *J Am Vet Med Assoc* 2013, **243:**689–695.
18. Bruce WJ, Rose A, Tuke J, Robins GM: **Evaluation of the triple tibial osteotomy. A new technique for the management of the canine cruciate-deficient stifle.** *Vet Comp Orthop Traumatol* 2007, **20:**159–168.
19. Drygas KA, McClure SR, Goring RL, Pozzi A, Robertson SA, Wand C: **Effect of cold compression therapy on postoperative pain, swelling, range of motion, and lameness after tibial plateau leveling osteotomy in dogs.** *J Am Vet Med Assoc* 2011, **238:**1284–1291.
20. Gordon-Evans WJ, Dunning D, Johnson AL, Knap KE: **Effect of the use of carprofen in dogs undergoing intense rehabilitation after lateral fabellar suture stabilization.** *J Am Vet Med Assoc* 2011, **239:**75–80.
21. Jandi AS, Schulman AJ: **Incidence of motion loss of the stifle joint in dogs with naturally occurring cranial cruciate ligament rupture surgically treated with tibial plateau leveling osteotomy: Longitudinal clinical study of 412 cases.** *Vet Surg* 2007, **36:**114–121.
22. Jerram RM, Walker AM, Warman CGA: **Proximal tibial intraarticular ostectomy for treatment of canine cranial cruciate ligament injury.** *Vet Surg* 2005, **34:**196–205.
23. Monk ML, Preston CA, McGowan CM: **Effects of early intensive postoperative physiotherapy on limb function after tibial plateau leveling osteotomy in dogs with deficiency of the cranial cruciate ligament.** *Am J Vet Res* 2006, **67:**529–536.
24. Mölsä SM, Hielm-Björkman AK, Laitinen-Vapaavuori OM: **Force platform analysis in clinically healthy Rottweilers: Comparison with Labrador Retrievers.** *Vet Surg* 2010, **39:**701–707.

25. Mostafa AA, Griffon DJ, Thomas MW: **Morphometric characteristics of the pelvic limbs of Labrador Retrievers with and without cranial cruciate ligament deficiency.** *Am J Vet Res* 2009, **70:**498–507.
26. DeRooster H, Van Bree H: **Use of compression stress radiography for the detection of partial tears of the canine cruciate ligament.** *J Small Anim Pract* 1999, **40:**573–576.
27. **International elbow protocol (Vancouver 2012)** [http://www.vet-iewg.org/joomla/index.php/archive/23-2001-international-elbow-protocol-vancouver]
28. Eichelberg H, Wurster H: **Untersuchungen an Boxern zum Verknöcherungsverlauf bei der Spondylosis deformans.** *Kleintierprax* 1983, **28:**393–444.
29. Herzog W, Nigg BM, Read LJ, Olsson E: **Asymmetries in ground reaction force patterns in normal human gait.** *Med Sci Sports Exerc* 1988, **21:**110–114.
30. Hyytiäinen HK, Mölsä SM, Junnila JT, Laitinen-Vapaavuori OM, Hielm-Björkman AK: **Ranking of physiotherapeutic evaluation methods as outcome measures of stifle functionality in dogs.** *Acta Vet Scand* 2013, **55**(29):1–9.
31. Hyytiäinen HK, Mölsä SM, Junnila JT, Laitinen-Vapaavuori OM, Hielm-Björkman AK: **Use of bathroom scales in measuring asymmetry of hindlimb static weight bearing in dogs with osteoarthritis.** *Vet Comp Orthop Traumatol* 2012, **25:**390–396.
32. Arnoczky SP, Tarvin GB, Marshall JL, Salzman B: **The over-the-top procedure: a technique for anterior cruciate ligament substitution in the dog.** *J Am Anim Hosp Assoc* 1979, **15:**283–290.
33. Flo GL: **Modification of the lateral retinacular imbrications technique for stabilizing cruciate ligament injuries.** *J Am Anim Hosp Assoc* 1975, **11:**570–576.
34. Slocum B, Devine Slocum T: **Tibial plateau leveling osteotomy for repair of cranial cruciate ligament rupture in the canine.** *Vet Clin North Am Small Anim Pract* 1993, **23:**777–795.
35. Lafaver S, Miller NA, Stubbs WB, Lanz OI, Martin RA, Shires PK: **Tibial tuberosity advancement for stabilization of the canine cranial cruciate ligament-deficient stifle joint: surgical technique, early results, and complications in 101 dogs.** *Vet Surg* 2007, **36:**573–586.
36. Rumph PF, Kincaid SA, Visco DM, Baird DK, Kammermann JR, West MS: **Redistribution of vertical ground reaction force in dogs with experimentally induced chronic hindlimb lameness.** *Vet Surg* 1995, **24:**384–389.
37. Hielm-Björkman AK, Kapatkin AS, Rita HJ: **Reliability and validity of a visual analogue scale used by owners to measure chronic pain attributable to osteoarthritis in their dogs.** *Am J Vet Res* 2011, **72:**601–607.
38. Voss K, Galeandro L, Wiestner T, Haessig M, Montavon PM: **Relationships of body weight, body size, subject velocity, and vertical ground reaction forces in trotting dogs.** *Vet Surg* 2010, **39:**863–869.
39. Voss K, Wiestner T, Galeandro L, Hässig M, Montavon PM: **Effect of dog breed and body conformation on vertical ground reaction forces, impulses, and stance times.** *Vet Comp Orthop Traumatol* 2011, **24:**106–112.
40. Hurley CR, Hammer DL, Shott S: **Progression of radiographic evidence of osteoarthritis following tibial plateau leveling osteotomy in dogs with cranial cruciate ligament rupture: 295 cases (2001-2005).** *J Am Vet Med Assoc* 2007, **230:**1674–1679.
41. Lineberger JA, Allen DA, Wilson ER, Tobias TA, Shaiken LG, Shiroma JT, Biller DS, Lehenbauer TW: **Comparison of radiographic arthritic changes associated with two variations of tibial plateau leveling osteotomy. A retrospective clinical study.** *Vet Comp Orthop Traumatol* 2005, **18:**13–17.

Permissions

All chapters in this book were first published in VR, by BioMed Central; hereby published with permission under the Creative Commons Attribution License or equivalent. Every chapter published in this book has been scrutinized by our experts. Their significance has been extensively debated. The topics covered herein carry significant findings which will fuel the growth of the discipline. They may even be implemented as practical applications or may be referred to as a beginning point for another development.

The contributors of this book come from diverse backgrounds, making this book a truly international effort. This book will bring forth new frontiers with its revolutionizing research information and detailed analysis of the nascent developments around the world.

We would like to thank all the contributing authors for lending their expertise to make the book truly unique. They have played a crucial role in the development of this book. Without their invaluable contributions this book wouldn't have been possible. They have made vital efforts to compile up to date information on the varied aspects of this subject to make this book a valuable addition to the collection of many professionals and students.

This book was conceptualized with the vision of imparting up-to-date information and advanced data in this field. To ensure the same, a matchless editorial board was set up. Every individual on the board went through rigorous rounds of assessment to prove their worth. After which they invested a large part of their time researching and compiling the most relevant data for our readers.

The editorial board has been involved in producing this book since its inception. They have spent rigorous hours researching and exploring the diverse topics which have resulted in the successful publishing of this book. They have passed on their knowledge of decades through this book. To expedite this challenging task, the publisher supported the team at every step. A small team of assistant editors was also appointed to further simplify the editing procedure and attain best results for the readers.

Apart from the editorial board, the designing team has also invested a significant amount of their time in understanding the subject and creating the most relevant covers. They scrutinized every image to scout for the most suitable representation of the subject and create an appropriate cover for the book.

The publishing team has been an ardent support to the editorial, designing and production team. Their endless efforts to recruit the best for this project, has resulted in the accomplishment of this book. They are a veteran in the field of academics and their pool of knowledge is as vast as their experience in printing. Their expertise and guidance has proved useful at every step. Their uncompromising quality standards have made this book an exceptional effort. Their encouragement from time to time has been an inspiration for everyone.

The publisher and the editorial board hope that this book will prove to be a valuable piece of knowledge for researchers, students, practitioners and scholars across the globe.

List of Contributors

Henri G. M. J. Bertrand and Aurelie A. Thomas
Comparative Biology Centre, Newcastle University, Framlington Place, Newcastle Upon Tyne NE2 4HH, UK

Yvette C. Ellen
Comparative Biology Centre, Newcastle University, Framlington Place, Newcastle Upon Tyne NE2 4HH, UK
School of Veterinary Medicine and Science, Nottingham University, Nottingham, UK

Paul A. Flecknell
Comparative Biology Centre, Newcastle University, Framlington Place, Newcastle Upon Tyne NE2 4HH, UK
Institute of Neurosciences, Newcastle University, Newcastle Upon Tyne, UK

Robert S. Dorward
School of Veterinary Medicine and Science, Nottingham University, Nottingham, UK

Verónica Vieitez, Víctor López Rámis, Massimo Santella and Luis Javier Ezquerra
Veterinary Teaching Hospital, University of Extremadura, Avda, Universidad s/n, 10003 Cáceres, Spain

Ignacio Álvarez Gómez de Segura
Department of Animal Medicine and Surgery, Veterinary Faculty, University Complutense of Madrid, Avda. Puerta de Hierro, 28040 Madrid, Spain

Adamu Abdul Abubakar and Hui Cheng Chen
Department of Veterinary Clinical Studies, Faculty of Veterinary Medicine, Universiti Putra Malaysia, 43400 Serdang, Selangor, Malaysia

Ubedullah Kaka
Department of Veterinary Clinical Studies, Faculty of Veterinary Medicine, Universiti Putra Malaysia, 43400 Serdang, Selangor, Malaysia
Department of Surgery and Obstetrics, Faculty of Animal Husbandry & Veterinary Sciences, Sindh Agriculture University Tandojam, Sindh 70060, Pakistan

Asmatullah Kaka
Department of Veterinary Clinical Studies, Faculty of Veterinary Medicine, Universiti Putra Malaysia, 43400 Serdang, Selangor, Malaysia
Faculty of Animal Husbandry & Veterinary Sciences, Sindh Agriculture University Tandojam, Sindh 70060, Pakistan

Bullo Saifullah
Material Synthesis and characterization laboratory, Institute of Advanced technology, Universiti Putra Malaysia, 43400 Serdang, Selangor, Malaysia

Mahdi Ebrahimi
Department of Veterinary Preclinical Sciences, Faculty of Veterinary Medicine, Universiti Putra Malaysia, 43400 Serdang, Selangor, Malaysia

Yong Meng Goh
Department of Veterinary Preclinical Sciences, Faculty of Veterinary Medicine, Universiti Putra Malaysia, 43400 Serdang, Selangor, Malaysia
Institutes of Tropical Agriculture, Universiti Putra Malaysia, 43400 Serdang, Selangor, Malaysia

Sharida Fakurazi
Laboratory of Vaccines and Immunotherapeutics, Institute of Bioscience, Universiti Putra Malaysia, 43400 Serdang, Selangor, Malaysia
Department of Human Anatomy, Faculty of Medicine and Health Science, Universiti Putra Malaysia, 43400 Serdang, Selangor, Malaysia

Atique Ahmed Behan
Department of Animal Sciences, Faculty of Agriculture, Universiti Putra Malaysia, 43400 Serdang, Selangor, Malaysia
Faculty of Animal Husbandry & Veterinary Sciences, Sindh Agriculture University Tandojam, Sindh 70060, Pakistan

Markus Horning
Alaska SeaLife Center, 301 Railway Avenue, Seward, AK 99664, USA
Oregon State University, 2030 SE Marine Science Drive, Newport, OR 97365, USA

Martin Haulena, Justin F. Rosenberg and Chad Nordstrom
Vancouver Aquarium, 845 Avison Way, Vancouver, BC V6G 3E2, Canada

Yu Moriguchi and Roger Härtl
Department of Neurological Surgery, Weill Cornell Medicine, New York-Presbyterian Hospital, Weill Cornell Brain and Spine Institute, 525 East 68th Street, New York, NY 10065, USA

Peter Grunert
Department of Neurological Surgery, Weill Cornell Medicine, New York-Presbyterian Hospital, Weill Cornell Brain and Spine Institute, 525 East 68th Street, New York, NY 10065, USA
Department of Neurological Surgery, Swedish Neuroscience Institute, Seattle, WA, USA

Brian P. Grossbard
Department of Orthopedics and Neurosurgery VCA-Animal Specialty, Yonkers, NY, USA

Rodolfo J. Ricart Arbona
Center of Comparative Medicine and Pathology, Memorial Sloan Kettering Cancer Center & Weill Cornell Medicine, New York City, NY, USA

Lawrence J. Bonassar
Department of Biomedical Engineering, Cornell University, Ithaca, NY, USA

Mohd Rafiq Mohd Ibrahim, Simmrat Singh, Azhar Mahmood Merican, Hanumantha Rao Balaji Raghavendran, Malliga Raman Murali and Sangeetha Vasudevaraj Naveen
Tissue Engineering Group (TEG), National Orthopaedic Centre of Excellence in Research and Learning (NOCERAL), Department of Orthopaedic Surgery, Faculty of Medicine, University of Malaya, Kuala Lumpur, Malaysia

Tunku Kamarul
Tissue Engineering Group (TEG), National Orthopaedic Centre of Excellence in Research and Learning (NOCERAL), Department of Orthopaedic Surgery, Faculty of Medicine, University of Malaya, Kuala Lumpur, Malaysia
Clinical Investigative Centre, Faculty of Medicine, University Malaya Medical Center, Kuala Lumpur, Malaysia

Matheus M. Mantovani, André M. Gimenes, Jacqueline R. de Castro and Denise S. Schwartz
Departamento de Clínica Médica, Faculdade de Medicina Veterinária e Zootecnia, Universidade de São Paulo, São Paulo, Brazil

Patrícia B. Flor
Departamento de Cirurgia, Faculdade de Medicina Veterinária e Zootecnia, Universidade de São Paulo, São Paulo, Brazil

Denise T. Fantoni
Departamento de Cirurgia, Faculdade de Medicina Veterinária e Zootecnia, Universidade de São Paulo, São Paulo, Brazil
Faculdade de Medicina Veterinária e Zootecnia da Universidade Federal de São Paulo, Av. Prof Dr Orlando Marques de Paiva 87, São Paulo, SP 05508-270, Brazil

Keila K. Ida
Laboratório de Investigação Médica 8, Anestesiologia, Faculdade de Medicina, Universidade de São Paulo, São Paulo, Brazil

Tsjester Huppes, Hanneke Hermans and Jos M. Ensink
Department of Equine Sciences, Faculty of Veterinary Medicine, Utrecht University, Yalelaan 114, 3584 CM Utrecht, Netherlands

Francesco Macrì, Simona Di Pietro, Cyndi Mangano, Michela Pugliese, Giuseppe Mazzullo, Nicola M. Iannelli, Vito Angileri, Simona Morabito and Massimo De Majo
Department of Veterinary Sciences, University of Messina, Polo Universitario Annunziata, 98168 Messina, Italy

Guillaume Leblond, Luis Gaitero, Noel M. Moens, Alex zur Linden, Fiona M. K. James and Gabrielle Monteith
Department of Clinical Studies, Ontario Veterinary College, University of Guelph, Guelph, ON N1G 2W1, Canada

John Runciman
School of Engineering, University of Guelph, Guelph, ON N1G 2W1, Canada

Umit Karademir and Cavit Kum
Department of Pharmacology and Toxicology, Faculty of Veterinary Medicine, University of Adnan Menderes, Isikli Koyu, Aydin, Turkey

Dilek Aksit
Department of Pharmacology and Toxicology, Faculty of Veterinary Medicine, Balikesir University, Balikesir, Turkey

Hasan Erdogan
Department of Internal Medicine, Faculty of Veterinary Medicine, University of Adnan Menderes, Isikli Koyu, Aydin, Turkey

Eyup Hakan Ucar and Cevdet Peker
Department of Obstetrics and Gynecology, Faculty of Veterinary Medicine, University of Adnan Menderes, Isikli Koyu, Aydin, Turkey

Cengiz Gokbulut
Department of Medical Pharmacology, Faculty of Medicine, Balikesir University, Balikesir, Turkey

Angela Briganti and Flavia Evangelista
Department of Veterinary Sciences, University of Pisa, Pisa, Italy

Antonio Crovace, Francesco Staffieri, Francesco Bentivegna, Paola Centonze and Annaliso Rizzo
Dipartimento delle Emergenze e Trapianti di Organo, Università degli Studi di Bari "Aldo Moro, " Sezione di Cliniche Veterinarie e P.A, Bari, Italy

Sebastian Schaub, Karsten Kemper, Kerstin H. Pueckler and Matthias A. Schneider
Department of Veterinary Clinical Sciences, Small Animal Clinic, Justus-Liebig-University Giessen, 35392 Giessen, Germany

Antje Hartmann
Department of Clinical Veterinary Medicine, Vetsuisse Faculty, University of Bern, 3012 Bern, Switzerland

Tobias Schwarz
Royal (Dick) School of Veterinary Studies, The University of Edinburgh, Roslin, Midlothian EH25 9RG, UK

Shebl E. Salem
Institute of Infection and Global Health, Department of Epidemiology and Population Health, University of Liverpool, Wirral CH64 7TE, UK
Department of Surgery, Faculty of Veterinary Medicine, Zagazig University, Zagazig, Egypt

Debra C. Archer
Institute of Infection and Global Health, Department of Epidemiology and Population Health, University of Liverpool, Wirral CH64 7TE, UK
Philip Leverhulme Equine Hospital, School of Veterinary Science, University of Liverpool, Wirral CH64 7TE, UK

Chris J. Proudman
School of Veterinary Medicine, University of Surrey, Guildford GU2 7TE, UK

Allison R Kenzig and James R Butler
Mississippi State University College of Veterinary Medicine, 240 Wise Center Drive, Mississippi State, MS 39762, USA

Lauren B Priddy, Kristen R Lacy and Steven H Elder
Mississippi State University College of Agricultural and Biological Engineering, 130 Creelman Street, Mississippi State, MS 39762, USA

B. Duncan X. Lascelles
Department of Clinical Sciences, Comparative Pain Research Laboratory, College of Veterinary Medicine, North Carolina State University, Raleigh, NC, USA
Department of Clinical Sciences, Comparative Medicine Institute, College of Veterinary Medicine, North Carolina State University, Raleigh, NC 27606, USA
Center for Pain Research and Innovation, Dental School, UNC Chapel Hill, Chapel Hill, NC, USA
Department of Anesthesiiology, Center for Translational Pain Medicine, Duke UniversityDurham, NC, USA

Lesley C. Rausch-Derra and Jessica A. Wofford
Aratana Therapeutics, Inc., Leawood, KS 66211, USA

Margie Huebner
ClinData Services, Inc., 6716 Holyoke Court, Fort Collins, CO 80525, USA

Selena Tinga, Stanley E. Kim, Scott A. Banks, Stephen C. Jones, Brian H. Park, Antonio Pozzi and Daniel D. Lewis
Comparative Orthopaedics and Biomechanics Laboratory, College of Veterinary Medicine and the Department of Mechanical & Aerospace Engineering, University of Florida, 2015 SW 16th Ave, Gainesville, FL 32610-0126, USA

Sebastiaan A. van Nimwegen and Jeffrey de Gier
Department of Clinical Sciences of Companion Animals, Faculty of Veterinary Medicine, Utrecht University, Yalelaan 108, 3584CM, Utrecht, the Netherlands

Jolle Kirpensteijn
Department of Clinical Sciences of Companion Animals, Faculty of Veterinary Medicine, Utrecht University, Yalelaan 108, 3584CM, Utrecht, the Netherlands
Hill's Pet Nutrition, 400 SW 8th Ave, Topeka, KS 66603, USA

Bart Van Goethem
Department of Small Animal Medicine, Faculty of Veterinary Medicine, Ghent University, Salisburylaan 133, 9820 Merelbeke, Belgium

Verónica Vieitez, Luis Javier Ezquerra, Víctor López Rámis, Massimo Santella and Ignacio
Veterinary Teaching Hospital, University of Extremadura, Avda, Universidad s/n, 10003 Cáceres, Spain

Álvarez Gómez de Segura
Department of Animal Medicine and Surgery, Veterinary Faculty, University Complutense of Madrid, Avda. Puerta de Hierro, 28040 Madrid, Spain

Gian Luca Rovesti and Laura Bertorelli
Clinica Veterinaria M. E. Miller, Cavriago, Italy

Veronica Devesa
Madrid, Spain

Jesus Rodriguez-Quiros
Department of Internal Medicine and Surgery, Veterinary Teaching Hospital, Veterinary School, Complutense University, Madrid, Spain

Abbie V. Viscardi and Patricia V. Turner
Department of Pathobiology, University of Guelph, 50 Stone Road E, Guelph, ON N1G 2W1, Canada

William McCartney
NOAH, 38 Warrenhouse Road, Baldoyle, Dublin 13, Ireland

Bryan MacDonald
Dublin City University, Glasnevin, Dublin 9, Ireland

Ciprian Andrei Ober
Department of Surgery, Faculty of Veterinary Medicine, University of Agricultural Sciences and Veterinary Medicine, Calea Manastur 3-5, Cluj-Napoca, Romania

Rubén Lostado-Lorza and Fátima Somovilla Gómez
Department of Mechanical Engineering, University of La Rioja, Avda. de la Paz, 93, 26006 Logroño, La Rioja, Spain

Matthew R. Field
Arkansas Veterinary Emergency & Specialists, 11619 Pleasant Ridge Road, Little Rock, AR 72212, USA

Ryan Butler and Robert W. Wills
Mississippi State University, College of Veterinary Medicine, 240 Wise Center Drive, Starkville, MS 39762, USA

Wilburn M. Maxwell
Memphis Veterinary Specialists, 555 Trinity Creek Cove, Cordova, TN 38018, USA

Yauheni Zhalniarovich, Marta Mieszkowska, Paulina Przyborowska-Zhalniarovich, Joanna Głodek and Zbigniew Adamiak
Department of Surgery and Radiologu with Clinic, Faculty of Veterinary Medicine, University of Warmia and Mazury in Olsztyn, Oczapowskiego 14, 10-718 Olsztyn, Poland

Andrzej Sobolewski and Grzegorz Waluś
ChM sp. z o. o, Lewickie 3b, 16-061 Juchnowiec Kościelny, Poland

Index